Biomedical Optics in Otorhinolaryngology

Biomedical Optics in Otorhinolaryngology

Head and Neck Surgery

Edited by

Brian J.-F. Wong

Department of Otolaryngology Head and Neck Surgery, Department of Biomedical Engineering, Division of Facial Plastic Surgery, The Beckman Laser Institute and Medical Clinic, University of California Irvine, Irvine, CA, USA

Justus Ilgner

Department of Otorhinolaryngology, Plastic Head and Neck Surgery, RWTH Aachen University Hospital, Aachen, Germany

Springer

Editors
Brian J.-F. Wong, M.D., Ph.D
Department of Otolaryngology Head and Neck Surgery
Department of Biomedical Engineering
Division of Facial Plastic Surgery
The Beckman Laser Institute and Medical Clinic
University of California Irvine
Irvine, CA, USA

Justus Ilgner, M.D
Department of Otorhinolaryngology
Plastic Head and Neck Surgery
RWTH Aachen University Hospital
Aachen, Germany

ISBN 978-1-4939-7966-0 ISBN 978-1-4939-1758-7 (eBook)
DOI 10.1007/978-1-4939-1758-7

Softcover reprint of the hardcover 1st edition 2016

Printed on acid-free paper

This Springer imprint is published by Springer Nature
The registered company is Springer Science+Business Media LLC New York

Foreword: Biomedical Photonics in Otorhinolaryngology

Efforts to explore human cavities began thousands of years ago. Physicians were interested in exploring the natural openings in the body, including the ear, nose, and throat for diagnostic and therapeutic purposes. The Edwin Smith Papyrus, the oldest known surgical text, described the situation in Ancient Egypt around 3000 BC. It describes Rhinoplasty for the reconstruction of a broken nose. The Ebers Papyrus is another one of the oldest medical texts and the situation in Ancient Egypt around 1700 BC. There is a detailed description of diseases of the ear, the nose, and the throat. Around 500 BC, physicians in Ancient Greece, belonging to the School of Hippocrates, used simple speculum for the first endoscopic imaging inside the rectum and the vagina.

The physicians in antiquity used their eyes to study these openings. Optical lenses were known in Greece and in other countries, but their magnification was relatively low ($\approx \times 2$) and therefore did not provide much help. Eye glasses (spectacles) were invented much later, around the thirteenth century, but again it is not clear that they offered much help to the practicing physician.

The first microscopes were invented in the sixteenth and seventeenth centuries and the ones developed around 1670–1690 by Leeuwenhoek and Malpigi and others could be used for observing blood cells. Leeuwenhoek used his microscope to observe bacteria from the mouth. All these microscopes could have been used for pathology, but they were not enthusiastically accepted by the medical world. First of all, they could only be used for small objects and, second, they exhibited strong chromatic aberration. An important progress was made with the development of the compound microscope (based on two convex lenses) around 1590–1600 by Hans and Zacharias Jannsen and by Galileo. Further developments by Carl Zeiss and Otto Schott led to the emergence of microscopes that were binocular, had much higher resolution, and had reduced chromatic aberration. This led to a wide use of these microscopes clinically in otolaryngology, starting around 1870.

The first practical camera was developed by Louis Daguerre in 1839 and was immediately used by physicians. George Eastman pioneered in 1885 the use of the flexible photographic film and then developed the KODAK still camera. At first, there was the monochrome (black and white) film and then color film, which was extensively used by the public and also made tremendous impact on practically all medical disciplines. The development of high-quality still camera was followed by the development of cine camera, both of which were extensively used in medicine till the twenty-first century.

A much later development involved the digitizing of images and storing them electronically. It started by the invention of the charge-coupled device (CCD) by George Smith and Willard Boyle in 1969. This led to the rapid development of digital cameras in the 1980s, and they were immediately used in medicine. It was followed by a plethora of rigid, compact cameras of exceptional picture quality and then the development of miniature cameras such as those used in smartphones and other popular devices. The various digital cameras have been used in all fields of medicine and in particular in otolaryngology

Electronic displays appeared in the 1920s, with the development of the cathode ray tube (CRT), and they were used in television sets and in computer monitors, which did have some effect on otolaryngology. Liquid crystals were studied since the early 1900s and were gradually used in liquid crystal displays (LCDs), which in the 2000s dominated the fields of large screen TV and computers and small screens of cameras and cellular phones. These displays made it possible to view instantaneously the image obtained with an electronic camera. A flat panel TV screen based on light-emitting diodes (LEDs) appeared in the 1980s, and it is likely that LED displays which give a much brighter screen and a much better picture quality will replace the LCD screens. These new display devices made an immediate effect on medicine, including otolaryngology.

The thoughts of examining the interior of the body date back to ancient times, but the main problem was how to illuminate that region. Bozinni invented the first working endoscope that could be used for this purpose. He used a candle as a light source and some mirrors illuminated the inside of the body and transmitted back an image. The first physician to use it clinically was ZZZ.

The first internally lit device used to inspect the interior of the human body was constructed by Philipp Bozzini of Mainz, Germany, in 1806. Bozzini called his device a "Lichtleiter" or light conductor. It was constructed of a tube, with various attachments, to be inserted into a body cavity. A candle and angled mirrors inside the device enabled the physician to see inside the cavity. Antoine Desormeaux was the first surgeon who introduced the Lichtleiter to a patient. Maximilian Nitze replaced the light source of the Lichtleiter by a miniature electrical light lamp around 1880 and got much better results. It was originally thought that the Lichtleiter would be most useful for examining the larynx, but the design later came to be adapted for urological and gynecological applications.

A major leap in endoscopy was made by Harold Hopkins who had originally developed the zoom lens. He developed a rigid endoscope based on a rod-lens system which provided images of very high quality, and these rigid endoscopes are still being used today.

Optical fibers are thin, flexible threads of transparent material (glass or plastic) that transmit light from side to side. Such fibers have been known for centuries, but Harold Hopkins and Narinder Kapany were the first to achieve in 1954 a good image using an ordered bundle of glass fibers in a flexible fiberscope. This was immediately used by Basil Hirschowitz for the development of a fiber-optic endoscope that was first used in gastroscopy and then in many other medical disciplines. Still cameras and video cameras were easily coupled to endoscopes for endoscopic imaging. In the beginning, the images were captured on a photographic film, and then it was possible to use digital cameras, instantaneously look at the images using electronic screens, and store them digitally on a computer or on an electronic chip. A more recent development was to attach a tiny digital camera at the tip of an endoscope, use it for endoscopic imaging, and use the fibers just for illumination. And, again, the image was shown on an electronic screen and stored electronically.

The first laser was demonstrated by Theodore Maiman in 1960. Shortly afterwards, it was first used in ophthalmology for the attachment of detached retina. The early lasers were not highly suitable for ENT work. In 1963, Kumar Patel invented the CO_2 laser whose radiation was highly absorbed by tissues, and it was very suitable for cutting tissues precisely and with little bleeding. It therefore led to a rapid development of the laser surgery in many medical disciplines. Geza Jako and Stuart Strong started using this laser in 1971 and used it for endoscopic surgery on a papillary lesion of the vocal cord.

Lasers are advanced sources or light, with unique properties such as very pure color, coherence, etc. There are pulsed lasers and CW lasers, covering the spectral range from the deep UV to the far IR. Low-intensity lasers were used for many diagnostic applications. Medium-intensity lasers were used for the treatment of diseased areas such as photothermal therapy or photodynamic therapy of cancer. Higher intensity lasers (including pulsed lasers) were used for surgery.

It was natural to couple laser beams into other optical elements, such as transmitting laser beams through optical fibers for surgery or for diagnosis. These fibers were easily inserted through endoscopes so that the medical procedures are carried out endoscopically.

As an example for more recent developments, we may mention that surgeons have been interested in natural orifice endoscopic surgery (NOTES) for surgical operations performed by an endoscope that is inserted through a natural orifice, such as the mouth or nose—thus reducing scarring.

During the last 60 years, there have been major developments in the fields of modern optics and electro-optics, and many of these developments found their way into medicine and in particular into otorhinolaryngology. The biomedical photonics applications in this field include the use of endoscopic techniques, microscopy, lasers for diagnosis, therapy, and surgery, optical imaging, optical coherent tomography (OCT), fiber optic sensors, etc.

Physicians working in otolaryngology may get the impression that these fantastic developments indicate that medicine today has made progress through the recent scientific/engineering developments and that the medicine of the past was highly inferior. This is a wrong impression. Medicine has slowly progressed for thousands of years, and today we benefit from all the contributions of generations of clever and innovative physicians. In this respect, we may use the metaphor attributed to Isaac Newton: If I have seen further it is by standing on the shoulders of giants.

Dr Katzir

Preface

Our objective in assembling this excellent series of chapters into one book was to provide an overview for scientists, engineers, and clinicians on the cutting-edge optical technologies used for the management of diseases of the head, neck, and upper airway as well as on traditional surgical photonic applications which have stood the test of time and yet provide enough potential for further development. It is by no means meant to be a comprehensive treatise on all uses of optical technologies in the head and neck. We have selected topics which we believe have significant potential for the innovation and evolution of technology.

The use of optical technologies in the otolaryngology—head and neck surgery started in the 1970s with the pioneering work of Jako, Strong, and Vaughn in Boston who introduced the laser as a tool for laryngeal and pharyngeal cancer operations. Later, with refinement in technology and delivery systems, surgical applications broadened to middle ear surgery, in particular for the surgical treatment of otosclerosis ("stapes surgery"). In the 1980s, unprecedented funding in the United States was available for fundamental research as a consequence of the Reagan administration's Strategic Defense Initiative. This was a windfall for the optics industry, and there was an immense spillover of technology into many civilian application areas including medicine. In 1988, at SPIE OE/LASE (then held in Los Angeles), biomedical optics was broken out as a separate session. A year later, the pioneering efforts of Abraham Katzir led to the formation of the Biomedical Optics Society. In 1995, the Biomedical Optics Symposium or "BiOS" as we know it today moved to San Jose forming Photonics West and has grown to include dozens of clinical disciplines, encompassing over 2000 oral presentations per year. The otolaryngology sessions have grown commensurately.

This book would not be possible without the input, contributions, and efforts from participants of the Otolaryngology—Head and Neck Surgery section at the SPIE Biomedical Optics Symposium. The winter "ENT" conferences at BiOS have grown and evolved over 20+ years originally focusing on purely surgical applications of lasers to the current emphasis on the broader use of optical technologies to study diseases of the head and neck, special senses and sensory organs, and the upper airway. Early leaders at BiOS include Stanley Shapshay, Hans Scherer, and Robert Ossoff. They fostered innovation in light-based therapies and diagnostics and saw the importance of creating a venue linking scientists, engineers, and clinicians. We have been honored to continue this tradition for the past 15 years.

Likewise, there is a second generation of clinicians and scientists who have contributed to the growth of optics in the management and study of head and neck disease. It is also important to recognize the contributions of many fellows of the Head and Neck Optical Diagnostics Society. "HNODS" was founded 7 years ago by Colin Hopper at University College London. HNODS is an umbrella organization through which the interest of those doing research in optical imaging and photodynamic related therapies could be further united as expertise and interest in diseases of the head and neck are spread across multiple specialties in Europe, unlike the United States, where Otolaryngology is dominant. Five international HNODS meetings (London, San Francisco (×2), Innsbruck, Orlando, Munich) have been held and a small international working group including Waseem Jerjes and Christian Betz has provided a venue for dissemination of information, collaboration, and growth particularly with photodynamic therapy, where regulatory issues in North America have made clinical evaluation and trial challenging.

Again, we view this volume as providing a cutting-edge review of emerging optical technologies for use in treating disorders of the head, neck, and upper airway. We hope that this provides scientists, engineers, and clinicians with an overview of this field and a starting point for future detailed study.

We would also like to acknowledge the participation of some key contributors to this volume who are also leaders in this field, in particular Colin Hooper, Waseem Jerjes, and Christian Betz. Finally, this volume would not have been possible at all without the support and guidance of Rebecca Amos and Daniel Dominguez at Springer.

Finally, we dedicate this book to our clinical teachers as well as our patients who have taught us so much about the need to develop better technologies to treat the most complex disorders that encompass the head and neck.

Irvine, CA, USA — *Brian J.-F. Wong*
Aachen, Germany — *Justus Ilgner*

Contents

Contributors

CHRISTOPH ARENS • *Department of Otorhinolaryngology, Head and Neck Surgery, University Hospital, Otto-von- Guericke-University, Magdeburg, Germany*

WILLIAM B. ARMSTRONG • *Department of Otolaryngology—Head and Neck Surgery, UC Irvine Medical Center, Orange, CA, USA; Department of Otolaryngology—Head and Neck Surgery, University of California, Irvine, CA, USA*

JAMES ATTRA • *The Tina and Rick Caruso, Department of Otolaryngology—Head and Neck Surgery, Keck School of Medicine of USC, Los Angeles, CA, USA*

FOUZI BENBOUJJA • *Department of Biomedical Engineering, Ecole Polytechnique, Montreal, QC, Canada*

CHRISTIAN STEPHAN BETZ • *Department of Otorhinolaryngology, Munich University Hospital, Munich, Germany*

MERRILL A. BIEL • *Department of Otolaryngology, University of Minnesota, Minneapolis, MN, USA; Virginia Piper Cancer Institute, Abbott Northwestern Hospital, Minneapolis, MN, USA*

CHRISTOPHER M. BINGCANG • *Department of Otolaryngology—Head and Neck Surgery, University of Nebraska Medical Center, Omaha, NE, USA*

ALEXANDER BLÖDOW • *Department of Otorhinolaryngology, Head and Neck Surgery and Communications Disorder, HELIOS Hearing Center Berlin-Brandenburg, Berlin, Germany*

CAROLINE BOUDOUX • *Department of Engineering Physics, Ecole Polytechnique Montréal, Montreal, QC, Canada*

MANFRED BOVI • *Institute of Pathology, Universitätsklinikum Aachen, Aachen, Germany*

JAMES A. BURNS • *Center for Laryngeal Surgery, Massachusetts General Hospital, Harvard Medical School, Boston, MA, USA*

ZHONGPING CHEN • *The Beckman Laser Institute, University of California Irvine, Irvine, CA, USA; Department of Biomedical Engineering, University of California Irvine, Irvine, CA, USA*

ARASH DARAFSHEH • *Department of Radiation Oncology, University of Pennsylvania, Philadelphia, PA, USA*

ROMAIN DETERRE • *Department of Biomedical Engineering, Ecole Polytechnique, Montreal, QC, Canada*

ADEL K. EL-NAGGAR • *Pathology and Head and Neck Surgery, The University of Texas MD Anderson Cancer Center, Houston, TX, USA*

ANNA ENGLHARD • *Department of Otorhinolaryngology, Munich University Hospital, Munich, Germany*

CSABA FARKAS • *Department of Medical Technology and Biophotonics, Fraunhofer Institute for Laser Technology, Aachen, Germany*

JAROD C. FINLAY • *Department of Radiation Oncology, University of Pennsylvania, Philadelphia, PA, USA*

ANN M. GILLENWATER • *Department of Head and Neck Surgery, University of Texas MD Anderson Cancer Center, Houston, TX, USA*

NICHOLAS J. GIORDANO • *Boston University School of Medicine, Boston, MA, USA*
NADIR GOULAMHOUSSEN • *Department of Engineering Physics, Ecole Polytechnique, Montreal, QC, Canada*
ELLEN GUDER • *Department of Otorhinolaryngology, Head and Neck Surgery, University of Rostock, Rostock, Germany*
CHRISTOPHER J. HARTNICK • *Department of Otolaryngology, Harvard Medical School, Massachusetts Eye and Ear Infirmary, Boston, MA, USA*
MIRIAM HAVEL • *Department of Otorhinolaryngology, Head and Neck Surgery, Munich University Hospital, Munich, Germany*
EMMANUEL HELIDONIS • *Arcuo Medical Inc., Nevada, USA; Professor Emeritus, Medical School, University of Crete, Heraklion, Crete, Greece*
MICHAEL L. HINNI • *Department of Otolaryngology—Head and Neck Surgery, Mayo Clinic, Phoenix, AZ, USA*
VANESSA VON HOLZSCHUHER • *Department of Ear, Nose and Throat Medicine, Martha-Maria Hospital, Munich, Germany*
COLIN HOPPER • *Eastman Dental Institute, University College London, London, UK*
GEREON HÜTTMANN • *Institute for Biomedical Optics, University of Lübeck, Lübeck, Germany*
JUSTUS ILGNER • *Department of Otorhinolaryngology, Plastic Head and Neck, RWTH Aachen University Hospital, Aachen, Germany*
AMEYA A. JATEGAONKAR • *University of Arizona College of Medicine-Phoenix, Phoenix, AZ, USA*
WASEEM JERJES • *Department of Surgery, University College London, London, UK; Health Education West Midlands, National Health Service, Worcestershire, UK*
JOSEPH JING • *The Beckman Laser Institute, University of California Irvine, Irvine, CA, USA; Department of Biomedical Engineering, University of California Irvine, Irvine, CA, USA*
TINO JUST • *Department of Otorhinolaryngology, Head and Neck Surgery, KMG Klinikum Güstrow GmbH, Güstrow, Germany*
M. BARIŞ KARAKULLUKCU • *Department of Head and Neck Surgery and Oncology, Netherlands Cancer Institute, Antoni van Leeuwenhoek Hospital, Amsterdam, The Netherlands*
NIELS KOKOT • *The Tine and Rick Caruso, Department of Otolaryngology—Head and Neck Surgery, Keck School of Medicine of USC, Los Angeles, CA, USA*
EVA LANKENAU • *Institute for Biomedical Optics, University of Lübeck, Lübeck, Germany*
FRANCES B. LAZAROW • *Department of Otolaryngology—Head and Neck Surgery, University of California, Irvine, CA, USA*
FRANCK MARIE LECLÈRE • *Centre of Expertise for Sex Reassignment Surgery, Department of Plastic & Transsexual Surgery, Burn Surgery, Hand Surgery, CHU University of Bordeaux, Centre François-Xavier-Michelet, Groupe Hospitalier Pellegrin, Bordeaux, France*
ACHIM LENENBACH • *Department of Medical Technology and Biophotonics, Fraunhofer Institute for Laser Technology, Aachen, Germany*
ANDREAS LEUNIG • *MVZ Bogenhausen, München, Germany*
STEEN J. MADSEN • *Department of Health Physics and Diagnostic Sciences, University of Nevada, Las Vegas, Las Vegas, NV, USA*
SERGE MORDON • *U1189-ONCO-THAI-Image Assisted Laser Therapy for Oncology, University of Lille, Lille, France*

Joachim Müller • *Department of Otorhinolaryngology, Hospital of University Munich, Munich, Germany*
Atilla Ovari • *Department of Otorhinolaryngology, Head and Neck Surgery, University of Rostock, Rostock, Germany*
Alpen B. Patel • *Department of Otolaryngology—Head and Neck Surgery, Mayo Clinic, Phoenix, AZ, USA*
Hans Wilhelm Pau • *Department of Otorhinolaryngology, Head and Neck Surgery, University of Rostock, Rostock, Germany*
James D. Phillips • *Department of Otolaryngology/Head and Neck Surgery, Vascular Anomalies Center, Arkansas Children's Hospital, Little Rock, AR, USA*
Friedrich Prall • *Institute of Pathology, University of Rostock, Rostock, Germany*
Chung-Ku Rhee • *Department of Otolaryngology, Medical Laser Research Center, Dankook University College of Medicine, Chungnam-do, Korea*
Rebecca R. Richards-Kortum • *Department of Bioengineering, Rice University, Houston, TX, USA*
Gresham T. Richter • *Department of Otolaryngology/Head and Neck Surgery, Vascular Anomalies Center, Arkansas Children's Hospital, Little Rock, AR, USA*
Claus-Peter Richter • *Department of Otolaryngology, Northwestern University Feinberg School of Medicine, Chicago, IL, USA*
Jan L.N. Roodenburg • *Department of Oral and Maxillofacial Surgery, University Medical Center Groningen, Groningen, The Netherlands*
Jennifer E. Rosen • *Department of Surgery, MedStar Washington Hospital Center, Washington, DC, USA*
Tara L. Rosenberg • *Department of Otolaryngology/Head and Neck Surgery, Baylor College of Medicine/Texas Children's Hospital, Houston, TX, USA*
Marc Rubinstein • *The Beckman Laser Institute, Department of Otorhinolaryngology, Klinikum der Universität München, Munich, Germany*
Florian Schrötzlmair • *Laser-Research-Laboratory, LIFE-Centre, Hospital of University, Munich, Germany; Department of Otorhinolaryngology, Hospital of University Munich, Munich, Germany*
Richard A. Schwarz • *Department of Bioengineering, Rice University, Houston, TX, USA*
Giriraj K. Sharma • *Department of Otolaryngology—Head and Neck Surgery, UC Irvine Medical Center, Orange, CA, USA*
V. Siedek • *Laser-Research-Laboratory, LIFE-Centre, Hospital of University, Munich, Germany; Department of Otorhinolaryngology, Hospital of University, Munich, Germany*
Emil Sobol • *Arcuo Medical Inc., Nevada, USA; Institute on Laser and Information Technologies, Moscow, Russia*
Ronald Sroka • *Laser-Research-Laboratory, LIFE-Centre, Hospital of University, Munich, Germany; Department of Otorhinolaryngology, Hospital of University, Munich, Germany*
Mathias Strupler • *Department of Engineering Physics, Ecole Polytechnique, Montreal, QC, Canada*
Benjamin von Stülpnagel • *Department of Otorhinolaryngology, Head and Neck Surgery, University of Rostock, Rostock, Germany*
Ahmed A. Sultan • *Department of Surgery, University College London, London, UK*

VALERY SVISTUSHKIN • *Department of Otorhinolaryngology, First Moscow State Medical University of I.M. Sechenov, Moscow, Russia*
XIAODONG TAN • *Department of Otolaryngology, Northwestern University Feinberg School of Medicine, Chicago, IL, USA*
TJOSON TJOA • *Department of Otolaryngology—Head and Neck Surgery, University of California, Irvine, CA, USA*
MARIO A. TRELLES • *Fundacion Antoni de Gimbernat, Instituto Médico Vilafortuny, Cambrils, Tarragona, Spain*
SUNIL VERMA • *Department of Otolaryngology—Head and Neck Surgery, UC Irvine Medical Center, Orange, CA, USA*
NADARAJAH VIGNESWARAN • *Diagnostic and Biomedical Sciences, The University of Texas School of Dentistry at Houston, Houston, TX, USA*
SEBASTIAAN A.H.J. DE VISSCHER • *Department of Oral and Maxillofacial Surgery, University Medical Center Groningen, Groningen, The Netherlands*
SUSANNE VOIGT-ZIMMERMANN • *Department of Otorhinolaryngology, Head and Neck Surgery, University Hospital, Otto-von-Guericke-University, Magdeburg, Germany*
VERONIKA VOLGGER • *Department of Otorhinolaryngology, Head and Neck Surgery, Klinikum Großhadern, Klinikum der Universität München, Munich, Germany*
MARTIN WEHNER • *Department of Medical Technology and Biophotonics, Fraunhofer Institute for Laser Technology, Aachen, Germany*
MARTIN WESTHOFEN • *Department of Otorhinolaryngology, Plastic Surgery of Head and Neck, Universitätsklinikum Aachen, Aachen, Germany*
MAX J.H. WITJES • *Department of Oral and Maxillofacial Surgery, University Medical Center Groningen, Groningen, The Netherlands*
GABRIELE WITT • *Department of Otorhinolaryngology, Head and Neck Surgery, University of Rostock, Rostock, Germany*
BRIAN J.-F. WONG • *Department of Otolaryngology Head and Neck Surgery, Department of Biomedical Engineering, Department of Facial Plastic Surgery, The Beckman Laser Institute and Medical Clinic, University of California Irvine, Irvine, CA, USA*
HUNTER YOUNG • *Department of Otolaryngology, Northwestern University Feinberg School of Medicine, Chicago, IL, USA*
PAMELA ZENGEL • *Laser-Research-Laboratory, LIFE-Centre, Hospital of University, Munich, Germany; Department of Otorhinolaryngology, Hospital of University, Munich, Germany*
KEN ZHAO • *Department of Otolaryngology, Chicago, USA*

Part I

Contemporary Laser Surgical Procedures in the Head and Neck

Chapter 1

Practical Endoscopy for Laser Interventions of the Upper Aerodigestive Tract

Frances B. Lazarow and William B. Armstrong

Introduction

This chapter will cover the fundamentals of endoscopy in otolaryngology, beginning with a history of the substantial progress that has been made since endoscopy was first developed in the 1800s, followed by a brief overview of the anatomy of the upper aerodigestive tract, and concluding with a discussion of contemporary office-based and surgical endoscopic practices. Knowledge of the fundamentals of endoscopy both in the office and the operating room is critical to understanding our current capabilities for visualizing and manipulating structures within the upper aerodigestive tract.

A Brief History of Endoscopy

Today, we take for granted the ability to visualize the airway, digestive tract, and genitourinary tract. While today's otolaryngologist regards endoscopy as a regular and necessary part of any clinical examination, there was a time when even visualizing the airway of a living patient was science fiction. The dramatic evolution of endoscopy has depended on the convergence of technological advances within and outside the field of medicine. Over the last two centuries, developments in lighting, optics, biomaterials, anesthesia, image documentation, and computer technology have transformed our ability to image internal anatomy and pathology. A few of the major advances are highlighted here.

Brian J.-F. Wong and Justus Ilgner (eds.), *Biomedical Optics in Otorhinolaryngology: Head and Neck Surgery*, DOI 10.1007/978-1-4939-1758-7_1,

The era of endoscopy began in the early 1800s, when Philip Bozzini became the first person to use an external light source (a candle reflected by mirrors), to visualize structures inside living human patients (primarily the esophagus, bladder, and rectum) [1, 2]. However, his device was so heavy and awkward that it was almost unusable in regular clinical practice [3]. By 1853, urologist Antonin Desormeaux developed the first functional endoscope to visualize the urethra, performed the first successful endoscopic operations, and coined the term "endoscopy" [4, 5]. Another urologist, Maximilian Carl-Friedrich Nitze, used a series of lenses to increase magnification and is credited with creating the first usable cystoscope in 1877 [2]. Adolph Kussmaul adapted Desormeaux's endoscope for the first esophagoscopies in 1867–1868 [4], although it was not until 1880 that Jan Mikulicz and Joseph Leiter were able to build the first gastroscope [2]. Initially, these new devices were primarily used for genitourinary and gastrointestinal applications, but physicians had harbored a keen interest in using endoscopy to more thoroughly visualize the airway since Manuel Garcia, Ludwig Turck, and Johann Czermak first used mirrors to examine the living larynx in the early 1850s. A major hurdle was overcome in 1884, with the discovery of cocaine as a topical anesthetic [1]. Prior to this, physicians had to use habituation to overcome the patient's gag reflex, an unpleasant process that required weeks of preparation to tolerate the procedure [1]. In 1895, Alfred Kirstein developed the first true direct laryngoscope, and soon after, Gustav Killian was able to perform the first bronchoscopy [1]. In 1910, Sidney Yankauer introduced the first laryngoscope that could accommodate binocular vision [1]. The next year, Killian introduced suspension laryngoscopy, an operative setup in which the laryngoscope is supported by a rigid platform affixed to the operating table, rather than held by the surgeon [1]. Binocular vision and the ability to use instruments with both hands made operative procedures on the larynx a reality. In 1953, the Zeiss Optical Company introduced the first binocular microscope, opening the door for Oskar Kleinsasser to develop and utilize specialized microsurgical instruments and pioneer the field of microlaryngoscopy and larynx microsurgery in the 1960s [2, 6]. In the early 1970s, M. Stuart Strong and Geza Jako coupled a carbon dioxide laser to a surgical microscope for use through a laryngoscope [7]. Since that time, numerous surgeons, especially Wolfgang Steiner, continued to develop endoscopes with better exposure and refined endoscopic instruments and surgical techniques, to allow effective manipulation of bulky specimens and obtain effective hemostasis to resect larger tumors [8–11].

Thomas Edison's invention of the light bulb in 1879 made possible the utilization of advances in endoscope design and anesthesia. Previous light sources such as candles, gas flames, and galvanized wires were dim, exothermic, and dangerous. As the twentieth century dawned, the incandescent light bulb was smaller, ran cooler, and shone brighter, which pushed the march of progress in endoscopy forward. Mikulicz was the first to use a miniature electric bulb in the esophagogastroscope [12]. However, distal incandescent bulbs were still problematic because of their propensity to burn out during the case, a potentially devastating event. In 1930, gynecologist Heinrich Lamm introduced the concept of flexible fiber optics to endoscopy by showing that fine threads of glass fibers could be bundled together to act as a conduit for a light source, and these bundles could be bent [2]. Fiber-optic light carriers brightened images even more than incandescent bulbs, without a corresponding increase in heat output [2]. In the late 1950s, fiber-optic cables were further manipulated to transmit images, allowing for completely flexible instruments [2]. By 1968, Sawashima and Hirose described the first flexible transnasal laryngoscope [1]. While flexible fiber-optic endoscopes were a major advance, their image quality did not approach that of the Storz-Hopkins rigid endoscope. This scope design used glass rods instead of the traditional air interspace between lenses, which absorbed less light along the length of the scope and provided a wider viewing angle [1, 2]. This technology was invented by Harold Hopkins in the 1950s and improved when Hopkins and Karl Storz collaborated in 1965 [1]. An updated version of this scope remains widely used in clinical practice today.

Documentation of image findings historically relied on notes or diagrams drawn by the clinician. With improved lighting and image delivery, photography could now be used to permanently record images and document findings objectively for comparison over time. Film and, later, videotape recordings of examinations became possible. In 1969, charge-coupled devices (CCD) were invented [1]. A CCD is an integrated circuit that contains light-sensitive capacitors aligned in a two-dimensional array, with each capacitor representing one picture element (pixel). When photons contact the CCD, they generate electric signals that are digitally processed to produce high-quality color digital image data that can be displayed on video monitors, printed, or saved on computer media. The CCD enabled development of cameras that directly connect to the endoscope so multiple people could view the examination at once and digital recordings could be made to facilitate comparison of exams over time.

Improvements continued to be made to endoscopic visualization throughout the close of the twentieth century and the dawn of the twenty-first century. CCDs were progressively miniaturized and moved from camera heads to the distal tip of the endoscope. They were put into gastrointestinal flexible endoscopes in 1984, creating what would be known as "chip on the tip" endoscopes [1]. The first "chip on the tip" transoral flexible bronchoscope became available in 1990 [1]. In 1999, CCD technology was miniaturized sufficiently to allow the development of a "chip on the tip" endoscope that could be passed through the nose, allowing endoscopy to occur without sedation. This scope used a CCD camera for image transfer and fiber-optic technology for light delivery [1]. By the beginning of the twenty-first century, "chip on the tip" technology had improved to the point that the resolution of a flexible scope was very close to that of a rod-lens telescope, the gold standard of endoscopic image production [1].

The numerous advances in endoscope design and optics have enabled today's surgeon to perform many therapeutic procedures, from biopsies and balloon dilations to laser ablation of tumors, on unsedated patients in the ambulatory office setting. Office procedures in the awake patient allow dynamic assessment of function and treatment results, especially of the vocal cords (*see* Table 1). Performing procedures in the office also eliminates the medical risks of general anesthesia, decreases direct (expense of the medications, monitors, facility, nursing/anesthesia staff, etc.) and indirect (lost work time for both the patient and the companion who must drive the patient home from the procedure) costs of general anesthesia or moderate sedation, and increases surgeon productivity because of more rapid turnover of procedures. With the growing focus on containing healthcare expenditures and increasing patient demand for minimally invasive care, it can be expected that existing office procedures will become a mainstay of clinical practice, and as

Table 1
Comparison of office endoscopy and operating room endoscopy

	Office endoscopy	OR endoscopy
Advantages	• Ability to see dynamic function • No tissue collapse • Avoid medical risks of general anesthesia • Lower cost • Increased surgeon efficiency due to shorter turnover time	• No risk of limitation due to patient discomfort • Ability to control bleeding • Physician has greater opportunity to palpate and manipulate structures
Disadvantages	• Patient discomfort • Limited extent of procedures • More difficult to control bleeding	• Higher cost • Risks of general anesthesia • Tissue collapse/difficult exposure • No ability to see function

technology improves and surgeons gain more experience in the ambulatory setting, even more procedures will be transferred from the operating room to the office.

While these improvements in endoscopic image quality have enabled physicians to see tissue surfaces with exceptional clarity, endoscopes cannot see into the tissue and provide details about changes occurring below the surface. Imaging modalities such as CT and MRI are important adjuncts to endoscopy and are primarily useful for determining the depth of tumor invasion. This information can have important implications for cancer staging and prognosis. Other imaging technologies, such as high-frequency ultrasound, confocal microscopy (*see* Chaps. 38 and 39), tissue spectroscopy, and optical coherence tomography (*see* Chaps. 41–45), are being investigated or used to analyze the subsurface structure of tissues.

Today, the otolaryngologist's office is equipped with a variety of rigid and flexible endoscopes, which are used multiple times daily and are invaluable to clinical practice. These endoscopes have a variety of applications, which will be discussed later in this chapter. While distal chip endoscopy provides superb images, this technology is still very expensive, which has limited its utilization until now. However, these costs are decreasing, so it is likely distal chip endoscopes will be more widely adopted in the future.

Basic Anatomy of the Upper Aerodigestive Tract

The following sections are not meant to be a comprehensive overview of anatomy but rather a brief discussion of the most important and frequently seen structures and conditions encountered during endoscopy. In general, regardless of anatomic site, the examiner should note the quality and color of the mucosa, identify the precise location of abnormalities, and obtain measurements of the dimensions of anatomic lesions. Special note is made of any masses, swollen or asymmetric tissues, friable lesions, bleeding, edema, or inflammation (*see* Fig. 1).

Nasal Cavity

Structures seen in the nasal cavity include the turbinates, nasal septum, and sinus ostia (sinus drainage pathways). Large turbinates or a deviated septum can impair airflow and sinus drainage. It is also important to note the color and quality of the nasal mucosa, diagnose polyps, recognize purulent sinus drainage, and identify prominent blood vessels. The examiner generally cannot directly examine the sinuses as the natural ostia are too small to allow passage of an endoscope.

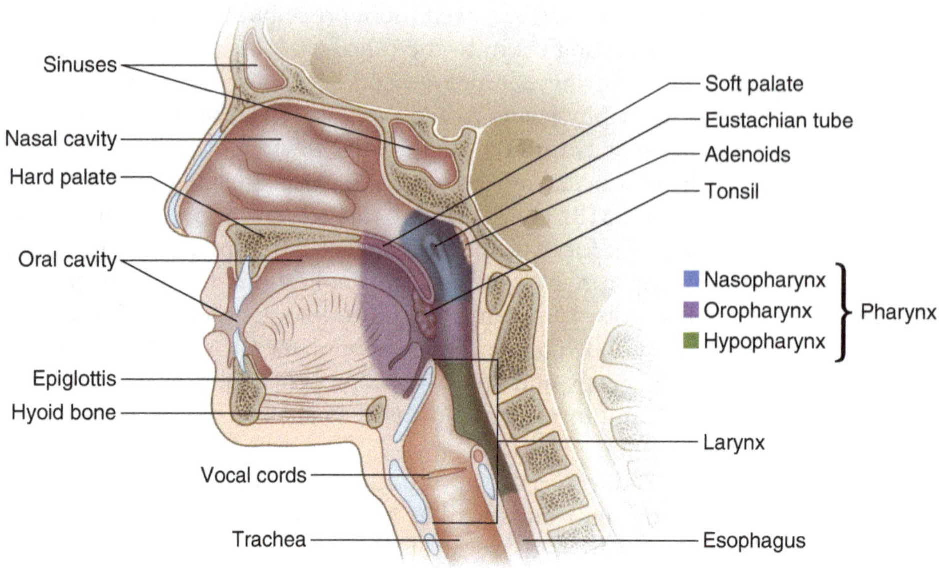

Fig. 1 Basic anatomy of the head and neck. Key structures in the head and neck. Note the delineation of the pharynx into the nasopharynx, oropharynx, and hypopharynx

Oral Cavity

The oral cavity can be visualized with good lighting and mirrors when necessary. Endoscopy is not required for even the most thorough exams. The oral cavity is bounded by the skin-vermillion junction of the lips and includes the hard palate, anterior two-thirds of the tongue, buccal membranes, upper and lower alveolar ridge, and retromolar trigone to the floor of the mouth [13]. It is important to note the condition of the teeth, gums, and tongue.

Nasopharynx

The nasopharynx begins anteriorly at the posterior choanae of the nasal cavity, encompasses the space beneath the sphenoid sinus, extends posteriorly to the posterior pharyngeal wall, and extends inferiorly to the plane forming the superior surface of the soft palate. Its contents include the adenoids and the openings to the Eustachian tubes.

Oropharynx

The oropharynx extends vertically from the plane of the soft palate to the epiglottic vallecula. The anterior border is the junction of the anterior two-thirds and posterior one-third of the tongue at the circumvallate papillae and the junction of the hard and soft palate. It contains the base of tongue, palatine tonsils, tonsillar pillars, and soft palate [13]. The majority of the oropharynx can be visualized directly with the exception of the tongue base, which requires mirror or endoscopic visualization because it is hidden from view by the anterior portion of the tongue.

Hypopharynx

The hypopharynx connects the oropharynx to the esophagus and lies behind and around the larynx. Radiographically, it runs from the level of the hyoid bone superiorly to the lower level of the cricoid cartilage [14]. On examination, the level of the vallecula approximates that of the hyoid bone. The hypopharynx can be divided into three sites: the piriform sinus, the postcricoid area, and the posterior pharyngeal wall. The hypopharynx is lined with stratified squamous epithelium and has a rich network of lymphatics.

Larynx

The larynx connects the hypopharynx to the trachea. It extends from the tip of the epiglottis to the inferior border of the cricoid cartilage. The larynx consists of the hyoid bone, thyroid cartilage, and cricoid cartilage as well as paired arytenoid, corniculate, and cuneiform cartilages with associated muscles, fat, connective tissues, and blood supply. The major anatomic structures seen on endoscopy are the epiglottis, aryepiglottic folds, false vocal folds, true vocal folds, and subglottis. It is important to visualize the larynx when the patient reports any voice changes, such as hoarseness. Changes to the mucosa of the larynx, or in the amount or quality of secretions, can also indicate pathology.

Trachea

The trachea is a semirigid tubular structure containing 15–20 C-shaped cartilaginous rings held together by connective tissue and lined with pseudostratified columnar epithelium [15]. The trachea is 4–6 in. long, begins at the larynx, and splits into the primary bronchi, which lead into the lungs. The trachea is not routinely assessed during a typical office exam, but it can be examined after administering topical anesthesia and passing the endoscope past the vocal cords.

Esophagus

The esophagus is connected to the oropharynx via the hypopharynx. It consists of layers of mucosa, circular and longitudinal muscle, and adventitia. The upper third of the esophagus is striated muscle, the middle third is a mix of striated and smooth muscle, and the lower third is smooth muscle. The esophagus is also not routinely assessed during a routine office exam.

Flexible Endoscopy

Introduction

Flexible endoscopy is a fundamental tool for the otolaryngologist in the ambulatory setting. In addition to being an exceptionally safe and efficient diagnostic device to assist evaluation of numerous complaints such as voice changes, dysphagia, neoplasms, and reflux, advances in endoscope design and optics have enabled the surgeon to perform many therapeutic procedures via flexible endoscopy on unsedated patients in the office. These interventions include biopsies, dilations, laser ablations, and vocal fold injections. A typical flexible endoscope is seen in Fig. 2.

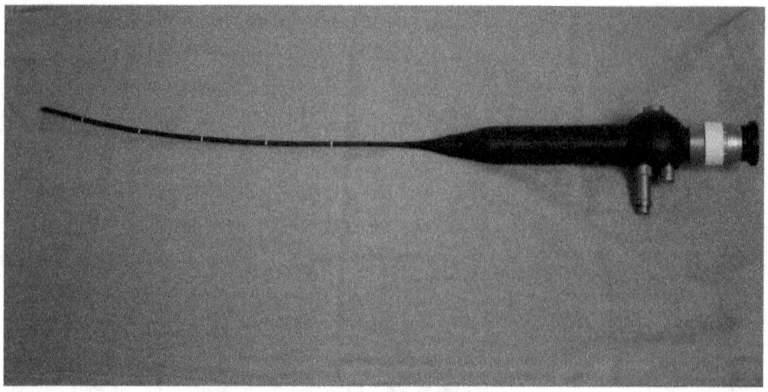

Fig. 2 Flexible endoscope. An example of a flexible fiber-optic endoscope. This endoscope is inserted transnasally and used to examine the nasal cavity, pharynx, and larynx of awake patients in the office. The tip can be manipulated by the physician via a mechanism at the proximal end (not shown) in order to better guide the endoscope through the upper airway and more thoroughly inspect particular areas of interest

Nasal Cavity, Nasopharynx, Oropharynx, and Larynx

Rigid endoscopy is generally preferred over its flexible counterpart because image quality is superior with a rigid endoscope (*see* Table 2). Magnification and light transport are inferior with flexible endoscopy [16]. With flexible endoscopy, there are distortions at the periphery of the viewing field, and when the image is in focus, there is a honeycomb effect that is increased by the edge-detection software of digital imaging systems [16]. Flexible endoscopes are less often used in the operating room (where patients are under general anesthesia) for these reasons. However, advantages of a flexible endoscope over a rigid endoscope include the ability to evaluate the larynx while the patient speaks or sings. In the larynx, flexible endoscopy is generally preferred when the clinical question is one of movement rather than structure and is better for assessing neurologic function, connected speech, and movement disorders. Additionally, flexible endoscopy allows more accurate assessment of arytenoid mobility and the glottic gap because of the neutral tongue and neck positions. Flexible endoscopy also allows inspection of the nasal cavity, nasopharynx, oropharynx, hypopharynx, and larynx in the same exam, which is useful in a patient with several complaints or one who poorly tolerates multiple exams [16].

Prior to undergoing flexible endoscopy, the patient's nasal cavity is anesthetized and decongested with a topical spray. The endoscope is inserted through the nasal cavity and directed into the nasopharynx and down to the larynx. The patient can be directed to phonate, repeat passages, swallow, cough, and perform Valsalva or other maneuvers to evaluate the anatomy and function of the structures in view (*see* Fig. 3a, b).

Table 2
Comparison of methods to visualize the larynx

	Mirror	Flexible fiber-optic endoscope	Flexible distal chip endoscope	Rigid endoscope
Difficulty of exam	+++	+	+	++
Optical image quality	++++	++	+++	++++
Dynamic function/phonation “eee”	+	+	+	+
Connected speech/conversation	–	+	+	–
Ability to photograph/record	–	+	+	+

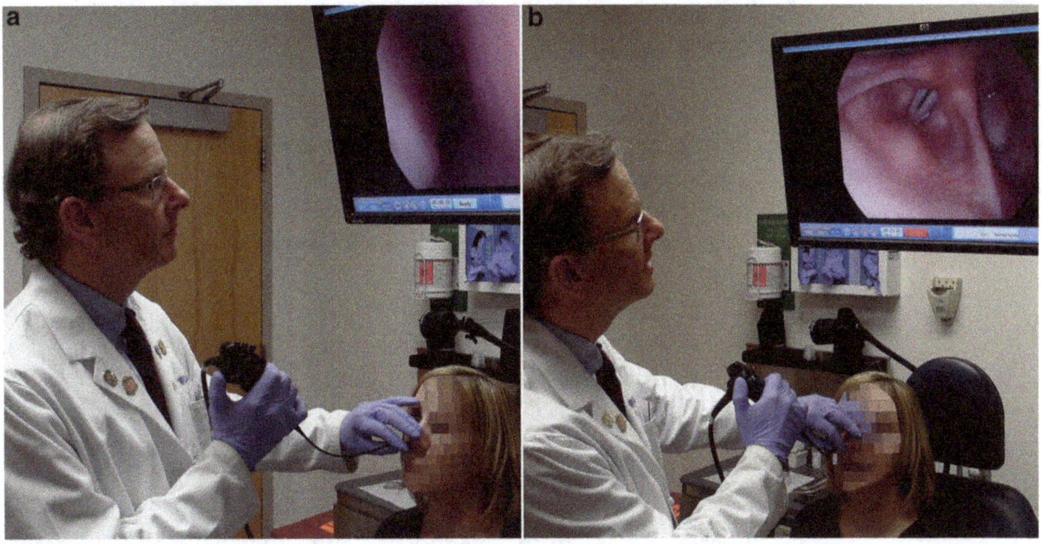

Fig. 3 (a–b) Flexible laryngoscopy. A patient being examined with a flexible endoscope. (**a**) The physician advances the endoscope through the patient's nasal cavity, which can be seen on the screen above the patient's head. (**b**) The physician has now advanced the scope through the nasal cavity to the pharynx, bringing the larynx into view. The patient has been directed to say “eee” to evaluate the motion of the vocal cords

Esophagus

Esophagoscopy was one of the first applications for flexible endoscopes, and the instruments have been miniaturized to allow passage through the nasal cavity. Historically, flexible esophagoscopy was first performed transorally, generally with sedation, but miniaturization of scope diameter and placement of the camera on the distal end of the endoscope has allowed insertion of the endoscope through the nasal passage. Transnasal esophagoscopy (TNE) is very similar to flexible laryngoscopy, with the additional step of passing the scope beyond the larynx into the esophagus. TNE elicits less gag reflex because it avoids the oral cavity, so it does not require the patient to be sedated. These esophagoscopes are small diameter (3–5 mm) but still have a working channel to pass biopsy forceps, laser fibers, and dilators, as well as having suction capability. This allows the physician to perform a variety of procedures in the office without the risks or costs that accompany sedation. Transoral flexible esophagoscopy generally requires moderate sedation and is used for more extensive procedures or in patients who cannot tolerate procedures in the office due to anxiety or discomfort.

Flexible esophagoscopy has been adopted to evaluate and manage a variety of clinical conditions including dysphagia, chronic cough, refractory or long-standing gastroesophageal reflux, laryngopharyngeal reflux, confirmation of findings on an abnormal radiographic study, screening for Barrett's metaplasia, evaluation of strictures, and evaluation for a second primary tumor in the workup of head and neck cancer. Interventional indications include biopsy, treatment of bleeding lesions, prophylactic banding of esophageal varices, foreign body removal, removal or ablation of lesions, and dilation of stenotic regions [12].

Trachea/Bronchi

In the office setting, the proximal trachea is often visualized from above the larynx with rigid or flexible endoscopes. Passage of the endoscope through the glottis generally elicits a violent cough reflex and spasmodic closure of the larynx. Topical anesthesia applied to the larynx and trachea allows passage of a flexible endoscope into the trachea and bronchi.

Flexible bronchoscopy is a method of visualizing the lower airway and lungs. It can be performed via the oral or nasal route [17]. Although flexible bronchoscopy can be performed without sedation (similar to TNE), many physicians elect to use moderate sedation, and a few use general anesthesia, especially for more advanced procedures with larger endoscopes [17].

Similar to TNE performed in the office setting, flexible bronchoscopy has both diagnostic and therapeutic indications. Indications for diagnostic bronchoscopy include hemoptysis, suspected stricture or obstruction, suspected or known cancer, foreign body aspiration, and evaluation of burns or chemical injury to the airways [17]. Flexible bronchoscopes have a channel that allows passage of suction, medication, and other instruments, which allow for removal of a mass, dilation of strictures, stent placement, and foreign body removal [17]. Small biopsies, balloon dilations, and laser ablations can be performed in the properly equipped ambulatory suite.

Rigid Endoscopy

Rigid Endoscopy in the Office

Flexible endoscopy is convenient, efficient, and well tolerated by patients, elicits less gag reflex, and is essential for exams in patients with certain anatomic variants. Rigid endoscopy, however, is considered the gold standard for image quality and is occasionally necessary for obtaining an accurate diagnosis. In the office setting, rigid telescopes are used to evaluate the nasal cavity, nasopharynx, and larynx. It provides high resolution, bright, clear images with excellent contrast [16]. There is minimal optical distortion, and images are more accurately magnified than with a flexible endoscope [16].

Nasal Cavity/ Nasopharynx

Rigid endoscopes have been developed to evaluate the nasal cavity and nasopharynx in the office. Rigid nasal endoscopes come in diameters of 2.7–4 mm and in multiple angles from 0° to 90° [18]. The portion of the scope that can be inserted into the patient's nose is approximately 20 cm long, with additional length at the proximal end for attachment of a light source and a camera (*see* Fig. 4). Nasal endoscopy is an office procedure that requires light topical anesthetic and mucosal vasoconstriction. It is generally well tolerated by patients and can visualize the nasal passages, drainage pathways from the sinuses, and the nasopharynx. Biopsies of the nasal cavity and nasopharynx can also be taken with endoscopic guidance.

Larynx

Examination of the larynx is performed by having the patient in the "sniffing position" with the examiner grasping the tongue. An angled telescope (70° or 90°) is passed over the tongue and aimed to visualize the larynx (*see* Fig. 5). Laryngeal anatomy and vocal cord motion are well visualized, but examination of phonation is limited to producing sustained vowels (e.g., "eee") [16].

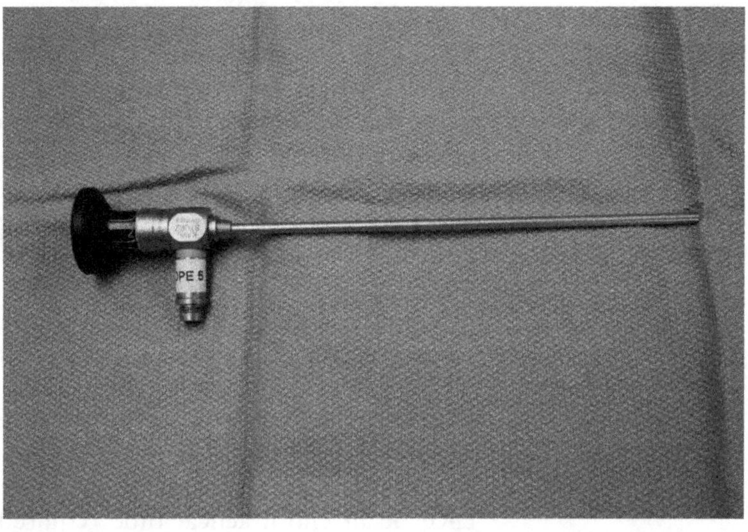

Fig. 4 Rigid endoscope. 0° (degree) rigid endoscope, 18 cm long and 4 mm in diameter. Rigid endoscopes such as this are used in the office and the operating room. It is inserted transnasally and used for inspection of the nasal cavity, sinus drainage pathways, and nasopharynx

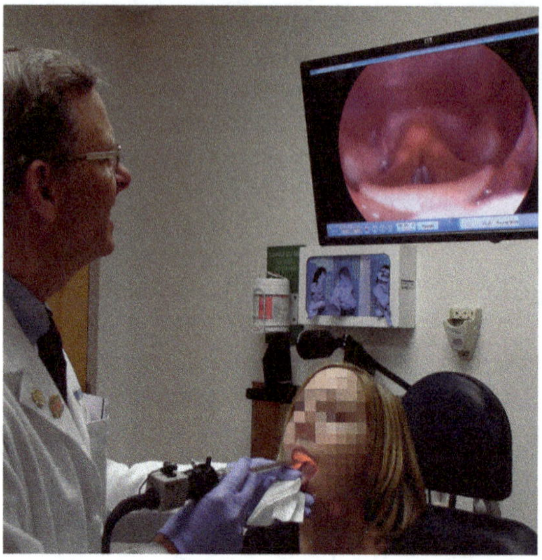

Fig. 5 Rigid laryngoscopy. A patient undergoing rigid laryngoscopy. The patient sits in the "sniffing position" with the neck extended. The physician grasps the patient's tongue with one hand and guides the angled, rigid telescope over the tongue with the other hand. The physician can see the vocal cords come in to view on the screen above the patient's head as he advances the endoscope

Many neurologic or functional disorders require use of a flexible endoscope to evaluate function with connected speech, coughing, swallowing, and other maneuvers not possible when using the rigid endoscope [16].

Rigid Endoscopy in the Operating Room

While office-based endoscopy is essential to every otolaryngologist's outpatient practice, surgical endoscopy also has an equally important role in the operating room. Surgical endoscopy is most often performed under general anesthesia, although some procedures can be accomplished with moderate sedation. Rigid direct laryngoscopy performed in the operating room is often performed to more precisely characterize lesions identified in the office setting and to obtain biopsies and tissue palpation for staging of tumors. Surgical endoscopy provides unimpeded access for biopsies, injections, excisions, and other procedures that would not be tolerated in the awake patient, especially if the possibility of significant bleeding or airway compromise is anticipated. However, it generally does not allow assessment of dynamic movement, and visualization can sometimes be impaired by airway collapse or presence of an endotracheal tube required to support ventilation during general anesthesia.

Operative endoscopy is also performed as part of the staging of head and neck cancers. Rigid operative endoscopy is performed to visualize and biopsy the primary tumor and to evaluate the larynx, esophagus, trachea, and bronchi for second primary tumors. Studies have shown that panendoscopy (laryngoscopy, bronchoscopy, and esophagoscopy) reveals a 2.4–4.5 % incidence of second primary tumors of the upper aerodigestive tract [19–21]. However, others have determined that screening panendoscopy only shows second primary tumors in patients with a smoking history [22]. While the incidence of a synchronous primary tumor is low, it has a dramatic impact on the treatment of the patient.

Anesthesia for Surgical Endoscopy

Although local anesthesia can be used to anesthetize the larynx for some surgical procedures, the vast majority of surgical cases are performed under general anesthesia. While a complete discussion of surgical anesthesia is beyond the scope of this text, it is useful to understand a few basic principles, especially when considering laryngeal surgery. It is critical to maintain a patent airway and preserve ventilation to the lungs. This is most commonly performed using a flexible tube (endotracheal tube) passed through the nose or mouth and through the vocal folds into the trachea. This tube often impairs visualization of the larynx, making it difficult or impossible to perform delicate surgery on the larynx. Use of smaller endotracheal tubes can improve visualization of critical structures. Alternatively, removal of the tube for short periods of time can be performed [23]. A third technique is to use jet ventilation where a small diameter tube is placed either above or below the vocal folds, and high velocity oxygen is blown into the lungs to provide ventilation [23]. These techniques require close cooperation with the anesthesiologist to ensure adequate ventilation and prevent catastrophic complications.

Nasal Cavity and Nasopharynx

The majority of diagnostic nasal endoscopies and minor procedures can be performed in the office setting. More invasive surgical procedures or examinations in patients who cannot tolerate office endoscopy (e.g., young children) require a trip to the operating room to provide adequate anesthesia, instrumentation, and control of analgesia and hemorrhage. Advances in endoscope design and instrumentation have revolutionized surgery of the paranasal sinuses and skull base [24]. Surgical procedures have advanced from control of nasal hemorrhage and endoscopic drainage of the sinuses to advanced skull base approaches to the anterior and middle cranial fossae [24]. As discussed earlier, there are several endoscopes available in a variety of differing diameters and angles in order to provide the best visualization.

Oropharynx

The oropharynx can be visualized well with office endoscopy, as discussed previously. Invasive procedures that will cause pain, gagging, or bleeding are treated in the operating room but do not require endoscopes for visualization of these structures.

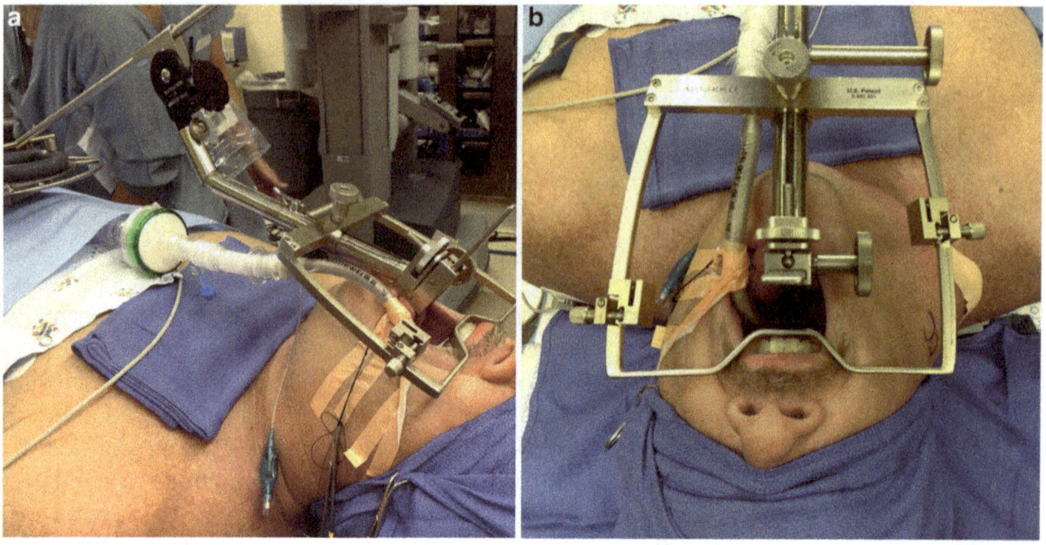

Fig. 6 Suspension laryngoscopy. Two viewpoints of a patient undergoing suspension laryngoscopy in the operating room: (**a**) oblique view and (**b**) top view (surgeon's view). The laryngoscope is fixed by an external structure, so the surgeon is free to operate with both hands. The patient also has an endotracheal (breathing) tube in place to maintain oxygenation throughout the procedure

Larynx and Hypopharynx

While many laryngeal procedures are successfully performed in the properly equipped office setting, most still require a trip to the operating room with sedation or general anesthesia. The operative laryngoscope is a bladed, rigid tube that is inserted through the mouth and into the pharynx to expose the larynx and hypopharynx for direct, line-of-sight view. A fiber-optic light carrier placed within the laryngoscope provides illumination. The laryngoscope can be suspended to fix the operative field and free the surgeon to work with both hands for operative manipulation (suspension laryngoscopy) (*see* Fig. 6a, b). A variety of laryngoscopes have been designed to meet the variability in patient anatomy and differing exposures required for various surgical procedures. They have in common increased diameter of the barrel to allow insertion of telescopes and surgical instruments and allow binocular microscopic visualization of anatomy beyond the lumen of the endoscope. Suspension laryngoscopy can also be performed in conjunction with a microscope or rigid telescope (microdirect laryngoscopy). The ability to suspend or fix the laryngoscope and obtain a magnified view affords the surgeon the ability to clearly visualize the fine structures of the larynx and manipulate the tissues with instruments in both hands to perform precise surgical maneuvers or deliver laser energy to the larynx.

Lower Airway

Rigid bronchoscopy is used to visualize the lower airways. A rigid bronchoscope is an elongated metal pipe of variable diameter with length of up to approximately 40 cm with capability for passing instruments and suction, direct visualization, ventilation of the airway, and passage of rigid telescopes. It is placed transorally in a patient under general anesthesia [17, 25]. Rigid bronchoscopes can accommodate a variety of telescopes with viewing angles of 0°–180° for visualization of the various bronchial passages to the upper and lower lobes of the lungs. While flexible bronchoscopy has limited the indications for its rigid counterpart, rigid bronchoscopy is necessary when larger instruments must be used, as in the cases of foreign body removal, placement of airway stents, and control of brisk hemorrhage from the trachea or bronchi.

Esophagus

Rigid esophagoscopy is almost always performed in the operating room on patients under general anesthesia, although historically it was often performed in the awake patient. The rigid esophagoscope, like the rigid bronchoscope, must be inserted transorally. While TNE is useful for diagnostic and limited therapeutic procedures, rigid endoscopy is required for more advanced or difficult procedures such as foreign body removal, management of a difficult airway, or control of a bleeding tumor.

Adjuncts to Endoscopy

Stroboscopy

Standard optical examination and video recording can evaluate the opening and closing of the vocal folds, as well as the presence of gross lesions. However, more nuanced pathology must be addressed by looking at the vibration of the vocal folds. The vocal folds normally vibrate in a periodic, sine wave pattern, between 100 and 1000 cycles per second (Hz) (with normal speech production centered around 100–200 Hz), which is far too rapid for the human eye to discriminate [26]. The stroboscope produces very bright and very short bursts of light synchronized with the frequency of vocal fold vibration. This produces a stop action or slow motion view of the vibratory cycle of the vocal fold [16]. The light pulses from the stroboscope can be delivered through rigid or flexible telescope systems. Stroboscopy provides high-quality imaging of the vibratory dynamics of the laryngeal mucosa. It can provide information about vocal fold vibration patterns and mucosal pliability, identify subtle mucosal or submucosal lesions, and evaluate the lesions' impact on vocal fold vibration [16]. Although flexible stroboscopy is possible and used in patients who cannot tolerate insertion of a rigid telescope, the image quality is markedly inferior unless a distal chip endoscope is used.

High-Speed Digital Imaging

While stroboscopy is a powerful tool for analyzing vocal disturbances and can often provide an accurate diagnosis, a small proportion of laryngeal disorders have irregular or aperiodic vibratory function not captured by stroboscopy. High-speed cinematography has been used as a research tool to photograph the larynx with speeds of 2000–4000 (and higher) frames per second [16]. This is a very expensive technique available in only a few research laboratories. This allows the physician to see vocal fold vibration patterns regardless of their length and allows the examiner to analyze the onset and offset of phonation, vibration in surrounding structures (e.g., ventricular folds), intermittent vibration breaks, and differences in the frequency of vibration along different portions of the same vocal fold [27–30]. High-speed digital imaging (HSDI) is only available using rigid endoscopes because flexible endoscopes cannot provide enough light to capture images that are bright or clear enough [16]. However, challenges with HSDI exist as well. Because so much data is captured, currently available systems can only record for 2–4 s at a time, depending on image capture rate and image size [16]. Even this short duration of recording necessitates prolonged software processing time to save the images digitally. Additionally, the spatial resolution is inferior to that of stroboscopy, and there is no capability for synchronized audio playback. The financial cost of an HSDI system is still beyond the budgets of most clinical practices. Finally, there are not yet standard parameters for normal or pathologic observation of real-time vocal fold vibration [16], which limits the clinical utility of HSDI at the present time.

Narrow Band Imaging

Narrow band imaging (NBI) is a new endoscopic imaging technique that takes advantage of the differential absorption characteristics of tissue to allow for the detailed analysis of mucosal and vascular structures [16]. NBI uses mechanical light-filtering technology to pass only blue and green wavelengths of light. Hemoglobin's peak light absorption occurs at these blue and green wavelengths, making blood vessels appear very dark, which creates sharper contrast for better visualization of fine mucosal details [31].

NBI was originally developed for identifying Barrett's esophagus, a condition in which the normal stratified squamous epithelial lining of the esophagus is replaced with the simple columnar epithelium found elsewhere in the lower digestive tract (40). The condition is strongly associated with esophageal adenocarcinoma. NBI is now being used in research settings to determine its utility for lesions of the head and neck [27, 31].

Tissue Fluorescence and Reflectance

Oral cavity cancer is a significant health problem, with an incidence of around 500,000 new cases per year worldwide [28]. Most of these lesions are not diagnosed until symptomatic, which generally corresponds to late-stage disease and poor survival [30]. The current standard of care for oral cavity cancer screening is visual inspection under white light and palpation; however, successful identification is dependent on examiner experience [30]. Recently, new methods have been developed as more objective screening tools for oral cavity cancer, which rely on autofluorescence and reflectance of tissue. Oral cavity tissues contain fluorophores which absorb UV photons and emit longer wavelength photons, which can be visualized as fluorescence [30]. Neoplastic tissues have fewer fluorophores, leading to less fluorescence [30]. The VELscope System (LED Medical Diagnostics, Inc) and Identafi 3000 (Trimira) are two examples of devices developed to capitalize on these tissue properties [29]. Unfortunately, although FDA approved, these devices have not significantly improved the diagnosis of oral cavity cancer. One study found that the Identafi 3000 had lower specificity for disease detection than standard white light examination [30].

Conclusion

Since the origin of endoscopy, exceptional progress has been made in visualization of the interior architecture of the head and neck. The convergence of improvements in lighting, optics, mechanical instrumentation, and miniaturization has revolutionized, and still continues to advance, our ability to see and manipulate tissues in the upper airway and digestive tract. While rigid endoscopy is still the gold standard for image production, flexible endoscopy has become an important part of outpatient diagnosis and interventions. As technology advances, adjuncts are made to endoscopy to improve visualization and diagnostic capabilities even further. Endoscopy is now a mainstay of every otolaryngologist's clinic and operating room and will remain a permanent fixture for many years to come.

References

1. Clary MS, Courey MS. Development of procedures and techniques for the office. Otolaryngol Clin North Am. 2013;46(1):1–11.
2. Morgenthal CB, et al. The role of the surgeon in the evolution of flexible endoscopy. Surg Endosc. 2007;21(6):838–53.
3. Reuter MA, Reuter HJ, Engel RM. History of endoscopy. In: Nitze M, editor. Museum fur Medizinische Endoskopie. Zurich: V Stuttgart and Karl Kramer Verlag Stuttgart; 2003.
4. Becker HD. Bronchoscopy: the past, the present, and the future. Clin Chest Med. 2010;31(1):1–18. Table of Contents.
5. Nezhat C. Nezhat's history of endoscopy: a historical analysis of endoscopy's ascension since antiquity. Tuttlingen, Germany: EndoPress; 2011.
6. Kleinsasser O. Microlaryngoscopy and endolaryngeal microsurgery. Philadelphia, PA: W. B. Saunders; 1968.
7. Strong MS, Jako GJ. Laser surgery in the larynx. Early clinical experience with continuous CO 2 laser. Ann Otol Rhinol Laryngol. 1972;81(6):791–8.
8. Steiner W. Experience in endoscopic laser surgery of malignant tumours of the upper aero-digestive tract. Adv Otorhinolaryngol. 1988;39:135–44.
9. Steiner W. Results of curative laser microsurgery of laryngeal carcinomas. Am J Otolaryngol. 1993;14(2):116–21.
10. Steiner W, et al. Transoral laser microsurgery for squamous cell carcinoma of the base of the tongue. Arch Otolaryngol Head Neck Surg. 2003;129(1):36–43.

11. Steiner W, et al. Organ preservation by transoral laser microsurgery in piriform sinus carcinoma. Otolaryngol Head Neck Surg. 2001; 124(1):58–67.
12. Chheda NN, Postma GN. Transnasal esophagoscopy. In: Flint PW, editor. Cummings otolaryngology—head and neck surgery. Philadelphia, PA: Mosby Elsevier; 2010. p. 981–5.
13. Couch M. History, physical examination, and the preoperative evaluation. In: Flint PW, editor. Cummings otolaryngology—head and neck surgery. Philadelphia, PA: Mosby Elsevier; 2010.
14. Nabili V, Yoo G, Golub J, Pasha R. Head and neck cancer. In: Pasha R, editor. Otolaryngology head and neck surgery: clinical reference guide. San Diego, CA: Plural Publishing; 2011.
15. Husain A. The lung. In: Kumar V, Abbas AK, Fausto N, Aster JC, editors. Robbins and Cotran pathologic basis of disease. Professionalth ed. Philadelphia, PA: W. B Saunders, Elsevier; 2010.
16. Samlan RA, GArtner-Schmidt J, Kunduk M. Visualization of the larynx. In: Flint PW, editor. Cummings otolaryngology—head and neck surgery. Philadelphia, PA: Mosby Elsevier; 2010. p. 813–24.
17. Kupeli E, Karnak D, Mehta AC. Flexible bronchoscopy. In: Murray and Nadel's textbook of respiratory medicine. Philadelphia, PA: Saunders Elsevier; 2010.
18. Lawrason AE, Brown S, Tessema B, Myers AD. Nasal endoscopy. 2012 April 20 [cited 2013 Dec 15]. Available from: http://emedicine.medscape.com/article/1890999-overview
19. Rennemo E, Zatterstrom U, Boysen M. Synchronous second primary tumors in 2,016 head and neck cancer patients: role of symptom-directed panendoscopy. Laryngoscope. 2011;121(2):304–9.
20. Hujala K, Sipila J, Grenman R. Panendoscopy and synchronous second primary tumors in head and neck cancer patients. Eur Arch Otorhinolaryngol. 2005;262(1):17–20.
21. Strobel K, et al. Head and neck squamous cell carcinoma (HNSCC)—detection of synchronous primaries with (18)F-FDG-PET/CT. Eur J Nucl Med Mol Imaging. 2009; 36(6):919–27.
22. Rodriguez-Bruno K, Ali MJ, Wang SJ. Role of panendoscopy to identify synchronous second primary malignancies in patients with oral cavity and oropharyngeal squamous cell carcinoma. Head Neck. 2011;33(7): 949–53.
23. Feldman MA, Patel A. Anesthesia for eye, ear, nose, and throat surgery. In: Miller RD, editor. Miller's anesthesia. Philadelphia, PA: Churchill Livingstone, Elsevier; 2009.
24. Stamm AC, Pignatari SSN. Transnasal endoscopic-assisted surgery of the anterior skull base. In: Cummings CW, Flint PW, editors. Cummings otolaryngology—head and neck surgery. Philadelphia, PA: Mosby Elsevier; 2010.
25. Morris IR. Anesthesia and airway management of laryngoscopy and bronchocopy. In: Hagberg CA, editor. Benumof's airway management, Second edition. Philadelphia, PA: Mosby Elsevier; 2007.
26. American Academy of Otolaryngology—Head and Neck Surgery. How the voice works. 2014 [cited 2014 Jan 5].
27. Wen YH, et al. Narrow-band imaging: a novel screening tool for early nasopharyngeal carcinoma. Arch Otolaryngol Head Neck Surg. 2012;138(2):183–8.
28. Johnson NW, et al. Global oral health inequalities in incidence and outcomes for oral cancer: causes and solutions. Adv Dent Res. 2011;23(2):237–46.
29. Sweeny L, et al. Assessment of tissue autofluorescence and reflectance for oral cavity cancer screening. Otolaryngol Head Neck Surg. 2011;145(6):956–60.
30. Messadi DV. Diagnostic aids for detection of oral precancerous conditions. Int J Oral Sci. 2013;5(2):59–65.
31. Bertino G, Cacciola S, Fernandes WB Jr, Fernandes CM, Occhini A, Tinelli C, Benazzo M. Effectiveness of narrow band imaging in the detection of pre-malignant and malignant lesions of the larynx: validation of a new endoscopic clinical classification. Head Neck. 2015;37(2):215–22. doi: 10.1002/hed.23582

Chapter 2

Laser Interventions for Early Cancer in the Upper Aerodigestive Tract

Christopher M. Bingcang and Sunil Verma

Introduction

The glottis is a unique subsite of the aerodigestive tract where cancer often presents early. A small lesion of the vocal fold often causes a marked change in an individual's voice, leading to the discovery of early glottic cancer. Further, the glottis is a unique subsite of head and neck cancer as its lymphatic drainage is sparse. This combination of factors causes a large number of glottic cancers to present early without spread to adjacent lymph nodes.

Due to this unique presentation of early glottic cancer, diverse treatment methods have been developed. Historically treatments have been in the form of open transcervical surgery, endoscopic transoral surgery using cold steel instrumentation, and external beam radiation therapy. However, the introduction of lasers to the management of early glottic cancer has revolutionized management of this disease. Lasers offer unique benefits in terms of accurate ability to cut and simultaneously coagulate tissue.

The challenge in surgically treating laryngeal cancer is that there is little space to work and stray damage can result in loss of function. Lasers have been used to increase accuracy of surgery in a confined space. Other advantages of lasers include decreased postoperative edema and the ability to seal small blood vessels and lymphatics thereby minimizing potential metastatic spread [1].

The laser has revolutionized the way in which early glottic carcinoma is treated. Prior to the widespread use of the laser, patients with early glottic carcinoma would require open transcervical surgery with laryngofissure and cordectomy, or endoscopic

Brian J.-F. Wong and Justus Ilgner (eds.), *Biomedical Optics in Otorhinolaryngology: Head and Neck Surgery*, DOI 10.1007/978-1-4939-1758-7_2, cold steel-assisted resection, which was fraught with decreased visibility due to the propensity of the tissue to bleed. In the mid-twentieth century, radiation therapy became an option for treating patients with laryngeal cancer, but this has been associated with higher cost, as well as acute and late side effects of radiation [2]. Additionally, patients that live far away from a city that has radiation therapy centers can ill afford to make the daily travel to the center over the required 7 weeks. As the laser became more available and affordable, patients now have another excellent option for treatment for their laryngeal cancer. Understanding the role of lasers and the challenges in the use of lasers may help engineers to design improved lasers that could increase efficacy of treatment, decrease complications of treatment, decrease costs, and increase availability of technology.

Definition of Early Laryngeal Cancer

Laryngeal cancer is prevalent worldwide, and in the United Stated is expected to affect over 12,000 new persons in 2014, while 3600 people with laryngeal cancer are expected to die in 2014 [3]. An estimated 3400 new cases of hypopharyngeal cancer will develop in 2014. Of laryngeal cancer, 60 % will affect the glottis, 35 % will affect the supraglottis, and the remaining 5 % will affect the subglottis.

The most common type of malignancy that presents in the larynx is squamous cell carcinoma, and the discussion of this chapter will focus on management of this disease. Tables 1 and 2 show the American Joint Committee on Cancer staging of supraglottic and glottic cancer, recently updated in 2010 [4]. T1a lesions may involve the superficial lamina propria layer, vocal ligament, or vocalis muscle of one vocal fold. Both surgical and radiation treatment create defects or scarring that adversely affect normal laryngeal function, namely, voice and swallow. As the depth of invasion increases, surgical resection creates glottic incompetence with resulting dysphonia [5].

The unique challenge with management of glottic malignancies is maintenance of vocal fold microstructure. Hirano's seminal description of the cover-body model of phonation led to further understanding about relation of depth of invasion and vocal outcomes [6, 7]. The goal for treatment is the removal of all cancerous tissue with a small margin of normal tissue, while preserving maximal normal tissue to optimize vocal function. The laser, with its ability to remove submillimeter segments of tissue, allows the surgeon the precision to balance the complete removal of cancerous tissue while avoiding removing excess noncancerous tissue that could adversely affect the functions of the larynx.

Table 1
Primary tumor (T)

TX	Primary tumor cannot be assessed
T0	No evidence of primary tumor
Tis	Carcinoma in situ
Supraglottis	
T1	Tumor limited to one subsite of supraglottis with normal vocal cord mobility
T2	Tumor invades mucosa of more than one adjacent subsite of supraglottis or glottis or region outside the supraglottis (e.g., mucosa of base of tongue, vallecula, medial wall of pyriform sinus) without fixation of the larynx
T3	Tumor limited to larynx with vocal cord fixation and/or invades any of the following: postcricoid area, preepiglottic space, paraglottic space, and/or inner cortex of thyroid cartilage
T4a	Moderately advanced local disease
	Tumor invades through the thyroid cartilage and/or invades tissues beyond the larynx (e.g., trachea, soft tissues of neck including deep extrinsic muscle of the tongue, strap muscles, thyroid, or esophagus)
T4b	Very advanced local disease
	Tumor invades prevertebral space, encases carotid artery, or invades mediastinal structures
Glottis	
T1	Tumor limited to the vocal cord(s) (may involve anterior or posterior commissure) with normal mobility
T1a	Tumor limited to one vocal cord
T1b	Tumor involves both vocal cords
T2	Tumor extends to supraglottis and/or subglottis and/or with impaired vocal cord mobility
T3	Tumor limited to the larynx with vocal cord fixation and/or invasion of paraglottic space and/or inner cortex of the thyroid cartilage
T4a	Moderately advanced local disease
	Tumor invades through the outer cortex of the thyroid cartilage and/or invades tissues beyond the larynx (e.g., trachea, soft tissues of neck including deep extrinsic muscle of the tongue, strap muscles, thyroid, or esophagus)
T4b	Very advanced local disease
	Tumor invades prevertebral space, encases carotid artery, or invades mediastinal structures

Nodal and distant metastatic staging have been omitted as early laryngeal cancer features neither nodal nor distant metastasis

As long as the contralateral vocal fold is without significant disease, then vocal function will be largely preserved if glottic closure is complete [8]. For this reason, T1b lesions and lesions of the anterior commissure create defects in the contralateral vocal fold that result in significantly decreased vocal function. T2 lesions

Table 2
Anatomic stage/prognostic groups

Stage	T	N	M
0	Tis	N0	M0
I	T1	N0	M0
II	T2	N0	M0
III	T3	N0	M0
	T1	N1	M0
	T2	N1	M0
	T3	N1	M0
IVA	T4a	N0	M0
	T4a	N1	M0
	T1	N2	M0
	T2	N2	M0
	T3	N2	M0
	T4a	N2	M0
IVB	T4b	Any N	M0
	Any T	N3	M0
IVC	Any T	Any N	M1

likewise require deeper resections thereby causing larger glottic gaps. The surgeon must counsel the patient regarding these effects as goals for treatment are discussed.

Mechanisms of Lasers Used in Laryngeal Cancer

Two lasers have been described to commonly manage laryngeal cancer: carbon dioxide (CO2) and potassium titanyl phosphate (KTP). The first description of the carbon dioxide laser in laryngeal surgery was in 1972 when Jako and Strong treated benign and premalignant laryngeal lesions [9]. In 1975, Strong described the use of the CO2 laser for excising carcinoma [10]. To date the carbon dioxide laser is the most commonly used laser for excision of glottic cancer. The carbon dioxide laser, with its 10,600 nm wavelength, is preferentially absorbed by water. Traditionally carbon dioxide laser beam is delivered into the larynx during direct microlaryngoscopy using a micromanipulator to target the tissues of interest. The laser spot size can be focused to 250 μm with recent technological advances [11], and a very precise cut may be made with this laser while decreasing thermal injury to surrounding tissue. This precision is critical in the larynx where

Table 3
Summary of lasers used to treat laryngeal cancer

Laser	Wavelength	Chromophore	Delivery
KTP	532 nm	Oxyhemoglobin	0.4 and 0.6 mm fiber optic
CO2	10,600 nm	Water	(1) 1.2 mm hollow core with dielectric mirror (photonic band-gap fiber) (2) Line-of-site/micromanipulator

preservation of tissues leads to dramatic improvement in voice after surgery.

Recently, a hollow fiber has been developed that delivers the energy from the carbon dioxide laser. (currently manufactured by OmniGuide and Clinicon). The fiber consists of a hollow-core tube surrounded by a dielectric mirror, which allows the use of CO2 either within a flexible endoscope or delivered through a handpiece. The fiber-based delivery permitted improved angulations for tangential surfaces that were difficult for line-of-site lasers [12].

The 532 nm KTP laser is the other laser commonly used to treat early glottic cancer. This differs from the carbon dioxide laser in that its energy is transmitted through a glass fiber. Additionally, the energy from this laser is preferentially absorbed by oxyhemoglobin. This also preferentially targets hypervascular lesions [13], which includes cancerous lesions [14]. It also may result in improved hemostasis over CO2 laser due to preferential absorption and destruction of the target lesion's supporting microvasculature. Unlike the CO2 laser, the KTP laser has only recently seen use for treating glottic cancer. Initially it was used in the larynx for benign disease [13, 15, 16]. In 2008, Zeitels and colleagues described the use of the potassium titanyl phosphate laser (KTP) to treat carcinoma [14]. Table 3 summarizes key KTP laser characteristics compared to other lasers used in excising laryngeal carcinoma.

Surgical Technique

Before undergoing surgery, patients must be counseled with a thorough discussion of surgery and its alternatives. The surgeon must be able to counsel patients regarding the cure rates, the treatment effects on voice and swallow, and treatment complications. Patients must also have the cardiopulmonary reserve to handle the risks of general anesthesia. Finally, the surgeon must be able to adequately expose the larynx with the laryngoscope and be prepared to perform an open resection if the larynx cannot be exposed endoscopically. Mandibular anatomic problems, such as retrognathia, enlarged tori, trismus, or problems with neck extension may prevent placement of the laryngoscope, thus requiring patients to undergo transcervical surgery or radiation instead.

Intraoperatively, the surgeon must take precautions to avoid potential fire. Flammable gases and potential fuel sources such as the endotracheal tube are within the line of site of the laser. First, the door to the room is closed and signage to alert potential incomers of laser use is placed on the door. Personnel in the room are distributed with appropriate laser-safe eyewear. Each laser has specific protective eyewear that filters the corresponding wavelength of light, and therefore eyewear for different lasers should not be used. A laser-resistant endotracheal tube is used in the patient. Because the tip of the endotracheal tube is susceptible to laser fire, it should be covered with saline-soaked cottonoid pledgets. Suction is used to evacuate laser plume, which allows improved visualization and decreases toxic and carcinogenic fumes that may inadvertently be inhaled by operating room personnel. The anesthesiologist must reduce use of flammable gases and decrease the percentage of supplementary oxygen below 30 %. Finally, the patient's face is covered in saline-soaked towels, and OR staff should always be at the ready to immediately douse any flames that start.

Endoscopic Laser Resection of Early Glottic Carcinoma

The patient is placed under general anesthesia and is intubated with a laser-safe endotracheal tube. A tooth guard is used to protect the upper dentition, and a laryngoscope placed through the oral cavity and positioned to fully expose the endolarynx and the lesion. The largest laryngoscope that fits within the patient's oral cavity and oropharynx should be used in order to permit wide binocular visualization. Univalve or bivalve laryngoscopes may be used. Regardless of the choice, the anterior commissure must be exposed; laryngoscopes such as the Storz Triangle laryngoscope or the Endocraft Zeitels Universal Modular Glottiscope permit excellent anterior commissure exposure. The laryngoscope is placed on fulcrum or gallows suspension to allow bimanual technique. The binocular microscope is used for magnification and allowing depth perception. Laser safety precautions are followed as previously discussed. In many cases, the vestibular fold may be resected to optimize exposure for surgery as well as for future cancer surveillance [17]. Saline with epinephrine is injected into the superficial lamina propria to provide vasoconstriction, hydrodissection, and to establish depth of tumor invasion; it also acts as a heat sink to decrease thermal damage to noncancerous tissue [18]. Laser-assisted resection of the cancer may then be performed by one of several techniques. Three methods will be described.

The extent of resection has been classified by the European Laryngological Society [19]. Such a classification has been developed

Table 4
Endoscopic cordectomy: classification by European laryngological society

Subepithelial cordectomy	Type I
Subligamental cordectomy	Type II
Transmuscular cordectomy	Type III
Total or complete cordectomy	Type IV
Extended cordectomy encompassing	
Contralateral fold	Type IVa
Arytenoids	Type IVb
Ventricular fold	Type IVc
Subglottis	Type IVd

in order to help better relate extent of resection to outcomes. Table 4 shows ELS type for depth of excision. The type of resection is determined postoperatively rather than as preoperative plan. The first three types describe successive layers. Type I is performed during an excisional subepithelial resection, whose biopsy reveals carcinoma in situ and thus deeper resection is not needed. Types III and IV include cordectomies for carcinomas that invade the superficial lamina propria and the vocalis ligament, respectively; these may be T1 or T2 carcinomas, but spare the contralateral vocal fold.

Partial Cordectomy: En Bloc Resection

The CO2 laser has been traditionally used for performing a laser-assisted endoscopic partial cordectomy technique as described by Strong [10], Eckel and Thumfart [20], and Ossoff et al. [5]. Once laryngeal exposure is achieved, the lesion is grasped by the surgeon with forceps in one hand while the other hand operates the micromanipulator. Retraction forces are placed on the lesion while the laser is fired around the margins of the lesion. The margin is initially outlined superficially and is continued into deeper planes layer by layer. The lesion is excised en bloc down to the vocalis muscle or deeper if the lesion is larger. Once the lesion is excised, small specimens are removed from the periphery and deep layers to be sent for frozen section. Any positive margins may thus be treated by additional laser resection. During the procedure, any excessive hemorrhage may be treated by a defocused beam. Rarely does laryngeal edema from surgery result in airway obstruction, and therefore the patient in most cases can be extubated immediately after surgery.

Partial Cordectomy-Piecemeal Resection

Although oncologically successful, en bloc resection may increase the risk of excising excessively large margins, thereby resulting in worse vocal outcomes. Steiner described a piecemeal resection method that excised the lesion in successive fashion, allowing the surgeon to preserve as much normal tissue as possible [21, 22]. The tumor is bisected, which allows accurate assessment of depth of tumor. The technique demands maintaining correct orientation of the specimen as well as having excellent surgical pathology that can accurately assess frozen sections. Performed correctly, the surgeon is able to avoid excising excessive noncancerous tissue, while preserving adequate margins.

Photoangiolytic Laser Cordectomy

The photoangiolytic lasers such as KTP and PDL have recently begun to be used to treat carcinomas. This technique was initially described by Zeitels et al. in 2008 [14]. His group used the KTP and PDL to treat 13 T1 and 9 T2 lesions and at the time of the report, none of the patients had recurrence of cancer. Rather than excising the lesion en bloc, the surgeon ablates the lesion with a 3 mm peripheral margin layer by layer until normal tissue is reached. This technique takes advantage of the increased density of vascularity of cancerous lesions, as the energy from the photoangiolytic lasers is preferentially absorbed by blood vessels. Success of this operation is predicated on the surgeon's ability to recognize the interface between cancerous and normal tissue, which can be challenging. Depth and width of treatment are thus determined by the exact interface with normal tissue, which is progressively seen as each layer is ablated. This results in avoidance of removing excessive normal tissue and thus optimizes vocal function. Intraoperative frozen histopathologic sections are obtained at the periphery as well at the deep margins to confirm complete treatment.

Importance of Intraoperative Frozen Sections

Frozen sections are essential for determining extent of resection, while preserving noncancerous tissue. In the past, there has been concern that the thermal effect of the laser on tissue decreases the reliability of frozen section. However, Remacle et al. retrospectively reviewed multiple patients undergoing endoscopic CO2 laser cordectomies for T1 through T3 glottic cancers [23]. This group found that frozen sections were concordant with permanent sections in nearly 95 % of cases.

Endoscopic Laser Resection of Supraglottic Carcinoma

Early supraglottic carcinoma may also be resected with endoscopic approach and laser. Laser resection for supraglottic cancer was first reported by Vaughan in 1978 [24]. Zeitels et al. reported on a series of 45 patients who had T1 to T3 lesions of the supraglottic larynx or posterior pharyngeal wall without any neck disease [25]. T1 and smaller T2 tumors were easily resected with negative intraoperative margins and did not undergo radiotherapy, and only one patient had developed a neck recurrence, subsequently undergoing neck dissection and postoperative radiation. The 23 patients with larger tumors all received postoperative radiation, and despite this, four patients had recurrence, eventually requiring total laryngectomy, and a total of four patients died from their disease. This study as well as early works by Rudert [26], Eckel [27], Steiner [28], and Davis [29] has established endoscopic laser resection for supraglottic carcinoma as a viable option for selected patients. Because of the propensity of epiglottic lesions to spread to the preepiglottic space, especially with infrahyoid epiglottic lesions, this space must be resected as well. In fact, Zeitels' group did not perform endoscopic resection at all if this space was involved [25].

Complications of Endoscopic Laser Surgery

Complications directly related to use of the laser are rare, but potentially devastating. Healy et al. described nine complications in 4416 CO2 laser cases of the aerodigestive tract for a rate of 0.2 % [30]. Six of these complications were fires, and of these four were fires from ignition of the endotracheal tubes that were not laser protected. Two complications were due to excessive bleeding from bronchial tumors. One complication resulted in a facial burn from an overheated rigid bronchoscope resting on a patient's cheek. Other potential complications related to endoscopic resection are granuloma from exposed cartilage or char left after the operation. Chondritis may also develop from exposed cartilage and may be prevented by perioperative antibiotics and steroids. Hemorrhage should be controlled by a return to the operating room and defocused beam or electrocautery to site of bleeding.

Outcomes of Endoscopic Laser Surgery

Voice Quality with Endoscopic Laser Surgery versus Radiation Therapy

Early studies contrasting radiation versus surgery for early glottic carcinoma found that although disease control was similar, voice quality was significantly worse for surgical resection [31–33]. A meta-analysis by Higgins et al. of 7600 patients with early glottic cancer showed a trend for better voice quality with radiation over endoscopic laser surgery. In contrast, some recent studies suggest that voice outcomes after endoscopic laser surgery for glottic carcinoma are no worse than radiation therapy [34, 35]. One study found that voice was better with endoscopic laser surgery, but patients undergoing surgery were selected due to a more superficial involvement of the tumor, and therefore only required either ELS type I or type II cordectomy [36]. Indeed, while ELS type I and II resections showed better voice compared to radiation, ELS type III and type IV, sub-ligamentous and submuscular resections, had significantly worse voices compared to radiation [32]. This suggests that depth of invasion and deeper resection worsens voice quality. Additionally significant worsening was noted when the anterior commissure was involved [34, 37].

Oncologic Efficacy of Endoscopic Laser Surgery

Surgeons must guide patients deciding between radiation and surgery for early glottic carcinoma as both modalities have been shown to be essentially equivalent in terms of disease control [2, 38–41]. The most important factors to consider in determining modality of treatment are efficacy of removing disease, maintenance of voice and quality of life, and costs of care. Disease control as well as overall survival is established to be high for early glottic carcinoma. Lucioni and colleagues found that overall survival was 90 %, and when excluding mortality not related to laryngeal carcinoma, disease-free survival was 98.8 % [42]. Indeed most studies performed to date support that endoscopic laser resection of early glottic carcinoma is equivalent and in some cases superior to radiation therapy regarding control of disease. Remmelts et al. found that 5-year laryngeal preservation for T1 glottic cancers treated with laser was 93 %, which was statistically significantly better than those treated by radiation therapy versus 83 % for radiation therapy [37]. Additionally Krengli et al. found that local control over 60 months was 95.6 % with endoscopic laser surgery while 91.2 % for radiation therapy [32]. The meta-analysis by Higgins et al. examined local control and laryngectomy-free survival in 7600 patients with T1 or T2 glottic cancer and found that there was no difference between endoscopic laser surgery and radiation therapy, although there was a trend toward better survival in endoscopic laser surgery [43].

Costs of Endoscopic Laser Resection Compared to Radiation Therapy

Several studies in Europe and North America suggest that endoscopic laser resection is less costly than radiotherapy for Tis and T1 cancers. Goor et al. reviewed 89 patients with T1a glottic carcinoma over 2 years. 35 were treated with 6000 cGy whereas 54 were treated with endoscopic laser resection. Radiotherapy cost 8322 euros per case versus 4434 euros per case for surgery. Furthermore, disease control and voice quality were not found to be different [40]. Similarly Higgins performed a meta-analysis comparing radiotherapy versus endoscopic laser resection for T1 glottic cancers [2]. Average costs of radiotherapy were found to be $4829 whereas endoscopic laser resection cost $2407.

Endoscopic KTP Laser Surgery Efficacy

Although not used as extensively as CO2 laser, the KTP laser is showing some promise as an excellent tool for treating early glottic carcinoma. Murono et al. performed KTP endoscopic KTP laser surgery for T1a glottic carcinoma in 24 patients. Tumor was excised with KTP laser, followed by circumferential ablation surrounding the surgical margin, and found local control in 22 of the 24 patients (91.7 %). This is comparable to the local control rate noted in the literature [44]. Additionally voice results were found to be excellent as patients had significant improvement from pre- to postoperative voice after KTP laser surgery in T1 and T2 glottic carcinomas [45].

Summary

Laser laryngeal surgery is a powerful tool for management of early glottic cancer. Laser surgery may offer patients improved cancer-free and voice outcomes as well as cost much less to perform.

References

1. Ossoff RH, Duncavage JA, Fried MP, Courey MS. Laser laryngoscopy. In: Fried MP, editor. The larynx: a multidisciplinary approach. St. Louis, MO: CV Mosby; 1996. p. 397–411.
2. Higgins KM. What treatment for early-stage glottic carcinoma among adult patients: CO2 endolaryngeal laser excision versus standard fractionated external beam radiation is superior in terms of cost utility? Laryngoscope. 2011;121(1):116–34.
3. American Cancer Society. Cancer facts & figures 2014. 2014. http://www.cancer.org/acs/groups/content/@research
4. Edge SB, Byrd DR, Compton CC, Fritz AG, Greene FL, Trotti A, eds. Larynx. In: AJCC Cancer Staging Manual. 7th ed. New York, NY: Springer; 2010. p. 57–62.
5. Ossoff RH, Sisson GA, Shapshay SM. Endoscopic management of selected early vocal cord carcinoma. Ann Otol Rhinol Laryngol. 1985;94(6 Pt 1):560–4.
6. Hirano M. Morphological structure of the vocal cord as a vibrator and its variations. Folia poniatr. 1974;26:89–94.
7. Hirano M, Hirade Y. CO2 laser for treating glottic carcinoma. Acta Otolaryngol Suppl. 1988;458:154–7.
8. Jiang JJ, Titze IR. A methodological study of hemilaryngeal phonation. Laryngoscope. 1993;103(8):872–82.
9. Strong MS, Jako GJ. Laser surgery in the larynx. early clinical experience with continuous CO2 laser. Ann Otol Rhinol Laryngol. 1972;81(6):791–8.
10. Strong MS. Laser excision of carcinoma of the larynx. Laryngoscope. 1975;85(8):1286–9.
11. Ossoff RH, Werkhaven JA, Raif J, Abraham M. Advanced microspot microslad for the CO2 laser. Otolaryngol Head Neck Surg. 1991;105(3):411–4.
12. Zeitels SM, Kobler JB, Heaton JT, Faquin W. Carbon dioxide laser fiber for laryngeal cancer surgery. Ann Otol Rhinol Laryngol. 2006;115(7):535–41.
13. Hirano S, Yamashita M, Kitamura M, Takagita S. Photocoagulation of microvascular and hemorrhagic lesions of the vocal fold with the KTP laser. Ann Otol Rhinol Laryngol. 2006;115(4):253–9.
14. Zeitels SM, Burns JA, Lopez-Guerra G, Anderson RR, Hillman RE. Photoangiolytic laser treatment of early glottic cancer: a new management strategy. Ann Otol Rhinol Laryngol Suppl. 2008;199:3–24.
15. Zeitels SM, Akst LM, Burns JA, Hillman RE, Broadhurst MS, Anderson RR. Office-based 532-nm pulsed KTP laser treatment of glottal papillomatosis and dysplasia. Ann Otol Rhinol Laryngol. 2006;115(9):679–85.
16. Hsiung MW, Kang BH, Su WF, Pai L, Wang HW. Clearing microvascular lesions of the true vocal fold with the KTP/532 laser. Ann Otol Rhinol Laryngol. 2003;112(6):534–9.
17. Kerrebijn JD, DeBoer MF, Knegt PP. CO2-laser treatment of recurrent glottic carcinoma. Clin Otolaryngol. 1992;17(5):430–2.
18. Zeitels SM. Vocal fold dysplasia/atypia and carcinoma. In: Zeitels SM, editor. Atlas of phonomicrosurgery and other endolaryngeal procedures for benign and malignant disease. San Diego, CA: Singular-Thomson Learning; 2001. p. 177–218.
19. Remacle M, Eckel HE, Antonelli A, et al. Endoscopic cordectomy. a proposal for a classification by the working committee, European laryngological society. Eur Arch Otorhinolaryngol. 2000;257(4):227–31.
20. Eckel HE, Thumfart WF. Laser surgery for the treatment of larynx carcinomas: indications, techniques, and preliminary results. Ann Otol Rhinol Laryngol. 1992;101:113–8.
21. Steiner W. Experience in endoscopic laser surgery of malignant tumours of the upper aero-digestive tract. Adv Otorhinolaryngol. 1988;39:135–44.
22. Steiner W, Ambrosch P. The role of the phoniatrician in laser surgery of the larynx. In: Steiner W, Ambrosch P, editors. Endoscopic laser surgery of the upper aerodigestive tract. New York, NY: Thieme; 2000. p. 124–9.
23. Remacle M, Matar N, Delos M, Nollevaux M-C, Jamart J, Lawson G. Is frozen section

reliable in transoral CO(2) laser-assisted cordectomies? Eur Arch Otorhinolaryngol. 2010;267(3):397–400.

24. Vaughan CW. Transoral laryngeal surgery using the CO2 laser: laboratory experiments and clinical experience. Laryngoscope. 1978; 88(9 Pt 1):1399–420.
25. Zeitels SM, Koufman JA, Davis RK, Vaughan CW. Endoscopic treatment of supraglottic and hypopharynx cancer. Laryngoscope. 1994; 104(1 Pt 1):71–8.
26. Rudert H, Werner JA. Endoscopic resections of a glottic and supraglottic carcinomas with the CO2 laser. Eur Arch Otorhinolaryngol. 1995;252(3):142–6.
27. Eckel HE. Endoscopic laser resection of supraglottic carcinoma. Otolaryngol Head Neck Surg. 1997;117(6):681–7.
28. Steiner W. Results of curative laser microsurgery of laryngeal carcinomas. Am J Otolaryngol. 1993;14(2):116–21.
29. Davis RK, Shapshay SM, Strong MS, Hyams VJ. Transoral partial supraglottic resection using the CO2 laser. Laryngoscope. 1983; 93(4):429–33.
30. Healy GB, Strong MS, Shapshay SM, Vaughan CW, Jako GJ. Complications of CO2 laser surgery of the aerodigestive tract: experience of 4416 cases. Otolaryngol Head Neck Surg. 1984;92(1):13–8.
31. Rydell R, Schalén L, Fex S, Elner A. Voice evaluation before and after laser excision vs. radiotherapy of T1A glottic carcinoma. Acta Otolaryngol. 1995;115(4):560–5.
32. Krengli M, Policarpo M, Manfredda I, et al. Voice quality after treatment for T1a glottic carcinoma: radiotherapy versus laser cordectomy. Acta Oncol (Madr). 2004;43(3): 284–9.
33. Núñez Batalla F, Caminero Cueva MJ, Señaris González B, et al. Voice quality after endoscopic laser surgery and radiotherapy for early glottic cancer: objective measurements emphasizing the voice handicap index. Eur Arch Otorhinolaryngol. 2008;265(5):543–8.
34. McGuirt WF, Blalock D, Koufman JA, et al. Comparative voice results after laser resection or irradiation of T1 vocal cord carcinoma. Arch Otolaryngol Head Neck Surg. 1994;120(9): 951–5.
35. Sjögren EV, van Rossum MA, Langeveld TP, et al. Voice outcome in T1a midcord glottic carcinoma: laser surgery vs. radiotherapy. Arch Otolaryngol Head Neck Surg. 2008;134(9): 965–72.
36. Peeters AJGE, van Gogh CDL, Goor KM, Verdonck-de Leeuw IM, Langendijk JA, Mahieu HF. Health status and voice outcome after treatment for T1a glottic carcinoma. Eur Arch Otorhinolaryngol. 2004;261(10):534–40.
37. Remmelts AJ, Hoebers F, Klop WM, Balm AJ, Hamming-Vrieze O, van den Brekel MW. Evaluation of laser surgery and radiotherapy as treatment modalities in early stage laryngeal carcinoma: tumour outcome and quality of voice. Eur Arch Otorhinolaryngol. 2013; 270(7):2079–87.
38. Cragle SP, Brandenburg JH. Laser cordectomy or radiotherapy: cure rates, communication, and cost. Otolaryngol Head Neck Surg. 1993;108(6):648–54.
39. Gallo A, de Vincentiis M, Manciocco V, Simonelli M, Fiorella ML, Shah JP. CO2 laser cordectomy for early-stage glottic carcinoma: a long-term follow-up of 156 cases. Laryngoscope. 2002;112(2):370–4.
40. Goor KM, Peeters AJGE, Mahieu HF, Langendijk JA, Rene C. Cordectomy by CO2 laser or radiotherapy for small T1a glottic carcinomas: costs, local control, survival, quality of life, and voice quality. Head Neck. 2007;29(2):128–36.
41. Higgins KM, Punthakee X. Meta-analysis comparison of open versus percutaneous tracheostomy. Laryngoscope. 2007;117(3):447–54. doi:10.1097/01.mlg.0000251585.31778.c9.
42. Lucioni M, Marioni G, Bertolin A, Giacomelli L, Rizzotto G. Glottic laser surgery: outcomes according to 2007 ELS classification. Eur Arch Otorhinolaryngol. 2011;268(12):1771–8.
43. Higgins KM, Shah MD, Ogaick MJ, Enepekides D. Treatment of early-stage glottic cancer: meta-analysis comparison of laser excision versus radiotherapy. J Otolaryngol Head Neck Surg. 2009;38(6):603–12.
44. Murono S, Endo K, Kondo S, Wakisaka N, Yoshizaki T. Oncological and functional outcome after transoral 532-nm pulsed potassium-titanyl-phosphate laser surgery for T1a glottic carcinoma. Lasers Med Sci. 2013;28(2):615–9.
45. Friedman AD, Hillman RE, Landau-Zemer T, Burns JA, Zeitels SM. Voice outcomes for photoangiolytic KTP laser treatment of early glottic cancer. Ann Otol Rhinol Laryngol. 2013;122(3):151–8.

Chapter 3

Laser Resection of Pharyngeal Cancer

Ameya A. Jategaonkar, Alpen B. Patel, and Michael L. Hinni

Introduction

Transoral laser microsurgery (TLM) is a surgical treatment method for primary cancers of the mouth, pharynx, and larynx and offers decreased morbidity when compared to traditional open approaches. TLM typically utilizes a carbon dioxide (CO_2) laser for resection of tissues. An operating microscope supplies the illumination and magnification. Access is gained via the natural anatomy of the upper aerodigestive tract. TLM differs from open surgery in two significant ways: the tumor block can be transected into manageable units by the laser (in situ), permitting margin mapping. And healing is allowed to occur by secondary intention. While this "piecemeal" removal of the tumor deviates from the "en bloc" principle of conventional oncologic surgery, it adds a diagnostic dimension to TLM.

It is important to note that TLM is excision, not vaporization. TLM requires a specimen from which meaningful frozen section margins can be obtained. While individual specimens extracted by this piecemeal approach may be small, in total, their volume is comparable to that of an open resection.

The name transoral laser microsurgery can be misleading. TLM is not wholly transoral. Open surgery may be required for neck dissections to treat regional lymph node metastases. Furthermore, TLM is not entirely a laser procedure either. Hemostasis depends on electrocautery and vascular clips; additionally blunt and sharp dissection is regularly employed. Finally, TLM is not exclusively surgical. Radiation therapy (RT) or chemoradiotherapy (CRT) may be added as adjuvant therapy for advanced cancers.

Brian J.-F. Wong and Justus Ilgner (eds.), *Biomedical Optics in Otorhinolaryngology: Head and Neck Surgery*, DOI 10.1007/978-1-4939-1758-7_3, © Springer Science+Business Media New York 2016

There is a spectrum of disease within otolaryngology that is treated with lasers.

TLM is a strategy that is typically reserved for the treatment of neoplastic processes. This chapter focuses on the utilization of TLM for the treatment of pharyngeal (specifically oropharyngeal) cancer.

Conventional Approaches and Their Outcomes

The pharynx can be roughly divided into three components: the nasopharynx, oropharynx, and hypopharynx. Malignancies of each of these regions are treated somewhat differently given the varying regional anatomy. Conventional surgical oncology requires sufficient access to enable "en bloc" tumor resection. Access is a challenge in tumors of the oropharynx, particularly the distal oropharynx. Here the mandible is the source of greatest impediment. Therefore, treatment methods center on getting "around" the mandible. Conventional open operations involve lip-splits, mandibulotomies, and/or pharyngotomies to gain adequate exposure. While these open operations have yielded satisfactory oncologic outcomes, the morbidities often result in diminished functional results [1, 2]. With modern patients increasingly resistant to such measures, RT and CRT began to emerge as alternative primary treatment methods. In a comparison of patients receiving primary radiation vs. primary surgery (open resection) for treatment of base of tongue squamous cell carcinoma (SCCA), surgical patients had significantly poorer quality of life (functional) outcomes. Surgical patients scored significantly poorer in their ability to eat in public, have understandable speech, and normalcy of diet [3]. Additionally, work by Parsons et al. had a significant impact on the treatment of oropharyngeal cancer. Parsons conducted a review of 51 studies reporting on 6400 patients with oropharyngeal SCCA. The work compared patients who were treated with primary surgery (open operations) with or without RT or primary RT without neck dissections [4]. This review revealed similar oncologic results between the two treatment modalities (5-year cause-specific survival rates were statistically the same). However, the review demonstrated a severe complication rate of 23 % in the surgical intervention group versus a 6 % complication rate in the radiotherapy group. Ultimately, this resulted in a shift in the treatment of oropharyngeal SCCA away from surgery and toward RT. As a result, treatment of most oropharyngeal cancers, particularly locoregionally advanced disease (stages III and IV), has fallen within the domain of radiation and medical oncology.

Surgery, in general, has moved toward minimally invasive methods over the last several decades. Otolaryngology has been no different, and TLM reflects this new paradigm. Transoral laser microsurgery presents an alternative to conventional surgery and RT that has excellent oncologic and functional results.

Transoral Laser Microsurgery: Functional and Oncologic Outcomes

Transoral approaches for the treatment of head and neck cancers have existed for decades [5]. Lasers have been used in the oropharyngeal and laryngeal surgeries since the 1970s as well [6–8]. Nevertheless, surgical treatment of oropharyngeal cancer has been hindered most by poor access to the anatomy of the distal oropharynx. As discussed earlier, due to the morbidities of traditional lip-split/mandibulotomy approaches, much of the world moved toward RT and CRT as the preferred primary treatment method. Wolfgang Steiner approached the issues of accessibility from another direction. Steiner is credited with developing the surgical technique of TLM. He utilized a distending bivalved laryngoscope to provide appropriate exposure of tumors of the inferior oropharynx [9]. With sufficient exposure, the tumor can be grasped using a tenaculum with one hand and a laser utilized to cut the tumor with the other hand.

Ultimately TLM and breakthroughs within TLM have allowed surgery to be primary treatment for disease that would otherwise not have been amenable to surgical interventions [10]. The magnification and illumination that is used during TLM exceeds that provided by loupes and a headlamp. This allows the surgeon to carefully assess normal and abnormal tissues as he or she operates and carefully resect the tumor with margins. The ability of the surgeon to operate with this precision optimizes the preservation of normal anatomy and function. As a result, TLM has demonstrated excellent functional outcomes. Cancer and subsequent surgery of the pharynx has the potential to result in dysphagia and aspiration, which can detrimentally affect a patient's quality of life. Thus, preservation of swallowing function is a prominent goal of any treatment modality for head and neck cancer [11]. In early work with TLM for base of tongue carcinoma, Steiner reported that 73 % of patients enjoyed undisturbed oral intake of all food consistencies. Only 6 % of patients had dysphagia that was severe and unimproving and thus resulted in permanent gastronomy tube feeding [10]. Several other studies have demonstrated comparable functional outcomes [12, 13]. Grant et al. also utilized TLM as the primary treatment method for base of tongue carcinoma. Only 8 % of patients in this study required permanent tube feeding, and all eight patients received adjuvant RT [14]. Overall, Grant et al. reported that the median outcome for patients was normal, asymptomatic swallowing function. Rich et al. specifically looked at the swallowing function of patients following primary TLM (with adjuvant therapy) for advanced stage oropharyngeal cancer (stage III or IV). They reported 55 % of patients had good swallowing function during and consistently after treatment. An additional 32 % had poor swallowing function during the course of their treatment, which recovered. Ultimately only 8 % of patients who presented with advanced oropharyngeal cancer had poor swallowing function after treatment [15].

The oncologic outcomes of TLM have also been excellent. Steiner was able to achieve a Kaplan–Meier 5-year local control rate of 85 %. Additionally there were no local recurrences in lower grade tumors (T1 and T2). The 5-year recurrence-free survival in Steiner's work was 73 % [10]. Grant et al. in a study of 59 patients who received primary TLM for SCCA of the base of tongue (representing all 4 T stages) achieved 5-year Kaplan–Meier local control estimates of 90 % [14]. In a study of 128 patients treated with TLM for SCCA of the palatine tonsil, Hinni et al. had a local control rate of 95.4 %. Moreover, Kaplan–Meier 2-, 5-, and 10-year disease-free survival estimates were 96.5 %, 94.5 %, and 94.5 %, respectively [16]. TLM's effectiveness as the primary treatment method for advanced oropharyngeal tumors (T3 and T4) has also been demonstrated. In addition to treating larger tumors directly, TLM can be done with a neck dissection to treat neck metastases. TLM can also be coupled with adjuvant RT (or CRT). TLM with adjuvant therapy has demonstrated efficacy in treating locoregionally advanced disease [17, 18]. Haughey et al. studied 214 patients with stage III or IV disease. TLM with neck dissection was the primary treatment modality. Of these 214, 77 % received adjuvant therapy. Ultimately, Haughey et al. achieved 5-year Kaplan–Meier overall survival and disease-specific survival rates of 78 % and 84 %, respectively [18]. Figures 1, 2, 3, 4, 5, and 6 illustrate a typical TLM case.[1]

Cost considerations are becoming an increasing component of the calculus of healthcare. A substantial financial investment is needed to enable TLM. The institution will incur the costs of training and equipment. And, TLM adds to the workload of pathologists and cyto-technicians. TLM can also require patients to travel since its availability is limited in the United States. Nevertheless,

[1] These figures are of a 51-year-old male who presented with 6 months of left jaw pain and otalgia. He was initially diagnosed and treated for temporomandibular joint dysfunction. Subsequently, a dentist noted a tonsillar mass and referred the patient to otolaryngology. He underwent a tonsillectomy that failed to remove the entire lesion. The patient then presented for evaluation and treatment.

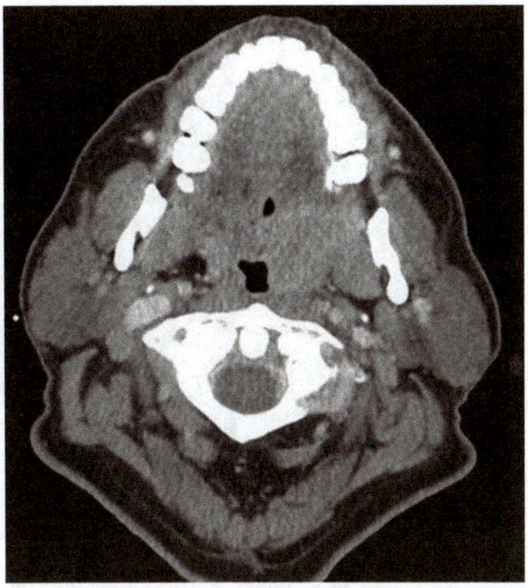

Fig. 1 CT scan of the left-sided T3 oropharyngeal tumor

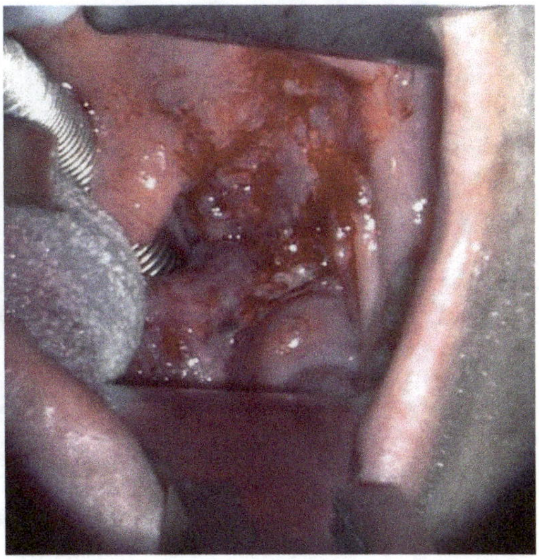

Fig. 2 Left-sided oropharyngeal tumor seen intraoperatively, prior to resection

despite these additional expenditures, TLM reduces costs considerably [19, 20]. In a study of the costs associated with treatment of oropharyngeal cancer, Moore et al. reported that CRT alone is 2.4 times more costly than transoral surgery with adjuvant RT and 5.29 times more expensive than surgery alone [20]. When several treatment options exist that are equivalent in their resultant quality of life and oncologic capabilities, costs can and will be considered. TLM results in shorter hospital stays and fewer complications.

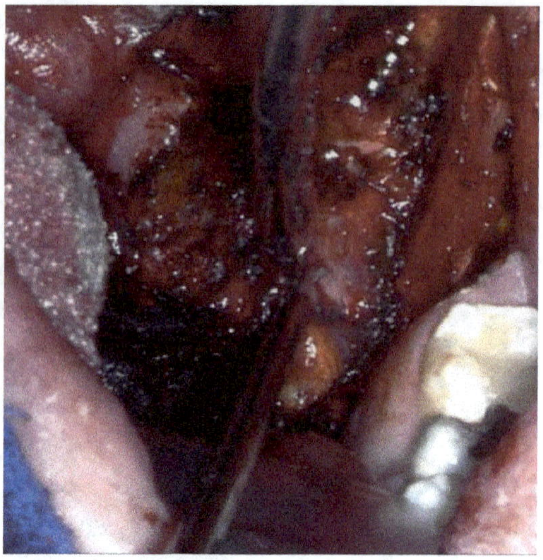

Fig. 3 Tumor shown intraoperatively during resection. Vascular clips used for hemostasis also seen

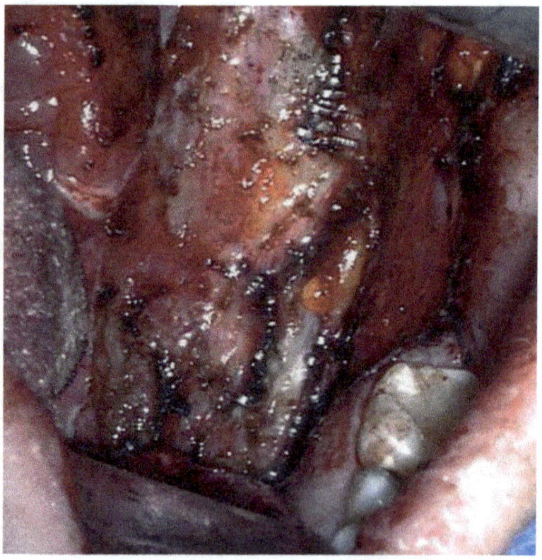

Fig. 4 Defect following TLM for left oropharyngeal squamous cell carcinoma

History of Lasers in Otolaryngology

The laser began in the microwave spectrum as the MASER (Microwave Amplification by Stimulated Emission of Radiation). Schawlow and Townes proposed that this concept could be translated into the visible spectrum [21]. Theodore Maiman utilized a ruby to do just this when he constructed the first laser in 1960

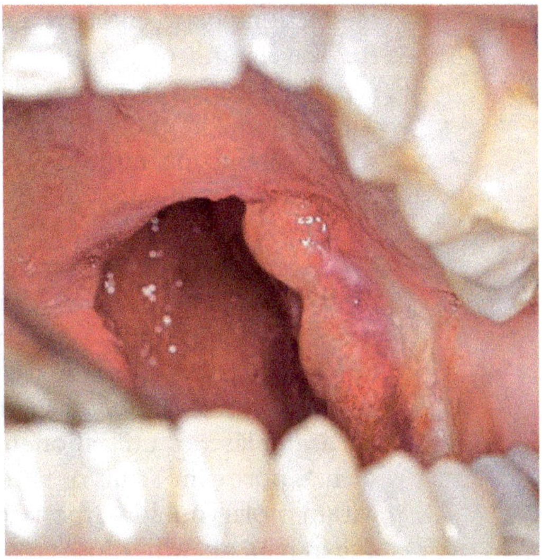

Fig. 5 Defect shown healing by secondary intention with granulation tissue 2 weeks after TLM

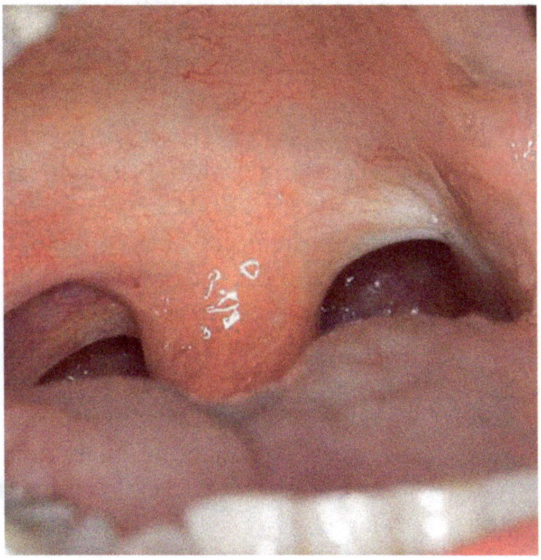

Fig. 6 Healed defect site, 1 year after resection

[22]. Lasers quickly found their way into the medical field. Ritter, Campbell, and Koester did early work, utilizing a ruby laser for photocoagulation in retinal surgeries [23, 24]. McGuff et al. ablated atherosclerotic plaques with the same ruby laser [25]. As lasers continued to evolve, their applications grew more varied, including within otolaryngology.

Lasers have varied impacts on tissues. The laser radiation can be absorbed, reflected, scattered, or transmitted. The surgically relevant interactions of lasers are mediated by absorption. The interactions between lasers and tissues are largely determined by the wavelength of a given laser. As a result, the surgeon should account for the properties that are unique to each wavelength. This will enable the surgeon to optimize the efficacy of the laser while minimizing morbidity. Some of the more commonly used lasers in otolaryngology are discussed here.

Argon Laser

The Argon (Ar) laser produces light at various wavelengths. The most commonly used wavelengths are 488 and 514 nm. The extinction length of the Argon laser in water is very lengthy, and water only poorly absorbs argon laser radiation. However, Argon lasers are absorbed well by pigmented tissue. These properties lend the argon laser to utilization in the treatment of pigmented lesions such as port wine stains or tattoo removal. Among the various uses within otolaryngology, the argon laser has been shown to be effective in patients with otosclerosis undergoing stapedotomy [26].

Neodymium–Yttrium Aluminum Garnet Laser

The Neodymium–Yttrium Aluminum Garnet (Nd:YAG) laser utilizes a Yttrium Aluminum garnet that has been doped with Neodymium (Nd), i.e., some of the Yttrium ions have been replaced by Nd. This has a wavelength of 1064 nm and an extinction length of 40 mm. The absorbance of an Nd:YAG laser varies based on the color of the tissue/substance. Water only weakly absorbs this 1064 nm laser. The Nd:YAG laser exhibits notable scattering within biological tissues. As a result, the Nd:YAG laser produces a zone of damage that extends 4 mm laterally and deep from the point of laser contact. This wider zone makes particularly fine and precise operation difficult with the Nd:YAG laser, particularly if the laser is operated continuously (as opposed to pulsed). This laser is used in otolaryngology predominantly in the ablation of obstructive lesions of the tracheobronchial tree and esophagus and in the treatment of vascular malformations. The Nd:YAG laser's deeper zone of thermal and coagulative damage gives the operator more reliable hemorrhage management than some other lasers.

Potassium Titanyl Phosphate Laser

Potassium titanyl phosphate (KTP) lasers are modified Nd:YAG lasers. KTP is used as a frequency doubling diode in a Nd:YAG laser. The resultant laser radiation, with its frequency doubled, has a wavelength of 532 nm. Due to the similar wavelengths, a KTP laser exhibits properties similar to those of an Argon laser. However, the 532 nm radiation of the KTP laser is strongly absorbed by oxyhemoglobin. The result is secure hemorrhage management during an operation. When coupled with endoscopes and flexible probes, the KTP laser has many utilities within otolaryngology. The KTP laser is used in the treatment of various sinus and tracheal lesions ranging from papillomas and dysplasia to head and neck cancer. This laser is used in an operative and office setting [27–29].

Carbon Dioxide Laser

Carbon dioxide (CO_2) as the gain medium produces a laser with a wavelength of 10.6 μm (10,600 nm). This places the radiation within the infrared (invisible) region of the electromagnetic spectrum. In clinical settings, this laser is coupled with a helium neon laser that has a wavelength within the visible (red) spectrum. This coaxial helium neon laser guides the surgeon. The 10,600 nm radiation is strongly absorbed by water. The CO_2 laser has an extinction length less than 0.05 mm in soft tissues and exhibits minimal scattering. The interaction between the laser and tissues produces a characteristic wound with a region of vaporization and thermal necrosis that is 100 μm wide. Therefore, the CO_2 laser cuts with minimal collateral tissue damage and the surgeon can use the CO_2 laser to precisely cut tissues. When coupled with a flexible fiber, the CO_2 laser becomes handheld and can be used at angles, increasing versatility for some situations. These properties and capabilities have made the CO_2 laser widely used within otolaryngology.

Bleeding is an important consideration during TLM using a CO_2 laser. Due to the small depth of penetration and excellent absorption by water, anything but minimal bleeding stops laser surgery in its tracks. The laser simply boils blood as it appears, producing an expanding mass of charred blood. This charring shields the bleeding tissue from the laser. Therefore, hemostasis of blood vessels, larger/beyond the laser's 100-μm zone of efficacy, must be attained with electrocautery or vascular clips.

Margin Mapping

TLM defies a fundamental principle of surgical oncology, that of "en bloc" resection. Removal of a tumor en bloc has been a prudent means of preventing inadvertent and unseen dispersion of viable cancer cells. Should a scalpel penetrate the cancer it will expose cells that are alive. Moreover, viable cancerous cells may adhere to the blade. Nothing would then prevent the surgeon from transplanting these viable cells with subsequent incisions. Thus, when the wound is closed, transferred malignant cells increase the chance of recurrence. This is particularly likely with the reconstruction methods that follow conventional open resection. Healing by primary intention, with a flap or otherwise, would place any inadvertently dispersed cancer cells within healthy tissue, an environment favorable to proliferation. In open surgery, to prevent this chain of events, the surgeon isolates the cancer in an unbroken package of normal tissue. This prevents contact between any surgical instrument and viable cancer cells.

TLM does not use a scalpel to cut, rather a CO_2 laser. Cancer cells cannot adhere to this beam. Furthermore, any cells that are exposed by the laser are thermocoagulated, not viable. So, assuming that the specimen does not tear, forceps and clamps never contact viable cells. Therefore, in TLM there is no device of physical transplantation of malignant cells. Additionally in TLM the wound is not closed, but allowed to heal by secondary intention. Thus, any unseen cancer cells fall on a layer of coagulum, not in the favorable confines of healthy tissue [30]. Finally, Werner et al. showed that the CO_2 laser seals off lymphatic vessels as it cuts. And, these lymphatics remain closed for 10 days [31]. This theoretical basis for TLM has been validated by excellent local control rates ranging from 85 to 99 % [9, 10, 16].

The CO_2 laser's ability to cut with minimal thermal necrosis gives it a unique advantage over another laser or bovie. Using this ability to make clean, precise incisions the surgeon can carefully observe the tumor–host interface. This ability, coupled with the magnification of the operating microscope, permits microscopically driven piecemeal tumor resection. As the surgeon resects, piece by piece, he must orient and ink each resected specimen for the pathologist. It is paramount that the surgeon maintains orientation of the specimen. Moreover, as the tumor is further subdivided, the surgeon must keep track of the sites and sources of the various specimens. This can be accomplished with the use of differing color of ink, maps, lists, etc. The head and neck pathologist can use frozen section techniques to inform the surgeon of the presence of tumor within margins. The operation can therefore be tailored based on the pathology results. Excellent communication between the surgeon and the pathologist allows the operating surgeon to obtain a map of the tumor and its margins. This process is known as margin mapping and adds a diagnostic component to TLM. An illustration of the technique of tumor mapping can be seen in Fig. 7.

The oncologic results of TLM have been discussed earlier; in addition to that, margin mapping itself has been validated. In a case series of 128 patients who received TLM (with microscopically driven margin mapping) for tonsillar SCCA, Hinni et al. reported 2- and 5-year disease-free survival rates of 96.5 % and 94.5 %, respectively, and a local control rate of 99 % [16].

Contraindications to TLM

TLM, like any surgery, requires adequate access and exposure. Therefore, inability to expose is an absolute contraindication to TLM. The predominant limitations to exposure in TLM are known as the 10 Ts of access and exposure. These are teeth, tongue, tilt, transverse dimensions (mandibular), tori (mandibular), trismus, treatment (previous radiotherapy), tumor, tethering, and time (modified from Rich et al.) [17]. If the upper teeth are the only impairment, an extraction may be considered to avoid an open procedure.

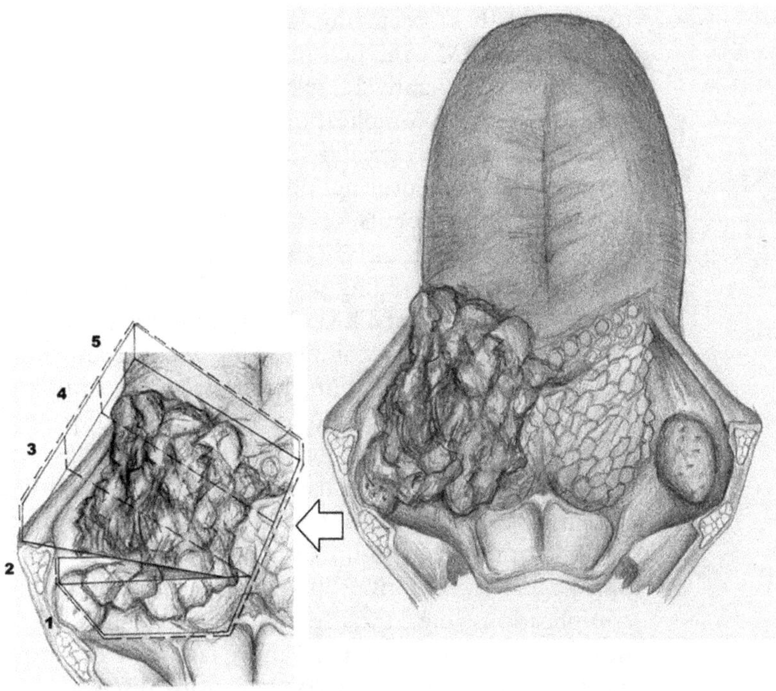

Fig. 7 Illustration of tumor mapping. Tumor can be seen removed in five separate slices sequentially. A deep margin for each slice is inked in the operating room to preserve orientation for pathology

Very advanced disease can also be a contraindication to TLM. Extensive spread to the neck, i.e., disease involving the great vessels or mandibular cortical penetration, is an absolute contraindication to TLM. TLM is also contraindicated in cases of unresectable cancer or advanced cancer needing reconstruction. If patients have significant functional impairments (e.g., severe persistent aspiration) or overwhelming comorbidities, then TLM is also not advisable. Recurrent cancer in a previously irradiated bed is also a relative contraindication to TLM, especially for the inexperienced surgeon [30].

It is also important to maintain realistic patient expectations. Lasers can be perceived as an especially novel tool. Thus, on occasion patients will place too much faith in lasers, i.e., the "laser myth." Here it is important to recall the limitations of TLM. TLM cannot restore the function or anatomy of tissues that have already been lost to cancer, RT, or previous surgery.

Complications of TLM

As with any surgery, complications do occur with primary transoral laser resections of head and neck tumors. While it is impossible to completely avoid complications, steps can be taken to minimize the risk of these occurring. Such precautions can be taken in all stages of a TLM case, i.e., preoperative, intraoperative, and postoperative. Preoperatively, selecting appropriate patients can mitigate the risk of complications. For example, previously treated patients are at a greater risk of having complications [32]. Intraoperatively, ensuring optimal exposure and hemostasis are important components of safe intraoperative execution. In the perioperative arena, airway management and monitoring for aspiration are key to avoiding postoperative complications.

Complications of TLM can be separated into minor and major complications. Minor complications include any and all forms of dental trauma, tongue contusions, oral cavity or pharyngeal tears/lacerations, mandibular trauma, nerve (lingual) paresis, and minor burns from the electrocautery or laser deflections. Transoral laser surgery very clearly puts structures of the oral cavity and oropharynx at risk. Manipulations of the laryngoscope and other steps taken to optimize exposure can damage dentition or cause tongue/pharyngeal lacerations. While steps are taken to minimize such complications (e.g., the use of Aquaplast splints to protect dentition), these complications are more favorable outcomes than compromised margins. Major complications discussed in this chapter are those we feel to be most salient: hemorrhage, airway fires, airway obstruction, and aspiration.

Hemorrhage

Hemorrhage following TLM is an unpredictable and potentially life-threatening complication. Bleeding from laser resections of oropharyngeal tumors is a particular concern due to the complex network of named vessels within the lateral pharyngeal anatomy. TLM's "inside-out" approach also reverses the traditional perception of anatomy. This has the potential to add another variable as the surgeon operates. As the surgeon progresses with the resection into deeper lateral pharyngeal tissues, larger and larger blood vessels may be encountered. Smaller vessels may be managed with electrocautery (bipolar). However, larger vessels, especially all named vessels, must be clipped or ligated. TLM can leave patients with impaired swallowing function and airway protection. This is particularly the case during the several weeks to months that are needed for healing. Postoperative bleeding in such patients can be catastrophic. In the event of a catastrophic bleed, the potential for death is not from exsanguination; rather aspiration and asphyxiation are the cause of death.

While postoperative bleeding is a very serious concern, it is a rare complication. Pollei et al. studied 906 patients treated with oropharyngeal SCCA who were treated with transoral surgical methods. Their work demonstrated an overall postoperative bleed rate of 5.4 % [33]. Furthermore, in a review of 701 cases, Salassa et al. identified 10 patients who experienced major postoperative hemorrhage. A catastrophic bleed occurred in three of these patients, or 0.4 % of the 701 cases reviewed [34].

Transoral surgery results in an "inside-out" perception of anatomy that can present a new variable when operating. However, with a thorough knowledge of anatomy the surgeon can anticipate major blood vessels while operating. Hemostasis can be obtained with electrocautery or vascular clips. Selected patients may also benefit from ligation of vessels within the neck. Ultimately, proper precautions enable TLM to represent a safe treatment modality.

Airway Fire

Fire within the airway represents a very serious complication of TLM. These fires are extremely rare in North America. The ignition of such a fire requires high temperatures (or a spark), flammable materials, and adequate oxygen. Laser surgery can certainly result in temperatures high enough for combustion. Temperatures routinely approach 250 °C where tissues are vaporized when the laser is used to make incisions. This temperature carbonizes tissues. The carbonized tissue can then combust locally within the laser's focus. Resultant temperatures can exceed 1000 °C. Therefore, temperatures are more than sufficient to ignite flammable substances. Critically, the electrocautery as a source of ignition should not be overlooked since most ignitions are related to electrocautery [35, 36].

Materials of the endotracheal tube and its contents (oxygen and inhalable anesthetics) contribute to airway fires. Therefore, many institutions mandate "laser-proof" tubes. "Laser-Proof" endotracheal tubes often have an outer layer of aluminum or copper to shield the tube and its contents from the laser. Additionally avoiding the use of flammable gases (such as nitrous oxide) and limiting oxygen concentrations is imperative. The most important consideration when performing TLM is the FiO_2 (fraction of inspired oxygen) [37]. Maintaining the oxygen concentration below 27 % can minimize any risk of fire.

By taking the necessary precautions, the risk of airway fires can be virtually eliminated. A recent study at the Mayo Clinic Hospital in Phoenix, Arizona, reviewed 4000 sequential CO_2 laser procedures and failed to find a single laser fire [38]. Like many other inadvertent medical errors, laser airway fires can be avoided with focused and timely intraoperative communication.

Aspiration

The structures of the pharynx and larynx normally function by preventing foodstuffs, fluids, and solids from entering the airway but permit their entrance through the esophagus. Several coordinated movements of the tongue, palate, pharynx, and larynx are needed for safe and proper swallowing. Intact sensory innervation is needed to coordinate the motor components. If the requisite neural or muscular functions are lost, swallowing can be impaired. As discussed earlier, TLM cannot restore any anatomy or function that has been compromised by cancer or previous therapy (surgery or RT).

Following TLM most patients will experience some degree of aspiration. Therefore, it is often prudent to place a nasogastric feeding tube at the time of surgery. Should the patient not need the tube it can be removed the following day. This is easier than having to place a nasogastric tube when the patient is unable to swallow in the postoperative setting. Aspiration pneumonia is a relatively common complication affecting about 5–6 % of TLM patients [35, 39]. Elderly patients are particularly susceptible to this. Thus, it is important to recognize and treat a pneumonia. Also patients are encouraged to maintain an upright position until their swallowing function and management of oral secretions improve.

Preoperative and postoperative involvement of a swallowing therapist is also extremely valuable. A speech and language pathologist can assist patients and help them determine when it is safe to resume an oral diet. Additionally, the value of the emotional support provided to patients is incalculable.

Airway Obstruction

Intraoperatively, airway obstruction is unlikely unless the endotracheal tube is displaced. Once the patient has been extubated, significant edema or soft tissue herniation into the airway can obstruct the airway. Surgical resection can release remnant tissues from normal attachments. Freed soft tissue can then herniate and obstruct the airway. Obstruction related to tissue herniation is a somewhat bigger risk in supraglottic and hypopharyngeal surgeries.

Protracted tongue pressure can result in tongue edema. This can then occlude the airway following extubation. Loss of venous outflow during a neck dissection (resection of a jugular vein) and extensive fluid resuscitation can increase this risk. Significant surgical edema responds poorly to medication. Thus, an elective tracheostomy may be the best course of action in those patients receiving lengthy operations and/or bilateral neck dissections.

Airway obstruction is a substantial, but rare, complication of transoral surgery in the postoperative setting. Our temporary rate is 15 % with most patients also receiving simultaneous neck dissections. Permanent tracheostomy rates are extremely low, i.e., 0–1 % [13, 14, 40].

Conclusion

TLM represents a new paradigm in head and neck surgery. Unlike open approaches, TLM addresses anatomical impediments with a minimally invasive transoral approach. As a result, the disassembly and reconstruction of a conventional head and neck cancer operation can be avoided. This approach affords reduced morbidity, shorter hospital stays, and reduced overall costs.

When the careful and precise incisions of a CO_2 laser are coupled with the brilliant illumination and magnification of an operating microscope, an additional dimension of tumor resection is realized. A diagnostic dimension! Working with a head and neck pathologist TLM allows a surgeon to precisely map a tumor's extent and depth of invasion. The operation can then be tailored even more precisely to a given tumor and further minimize injury to otherwise healthy tissues. This piecemeal approach does violate a time-honored dictum of surgical oncology, the "en bloc" resection, but it has been convincingly demonstrated to be oncologically safe. In TLM healing by secondary intention and laser-mediated sealing of lymphatics may help prevent recurrence. Ultimately, TLM is a versatile and individualized surgical approach. It is an excellent primary treatment modality for both early and advanced pharyngeal cancer which should be made available to patients as an option by multidisciplinary cancer centers.

References

1. Harrison LB, Lee HJ, Pfister DG, et al. Long term results of primary radiotherapy with/without neck dissection for squamous cell cancer of the base of tongue. Head Neck. 1998;20(8):668–73.
2. Parsons JT, Million RR, Cassisi NJ. Carcinoma of the base of the tongue: results of radical irradiation with surgery reserved for irradiation failure. Laryngoscope. 1982;92(6 Pt 1): 689–96.
3. Harrison LB, Zelefsky MJ, Armstrong JG, Carper E, Gaynor JJ, Sessions RB. Performance status after treatment for squamous cell cancer of the base of tongue--a comparison of primary radiation therapy versus primary surgery. Int J Radiat Oncol Biol Phys. 1994;30(4): 953–7.
4. Parsons JT, Mendenhall WM, Stringer SP, et al. Squamous cell carcinoma of the oropharynx. Cancer. 2002;94(11):2967–80. doi:10.1002/cncr.10567.
5. Huet. Electrocoagulation in cancer of the tonsils. Discussion. Ann Otolaryngol. 1951; 68(5–6):406–8.
6. Jako GJ, Vaughan CW, Strong MS, Polanyi TG. Surgical management of malignant tumors of the aerodigestive tract with carbon dioxide laser microsurgery. Int Adv Surg Oncol. 1978;1:265–84.
7. Strong MS. Laser excision of carcinoma of the larynx. Laryngoscope. 1975;85(8):1286–9. doi:10.1288/00005537-197508000-00003.
8. Davis RK, Shapshay SM, Strong MS, Hyams VJ. Transoral partial supraglottic resection using the CO2 laser. Laryngoscope. 1983; 93(4):429–32.
9. Steiner W, Ambrosch P. Endoscopic laser surgery of the upper aerodigestive tract. New York: Thieme; 2000.
10. Steiner W, Fierek O, Ambrosch P, Hommerich CP, Kron M. Transoral laser microsurgery for squamous cell carcinoma of the base of the tongue. Arch Otolaryngol Head Neck Surg. 2003;129(1):36–43.
11. Salassa JR. A functional outcome swallowing scale for staging oropharyngeal dysphagia. Dig Dis. 1999;17(4):230–4.
12. Canis M, Ihler F, Wolff HA, Christiansen H, Matthias C, Steiner W. Oncologic and functional results after transoral laser microsurgery of tongue base carcinoma. Eur Arch Otorhinolaryngol. 2012;270(3):1075–83. doi:10.1007/s00405-012-2097-1.
13. Henstrom DK, Moore EJ, Olsen KD, Kasperbauer JL, McGree ME. Transoral resection for squamous cell carcinoma of the base of the tongue. Arch Otolaryngol Head Neck Surg. 2009;135(12):1231–8. doi:10.1001/archoto.2009.177.
14. Grant DG, Salassa JR, Hinni ML, Pearson BW, Perry WC. Carcinoma of the tongue base treated by transoral laser microsurgery, part one: untreated tumors, a prospective analysis of oncologic and functional outcomes. Laryn-

goscope. 2006;116(12):2150–5. doi:10.1097/01.mlg.0000244159.64179.f0.

15. Rich JT, Liu J, Haughey BH. Swallowing function after transoral laser microsurgery (TLM) ± adjuvant therapy for advanced-stage oropharyngeal cancer. Laryngoscope. 2011; 121(11):2381–90. doi:10.1002/lary.21406.
16. Hinni ML, Zarka MA, Hoxworth JM. Margin mapping in transoral surgery for head and neck cancer. Laryngoscope. 2013;123(5):1190–8. doi:10.1002/lary.23900.
17. Rich JT, Milov S, Lewis Jr JS, Thorstad WL, Adkins DR, Haughey BH. Transoral Laser Microsurgery (TLM) ± adjuvant therapy for advanced stage oropharyngeal cancer. Laryngoscope. 2009;119(9):1709–19. doi:10.1002/lary.20552.
18. Haughey BH, Hinni ML, Salassa JR, et al. Transoral laser microsurgery as primary treatment for advanced-stage oropharyngeal cancer: a united states multicenter study. Head Neck. 2011;33(12):1683–94. doi:10.1002/hed.21669.
19. Pearson BW, Salassa JR. Transoral laser microresection for cancer of the larynx involving the anterior commissure. Laryngoscope. 2003;113(7):1104–12.doi:10.1097/00005537-200307000-00002.
20. Moore EJ, Hinni ML, Olsen KD, Price DL, Laborde RR, Inman JC. Cost considerations in the treatment of oropharyngeal squamous cell carcinoma. Otolaryngol Head Neck Surg. 2012;146(6):946–51. doi:10.1177/0194599812437534.
21. Schawlow AL, Townes CH. Infrared and optical masers. Phys Rev. 1958;112(6):1940.
22. Maiman TH. Stimulated optical radiation in ruby. Nature. 1960;187(4736):493–4.doi:10.1038/187493a0.
23. Noyori KS, Campbell CJ, Rittler MC, Koester C. Ocular thermal effects produced by photocoagulation. Arch Ophthalmol. 1963;70:817–22.
24. Campbell CJ, Rittler MC, Koester CJ. The optical maser as a retinal coagulator: an evaluation. Trans Am Acad Ophthalmol Otolaryngol. 1963;67:58–67.
25. McGuff PE, Bushnell D, Soroff HS, Deterling RA. Studies of the surgical applications of LASER (Light Amplification by Stimulated Emission of Radiation). Surg Forum. 1963;14:143–5.
26. Strunk CL, Quinn FB. Stapedectomy surgery in residency: KTP-532 laser versus argon laser. Am J Otol. 1993;14(2):113–7.
27. Zeitels SM, Akst LM, Burns JA, Hillman RE, Broadhurst MS, Anderson RR. Office-based 532-nm pulsed KTP laser treatment of glottal papillomatosis and dysplasia. Ann Otol Rhinol Laryngol. 2006;115(9):679–85.
28. Sridharan S, Achlatis S, Ruiz R, et al. Patient-based outcomes of in-office KTP ablation of vocal fold polyps. Laryngoscope. 2013; 124(5):1176–9. doi:10.1002/lary.24442.
29. Nagel TH, Hinni ML, Hayden RE, Lott DG. Transoral laser microsurgery for the unknown primary: a role for lingual tonsillectomy. Head Neck. 2013;36(7):942–6. doi:10.1002/hed.23372.
30. Hinni LM, Salassa JR, Pearson BW. Transoral laser microresection of advanced laryngeal tumors. In: Flint P, Haughey BH, Lund VJ, et al., editors. Cummings otolaryngology head and neck surgery, vol. 5. Philadelphia, PA: Mosby; 2010. p. 1525–38. doi:10.1016/B978-0-323-05283-2.00110-5.
31. Werner JA, Lippert BM, Schünke M, Rudert H. Animal experiment studies of laser effects on lymphatic vessels. A contribution to the discussion of laser surgery segmental resection of carcinomas. Laryngorhinootologie. 1995;74(12):748–55. doi:10.1055/s-2007-997838.
32. Grant DG, Salassa JR, Hinni ML, Pearson BW, Hayden RE, Perry WC. Transoral laser microsurgery for recurrent laryngeal and pharyngeal cancer. Otolaryngol Head Neck Surg. 2008;138(5):606–13. doi:10.1016/j.otohns.2007.12.046.
33. Pollei TR, Hinni ML, Moore EJ, et al. Analysis of postoperative bleeding and risk factors in transoral surgery of the oropharynx. JAMA Otolaryngol Head Neck Surg. 2013;139(11):1212–8. doi:10.1001/jamaoto.2013.5097.
34. Salassa J, Hinni ML, Grant D, Hayden R. Postoperative bleeding in transoral laser microsurgery for upper aerodigestive tract tumors. Otolaryngol Head Neck Surg. 2008;139(3):453–9. doi:10.1016/j.otohns.2008.06.010.
35. Vilaseca-González I, Bernal-Sprekelsen M, Blanch-Alejandro J-L, Moragas-Lluis M. Complications in transoral CO2 laser surgery for carcinoma of the larynx and hypopharynx. Head Neck. 2003;25(5):382–8. doi:10.1002/hed.10207.
36. Ellies M, Steiner W. Peri- and postoperative complications after laser surgery of tumors of the upper aerodigestive tract. Am J Otolaryngol. 2007;28(3):168–72. doi:10.1016/j.amjoto.2006.08.008.

37. Roy S, Smith LP. What does it take to start an oropharyngeal fire? Oxygen requirements to start fires in the operating room. Int J Pediatr Otorhinolaryngol. 2011;75(2):227–30. doi:10.1016/j.ijporl.2010.11.005.
38. Rayon MM, McCormick S, Schaitberger S, Baldea B, Hinni ML. The last time out: ensuring safe operation of lasers in the operating room suite. Presented at: International Laser Safety Conference, 2013 Conference Program Proceedings; March 18–21, 2013; Orlando, FL
39. Bernal-Sprekelsen M, Vilaseca-González I, Blanch-Alejandro J-L. Predictive values for aspiration after endoscopic laser resections of malignant tumors of the hypopharynx and larynx. Head Neck. 2004;26(2):103–10. doi:10.1002/hed.10363.
40. Camp AA, Fundakowski C, Petruzzelli GJ, Emami B. Functional and oncologic results following transoral laser microsurgical excision of base of tongue carcinoma. Otolaryngology—Head and Neck Surgery. 2009;141(1):66–9. doi:10.1016/j.otohns.2009.02.028.

Chapter 4

Transoral Laser Microsurgery for Laryngeal Cancer

Tjoson Tjoa and William B. Armstrong

Introduction

Cancer of the larynx is the third most common malignancy of the upper aerodigestive tract [1]. 85–95 % of these are squamous cell carcinoma, a result of malignant transformation of the epithelial layer of the larynx [2]. In the United States, 60 % of laryngeal cancer will affect the glottis, 35 % will affect the supraglottis, and the remaining 5 % will affect the subglottis. Historically, treatment of laryngeal cancer has been in the form of open transcervical surgery, endoscopic transoral surgery using cold steel instrumentation, and external beam radiation therapy (RT). The advances of direct laryngoscopy, microscopic instrumentation, and lasers in the twentieth century have paved the way for transoral laser microsurgery (TLM), which now competes with, and often replaces, the traditional modalities to treat laryngeal cancer (Fig. 1).

Alfred Kirstein developed the first direct laryngoscope with electric lighting in 1895 [3]. 20 years later, Chevalier Jackson reported the endoscopic resection of an epiglottic cancer with punch biopsy forceps. In the mid-twentieth century, Scalco described the use of the microscope in conjunction with the suspension laryngoscope, which, along with the use of general endotracheal anesthesia, allowed for a leap in precision with regard to surgery of the vocal cords. Shortly thereafter, Kleinsasser designed further instrumentation and introduced the 400-mm lens [4], which increased the working distance between the microscope and the laryngoscope, allowing for the use of long-shafted laryngeal instruments [5].

The development of lasers in the late 1950s in many ways revolutionized the management of laryngeal disease. Michael Polanyi coupled the CO_2 laser to a microscopic attachment [6], which was used by Jako to evaporate discrete areas of tissue on the vocal cord

Brian J.-F. Wong and Justus Ilgner (eds.), *Biomedical Optics in Otorhinolaryngology: Head and Neck Surgery*,
DOI 10.1007/978-1-4939-1758-7_4,

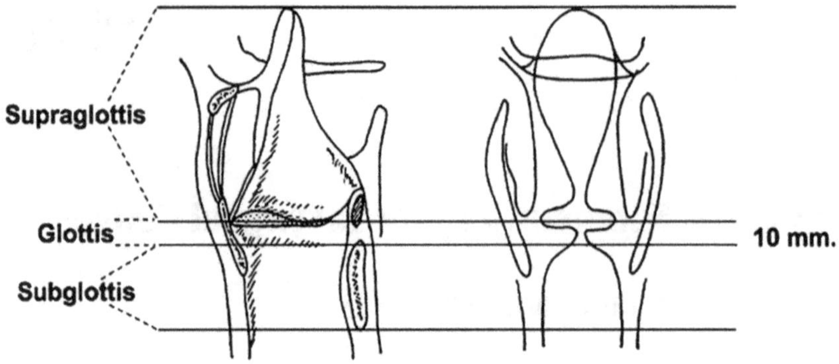

Fig. 1 Sagittal and coronal sections of the larynx showing the cancer subsites (adapted from Coates GM, Schenck HP. Otolaryngology. W.F. Prior Co., Hagerstown, MD. 1966, Vol. 5, Chapter 7, page 4)

surface in a rapid and bloodless manner [7]. The development of the micromanipulator by Polanyi and Jako was a landmark development that allowed for microscopic precision on the vocal cord target with a no-touch technique, the other hand being free to grasp the pathology and/or suction the operative field free of secretions or debris [8]. The concurrent use of CO_2 laser with microlaryngoscopy by Polanyi, Jako, and Strong has greatly facilitated the now common practice of endoscopic excision of papillomas and early carcinomas [9].

With relatively little change in mortality since the 1970s, current clinical focus is not simply on improving survival, but on expanding the application of and indications for laryngeal preservation modalities to improve function and quality of life. Transoral laser microsurgery (TLM) is now a readily accepted modality of treatment of early stage laryngeal carcinoma, with indications for advanced stage tumors as well. It allows for the resection of tumor through a transoral approach with or without endoscopes using operating microscope visualization and laser tissue excision. It has provided a useful alternative to open laryngeal surgery and external beam radiation.

Principles of TLM

The term "LASER" was introduced as an acronym for light amplification by stimulated emission of radiation. The carbon dioxide laser was developed in 1963 by Kumar Patel (Bell Labs) and has become the workhouse for TLM of the larynx. The CO_2 laser functions primarily as a hemostatic scalpel when the beam is focused, with the ability to simultaneously cut and coagulate tissue. When the beam is defocused, the CO_2 laser can also be used effectively to ablate and cytoreduce epithelial disease such as diffuse papillomatosis [10]. Operating at a wavelength 10.6 μm in the infrared region, CO_2 lasers deliver nonionizing electromagnetic radiation that is well absorbed by water, which is ubiquitous in the laryngeal soft tissues.

The goal of TLM is no different than that of traditional open and endoscopic surgical techniques: to remove tumor completely with clear surgical margins. What distinguishes TLM from open surgery is that healing is allowed to occur by secondary intention and the tumor block can be subdivided into manageable units by the laser (in situ). While this violates the classic Halstedian principle of en bloc resection, extensive study by Steiner [11, 12] and others [13–15] has demonstrated that there is no sacrifice of oncologic control using a blockwise resection of the tumor in discrete segments. Successful oncologic and functional outcomes are routinely achieved, as long as several guiding principles are followed.

The first is that high powered magnification and bright illumination are used to visualize the cut surface. This represents a stark advantage over open surgery, in which tumor margins are grossly visualized with the naked eye or under minimal loupe magnification with a headlight. Under microscopic visualization, tissues reveal subtle information about their consistency as they are retracted. Cancer is either stiff or soft and friable, with dysmorphic architecture. Beyond the tumor, the expected microarchitecture is striated muscle, fat, seromucinous glands, fibrous perichondrium, cartilage, or bone, which can be distinguished by an experienced surgeon [16]. Additionally, tumor tissue takes on a different appearance than normal tissue after laser ablation, with more char on the tumor tissue. The ability to see these subtle differences in tissue content and vascularity allows for detailed real-time assessment of margins.

The second principle is that laser cutting with a spot size that can be focused to 250 μm and emitted in brief, microsecond pulses can be used to make precise cuts while allowing the tissue to cool in between pulses, thereby minimizing thermal damage to the surrounding tissue. Within the past decade, the development of the flexible fiber to deliver the CO_2 laser beam has added to the precision and also allowed for the ability to make tangential cuts out of the line of sight of straight laryngoscope delivery. The fiber consists of a hollow-core tube surrounded by a dielectric mirror, which allows the use of CO_2 either within a flexible endoscope or delivered through a hand-piece. Use of the CO_2 laser has been shown to seal the lymphatic vessels of the wound margin, which remain sealed for about 10 days after laser surgery [17, 18].

A third principle is to perform stepwise resection of blocks of tumor with clearance at each region or subsite before proceeding to the next area (Fig. 2). It is particularly important to carefully label and orient each specimen. Once the pathologist evaluates the

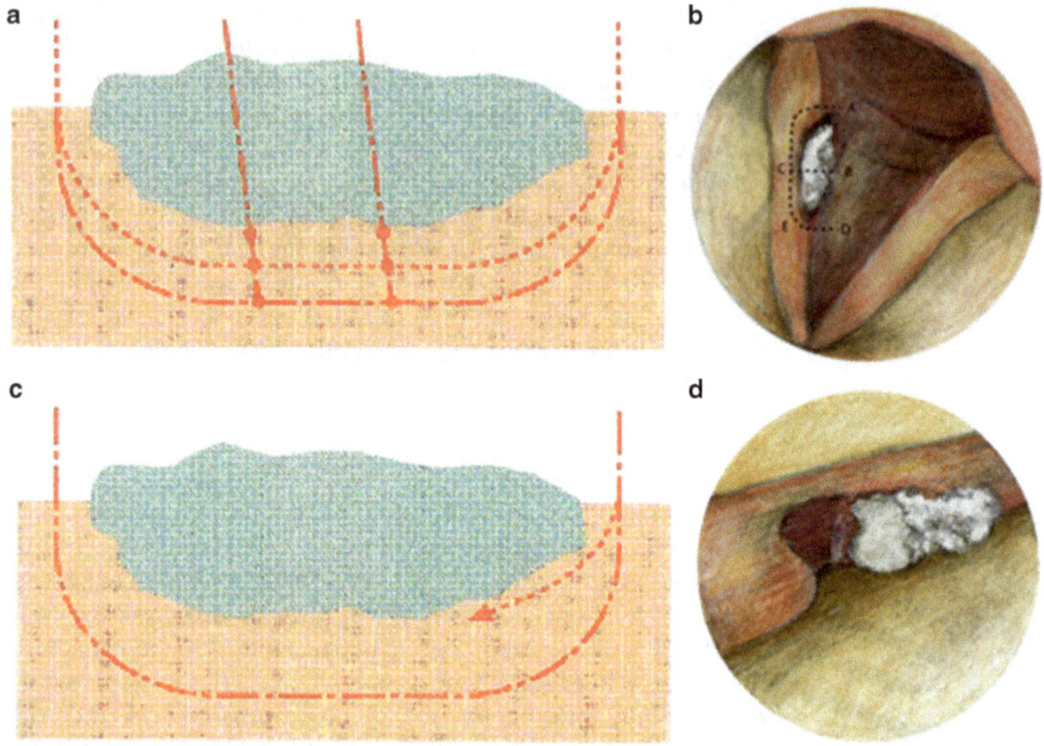

Fig. 2 Schematic and drawings showing (**a**, **b**) piecemeal removal of tumor and (**c**, **d**) en bloc resection

depth of tumor infiltration, basal clearance, and margins, re-excision of tissue at any positive or close margins can occur incrementally. This can be done at any time, since the wound is left open to heal and there is no risk of burying tumor under a reconstructive flap.

There are a number of reasons why en bloc resection is not required. First of all, cancer in the airway is already exposed. There is an open surface that allows direct visualization of an entire border of the cancer. Also, as the laser beam cuts through the tissue, there is no adherence of the cancer cells to it. With cold steel instrumentation, one of the concerns is that cancer cells can be seeded by the passage of the knife from diseased to healthy tissue. As mentioned above, lymphatics and small blood vessels are sealed with the laser cut, helping to prevent spread of cancer through those channels. The laser itself allows for photocoagulation of surface tumor cells and leaves a hostile environment for any cells that do get seeded.

The advantages of TLM are multiple. First, treatment of the larynx with TLM does not preclude any future possibilities for treatment, should there be recurrence or a second primary tumor. Re-excision with the laser, open excision, and radiation all remain treatment options. This is in contrast to external beam radiation, which leaves a salvage total laryngectomy as the only possibility in cases of recurrence [19].

Second, TLM has less morbidity than open approaches, which in many cases requires a temporary tracheostomy and possible feeding tube. With an approach to the tumor from inside the airway, there is no dissection through normal muscle, nerves, and cartilage, and the laryngeal framework continues to support and provide structure to the airway. This results in decreased rates of postoperative stenosis and allows for healing by secondary intention. There is also a decreased risk of fistula formation and lower chance of postoperative infection. All of this contributes to improved functional outcome and decreased length of hospital stay.

The precision of TLM results in minimal damage to adjacent tissue, which reduces healing time, wound contraction, scarring, and postoperative edema [20, 21]. There is also a delayed acute inflammatory reaction and reduced myofibroblast activity, which results in improved postoperative function with swallowing and speech [21]. Initial concerns about the accuracy of pathologic assessment of margins in TLM have largely been alleviated by studies that have shown that thermal damage on the borders of biopsy specimens does not interfere with the pathologist's establishment of a firm diagnosis [21].

Operative Technique

A thorough preoperative evaluation with accurate staging is critical for operative success. The lesion must be accurately visualized either in the office or through operative endoscopy, and histological confirmation of malignancy is mandatory. For larger tumors, preoperative MRI or CT scan imaging should be performed to evaluate depth of tumor invasion and presence of nodal metastases. Once the patient is in the operating room under general anesthesia, a confirmatory direct laryngoscopy is performed.

Prior to starting the laser resection, several laser safety measures should be implemented to minimize the risk of complications (Fig. 3a). The primary risks of the laser are burns to the patient and members of the operative team, so it is important to protect the patient's eyes with protective eye pads moistened with saline. Likewise, all operative personnel must wear protective eyeglasses. Signs are placed outside the operating room to indicate that a laser is in use. The facial skin is protected using surgical towels soaked in saline solution, and these towels need to be kept moist during the entire procedure. A smoke evacuator is used to remove laser plume created by the laser. A protected endotracheal tube designed to decrease the risk of ignition from laser impact is used. The cuff of the laser-protected tube is inflated using saline with methylene blue dye to help identify endotracheal tube cuff rupture and help prevent tube

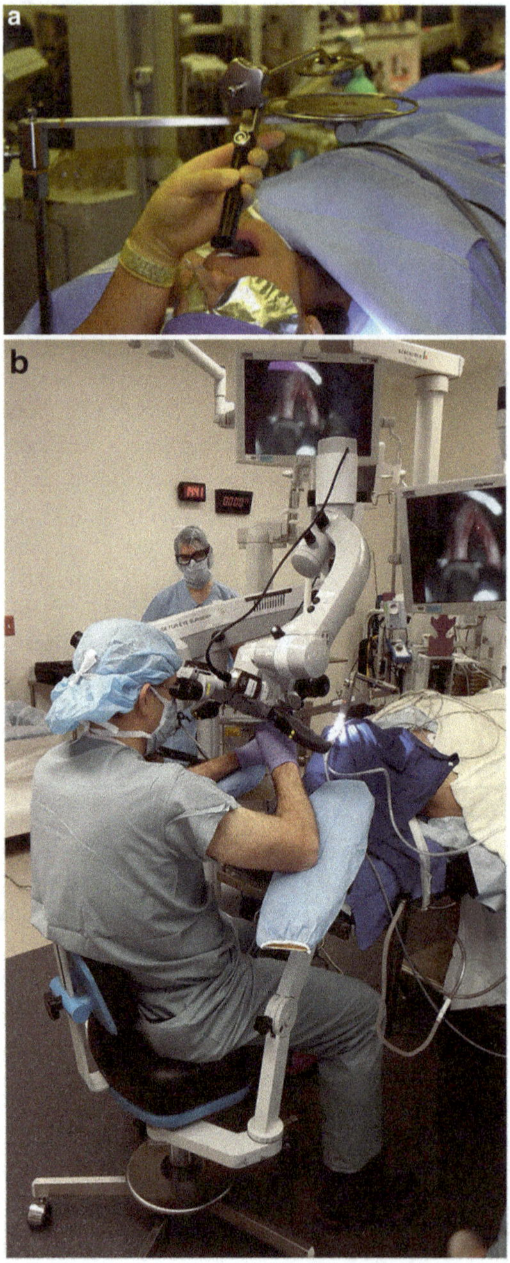

Fig. 3 (**a**) Setup of patient with laser-safe eye protection and insertion of laryngoscope. (**b**) Laser surgery being performed under visualization with the operating microscope. Moist towels are used around the face to protect from the laser

ignition if there is cuff damage during the procedure. Irrigation solution is immediately available in the event of ignition of the drapes or other flammable materials. The oxygen concentration is also lowered to below 30 % FiO_2 when using the laser to decrease the likelihood of airway fire [22]. In the event of an airway fire, the endotracheal tube is immediately removed, the flow of airway gases halted, flammable material such as sponges are removed, and saline poured into the airway [23]. Once the fire is extinguished, the airway is re-secured, the endotracheal tube examined for missing fragments, bronchoscopy is performed, and the procedure is terminated.

Once the patient is prepared, the patient is placed in a supine position with the head fully extended. Upper dentition is protected using either a plastic or metal tooth guard. Using one of a variety of rigid laryngoscopes selected to visualize the desired structures, the larynx is visualized. Once adequate exposure of the tumor and surround structures is obtained, the laryngoscope is fixed using a suspension arm, which frees both hands for operative manipulation. The microscope is brought into position and the laser is coupled to the micromanipulator (Fig. 3b). Along with the invisible CO_2 laser beam, a coaxial helium–neon (He–Ne) laser aiming beam is used to align the laser to the target. Prior to surgery, the laser is tested to ensure both proper function and alignment of the CO_2 and He–Ne beams.

The procedure is begun by marking the peripheral margins using the CO_2 laser. The size of the margin depends on the location and stage of the tumor and whether the patient is undergoing primary treatment or resection of recurrent disease. If there has been prior RT, wider margins are taken because of the higher risk of an infiltrative pattern of spread through the tissues. For small glottic tumors, a margin of as little as 1 mm is necessary. For deep margins, several millimeters, and ideally a connective tissue barrier, are chosen for margins of resection.

Successful resection of tumors requires different techniques, laser energies, spot sizes, and pulse modes in order to perform the various tasks of tissue ablation, precise cutting, and coagulation of tissues. It is important to emphasize that for a given application, there are no fixed settings, and that practice patterns vary significantly by physician. Several laser parameters are selected for each particular case, including (a) power, (b) spot size, (c) exposure time, and (d) power (pulse) delivery. Laser energy can be delivered through intermittent pulses, repeated pulses, continuous wave (CW), or the use of very rapid (millisecond) pulse delivery in the form of ultrapulse or superpulse mode.

CW mode produces surrounding tissue damage from thermal spread of the laser energy. In order to produce adequate cutting and hemostasis with limited char formation and thermal spread, alternative pulse delivery modes have been developed to allow tissue cutting and hemostasis while limiting thermal damage to surrounding tissues. By producing high-energy, short-duration pulses in rapid succession, tissue ablation can occur with limited heat damage to surrounding tissues. The two most common modes, ultrapulse and superpulse, utilize slightly different strategies to produce rapidly pulsed waves that incorporate high peak power delivered in millisecond pulses.

Superpulse mode delivers short bursts (less than 1 ms) in rapid succession. The energy profile of the beam is characterized by a high initial peak energy spike with rapid drop in energy over duration of the pulse. The ultrapulse mode delivers a short pulse with a rapid peak onset, relatively constant energy delivery for the duration of the pulse, and rapid decline in power at the end of the pulse, approximating a square wave. The superpulse mode has higher peak energy but less total energy delivery per pulse and more rapid pulse delivery, while ultrapulse mode has lower peak energy in each pulse, higher energy delivered with each pulse, and longer duration between pulses [24, 25]. From a practical standpoint, the clinical differences between the two pulse modes are subtle, although the thermal damage from the superpulse mode is reported to be slightly greater than with ultrapulse mode [25].

Specially designed instrumentation, including microlaryngeal forceps, scissors, and insulated suction cannulae for cution and unipolar coagulation, are used to retract tissue or remove debris as the surgeon uses the micromanipulator to excise tissue (Fig. 4). As the tumor is removed in sections, the specimens are carefully labeled and oriented for the pathologist. Often, the marking ink used by pathologists is placed on the true margins in the operating room by the surgeon. Precise communication and collaboration with the pathologist is key in correctly interpreting margin status for these complex, three-dimensional specimens. In complicated cases, the specimen should be delivered to the pathologist by the surgeon to ensure correct orientation of the specimen.

Frozen-section margins are sent based on the surgeon's judgment of areas at greatest risk for recurrence. If positive margins are reported by the pathologist, additional tissue is removed until the margins are clear. Following resection, hemostasis is ensured, and the wound is left open without reconstruction to heal by secondary intention.

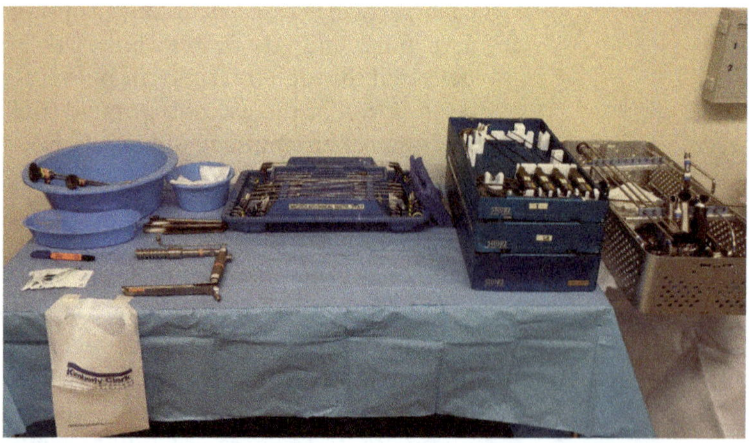

Fig. 4 Laser instrument table setup, with microlaryngeal instrumentation, endoscopes, insulated cannula suctions, and laryngoscope

Treatment of Glottic Cancer

Currently, regardless of treatment modality, the prognosis for Carcinoma in situ (Tis) and T1 lesions of the vocal cords is very good. Because of that, the goal of treatment has moved beyond simply cure and laryngeal preservation to include optimizing voice outcomes and minimizing cost and postoperative complications [19].

Small mid-cord tumors can be resected en bloc. When excised with narrow margins, the effect on the voice is comparable to treatment with RT. More extensive lesions are removed in sections with 1–3 mm margins (Fig. 5). A review performed by Ambrosch in 2007 revealed a 5-year local control rate of 80–94 % for Tis-T2a glottic carcinomas [19]. This is comparable to the local control rate of open partial laryngectomy (90–98 %) and avoids the short-term complications of open surgery [26, 27]. Because the approach to the tumor is from the inside of the airway, no breach of the laryngeal framework is needed for access. This allows for preservation of the strap muscles and obviates the need for a tracheostomy, thus resulting in shorter hospital stays and improved swallowing outcomes postoperatively.

The 5-year local control rate for TLM is also equivalent to that of external beam RT (approximately 81–90 %). Additionally, postoperative voice quality of life is comparable between the two treatment modalities [28]. However, TLM has been shown to be a much more cost-effective option [29, 30]. Furthermore, for T1 tumors, occasionally the tumor is removed with the initial diagnostic biopsy. TLM allows for assessment of residual tumor intraoperatively, thus avoiding unnecessary radiation in such cases. With organ preservation rates being similar (>94 %) in all three modalities, TLM remains a very attractive option for treatment of Tis and T1 tumors of the glottis. With regard to T2 lesions, the local control rate of TLM is actually higher than XRT (64–87 %), with better organ preservation rates (75–87 %) [26, 31, 32].

When early glottic carcinoma involves the anterior commissure, there is conflicting data about the effectiveness of TLM [33]. Steiner reviewed 263 cases and found that involvement of the anterior commissure affects local tumor control and organ preservation in T1/2 lesions, but does not affect overall survival [34]. Others have shown much higher recurrence rates than reported by Steiner after TLM in cases with anterior commissure involvement and recommended supracricoid partial laryngectomy as the treatment of choice in those cases [35].

While this may partially be attributed to inadequate tangential exposure at the anterior commissure, it is thought that inadequate diagnostic (under)-staging plays a contributing role to high recurrence rates. RT has also been shown to have high recurrence rates in anterior commissure involvement 57–85 % [36], supporting the

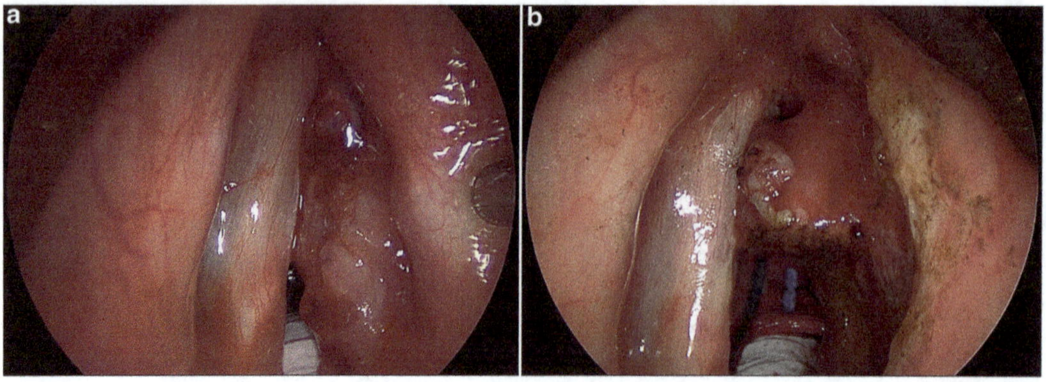

Fig. 5 (**a**) T1 right true vocal cord squamous cell carcinoma prior to laser excision, as viewed through laryngoscope. (**b**) Undergoing piecemeal excision, with the posterior portion removed. Laser-safe endotracheal tube is in view

notion that recurrence is not simply a matter of obtaining surgical exposure and proper operative technique.

Other studies have demonstrated that initial clinical evaluation failed to identify tumor invasion of the laryngeal cartilages and extra-laryngeal soft tissues resulting in a low staging accuracy of 45 %. The combination of clinical evaluation, endoscopic evaluation, and either CT or MRI imaging resulted in significantly improved staging accuracy of 80–87 % [37–39]. Because of this, it is recommended that tumors involving the anterior commissure receive axial helical CT scans reformatted with sagittal and coronal 1.0 mm cuts as part of the diagnostic workup [39].

For more advanced glottic carcinomas (T2b-3), published data on TLM is more scarce. If there is invasion into the paraglottic space, incisions are made laterally into the thyroid cartilage and inferiorly to the cricoid cartilage in order to clear disease. Ambrosch et al. published the largest series of T2b-3 lesions ($n = 167$) and found the 5-year local control rate was 74 % for pT2b carcinomas and 68 % for pT3 carcinomas. The respective secondary laryngectomy rates were 13.4 and 14.3 % [40]. The 5-year disease-free survival rate for both groups was 62 %. No patients required tracheostomy during the initial surgery, and postoperative speech and swallow function was fully rehabilitated.

Treatment of Supraglottic Cancer

Early stage supraglottic cancers have a tendency to be contained to within the boundaries of the supraglottic larynx and pre-epiglottic space. The traditional open approaches to these tumors have been the horizontal supraglottic laryngectomy, developed in 1939 by Alonso [41], and the supracricoid partial laryngectomy with cricohyoidopexy (SCPL-CHP), popularized within the last 25 years by Laccourreye [42]. For T1 lesions, the local control rates are reported to be 90–100 %, and 80–97 % for T2 lesions with open surgery. External beam radiation has shown local control rates of 77–100 % for T1 and 62–83 % for T2 lesions [19]. Tumor volume as assessed by preoperative CT imaging was the most significant prognostic factor involved in local control [43].

The first description of TLM for supraglottic cancer was by Vaughan in 1978 [44]. Subsequent refinement of the laryngoscopy equipment over the next 15 years, led by Steiner and his Goettingen University group, allowed for maximal exposure of the surgical working field. Working with Karl Storz, Inc, he helped to develop instruments that were robust enough to grasp tissue, coagulate, and apply clips endoscopically. Typically, ordinary tubular laryngoscopes are not suitable for procedures in this area and bivalved laryngoscopes with spreadable blades are used [45]. With increasing experience and meticulous follow-up, Steiner and his group were able to expand the indications of TLM from early glottic carcinoma to more advanced T stages of all sites of the larynx [11]. Based on the extent of resection that can be safely performed, most authors currently consider T1, T2, and selected T3 supraglottic cancers as indications for TLM.

Smaller tumors along the free margin of the epiglottis and the aryepiglottic fold can be excised en bloc. In fact, excisional biopsy alone of suspicious lesions may be curative in some cases of T1 and T2 tumors [46]. A review by Rodrigo et al. in 2008 revealed a 5-year local control rate of 88 % in T1 lesions and 89 % in T2 lesions [47], with a number of studies showing 100 % control in either T1 or T2 lesions using TLM [14, 48, 49].

Larger tumors require resection of the tumor in multiple sections with intraoperative frozen-section analysis. However, local control rates for T3 lesions are somewhat less favorable after treatment with TLM. Iro et al. found a 33.3 % recurrence rate in a series of 15 T3 lesions [50]. Rudert found a 22 % recurrence rate in a series of 9 T3 lesions [14] and concluded that those tumors that are upstaged due to pre-epiglottic space invasion are amenable to endoscopic resection. This was corroborated by Ambrosch et al., who reviewed a series of 41 T3 lesions, mostly as staged as a result of pre-epiglottic space invasion. 13 (26 %) of these required postoperative external beam radiotherapy due mostly to cervical metastases. The 5-year local control rate was 86 %, though 4 % of patients required total laryngectomy for recurrent disease [40].

With open supraglottic laryngectomy, local control rates exceed 90 % for T1 and T2 cancers, but the results drop to between 70 and 90 % for T3 cancer [19, 51]. The SCPL-CHP has been shown to have very low recurrence rates for T3 lesions (0–7 %) and may be an oncologically more effective alternative to TLM and standard open approaches when available. In the last 25 years, it has broadened the options available for treating larynx cancer by bridging the gap between the partial supraglottic laryngectomy and total laryngectomy [52]. SCPL-CHP includes resection of the entire epiglottis and the pre-epiglottic space, anterior vocal folds, and anterior commissure. In order for speech and swallow to be possible after this surgery, the resection must allow for preservation of at least one intact cricoarytenoid unit and an intact cricoid cartilage. However, even with this, voice outcome is poor, with a rough, low-frequency phonation from vibration of the arytenoids against the tongue base impacted onto the cricoid. Aspiration, which can be intractable, is more likely with this procedure, especially when arytenoid function and height is affected. Data has shown primary radiotherapy to be an inferior treatment alternative to either open or TLM surgery for early supraglottic lesions, with local control rates of 77–100 % for T1 cancers and 62–83 % for T2 cancers.

The endoscopic approach of TLM provides several distinct advantages over open resection: tracheotomies can generally be avoided, the incidence of pharyngocutaneous fistulas is markedly reduced, rehabilitation of swallowing is faster, the incidence of aspiration pneumonia is lower, and hospital stay is shorter [47]. Regardless of the surgical technique employed, negative margins are essential in limiting local recurrence. Additionally, supraglottic carcinomas have a high incidence of regional lymph node metastasis, ranging from 25 to 50 %. Lymph node metastasis is the most important prognostic factor in supraglottic cancer [47]. Because of this, most authors recommend that selective neck dissection be performed even in patients with stage I and II disease. In patients with known cervical metastasis, neck dissection combined with postoperative external beam radiotherapy offers the best chance of regional control.

Complications

In general, TLM is well tolerated with low complication rates and generally improved functional outcome compared to corresponding open procedures resecting the same size tumor. Early postoperative hemorrhage is a potentially lethal complication. The incidence of postoperative hemorrhage is similar in both endoscopic and open approaches and ranges from 3 to 14 % [47]. Often there will be a small amount of bleeding, but significant bleeding from a major artery in the larynx can result in aspiration of blood into the airway. Because TLM patients typically do not undergo a tracheotomy, endolaryngeal bleeding is especially concerning due to the risk of blood loss, aspiration, and hypoxia. It is thus recommended that larger vessels are clipped rather than cauterized intraoperatively. In the case of a severe postoperative bleed, it is critical to secure the airway, either by endotracheal intubation or by performing an urgent tracheostomy, followed by operative control of hemorrhage.

Airway obstruction is uncommon, as resection of the tumor generally provides an airway that is more widely patent following surgery. Since the neck is not incised, there is much less postoperative swelling and edema that characterizes open surgical procedures on the larynx. However, prolonged tongue retraction and compression during long operations can result in soft tissue ischemia and in tongue edema postoperatively. Additionally, prolonged displacement of the tongue by the laryngoscope during surgery can cause temporary lingual or hypoglossal paresis. In cases lasting more than 1–2 h, periodically releasing suspension to allow blood flow to the tongue markedly decreases the likelihood of developing postoperative tongue swelling or nerve dysfunction. The neuropathy caused by retraction is temporary and generally resolves over several weeks.

Aspiration can be caused by extensive resection, preexisting laryngeal impairment, advanced age, or poor health. Preoperative and postoperative assessment to determine the risk for aspiration is necessary to prevent development of aspiration pneumonia. Other complications encountered include mucosal burns of the lips, oral cavity, or oropharynx, dental injuries (loosened or chipped teeth), infection, dysphagia, chondroma or granuloma formation, and airway fires or burns.

Future Directions/Challenges

The functional and oncologic efficacy of TLM for early stage glottic lesions has been proven and is now well accepted as an effective treatment approach. Along with transcervical surgery, SCPL-CHP, and external beam radiation, it is an important piece of the surgeons' armamentarium against laryngeal carcinoma. There are extensive data on oncologic control and increasing data on voice outcome.

There is a steep learning curve for TLM. One of the keys to successful TLM surgery is exposure of the larynx, which requires both an adequate assortment of laryngoscope and advanced endoscopy skills. Additionally, time must be dedicated to becoming skillful at using the laser and microscope, whether it is with a micromanipulator or a handheld flexible fiber. TLM also necessitates an understanding of the detailed anatomy of the larynx from the "inside out." It requires the surgeon to be able to visualize and three dimensionally reconstruct endoscopic views.

An additional challenge of TLM is that it is difficult to teach to surgeons-in-training. The tactile feedback of dissecting tissues with the laser can only be honed with experience. Additionally, it can be difficult to maintain orientation of the three-dimensional (3-D) field when surgeons take turns alternating visualization through the primary lens. Visualization in a teaching arm or two-dimensional monitor does not capture the same views, and it is thus difficult to ensure oncologic resection.

Over the last decade, transoral robotic surgery (TORS) has emerged as a treatment option, with the ultimate goal of optimizing oncologic management while even further reducing treatment morbidity. Hockstein et al. demonstrated the ability of the robot to provide 3-D images through a dual endoscope mechanism within laryngeal mannequins [53]. Weinstein and O'Malley subsequently showed efficacy in humans with supraglottic laryngectomy and partial pharyngectomy [54–56]. In addition to 3-D images, robotic instrumentation provides a wide range of motions unavailable with traditional endoscopic instruments, scaling of movement, where large movements of the hands produce only small movements in the robotic instruments, and robotic dampening of hand tremors. Because of the maneuverability of the robotic arms, TORS has a benefit over traditional transoral laser surgery that is limited by the laser's line of sight. While it is commonly used in the oropharynx, it has yet to garner widespread acceptance in the larynx, where the ability to expose structures and manipulate instruments is limited by the size of the currently available robotic arms and the limited available instrumentation designed for prostate and gynecologic procedures. As advancements in robotics and optics continue to be made, further refinements will expand the indications and uses of robotic approaches.

Currently, TLM is a proven, minimally invasive alternative to open surgery for T1, T2, and selected T3 tumors of the glottis and supraglottis. The results of TLM are comparable to open partial laryngectomy procedures and RT in terms of local control and survival rates. With its low postoperative morbidity, TLM represents an attractive means to surgically remove cancer while preserving the laryngeal framework. In an era of emphasis on organ preservation and minimizing the cost of healthcare, TLM is an affordable option that allows for optimization of functional outcomes without sacrificing oncologic principles.

References

1. Siegel R, Naishadham D, Jemal A. Cancer statistics, 2013. CA Cancer J Clin. 2013;63(1):11–30.
2. Barnes L, Tse LY, Hunt JL, et al. Tumours of the hypopharynx, larynx and trachea: introduction. In: Barnes L, Eveson J, Reichart P, Sidransky D, editors. World Health Organization classification of tumours. Pathology and genetics of head and neck tumours. Lyon: IARC Press; 2005. p. 111–7.
3. Woodson GE. The history of laryngology in the United States. Laryngoscope. 1996;106(6): 677–9.
4. Kleinsasser O. Weitere technische Entwicklung und erste Ergebnisse der endolaryngealen Mikrochirurgie. Z Laryng Rhinol. 1965;44:711–27.
5. Zeitels SM. Universal modular glottiscope system: the evolution of a century of design and technique for direct laryngoscopy. Ann Otol Rhinol Laryngol Suppl. 1999;179:2–24.
6. Polanyi TG, Bredemeier HC, Davis Jr TW. A CO2 laser for surgical research. Med Biol Eng. 1970;8(6):541–8.
7. Jako GJ. Laser surgery of the vocal cords. An experimental study with carbon dioxide lasers on dogs. Laryngoscope. 1972;82(12):2204–16.
8. Shapshay SM, Jako GJ. Laser surgery of the vocal cords; an experimental study with carbon dioxide lasers on dogs. Laryngoscope.

1996;106(8):935–8 (Laryngoscope, 1972; 82:2204–2216).
9. Alberti PW. The history of laryngology: a centennial celebration. Otolaryngol Head Neck Surg. 1996;114(3):345–54.
10. Zeitels SM, Burns JA. Laser applications in laryngology: past, present, and future. Otolaryngol Clin N Am. 2006;39:159–72.
11. Steiner W. Results of curative laser microsurgery of laryngeal carcinomas. Am J Otolaryngol. 1993;14:116–21.
12. Steiner W, Ambrosch P. Endoscopic laser surgery of the upper aerodigestive tract. New York: Thieme; 2000.
13. Eckel HE. Endoscopic laser resection of supraglottic carcinoma. Otolaryngol Head Neck Surg. 1997;117:681–7.
14. Rudert HH, Werner JA, Höft S. Transoral carbon dioxide laser resection of supraglottic carcinoma. Ann Otol Rhinol Laryngol. 1999;108: 819–27.
15. Grant DG, Salassa JR, Hinni ML, Pearson BW, Hayden RE, Perry WC. Transoral laser microsurgery for carcinoma of the supraglottic larynx. Otolaryngol Head Neck Surg. 2007; 136(6):900–6.
16. Pearson BW, Salassa JR. Transoral laser microresection for cancer of the larynx involving the anterior commissure. Laryngoscope. 2003;113(7):1104–12.
17. Werner JA, Lippert BM, Schünke M, Rudert H. Animal experiment studies of laser effects on lymphatic vessels. A contribution to the discussion of laser surgery segmental resection of carcinomas. Laryngorhinootologie. 1995;74(12): 748–55.
18. Werner JA, Dunne AA, Folz BJ, Lippert BM. Transoral laser microsurgery in carcinomas of the oral cavity, pharynx, and larynx. Cancer Control. 2002;9(5):379–86.
19. Ambrosch P. The role of laser microsurgery in the treatment of laryngeal cancer. Curr Opin Otolaryngol Head Neck Surg. 2007;15(2) :82–8.
20. Burkey BB, Garrett G. Use of the laser in the oral cavity. Otolaryngol Clin North Am. 1996;29(6):949–61.
21. Jerjes W, Hamdoon Z, Hopper C. CO2 lasers in the management of potentially malignant and malignant oral disorders. Head Neck Oncol. 2012;4:17.
22. Ossoff RH. Laser safety in otolaryngology—head and neck surgery: anesthetic and educational considerations for laryngeal surgery. Laryngoscope. 1989;99(8 Pt 2 Suppl 48):1–26.
23. Apfelbaum JL, Caplan RA, Barker SJ, Connis RT, Cowles C, Ehrenwerth J, Nickinovich DG, Pritchard D, Roberson DW, Caplan RA, Barker SJ, Connis RT, Cowles C, de Richemond AL, Ehrenwerth J, Nickinovich DG, Pritchard D, Roberson DW, Wolf GL, American Society of Anesthesiologists Task Force on Operating Room Fires. Practice advisory for the prevention and management of operating room fires: an updated report by the American Society of Anesthesiologists task force on operating room fires. Anesthesiology. 2013;118(2):271–90.
24. Fisher JC. Basic biophysical principles of resurfacing of human skin by means of the carbon dioxide laser. J Clin Laser Med Surg. 1996;14(4):193–210.
25. Remacle M, Lawson G, Nollevaux MC, Delos M. Current state of scanning micromanipulator applications with the carbon dioxide laser. Ann Otol Rhinol Laryngol. 2008;117(4):239–44.
26. Fein DA, Mendenhall WM, Parsons JT, Million RR. T1–T2 squamous cell carcinoma of the glottic larynx treated with radiotherapy: a multivariate analysis of variables potentially influencing local control. Int J Radiat Oncol Biol Phys. 1993;25(4):605–11.
27. Cellai E, Frata P, Magrini SM, Paiar F, Barca R, Fondelli S, Polli C, Livi L, Bonetti B, Vitali E, De Stefani A, Buglione M, Biti G. Radical radiotherapy for early glottic cancer: results in a series of 1087 patients from two Italian radiation oncology centers. I. The case of T1N0 disease. Int J Radiat Oncol Biol Phys. 2005;63(5):1378–86.
28. Cohen SM, Garrett CG, Dupont WD, Ossoff RH, Courey MS. Voice-related quality of life in T1 glottic cancer: irradiation versus endoscopic excision. Ann Otol Rhinol Laryngol. 2006;115(8):581–6.
29. Brandenburg JH. Laser cordotomy versus radiotherapy: an objective cost analysis. Ann Otol Rhinol Laryngol. 2001;110(4):312–8.
30. Myers EN, Wagner RL, Johnson JT. Microlaryngoscopic surgery for T1 glottic lesions: a cost-effective option. Ann Otol Rhinol Laryngol. 1994;103(1):28–30.
31. Marshak G, Brenner B, Shvero J, Shapira J, Ophir D, Hochman I, Marshak G, Sulkes A, Rakowsky E. Prognostic factors for local control of early glottic cancer: the Rabin Medical Center retrospective study on 207 patients. Int J Radiat Oncol Biol Phys. 1999;43(5):1009–13.
32. Frata P, Cellai E, Magrini SM, Bonetti B, Vitali E, Tonoli S, Buglione M, Paiar F, Barca R, Fondelli S, Polli C, Livi L, Biti G. Radical radiotherapy for early glottic cancer: results in a series of 1087 patients from two Italian radiation oncology centers. II. The case of T2N0 disease. Int J Radiat Oncol Biol Phys. 2005;63(5):1387–94.
33. Bradley PJ, Ferlito A, Suárez C, Werner JA, Genden EM, Shaha AR, Leemans CR, Langendijk JA, Rinaldo A. Options for salvage after failed initial treatment of anterior vocal commissure squamous carcinoma. Eur Arch Otorhinolaryngol. 2006;263(10):889–94.
34. Steiner W, Ambrosch P, Rodel RMW, Kron M. Impact of anterior commissure involvement

on local control of early glottic carcinoma treated by laser microresection. Laryngoscope. 2004;114:1485–91.
35. Eckel HE. Local recurrences following transoral laser surgery for early glottic carcinoma: frequency, management, and outcome. Ann Otol Rhinol Laryngol. 2001;110:7–15.
36. Krespi YP, Meltzer CJ. Laser surgery for vocal cord carcinoma involving the anterior commissure. Ann Otol Rhinol Laryngol. 1989;98(2): 105–9.
37. Zäbren P, Becker M, Lang H. Staging of laryngeal cancer: endoscopy, computed tomography and magnetic resonance versus histopathology. Eur Arch Otorhinolaryngol. 1997;254 Suppl 1:S117–22.
38. Becker M, Zbären P, Casselman JW, Kohler R, Dulguerov P, Becker CD. Neoplastic invasion of laryngeal cartilage: reassessment of criteria for diagnosis at MR imaging. Radiology. 2008;249(2):551–9.
39. Barbosa MM, Araújo Jr VJ, Boasquevisque E, Carvalho R, Romano S, Lima RA, Dias FL, Salviano SK. Anterior vocal commissure invasion in laryngeal carcinoma diagnosis. Laryngoscope. 2005;115(4):724–30.
40. Ambrosch P, Rödel R, Kron M, et al. Transoral laser microsurgery for cancer of the larynx. A retrospective analysis of 657 patients [in German]. Onkologe. 2001;7:505–12.
41. Alonso Regules JE. Horizontal partial laryngectomy. Historical review and personal technique. In: Wigand ME, Steiner W, Stell PM, editors. Functional partial laryngectomy. Conservation surgery for carcinoma of the larynx. Berlin: Springer; 1984. p. 179–82.
42. Laccourreye H, Laccourreye O, Weinstein G, Menard M, Brasnu D. Supracricoid laryngectomy with cricohyoidopexy: a partial laryngeal procedure for selected supraglottic and transglottic carcinomas. Laryngoscope. 1990; 100(7):735–41.
43. Mancuso AA, Mukherji SK, Schmalfuss I, Mendenhall W, Parsons J, Pameijer F, Hermans R, Kubilis P. Preradiotherapy computed tomography as a predictor of local control in supraglottic carcinoma. J Clin Oncol. 1999;17(2):631–7.
44. Vaughan CW. Transoral laryngeal surgery using the CO2 laser. Laboratory experiments and clinical experience. Laryngoscope. 1978; 88:1399–420.
45. Zeitels SM, Vaughan CW. The adjustable supraglottiscope. Otolaryngol Head Neck Surg. 1990;103:487–92.
46. Zeitels SM, Vaughan CW, Domanowski GF, Fuleihan NS, Simpson GT. Laser epiglottectomy: endoscopic technique and indications. Otolaryngol Head Neck Surg. 1990;103(3): 337–43.
47. Rodrigo JP, Suárez C, Silver CE, Rinaldo A, Ambrosch P, Fagan JJ, Genden EM, Ferlito A. Transoral laser surgery for supraglottic cancer. Head Neck. 2008;30(5):658–66.
48. Zeitels SM, Koufman JA, Davis RK, Vaughan CW. Endoscopic treatment of supraglottic and hypopharynx cancer. Laryngoscope. 1994;104(1 Pt 1):71–8.
49. Ambrosch P, Kron M, Steiner W. Carbon dioxide laser microsurgery for early supraglottic carcinoma. Ann Otol Rhinol Laryngol. 1998;107:680–8.
50. Iro H, Waldfahrer F, Altendorf-Hofmann A, Weidenbecher M, Sauer R, Steiner W. Transoral laser surgery of supraglottic cancer: follow-up of 141 patients. Arch Otolaryngol Head Neck Surg. 1998;124(11):1245–50.
51. Prades JM, Schmitt TM, Timoshenko AP, Simon PG, de Cornulier J, Durand M, Guillot A, Martin C. Concomitant chemoradiotherapy in pyriform sinus carcinoma. Arch Otolaryngol Head Neck Surg. 2002;128(4):384–8.
52. Tufano RP, Stafford EM. Organ preservation surgery for laryngeal cancer. Otolaryngol Clin North Am. 2008;41(4):741–55.
53. Hockstein NG, Nolan JP, O'Malley Jr BW, Woo YJ. Robotic microlaryngeal surgery: a technical feasibility study using the daVinci surgical robot and an airway mannequin. Laryngoscope. 2005;115:780–5.
54. O'Malley Jr BW, Weinstein GS, Snyder W, Hockstein NG. Transoral robotic surgery (TORS) for base of tongue neoplasms. Laryngoscope. 2006;116:1465–72.
55. Weinstein GS, O'Malley Jr BW, Snyder W, Hockstein NG. Transoral robotic surgery: supraglottic partial laryngectomy. Ann Otol Rhinol Laryngol. 2007;116:19–23.
56. Weinstein GS, O'Malley Jr BW, Snyder W, Sherman E, Quon H. Transoral robotic surgery: radical tonsillectomy. Arch Otolaryngol Head Neck Surg. 2007;133:1220–6.

Chapter 5

Laser Applications for Nonmalignant Conditions of the Larynx

James A. Burns

Introduction

Laryngeal lesions such as papilloma, precancerous dysplasia, and vascular malformations can significantly impact voice production and patients' quality of life. These nonmalignant conditions of the larynx can disrupt glottic closure patterns and inhibit propagation of the mucosal wave during phonation. Surgical techniques for the management of these lesions have advanced exponentially with further understanding of the importance of preserving the superficial lamina propria (SLP) layer and advances in surgical technology. Laser applications for nonmalignant conditions of the larynx have allowed for lesions such as papilloma and precancerous dysplasia to be optimally treated with maximum preservation of the underlying layered vocal fold microstructure. Photoangiolytic lasers such as the 585 nm pulsed-dye laser (PDL) and 532 nm KTP laser specifically target the microvasculature associated with the growth of these nonmalignant lesions and offer a fiber-based delivery system that allows for office-based surgery using topical anesthesia. In general, the primary advantages of laser surgery for nonmalignant conditions of the larynx are extreme precision, hemostasis, and selectivity for certain tissue "targets" such as blood vessels, without harming surrounding tissue. Also, a 2013 nm diode-pumped thulium laser has been introduced into endoscopic laryngeal surgery for the treatment of certain benign conditions. This laser's chromophore is water, allowing for properties of hemostatic cutting on a fiber-based delivery system. This chapter will highlight salient principles of angiolytic laser use in the surgical management of vocal fold papilloma, precancerous dysplasia, and microvascular malformations both in the operating room under general anesthesia

Brian J.-F. Wong and Justus Ilgner (eds.), *Biomedical Optics in Otorhinolaryngology: Head and Neck Surgery*,
DOI 10.1007/978-1-4939-1758-7_5,

and in office-based settings with topical anesthesia. Additionally, office-based and microlaryngeal applications of the thulium laser in performing endolaryngeal surgery for benign conditions are reviewed.

Photoangiolytic Lasers: Overview

In the 1980s, Rox Anderson [1–3] proposed concepts of selective photothermolysis that allowed for specific targeted damage to cells by "suitably brief pulses" of optical radiation based on properties of the target tissue. Anderson, a dermatologist, applied selective photothermolysis to the development of yellow light (585–600 nm) pulsed-dye laser (PDL) for the treatment of vascular malformations by targeting oxyhemoglobin [3]. This concept eventually evolved into two angiolytic lasers: the 585-nm PDL and the 532-nm pulsed potassium titanyl phosphate (KTP) laser. These wavelengths are precisely selected to target absorbance peaks of oxyhemoglobin (~571 and ~541 nm) and can fully penetrate intraluminal blood and deposit heat uniformly into the vessel, thereby causing intravascular coagulation and "photoangiolysis" of the subepithelial microcirculation. The short pulse width is precisely selected to contain the heat to the vessel without causing collateral damage to the extravascular soft tissue from heat conduction. The output of these lasers is transmitted through a thin flexible glass fiber (≤0.6 mm).

When applied to vocal folds, the precise coagulation of subepithelial microcirculation within the layered microstructure of the phonatory mucosa has since been shown to be an effective strategy to treat laryngeal papillomatosis [4–9], precancerous dysplasia [4, 10, 11], and microvascular malformations [12–14]. Photoangiolytic lasers, which were originally introduced for endoscopic laryngeal surgery in 2002 to facilitate microflap resection of vocal fold precancerous dysplasia, are now used routinely in office-based laryngeal surgery to involute precancerous dysplasia and papilloma without resection [4, 5].

Photoangiolytic Lasers (PDL and KTP): Papilloma

Laryngeal papillomatosis (or recurrent respiratory papillomatosis, RRP) is a benign neoplastic process caused by the human papilloma virus (usually types 6 or 11) [15]. This disease remains challenging because of its propensity to recur after treatment and its characteristic location on the vibratory vocal fold surfaces that are vital for voice production. Optimal surgical management of papilloma includes aggressive ablation of disease to ensure the best possible local disease control along with precision that ensures maximum voice preservation. Photoangiolytic lasers such as the PDL and KTP lasers have been shown to effectively eradicate papilloma from the vocal fold surface with excellent voice preservation [4–9].

Pilot studies were performed using the 585 nm PDL for laryngeal papillomatosis in the late 1990s [6], followed shortly thereafter by large-scale investigations [4, 8]. The abundant microvasculature present in papilloma is a key feature when considering photoangiolysis for surgical management of this benign condition. The microcirculation could be targeted to involute the papillomatous growth or facilitate its "cold-instrument" resection while minimizing thermal trauma to the surrounding soft tissue, superficial lamina propria (SLP), and epithelium. In theory, this would be ideal for maintaining the pliability of the vocal folds' layered microstructure (SLP and epithelium) and glottal sound production. PDLs have been effective in treating papillomatosis without the associated clinically observed soft-tissue complications associated with the CO_2 laser (thermal damage, tissue necrosis, SLP scarring, and anterior commissure web formation). The presumed mechanism of disease regression is the selective destruction of the subepithelial microvasculature and separation of the diseased epithelium from the underlying SLP by denaturing the basement membrane zone-linking proteins. At this point, the papilloma can either be completely ablated or carefully resected from the underlying vocal fold layered microstructure. Typical energy settings for using the PDL to treat papilloma are 500–570 mJ per pulse and the endpoint of treatment is the characteristic white blanching of the papilloma which signifies adequate coagulation of the lesion's microcirculation.

A potential disadvantage of PDL treatment is that it can be difficult to accurately quantify the energy delivery and real-time tissue effects, despite the fact that this laser is unlikely to cause substantial soft-tissue injury to the vocal folds. Furthermore, given the extremely short pulse width (approximately 0.5 ms), it is not unusual for the vessel walls of the microcirculation to rupture, resulting in extravasation of blood into the surrounding tissue. In laryngeal lesions such as papillomatosis, the extravasated blood diverts the laser energy in the form of a heat sink, which diminishes the effectiveness and reduces the selectivity of the laser.

Another potential disadvantage of using the PDL to treat papilloma is that the smallest fiber size that can deliver the laser energy is 0.6 mm. This size fiber can easily cut and traumatize the channel of the flexible laryngoscope during office-based management of the disease. This problem has created a need for fiber sheaths to protect the laryngoscope channel. Using this additional sheath diminishes the usable space within the channel of the flexible laryngoscope, which is critical for effectively suctioning secretions during the procedure.

The 532 nm KTP laser overcomes many of the shortcomings of the PDL. Its 532 nm wavelength is more strongly absorbed by oxyhemoglobin than the 585 nm wavelength of the PDL. More importantly, the pulse width of the KTP laser is much longer than the PDL (15 ms as opposed to ~0.45 ms) and is adjustable. The longer pulse width distributes the laser energy over a time period approximately 30 times longer than that the PDL. In theory, this slower intravascular heating helps avoid the vessel wall rupture and extravasation that would commonly be observed with the PDL.

The longer pulse width of the KTP laser also takes advantage of the fact that the energy delivery time is less than the thermal relaxation time of the tissue. Consequently, there is minimal collateral extravascular thermal soft tissue trauma compared to using the same laser in a continuous mode.

Other advantages of the KTP laser as compared with the PDL are that the KTP laser is a solid-state instrument of which the output can be delivered through even smaller fibers (for example, 0.3 or 0.4 mm) and in a continuous wave mode for hemostatic cutting, if desired. Typical settings for using the KTP laser to treat papilloma are 525–675 mJ of fluence energy, which are obtained be varying the energy between 35 and 45 W at a constant pulse width of 15 ms and 2 pulses per second. The endpoint of treatment is the characteristic white blanching of the papilloma which signifies adequate coagulation of the lesion's microcirculation, and more exophytic areas of disease can be removed to expose the base of disease for further treatment.

The 585 nm PDL and the 532 nm KTP laser are both angiolytic lasers that provide safe and effective surgical management for laryngeal papillomatosis under general anesthesia [9]. Clinical results show that the majority of patients with papilloma can achieve 90 % or greater disease regression with Photoangiolytic laser surgery [8, 9]. The fiber-based delivery system for these lasers makes patients with recurrent papilloma candidates for office-based management under local anesthesia, thereby avoiding repeat trips to the operating room for general anesthesia.

Photoangiolytic Lasers (PDL and KTP): Precancerous Dysplasia

Precancerous dysplasia of the vocal folds has been related to chronic laryngeal irritation and inflammation. Etiologies include use of tobacco, exposure to inhaled irritants, reflux disease, and infectious conditions [16]. Laryngeal biopsies may show hyperplasia, keratosis, dysplasia, or carcinoma in situ, and patients should be carefully treated and followed up since invasive carcinoma may develop many years after the initial presentation. Vocal fold dysplasia has been described as localized areas of chalky white elevations on the vocal folds' surface, and designated as keratosis, hyperkeratosis, leukoplakia, and pachydermia larynges [17]. The phonatory mucosa of vocal folds is the laryngeal tissue most susceptible to the effects of inhaled irritants or carcinogens. Therefore, surgical management must consider preservation of the SLP and other layered microstructure of the vocal fold, especially given that these lesions can recur and require multiple treatments.

Photoangiolytic lasers such as the PDL and KTP provide safe and effective treatment for pre-cancerous dysplasia of vocal folds. Even though these lesions typically look white (as opposed to the red or speckled appearance of papilloma) they do contain a zone of erythroplasia and microvascular angiogenesis that attracts photoangiolytic laser energy. Clinical reports in the literature support that the 585-nm PDL [4, 11] and KTP laser [5] both successfully involute precancerous dysplasia [4, 11], revealing that 75–100 % of the visible disease will involute, and the procedure can be repeated as needed.

Typical energy settings for using the PDL to treat precancerous dysplasia are 500–570 mJ per pulse, and the endpoint of treatment is the characteristic white blanching of the surrounding area of the white lesion which signifies adequate coagulation of the lesion's microcirculation. Typical settings for using the KTP laser to treat precancerous dysplasia are 525–675 mJ of fluence energy, which are obtained by varying the energy between 35 and 45 W at a constant pulse width of 15 ms and 2 pulses per second. The endpoint of treatment is the characteristic white blanching or "bubbling" of the white lesion which signifies adequate coagulation of the lesion's microcirculation. The ultimate amount of energy delivered to the target tissue is determined by the fiber-to-tissue distance with less of an effect when the fiber is further away. A distance of about 2 mm is optimal for tissue effect using both the PDL and KTP lasers, but closer distances including direct contact with the lesion can be used.

Photoangiolytic Lasers (KTP): Microvascular Malformations

Microvascular malformation on vocal folds such as varices and ectasias are commonly the result of vocal overuse or abuse similar to that causing other benign vocal fold lesions such as nodules and polyps. Despite the structurally stabilizing characteristics of the walls of the microvasculature within the SLP, these vessels still develop altered conformations that can result in formation of varices and ectasias [12, 13]. Once present, ectasias and varices have been observed to rupture more easily than normal-appearing vessels, thereby causing symptoms of dysphonia.

Using angiolytic lasers coupled with high-powered magnification of the surgical microscope offers an ideal treatment strategy for ablating microvascular malformations of phonatory vocal fold

Table 1
KTP laser parameters for treating nonmalignant laryngeal conditions

	Energy (W)	Pulse width (ms)	Pulses/s	mJ delivered at fiber tip (mJ)
Papilloma	35–45	15	2	525–675
Dysplasia	35–45	15	2	525–675
Microvascular malformations	30–35	15–25	2	400–525

mucosa. This approach allows for the involution of aberrant microcirculation in a noncontact mode without disturbing the overlying epithelium and without creating thermal injury with subsequent scarring of the delicate vocal fold [14].

Although both angiolytic lasers (PDL, KTP) can effectively coagulate microvascular malformations, the 585-nm PDL potentially causes vessel wall disruption and rupture. This was presumed to be due to the violent percussive effect of the short pulse width of the PDL [13]. The longer pulse width of the KTP laser (15 ms) potentially distributes the laser energy over a time period approximately 30 limes longer than that of the PDL and allows for substantially more efficient and effective intravascular coagulation through slower intravascular heating without thermal injury to the vocal fold's layered microstructure. Typical settings for using the KTP laser to treat microvascular malformations are 400–525 mJ of fluence energy, which are obtained by varying the energy between 33 and 35 W at a typical pulse width of 15 ms and 2 pulses per second. Longer pulse widths up to 25 ms can be used when attempting to coagulate larger lesions, with more uniform heating of the vessel over a longer time leading to less rupture [18]. Table 1 summarizes the laser parameters used for KTP laser treatment of various non-malignant lesions of the larynx.

Hemostatic and Cutting Lasers (Thulium)

The thulium laser is a diode-pumped solid-state laser that has a thulium-doped YAG laser rod, which produces a continuous wave beam with a wavelength of 2.013 μm. This wavelength has a target chromophore of water and therefore simulates the hemostatic cutting properties of the CO_2 laser [19]. Similar to a CO_2 laser, efficient absorption of this laser's radiation by water facilitates its cutting and dissection characteristics. However, unlike a CO_2 laser, the energy is delivered by means of a fiber, which allows for tangential endoscopic dissection. The thulium laser can therefore be used to perform a number of endoscopic partial laryngectomy surgeries to remove benign laryngeal lesions. Typically, this involves removal of a variety of submucosal lesions such as cysts, congenital lesions, and connective tissue neoplasms. The thulium laser is also an effective ablator of laryngeal papillomatosis that involves the supraglottis or other nonvibratory areas of the vocal folds.

Although potentially causing more thermal damage on the soft tissues during cutting as compared with the CO_2 laser, the degree of thermal damage has not been shown to be excessive [19]. Typical settings of the thulium laser for hemostatic cutting with the larynx or ablating neoplasms on non-vibratory vocal fold tissue are 5–7 W of continuous cutting. The thulium laser can also be used through the side-port working channel of a flexible laryngoscope to perform ablation of a variety of benign and malignant epithelial lesions of the larynx in an office-based setting with topical anesthesia. The clinical indication for use of the thulium laser in this way can damage the delicate layered microstructure of phonatory membranes, so care must be taken to properly select patients who require less selective debulking of their disease [19].

Experiments Determining Laser Parameters for Photoangiolytic and Hemostatic/Cutting Lasers

A series of experiments evaluating the performance of photoangiolytic and hemostatic/cutting lasers in the same surgical model (chick chorioallantoic membrane or CAM [20]) helped to determine the laser parameters used for laryngeal lesions [18]. The results from this work can assist surgeons in selecting the appropriate laser and settings for a specific task and lesion. Since the inherent utility of any laser (or even the decision to use a laser) depends on a surgeons' perceived value for the clinical scenario, a thorough understanding of a laser's capabilities and limitations is helpful. This includes considerations of optimal thermal effect, energy output, tissue specificity, delivery system, hemostatic effect, cutting capability, and depth of penetration (among others). Other factors influencing the selection of a particular laser include the lesion, laryngeal site, and the treatment goal (selective photoangiolysis or cutting/ablation). Comparative experiments between KTP and PDL lasers using the chick chorioallantoic membrane to simulate vocal fold microvasculature reveal several advantages of the KTP laser over the PDL [20]. The longer pulse width of the KTP laser (15 ms) as compared to the PDL (~0.5 ms) created better coagulation and diminished vessel rupture, which had been experienced clinically with the PDL.

To determine the pulse width and power settings of the KTP laser that reliably produce vessel coagulation with and without cooling in larger vessels that simulate varices and ectasias, third order CAM vessels (0.5–0.98 mm) were targeted. Pulse width and power settings were varied through a range of energy outputs until optimal parameters were identified that reliably produced coagulation as opposed to rupture of the target vessel. Results showed that coagulation of microvascular malformations that are larger than normal, such as varices, is not expected to occur at pulse-width and power settings similar to those that effectively coagulate smaller caliber vessels [20]. This is seen clinically as a higher rupture rate when larger vessels are targeted during the treatment of papilloma, pre-cancerous dysplasia, and microvascular malformations. Coagulation of larger vessels (>0.5 mm) theoretically requires longer pulse-widths because temperature gradients around large vessels may result in local under heating of the intraluminal blood unless energy is delivered over a longer period of time [18].

A range of pulse width and power settings that reliably achieved vessel coagulation was identified, with no vessels were reliably coagulated at a pulse-width shorter than 35 ms, even at high power, and rupture occurred when the pulse-width was increased to 100 ms, even at low power [18]. As the power is increased at shorter pulse-widths (<35 ms), vessels are more likely to rupture than coagulate, and vessels also rupture as the pulse-width approaches a continuous mode even at very low power. Based on these results, a pulse width of 15 ms for the KTP laser is used with optimal coagulation during surgery for most benign laryngeal lesions.

To determine the optimal power settings for clinical use of the thulium laser, two pulses of laser energy were delivered to the CAM model with and without tissue cooling at a 20 ms pulse duration and a rate of 1 pulse per second with power settings of 2, 4, and 10 W [18]. Results showed that increasing the energy output through settings of 2, 4, and 10 W created greater thermal-damage zones. While only a minimal effect on the CAM was observed at the 2 W power setting, the thermal effect increased dramatically at 4 and 10 W [18].

This experiment demonstrated that the thermal-damage zone of the thulium laser is significant and that cooling the CAM effectively reduced this area [18]. The information obtained in this study allowed direct comparison of the zone of thermal damage created by each laser utilizing optimal clinical settings for hemostasis, with and without cooling, and provided guidelines for predicting tissue effects for surgeons who select these tools for laryngeal use. Based on these results, the recommended clinical settings for the thulium laser during endolaryngeal surgery are 5–7 W of continuous cutting with concurrent use of a cooling system.

Office-Based Laser Surgery of Benign Laryngeal Conditions

The primary reason that the endolaryngeal treatment of nonmalignant lesions of the larynx is usually performed in the operating room is for the administration of general anesthesia. This approach allows for precise and optimal management of the primary goals, which are diagnostic accuracy, regression of disease, and voice restoration. Some patients with recurrent vocal fold dysplasia and papillomatosis are followed with known disease until the adverse effects of the lesions' growth justifies the morbidity and costs of the surgical intervention. Essentially, readily observed disease is followed until one or more factors justify a decision to abandon the watchful-waiting model to embark on surgical intervention. These factors include airway restriction, voice deterioration, and worrisome appearance on clinical laryngoscopy. The fiber-based delivery of photoangiolytic provides the option of office-based management with topical anesthesia.

In 2002, office-based laser surgery using the PDL with local anesthesia for nonmalignant laryngeal lesions such as papilloma and dysplasia was first reported in the literature [4]. Office-based surgery with the PDL was often associated with procedural bleeding, which limited precision in a number of ways [4, 5]. Extravasated blood obscured visualization of the operative field and often precipitated coughing, both of which diminished the ability to precisely apply laser energy. This common sequence of events limited the effectiveness of the PDL by diminishing its selectivity for the disorder. The laser energy was inevitably absorbed by free blood, which was primarily on the surface of the epithelial lesion rather than in the sublesional or intralesional microcirculation. These factors reduced efficiency, which is important during the therapeutic window of local anesthesia of approximately 30 min with topical administration of lidocaine.

This type of bleeding that is particularly problematic in awake patients during office-based surgery is more likely to occur with the PDL due to its extremely short pulse width (approximately 0.5 ms). When blood within the vessel lumen heats too quickly, and not uniformly, vessel wall rupture can occur before complete intravascular coagulation. Thus, there is a narrow zone of optimal fluence to achieve complete intravascular coagulation, which is dependent on fiber-to-tissue distance, as well as the energy settings for each pulse. Office-based surgery with photoangiolytic lasers under local anesthesia through a flexible laryngoscope is unavoidably complicated by a moving laryngeal target. Furthermore, fiber-to-tissue distance cannot be determined accurately in the patient-awake setting, so tissue effect from the lasering is less precise. Although somewhat better for the KTP laser (in terms of the KTP laser being less likely to create rupture than the PDL), the lack of precision limits the office-based applications of photoangiolytic lasers to epithelial diseases involving neoplasms such as papilloma and precancerous dysplasia [5]. Studies have shown that patients tolerate office-based lasering with topical anesthesia quite well [4, 5, 21]. Microvascular malformations would likely rupture too readily (as often happens during their management in the operating room under general anesthesia) and are therefore not optimally treated in the office setting.

The surgical learning curve that exists in determining tissue effects of angiolytic lasers is difficult to determine and caution dictates that initial use of these lasers to treat papilloma and precancerous dysplasia be done in the operating room. In this way, variables such as patient movement during respiration and swallowing and patient tolerance to secretions and the overall procedure are controlled. Keeping a greater fiber-to-tissue distance initially also helps the surgeon gradually learn the laser effect on tissue. The fiber can be slowly advanced to the lesion with each pulse until the optimal degree of coagulation or ablation is being achieved. This approach limits the primary potential morbidity of treating any noncancerous lesion of the vocal fold and scarring of the superficial lamina propria (SLP).

There are a number of limitations with the flexible laryngoscopic approach. A specimen for histopathologic analysis is not obtained routinely as part of the decision-making process for treatment. This is considered to be acceptable for a number of reasons. Most importantly, all patients have previously undergone microlaryngoscopic biopsies in the operating room and the indication to obtain further postlaser intraoperative biopsies or treatment remained unchanged, based on laryngoscopic appearance during the office examination. Therefore, if the post-treatment clinical examination improved so that transparent normal-appearing epithelium was observed, a biopsy was unnecessary. However, if there was insufficient resolution or response to treatment after 3–4 weeks, the intraoperative option remained available. It is highly unlikely that there would be a clinically unrecognized new malignancy given the previous non-cancerous biopsy results and even less likely that a delay of several weeks would have a deleterious effect on long-term outcome. Another disadvantage of the local-anesthesia approach is that this treatment pathway may lead ultimately to more procedures [4, 5]. This is mainly because the threshold for intervention is decreased commensurate with the diminished morbidity associated with local anesthetic treatment. In addition, individual office-based operations are generally less effective compared with operative procedures under general anesthesia. The surgeon is understandably less aggressive using photoangiolytic lasers with local anesthesia because of reduced visual precision and the fact that the vocal folds are moving.

Summary

Since their introduction in laryngeal surgery over 40 years ago, lasers have facilitated critically important innovations, such as in the surgical management of nonmalignant laryngeal lesions. These advances have accommodated well to the specialty of otolaryngology—head and neck surgery. Lasers discussed in this chapter (PDL, KTP, Thulium) can provide new platform technologies that will likely lead to the enhanced treatment of a number of benign (and malignant) laryngeal disorders. There is an expanding acceptance for performing fiber-based laser surgery by means of local anesthesia in the clinic or office, especially for chronic diseases such as papilloma and precancerous dysplasia.

References

1. Anderson RR, Parrish JA. Selective photothermolysis: precise microsurgery by selective absorption of pulsed radiation. Science. 1983; 220(4596):524–7.
2. Anderson RR, Parrish JA. Microvasculature can be selectively damaged using dye lasers: a basic theory and experimental evidence in human skin. Lasers Surg Med. 1981;1(3):263–76.
3. Anderson RR, Jaenicke KF, Parrish JA. Mechanisms of selective vascular changes caused by dye lasers. Lasers Surg Med. 1983 ;3(3):211–5.
4. Zeitels SM, Franco Jr RA, Dailey SH, Burns JA, Hillman RE, Anderson RR. Office-based treatment of glottal dysplasia and papillomatosis with the 585-nm pulsed dye laser and local anesthesia. Ann Otol Rhinol Laryngol. 2004; 113(4):265–76.
5. Zeitels SM, Akst LM, Burns JA, Hillman RE, Broadhurst MS, Anderson RR. Office-based 532-nm pulsed KTP laser treatment of glottal papillomatosis and dysplasia. Ann Otol Rhinol Laryngol. 2006;115(9):679–85.
6. McMillan K, Shapshay SM, McGilligan JA, Wang Z, Rebeiz EE. A 585-nm pulsed dye laser treatment of laryngeal papillomas: preliminary report. Laryngoscope. 1998;108(7) :968–72.
7. Valdez TA, McMillan K, Shapshay SM. A new laser treatment for vocal cord papilloma—585-nm pulsed dye. Otolaryngol Head Neck Surg. 2001;124(4):421–5.
8. Franco Jr RA, Zeitels SM, Farinelli WA, Anderson RR. 585-nm pulsed dye laser treatment of glottal papillomatosis. Ann Otol Rhinol Laryngol. 2002;111(6):486–92.
9. Burns JA, Zeitels SM, Akst LM, Broadhurst MS, Hillman RE, Anderson RR. 532 nm pulsed potassium-titanyl-phosphate laser treatment of laryngeal papillomatosis under general anesthesia. Laryngoscope. 2007;117(8):1500–4.
10. Zeitels SM. Vocal fold atypia/dysplasia and carcinoma. Atlas of phonomicrosurgery and other endolaryngeal procedures for benign and malignant disease. San Diego, CA: Singular; 2001. p. 177–218.
11. Franco Jr RA, Zeitels SM, Farinelli WA, Faquin W, Anderson RR. 585-nm pulsed dye laser treatment of glottal dysplasia. Ann Otol Rhinol Laryngol. 2003;112(9 Pt 1):751–8.
12. Zeitels SM, Hillman RE, Desloge R, Mauri M, Doyle PB. Phonomicrosurgery in singers and performing artists: treatment outcomes, management theories, and future directions. Ann Otol Rhinol Laryngol Suppl. 2002; 190:21–40.
13. Hsiung MW, Kang BH, Su WF, Pai L, Wang HW. Clearing microvascular lesions of the true vocal fold with the KTP/532 laser. Ann Otol Rhinol Laryngol. 2003;112(6):534–9.
14. Zeitels SM, Akst LM, Bums JA, Hillman RE, Broadhurst MS, Anderson RR. Pulsed angiolytic laser treatment of ectasias and varices in singers. Ann Otol Rhinol Laryngol. 2006; 115(8):571–80.
15. Brandsma JL, Lewis AJ, Abramson A, Manos MM. Detection and typing of papillomavirus DNA in formaldehyde-fixed paraffin-embedded tissue. Arch Otolaryngol Head Neck Surg. 1990;116:844–8.
16. Jackson C. Cancer of the larynx: is it preceded by a recognizable precancerous condition? Trans Am Laryngol Assoc. 1922;44: 182–201.
17. Pierce NH. Leukoplakia Laryngis. Ann Otol Rhinol Laryngol. 1920;29:33–56.

18. Burns JA, Kobler JB, Heaton JT, et al. Predicting clinical efficacy of photoangiolytic and cutting/ablating lasers using the chick chorioallantoic membrane model: implications for endoscopic voice surgery. Laryngoscope. 2008;118(6):1109–24.
19. Zeitels SM, Burns JA, Akst LM, et al. Office-based and microlaryngeal applications of a fiber-based thulium laser. Ann Otol Rhinol Laryngol. 2006;115:891–6.
20. Broadhurst MS, Akst LM, Burns JA, et al. Effects of 532nm pulsed-ktp laser parameters on vessel ablation in the avian chorioallantoic membrane: implications for vocal fold mucosa. Laryngoscope. 2007;117:220–5.
21. Rees CJ, Halum SL, Wijewickrama RC, Koufman JA, Postma GN. Patient tolerance of in-office pulsed dye laser treatments to the upper aerodigestive tract. Otolaryngol Head Neck Surg. 2006;134(6):1023–7.

Chapter 6

Laser Myringotomy

Alexander Blödow

Anatomical Considerations and Historical Overview

The middle ear is an anatomic space medial of the eardrum which contains the ossicular chain and is covered with middle ear mucosa. It is aerated by the Eustachian tube in order to equalize the middle ear pressure to the normal environmental air pressure. The eardrum (synonymous to tympanic membrane) and the ossicular chain provide the transmission of sound energy to the inner ear, and their normal function is crucial for good hearing. Dysfunction of middle ear aeration results in reduced middle ear pressure and in its chronic situation fosters transformation of the respiratory middle ear mucosa to mucus-producing epithelium. This leads to a higher impedance of the sound transmitting system, as the reduced vibrational capability of the eardrum and the ossicular chain results in conductive hearing loss of variable extent. This problem can be resolved by creating a perforation in the tympanic membrane which has to remain patent for a couple of days to weeks. The procedure is called "myringotomy" and was first described in the seventeenth century by Riolan, who by accident penetrated the tympanic membrane and induced hearing improvement [1]. In 1800, Sir Astley Cooper published indications of myringotomy in the case of Eustachian tube dysfunction. In order to avoid damage to the ossicular chain, he suggested the anterior inferior part of the tympanic membrane to be best for puncturing and developed an instrument to perform myringotomy precisely [2]. In the following years, the widespread but uncritical use of myringotomy failed to gain hearing improvement in most cases, and the method fell into oblivion. In 1868, Hermann Schwartze clarified the indications when he proposed only persistent middle

Brian J.-F. Wong and Justus Ilgner (eds.), *Biomedical Optics in Otorhinolaryngology: Head and Neck Surgery*,
DOI 10.1007/978-1-4939-1758-7_6,

ear effusion or painful acute otitis media as cases suitable for myringotomy [3]. Already in the century, it turned out that the patency of the perforation was often too short to cure certain middle ear diseases. Many attempts have been undertaken to prolong the healing process of the tympanic membrane, e.g. application of foreign bodies like horsehairs or sulfuric acid in or on the perforation. In 1867 a galvanic device to perform thermic perforations was introduced, and in 1868, Politzer published the use of rubber tubes which were seated into the perforation [4]. All these methods were not successful and myringotomy was abandoned. In 1954, Armstrong reintroduced myringotomy with grommet insertion into the tympanic membrane as contemporary treatment of chronic middle ear effusion, and in 1978, Saito reintroduced burn perforations with tympanic membrane healing patterns of up to 6 months [5, 6]. In 1978, Wilpizeski introduced the CO_2 laser for myringotomy in squirrel monkeys, and in 1982, Goode was the first who introduced the CO_2 laser for myringotomy in humans [7, 8]. Since then, different laser and application systems for irradiation of tympanic membrane were launched in order to create a perforation with reliable handling and low risk in terms of inner ear damage.

Indications for Laser Myringotomy

Currently, there are different indications to create a perforation in the tympanic membrane in order to aerate the middle ear: acute otitis media (AOM), otitis media with effusion (OME), and middle ear barotrauma after hyperbaric oxygen therapy/scuba diving/airplane traveling (Fig. 1). The most important principle in treating all these conditions is ventilation of the tympanic cavity. By means of laser myringotomy, this can be achieved through a self-healing perforation.

AOM is one of most common diseases especially in early childhood and often treated with antibiotics. It is painful, it can cause conductive hearing loss and sometimes be complicated by affection of the inner ear with sensorineural hearing loss and vertigo.

A persistent Eustachian tube dysfunction, viral or bacterial load of the middle ear, disturbances of immune system, as well as genetic and environmental factors can lead to chronic otitis media with effusion (OME), which is the most common cause of hearing loss in young children. In some cases, chronic OME can also evolve from AOM. If after a 3–4-month surveillance period OME has not resolved spontaneously, surgical treatment is recommended in order to facilitate drainage of middle ear effusion [9]. The accepted standard surgical procedure is a conventional incisional knife

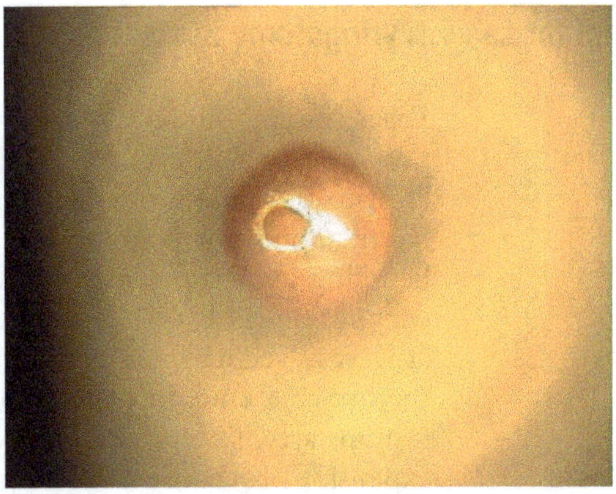

Fig. 1 CO_2 laser myringotomy (OPMI11/flashscanner, 5 W/0.2 s) in patient with OME, normal thickness of tympanic membrane; middle ear secretion was irrigated (×12)

myringotomy and insertion of ventilation tubes. The procedure is frequently performed under general anesthesia with or without additional adenoidectomy/tonsillotomy and has to be repeated in some cases for multiple times [10]. Since tube insertion may cause a certain number of adverse effects (persistent perforations, atrophic scars, purulent otorrhea, granulation tissue), it is important to verify its effectiveness [11]. Therefore, adenoidectomy with myringotomy was recommended as first-line therapy for children with chronic OME 4 years of age and older [12]. In order to avoid general anesthesia and insertion of ventilation tubes, CO_2 laser myringotomy was introduced as an option for office-based ventilation under topical anesthesia [13].

Barometric pressure changes like in hyperbaric oxygen therapy (HBO_2), descend underwater diving, or airplane traveling can cause middle ear disorders. In a hyperbaric environment, the negative pressure in the middle ear cavity in relation to the surroundings leads to a congestion of the tympanic membrane with ear bleeding and to conductive hearing loss due to transudate accumulation leaking from the middle ear mucosa. In scuba divers, middle ear barotrauma is more prevalent than inner ear barotrauma and can occur in up to 45 % 24 h after a dive [14]. In HBO_2 therapy, the cumulative risk to experience middle ear barotrauma is up to 36 % and the indication for VT insertion up to 14 % [15]. Laser myringotomy provides temporary middle ear ventilation, which offers significant potential benefits for patients since the procedure is tolerated without complications and patients can immediately return to HBO_2 treatment [16].

Requirement for Laser Myringotomy System

Laser systems suitable for laser myringotomy should have optical properties which ensure reliable transmission of the emitted laser light to the eardrum tissue. The laser has to be powerful and different application systems should be available, which are reliable in handling and have to work precisely in order to create a defined perforation. In clinical settings, the use of a laser system should be at least as secure for the structures of the middle and inner ear as the use of a knife in conventional incision myringotomy. All laser systems are of considerable cost, but laser myringotomy is not an expensive procedure as the equipment is commonly used also for laryngeal or ear surgery [17].

In literature, the laser most used frequently for myringotomy is the CO_2 laser. According to the high water content of the tympanic membrane, a CO_2 laser with a wavelength of 10,600 nm is highly suitable. CO_2 laser systems can either be connected to an operating microscope or to a laser otoscope. In order to create a hole of adequate size for patency, the laser spot can be defocused or a laser scanning system can be interconnected. These systems work in a noncontact mode. To a lesser extent, also diode lasers and erbium:YAG lasers have been used for myringotomy. Diode lasers with a wavelength of 810 to 980 nm have a high absorbance in pigmented molecules (hemoglobin). They can be transmitted via fiber-optic cables and work usually in contact mode when cutting or vaporization is needed; good coagulative properties have been observed in noncontact mode. The erbium:YAG laser is a pulsed, athermic crystal laser with a pulse duration in the microsecond range. Its short pulse duration and high peak power cause photoablation of tissue. The mechanism of ablation in erbium:YAG laser is based on the fact that its wavelength (2940 nm) hits the peak of optimal light absorption in water.

Tympanic Membrane Model for Laser Myringotomy

In order to examine ablative effects of different lasers or laser application systems and to determine power settings and threshold energy levels, laser myringotomy can be studied in animal models. Formalin-fixed human cadaveric eardrums lose water during fixation, and since most laser systems for myringotomy have high absorbance in water, fixed eardrums are less suitable for such investigation. Also tympanic membrane thickness has to be considered; since the average human tympanic membrane is about

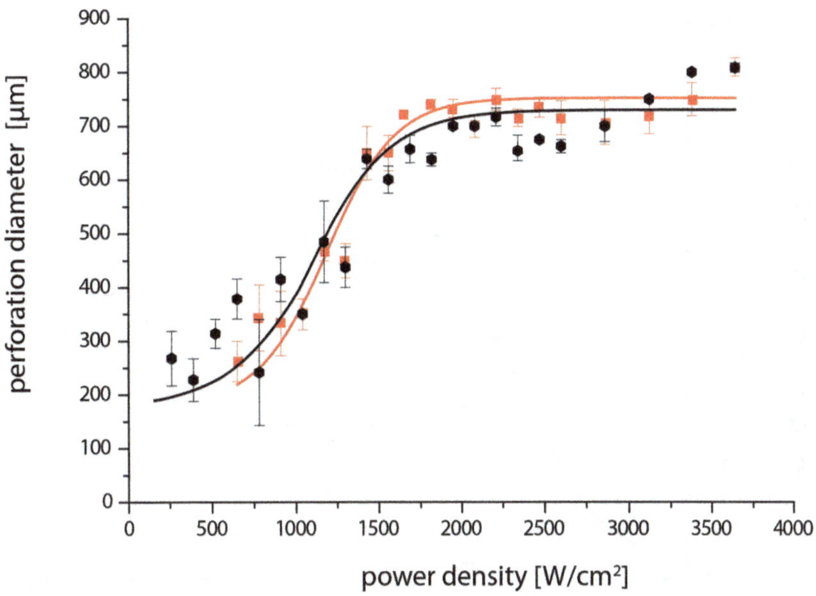

Fig. 2 Correlation of power density (W/cm^2) and perforation diameter (μm) for CO_2 laser myringotomy (operation microscope/MicroSlad®, focused spot size 700 μm, power settings 1–14 W, 0.05 s) in formalin-fixed human tympanic membrane (*red squares*) and unfixed horse tympanic membrane (*black dots*)

100 μm thick, animal models like mouse, rat, or guinea pig are inappropriate because their membrane thickness of 25–50 μm is considerably lower. Most suitable for experimental purposes is freshly harvested unfixed horse tympanic membrane. It is comparable in size, thickness, and histomorphological structure. Perforation diameters in relation to applied CO_2 laser power correlate between human tympanic membrane and horse tympanic membrane in the same manner (Fig. 2). Optimum parameters for laser myringotomy can be obtained from the point where the curve starts to saturate (Fig. 3). These parameters can then be transferred for use of laser systems on the eardrum in vivo [18, 19]. Furthermore, it is possible to examine changes according to laser irradiation in histological and electron microscopy studies in animal model (Figs. 4 and 5).

Parameters for Laser Myringotomy

In several clinical studies, different lasers and application systems have been used. Table 1 summarizes delivery parameters including power settings, pulse durations, spot size, and number of single shots for laser myringotomy. Parameters should to be sufficient in order to create a hole with only one shot (Figs. 6 and 7).

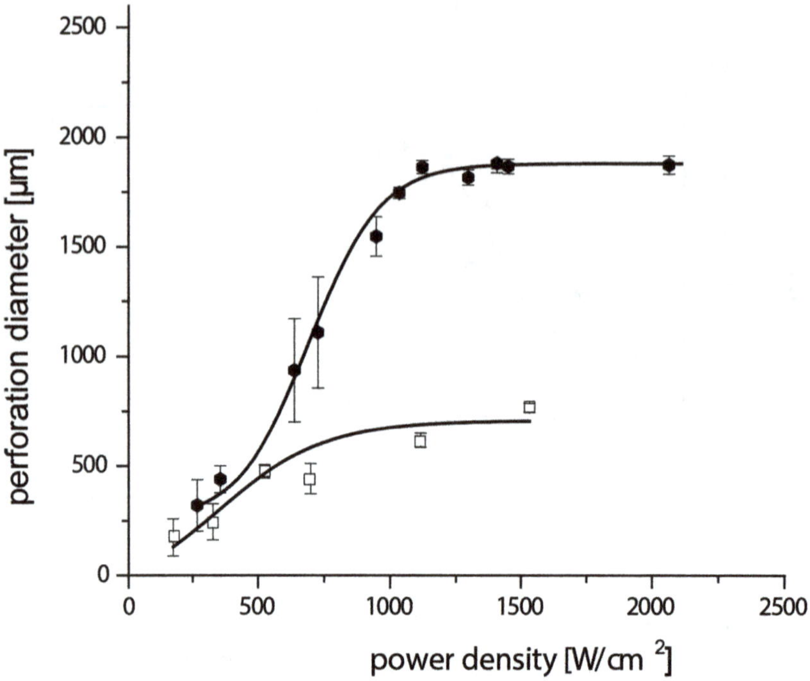

Fig. 3 Correlation of power density (W/cm²) and perforation diameter (µm) for CO_2 laser myringotomy (OPMI11/MicroSlad®) with focused technique (spot size 700 µm) and defocused technique (spot size 1800 µm) in unfixed horse tympanic membrane (*open squares* = focused, *black dots* = defocused); power settings for one-shot myringotomy are 5 W, 0.05 s/~1000 W/cm² (focused), and 32 W, 0.05 s/~1000 W/cm² (defocused)

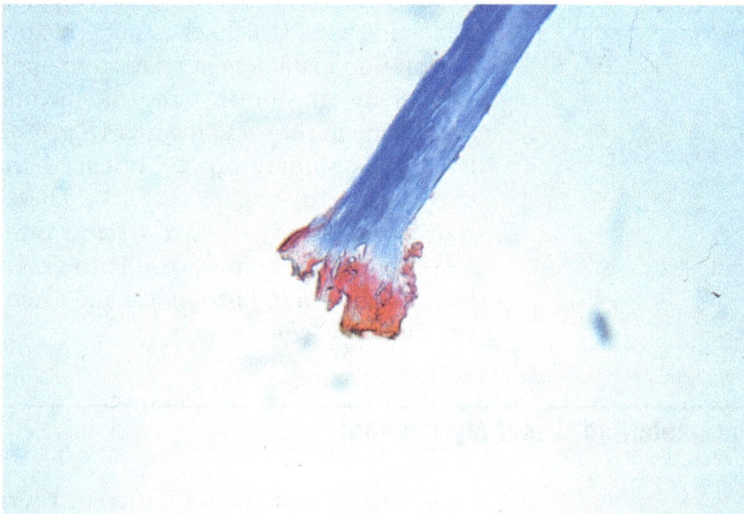

Fig. 4 Histological examination of a CO_2 laser myringotomy (5 W, 0.150 ms) in formalin-fixed human tympanic membrane stained with azan. Perforation margin shows carbonization dust (*black marginal spots*) and a coagulation zone of 100 µm (*red*), adjacent to damaged tympanic membrane tissue unchanged normal collagen fibers (*blue*) (×40)

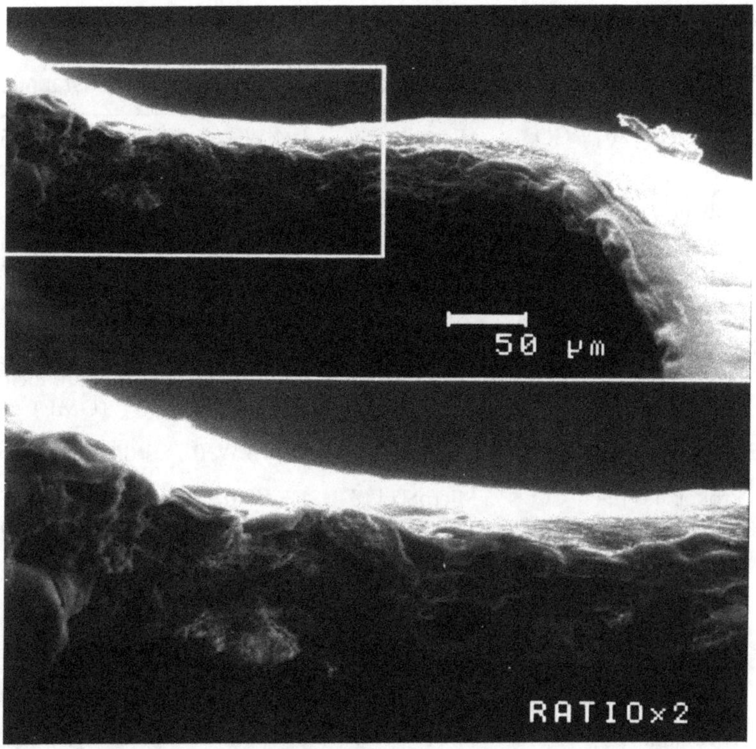

Fig. 5 Scanning electron microscopy of a CO_2 laser myringotomy in formalin-fixed human tympanic membrane (25 W, 0.1 s), *inset*: direct view on irradiated area at perforation margin, which appears molten; normal layers of collagen fibers are indiscernible (×200/×400)

Healing Patterns and Patency After Laser Myringotomy

Tympanic membrane perforations performed with CO_2 lasers in patients show a typical healing pattern. In a first stage, perforation margins show thickening and hyperemia, followed by generation of an onion skin-like membrane of keratinized material. It was confirmed in histologic studies that CO_2 laser myringotomies begin to close when the proliferating squamous epithelium reaches the edge of the perforation [29]. This proliferating keratinous membrane is formed at the perforation edge adjacent to the umbo, thus covering the perforation gradually and leading to eccentric residual perforation at the former myringotomy site. These parts of the tympanic membrane are then shifted in centrifugal way (from umbo toward the periphery) by epithelial migration. Carbonization dust from the former myringotomy site can be found in the external auditory canal in some patients at long-term follow-up [30]. For diode laser applications, it was shown that healing proceeded also from an initial onion-like productive scarring and ended up with an atrophic

Table 1
Power settings for different laser and application systems in laser myringotomy

Study	Laser	Optical delivery device	Laser settings	Focus/application/perforation size
Silverstein [20]	CO_2	MicroSlad®	1–4 W, 0.1 s/20 W	Focused 0.65 mm/defocused 2.2 mm/2 mm (OME)
Cohen [21]	CO_2	OtoScan®	10–30 W	1.6–2.6 mm (OME)
Coma [22]	CO_2	MicroSlad	0.8–1 W, 0.1 s	Spot 0.18 mm, multiple, circular orifice (OME)
Sedlmaier [23]	CO_2	OtoScan®	20 W, 0.08 s	Multiple, 1.4 mm (AOM)
Sedlmaier [23]	Er:YAG	Otoscope	100 mJ, 0.025 s	500 μm focus, 15 shots, circular, 2 mm (OME)
Sedlmaier [23]	CO_2	OtoScan®	12–15 W, 0.18 s	Focused, single, 2.2 mm (OME)
Prokopakis [24]	CO	MicroSlad®/ AcuSpot®	1.5 W, 0.2 s	Focused 0.65 mm, multiple, rosette circular (OME)
Cotter [25]	CO	OtoScan®	18–28 W	Single to multiple, 2.4 mm (AOM/OME)
Koopmann [26]	CO_2	Flashscanner	7–20 W	1.8–2.6 mm (OME)
Zanetti [27]	Diode	Fiber	18–35 W, 0.1 s	Contact mode, tip 0.6, three shots, 1.8 mm (OME)
D'Eredita [28]	Diode	Fiber	2 W, 0.5 s	Contact mode, five pulses, 2.5 mm (OME)
Lee [17]	CO_2	AcuSpot®	11–20 W, 0.10–0.15 s	Single, defocused pulse <2.5 mm (OME)

OME Otitis media with effusion, *AOM* acute otitis media

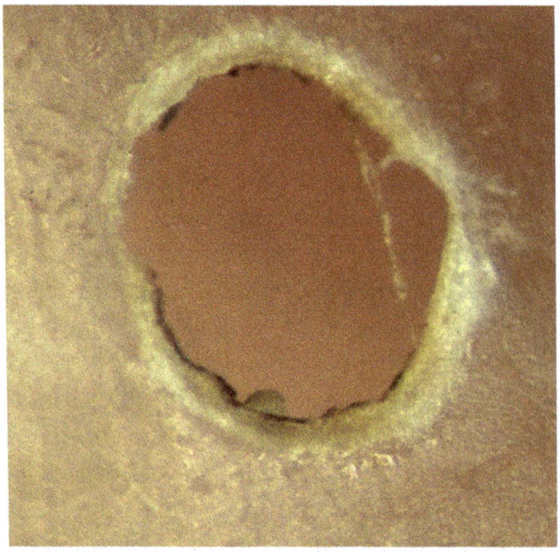

Fig. 6 CO_2 laser myringotomy in unfixed horse tympanic membrane with one shot of sufficient power settings (OPMI11/MicroSlad®, 10 W, 0.05 s), small zone of carbonization, which appears as black dust on the perforation margin, followed by a ~100 μm zone of coagulation (denatured collagen fibers = *gray*); perforation diameter corresponds to 700 μm (×40)

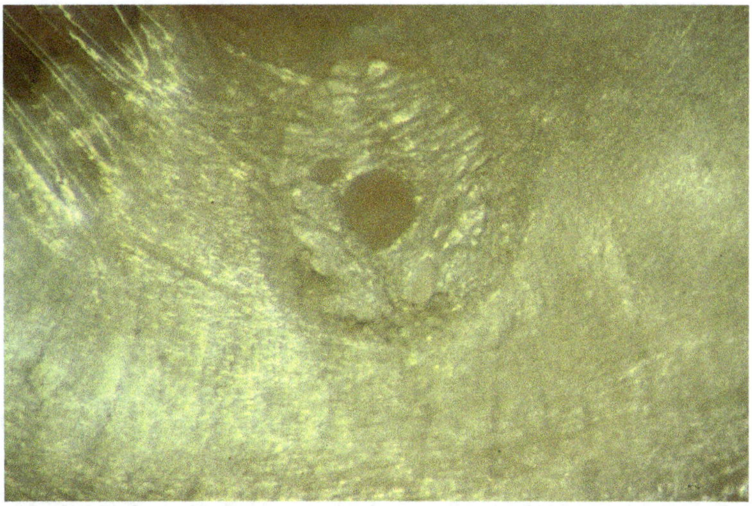

Fig. 7 CO_2 laser myringotomy in unfixed horse tympanic membrane, laser spot size of 2100 μm (OPMI11/flashscanner); power density (<1000 W/cm^2) was too low in order to create a hole within irradiated area; the perforation in the center corresponds to a diameter of 600 μm (×15)

membrane in the former perforation area. In long-term follow-up, this scar was barely noticeable in almost all treated eardrums [27].

In order to treat AOM, OME, and barotrauma, patency time of tympanic membrane perforation after laser myringotomy has to be sufficient to regain normal middle ear ventilation. Patency time can be influenced by the use of different laser and application systems and their delivery parameters, which might predict tympanostomy size.

In CO_2 laser myringotomy, Silverstein observed a direct correlation of patency time and tympanostomy size (1 mm/2 weeks, 1.5 mm/3 weeks, >2 mm/4 weeks) [20]. Cohen reported comparable data with closure time of 2–3 weeks after 1.6–2.6 mm myringotomies as did Coma with 30–40 days following 2–2.5 mm myringotomies [21, 22]. Sedlmaier found a mean closure time of 16 days for 2 mm perforations, although in patients submitted to additional adenoidectomy without tonsil surgery, perforation closure was slightly but significantly slower [23, 30]. Prokopakis created perforations of 2–2.5 mm size with an overall patency time ranging from 1 to 7 weeks (average 2.52 weeks). In a separate analysis, children with allergy or thick tympanic membrane and/or glue ear fluid had an average patency time of 3.2 weeks compared to nonallergic children or subjects with normal tympanic membrane with 2.1 weeks. A dependency between size and patency was not found [24]. In a study of Cotter, age, sex, microorganisms isolated, myringotomy size, laser power setting, and laterality did also not predict outcome [25]. Kuo found *Streptococcus pneumoniae* to be the most common pathogen in persistent AOM. The average eardrum healing time was significantly longer in those patients with positive cultures (22 days) than in those with negative cultures (16 days) [31].

In diode laser myringotomies, Zanetti showed that patency time ranged from 7 to 25 days (average 15 days) as smaller holes, as expected, healed earlier. The dimensions of the opening were influenced by power setting (18 vs. 35 W) and by the number of shots (1–6 shots) [27]. D'Eredità performed a perforation size of 2.5 mm with a diode laser. 50 % of perforations stayed open for 3.5 months, while this interval was prolonged to 6 months by insertion of a ventilation tube [32]. With the erbium:YAG laser otoscope, perforations of 2 mm diameter healed within 2 weeks and showed no atrophic scar formation at 6 months' follow-up [33].

Efficacy of Laser Myringotomy in Acute and Chronic Otitis Media

Conventional knife myringotomies heal within 2 days, which might be sufficient in AOM but is usually too short to achieve a therapeutic effect in OME. Gates et al. have shown that in children with OME, efficacy at 6 months' follow-up was 60 % for knife myringotomy and 10–15 % following additional insertion of tympanostomy tubes [12]. With laser myringotomy of 2–2.5 mm, the mean closure time is up to 3 weeks. This will usually be sufficient in most cases of AOM, but not in all OME cases [34]. The use of an anti-fibroblast agent such as mitomycin C has been shown to be ineffective to maintain patency of perforations after laser myringotomy in children for a longer time [28]. Reports of laser myringotomy efficacy differ considerably between study groups. In order to prolong middle ear aeration, laser myringotomy can be combined with VT insertion. This was investigated by Koopmann, who reported efficacy of CO_2 laser myringotomy in OME without VT to be only 40 % compared to with VT of 78 %. Adenoidectomy performed in combination with laser myringotomy as well as older age had a significantly positive influence on the success rate, whereas a significantly negative effect was found in patients with one or more siblings, parental smoking, and a parents' history of otitis media. No significant effect was found for history of tube insertion, sex, ethnic origin, history of adenoidectomy or adenotonsillectomy, season, breast-feeding, cleft palate, and tonsillectomy performed as combined procedure [26]. Cotter et al. presented data following 3 months' follow-up; overall, laser myringotomy efficacy was 43 % with a success rate of 46 % in recurrent AOM and 37 % in OME. Average time to myringotomy closure was nearly 4 weeks, and treatment failure with reappearance of middle ear effusion occurred within 2–7 weeks after the procedure. For children who failed initially, they did not offer to repeat the procedure. They considered the ideal patient to be a child older than 3 years of age with prolonged unilateral middle ear effusion and no other significant nasal symptoms [25]. A high incidence of treatment failure for CO_2 laser myringotomy in allergic children (49 %) was reported by Prokopakis: the addition of adenoidectomy did not improve the outcome. In a multivariate analysis on the factors related to a poor outcome of CO_2 laser myringotomies, they found a positive correlation with a greater thickness of the eardrum, with a high viscosity of the middle ear effusion, but could not demonstrate any influence of the myringotomy size or the laser device parameters [24]. In contrast, laser tympanic membrane fenestration in conjunction with adenoidectomy was effective in restoring normal middle ear function at 90 days posttreatment in more than 80 % of children in a study of Cook [35]. Garin demonstrated that a 2 mm CO_2 laser tympanic membrane fenestration avoids the need for ventilation tube insertion in 63 % of children and 75 % of adults [36]. Compared with 168 ears operated by tympanostomy with tube insertion, Coma showed that laser tympanostomy produced similar rates of auditive recovery by one month and only 15 % of recurrence of OME by 6 months [20]. Sedlmaier reported treatment failure also in only 15 %; OME recurrence was proved to be significantly higher in ears with mucous secretion (26 %) than with serous secretion (13.5 %) [30]. Recurrences were also reported in 40 % of the adult OME patients by Cohen and by Marchant within 2 and 3 months, respectively [21, 37]. Prokopakis reported a resolution rate of 47 % in adult OME and 100 % in adult AOM [38]. Deutsch demonstrated that a larger tympanostomy size and longer duration of fenestration patency were associated with greater incidence of cure for both AOM and OME [39]. Lee et al. concluded that laser myringotomy as only treatment had no advantage over watchful waiting or spontaneous resolution of OME since recurrence within the first 2 months was nearly 40 %. In their ear-to-ear matched pair analysis of 60 children with bilateral OME, efficacy at 6-month posttreatment was only 46 % in laser myringotomy versus 75 % in combined laser myringotomy plus ventilation tube insertion. While combined procedure reoperation was significantly less required, the interval until reoperation was significantly prolonged, and the need for subsequent procedure under general anesthesia was reduced. Therefore, with laser myringotomy-assisted ventilation tube insertion under topical anesthesia, frequent laser myringotomy failure was overcome, though it was less feasible in young children [17].

In diode laser myringotomy, Zanetti observed an OME recurrence in 92 % within 1 month from perforation closure, whereas in the group with ventilation tubes, OME recurrence was observed in 23 % [27]. D'Eredità confirmed that postoperative audiometric and office evaluations showed resolution of OME in both patient groups, diode laser myringotomy and knife myringotomy with ventilation tubes at 6 months' follow-up [32].

Complication Rate of Laser Myringotomy

Surgical complications occur only to a minor extent, since in most cases the middle ear is filled with fluid according to the disease process and laser energy is highly absorbed, so damage of middle ear structures can be avoided. Inner ear damage according to noise exposure due to laser energy application was reported only for repetitive, high-energy laser pulses, which will usually not be necessary for myringotomy in a clinical setting [40]. Application of CO_2 laser energy is performed in "no touch" technique, but also the tactile feedback provided by contact techniques is safe for trained oto-surgeons.

In all, complication rate is low (2–3 %); most studies report apparent otorrhea, atrophic scar formation, or persistent perforation [17, 30]. Otorrhea normally responds to topical antibiotic eardrops. However, myringoplasty for closure of a persistent perforation is less frequently required than following insertion of ventilation tubes. In a temporal bone study, it was shown that in laser myringotomy, damage of cochlear structures, in particular the round window membrane, is most unlikely [41]. Therefore, laser myringotomy is technically straightforward and minimally time-consuming, causes little discomfort, and can be easily performed under topical anesthesia on outpatient basis.

Conclusion

Laser myringotomy is a surgical procedure which can be used alternatively for temporary transtympanic ventilation of the middle ear. The feasibility, safety, and acceptance of laser myringotomy have been well established in many studies.

The CO_2 laser is a versatile instrument, which can be connected to different optical delivery systems in order to create a sufficient perforation. Diode lasers show an advantage as they deliver energy through a thin fiber-optic cable. The short-term functional benefit of improved hearing is immediate and comparable to conventional knife myringotomy, but long-term results with regard to resolution of effusion in glue ears in children and adults seem to be intermediate between knife myringotomy and tympanostomy with ventilation tube insertion. Selected indications could comprise situations in which short-time ventilation is sufficient to relieve symptoms, such as purulent AOM and barotrauma. Since efficacy data for laser myringotomy in OME differ in literature, the procedure remains a good option for office-based ventilation of the middle ear for families and patients where general anesthesia is a concern.

References

1. Brusis T, Luckhaupt H. Perforation of the eardrum. On the history of paracentesis and grommet insertion. Laryngorhinootologie. 1996;75:178–83.
2. Cooper A. Observations on the effects which take place from the destruction of the Membrana tympani of the ear. Philos Trans R Soc. 1800;Part 1:151.
3. Schwartze H. Studien und Beobachtungen über die künstliche Perforation des Trommelfells. Archiv für Ohrenheilkunde. 1868
4. Politzer, A. Über ein Verfahren zum Offenhalten künstlicher Perforationsöffungen im Trommelfelle. Wiener Medizinische Wochenschrift. 1868
5. Armstrong BW. A new treatment for chronic secretory otitis media. Arch Otolaryngol. 1954;59:653–4.
6. Saito H, Miyamoto K, Kishimoto S, Higashitsuji H, Kitamura H. Burn perforation as a method of middle ear ventilation. Arch Otolaryngol. 1978;104:79–81.
7. Wilpizeski C, Maioriello RP, Reddy JB. Biological applications of lasers: basic background. Trans Pac Acad Ophthalmol Otolaryngol. 1977;30:185–92.
8. Goode RL. CO_2 Laser myringotomy. Laryngoscope. 1982;92:420–3.
9. American Academy of Family Physicians, American Academy of Otolaryngology-Head and Neck Surgery, American Academy of Pediatrics Subcommittee on Otitis Media With Effusion. Otitis media with effusion. Pediatrics. 2004;113:1412–29. Review.
10. Rovers MM, Schilder AG, Zielhuis GA, Rosenfeld RM. Otitis media. Lancet. 2004;363:465–73.
11. Vlastarakos TP, Nikolopoulos S, Korres E, Tavoulari A, Tzagaroulakis E, Ferekidis E. Grommets in otitis media with effusion: the most frequent operation in children. But is it associated with significant complications? Eur J Pediatr. 2007;166:385–91.
12. Gates GA, Avery CA, Prihoda TJ, Cooper JC. Effectiveness of adenoidectomy and tympanostomy tubes in the treatment of chronic otitis media with effusion. N Engl J Med. 1987;317:1444–51.
13. Brodsky L, Brookhauser P, Chait D, Reilly J, Deutsch E, Cook S, Waner M, Shaha S, Nauenberg E. Office-Based Insertion of Pressure Equalization Tubes: The Role of Laser-Assisted Tympanic Membrane Fenestration. Laryngoscope. 1999;109:2009–14.
14. Uzun C. Evaluation of pre-dive parameters related to Eustachian tube dysfunction for symptomatic middle ear barotraumas in divers. Otol Neurotol. 2005;26:59–64.
15. Commons KH, Blake DF, Brown LH. A prospective analysis of independent patient risk factors for middle ear barotrauma in a multiplace hyperbaric chamber. Diving Hyperb Med. 2013;43:143–7.
16. Bent JP, April MM, Ward RF, Packard AM. Role of otoscan-assisted laser myringotomy in hyperbaric oxygen therapy. Undersea Hyperb Med. 2000;27:159–61.
17. Lee CH, Lee JH, Kim HM. Flexible integration of laser myringotomy and ventilation tube for bilateral Otitis media with effusion: analysis of laser tympanostomy versus ventilation tube. PLoS One. 2014;23, e84966.
18. Blödow A. Laser myringotomy with erbium:YAG laser and CO_2 laser. Doctoral thesis: Free University Berlin; 2003.
19. Sedlmaier B, Blödow A, Jovanovic S, Schönfeld U, Nagli L, Eberle HG. IR lasers and application systems for myringotomy. Lasers Med Sci. 2000;15:162–8.
20. Silverstein H, Kuhn J, Choo D, Krespi YP, Rosenberg SI, Rowan PT. Laser-assisted tympanostomy. Laryngoscope. 1996;106:1067–74.
21. Cohen D, Siegel G, Krespi J, Schechter Y, Slatkine M. Middle ear laser office ventilation (LOV) with a CO_2 laser flashscanner. J Clin Laser Med Surg. 1998;16:107–9.
22. Coma I, Aragon J, Rodriguez AF. CO_2 laser tympanostomy without ventilation tubes. Acta Otorrinolaringol Esp. 1999;50:101–5.
23. Sedlmaier B, Jivanjee A, Gutzler R, Huscher D, Jovanovic S. Duration of middle ear ventilation after laser myringotomy with the CO_2 laser otoscope Otoscan. HNO. 2001;49:447–53.
24. Prokopakis EP, Hajiioannou JK, Velegrakis GA, Velegrakis GA, Christodoulou PN, Scordalakis C, Helidonis ES. The role of laser assisted tympanostomy (LAT) in treating allergic children with chronic serous otitis media. Int J Pediatr Otorhinolaryngol. 2002;62:207–14.
25. Cotter CS, Kosko JR. Effectiveness of laser-assisted myringotomy for otitis media in children. Laryngoscope. 2004;114:486–9.
26. Koopman JP, Reuchlin AGN, Kummer EE, Boumans LJJM, Rijntjes E, Hoeve LJ, Mulder PG, Blom HM. Laser myringotomy versus ventilation tubes in children with otitis media with effusion: a randomized trial. Laryngoscope. 2004;114:844–9.

27. Zanetti D, Piccioni M, Nassif N, Campovecchi C, Redaelli de Zinis LO. Diode laser myringotomy for chronic otitis media with effusion in adults. Otol Neurotol. 2005;26:12–8.
28. D'Eredità R. Contact diode laser myringotomy and mitomycin C in children Otolaryngol. Head Neck Surg. 2004;130:742–6.
29. Gates GA, Avery CA, Cooper JC, Prihoda TJ. Chronic secretory otitis media: effects of surgical management. Ann Otol Rhinol Laryngol Suppl. 1989;138:2–32.
30. Sedlmaier B, Jivanjee A, Gutzler R, Huscher D, Jovanovic S. Ventilation time of the middle ear in otitis media with effusion (OME) after CO_2 laser myringotomy. Laryngoscope. 2002;112:661–8.
31. Kuo YL, Wang MC, Chu CH, Shiao AS. Re-evaluation of CO_2 laser myringotomy for managing children with persistent acute otitis media. J Chin Med Assoc. 2011;74:413–8.
32. D'Eredità R, Shah UK. Contact diode laser myringotomy for medium-duration middle ear ventilation in children. Int J Pediatr Otorhinolaryngol. 2006;70:1077–80.
33. Sedlmaier B, Tägl P, Gutzler R, Schönfeld U, Jovanovic S. Experimental and clinical experiences with the Er:YAG laser otoscope. HNO. 2000;48:816–21.
34. Sedlmaier B, Jovanovic S. Treatment of acute otitis media with the CO_2 laser. HNO. 2000;48:557–60.
35. Cook SP, Brodsky L, Reilly JS, Deutsch E, Waner M, Brookhouser P, Pizzuto M, Poje C, Nagy M, Shaha SH, Chait D, Bower C. Effectiveness of adenoidectomy and laser tympanic membrane fenestration. Laryngoscope. 2001;111:251–4.
36. Garin P, Ledeghen S, Van Prooyen-Keyser S, Remacle M. Office-based CO_2 laser-assisted tympanic membrane fenestration addressing otitis media with effusion. J Clin Laser Med Surg. 2001;19:185–7.
37. Marchant H, Bisschop P. Value of laser CO_2 myringotomy in the treatment of seromucous otitis. Ann Otolaryngol Chir Cervicofac. 1998;115:347–51.
38. Prokopakis EP, Lachanas VA, Christodoulou PN, Bizakis JG, Karatzanis AD, Velegrakis GA. Implications of laser assisted tympanostomy in adults. Otol Neurotol. 2005;26:361–3.
39. Deutsch ES, Cook SP, Shaha S, Brodsky L, Reilly JS. Duration of patency of laser-assisted tympanic membrane fenestration. Arch Otolaryngol Head Neck Surg. 2003;129: 825–8.
40. Pfalz R, Nagel D, Bald N, Hibst R. Vergleiche von Bera-Schwellen und cochleären Mikrofonpotentialen (CM) vor und nach der Laserung im Mittelohr narkotisierter Meerschweinchen. Eur Arch Otorhinolaryngol. 1993 Suppl:36–37
41. Bonabi S, Sedlmaier B. The risk of damaging the round window by CO2 laser myringotomy. A morphological experimental analysis of 61 human petrous bone specimens. HNO. 2008;56:1135–41.

Chapter 7

Laser-Based Stapes Surgery

Justus Ilgner, Martin Wehner, Manfred Bovi, and Martin Westhofen

Introduction and Historical Background

Otosclerosis was first described by Antonio Valsalva in 1741 who reported a bone alteration of the stapes footplate around the oval window. In 1841 Joseph Toynbee discovered otosclerosis to be one of the possible causes of hearing loss, as he interpreted the cause of the condition by inflammatory alteration of the middle ear mucosa, periosteum, or ostitis of the promontory wall. In contrast, Adam Politzer realized that otosclerosis was a primary disease of the labyrinthine capsule. His findings were confirmed by his own histologic examinations which showed osteoblasts and osteoclasts, as well as giant cells in various sections of pathologic bone [1].

The incidence of otosclerosis ranges between 6.1 and 8.3 per 100,000 and year. On postmortem examinations on human temporal bones, 12.3 % of female and 6.5 % of male specimens showed signs of focal sclerosis around the stapes footplate. The cause of otosclerosis is not fully understood. There is evidence for gender-specific factors, influenced by estrogen and progesterone as the disease may progress during pregnancy. Consequently, the female-to-male ratio is about 2– 1 [1, 2]. Recently, viral infections have been focused as major contributors to the disease, namely measles and rubella. There are epidemiological indicators that measles seem to play a major role in generating the disease, although pathogenetic mechanisms are yet unclear [3].

First therapeutic trials were performed by Kessel in 1878, Bucheron in 1888, and Minot in 1890 by mobilizing the fixed stapes. However, this procedure was only of limited success, as refixation occurred soon after surgery. First experiments in fenestrating the promontory or the labyrinth were described in 1897 by Passow and by Bárány in 1911. Following the onset of microscopic surgery in the 1950s, Shea first described successful removal

Brian J.-F. Wong and Justus Ilgner (eds.), *Biomedical Optics in Otorhinolaryngology: Head and Neck Surgery*, DOI 10.1007/978-1-4939-1758-7_7, © Springer Science+Business Media New York 2016

of the whole stapes and its replacement by a polyethylene stamp placed on a piece of vein graft in 1956 [4]. Later, modifications by Schuknecht et al. described a handmade prosthesis with a piece of connective tissue knotted into a string of 0.2 mm stainless steel wire, which was placed in the oval window and attached to the long Incus process [5]. Later, Fisch suggested not to remove the whole of the footplate, but to remove its suprastructure and drill a hole in its center instead, which acts as a cylinder for a prefabricated alloplastic prosthesis [6, 7].

Sataloff was the first to describe the experimental use of a Nd:YAG laser in otosclerosis in humans, although due to poor absorption of laser energy in bone, his technique with his particular laser system was not pursued further [8]. Better results, leading to clinical feasibility for laser use, were obtained with an Argon laser by Palva in 1979 [9] and by Perkins in 1980 [10]. Since then a great variety of laser systems has been used for stapes surgery, both in clinical and experimental settings. Although none of the existing laser systems show ideal properties, the use of lasers in otosclerosis has advanced both safety and reliability of the procedure compared to nonlaser operations, making lasers an indispensable tool for the otosurgeon.

Preoperative Diagnosis and Evaluation of Outcome Following Surgery

Among many diagnostic procedures, the most universally used are pure tone audiometry (PTA) and reflexes of the stapedius muscle [11]. The latter provides a more or less "direct" indicator for the disease process, as the reflex arch between auditory nerve, brainstem, and stapedial nerve branching off the facial nerve shows a distinct pressure change in the outer ear canal due to the force exerted by the stapedius muscle on the stapes. As in otosclerosis, the stapes footplate is partially or totally fixed, the movement of the stapes footplate is altered or absent, which can be read from the shape or total absence of reflexes. In postoperative follow-up, however, the reflex cannot be elicited as the stapes footplate is either removed or disconnected from its suprastructure, where the stapedius muscle is attached.

Pure tone audiometry (Fig. 1) is a subjective diagnostic method to assess hearing in awake and cooperative persons. It is measured over a frequency range usually between 125 and 8000 Hz in discrete steps, while hearing loss is assessed in 5 dB steps relative to the hearing threshold of healthy young persons, whose hearing is averaged to a baseline of zero. Thus, it provides a relative result in sound pressure levels [dB SPL]. Hearing is assessed by the use of headphones, requiring a patent and intact outer ear canal, tympanic membrane, and ossicular chain, which is summarized under the term "air conduction" (AC). The same test is performed with

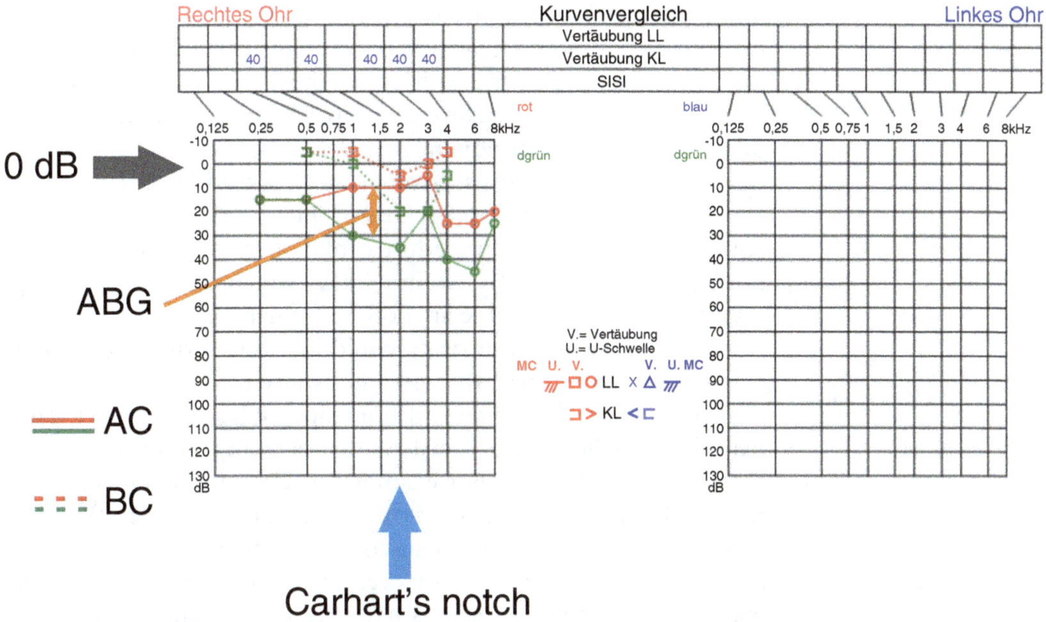

Fig. 1 Pure tone audiogram of the right ear preoperatively (*green lines*)—and postoperatively (*red lines*). X axis: scale of audible frequencies in octave steps. Y axis: logarithmic hearing level ranging from 0 to 130 dB. *Gray arrow*: Physiological hearing threshold in healthy humans, normalized to 0 dB. *Blue arrow*: Carhart's notch at 2 kHz, visible in bone conduction (*dotted line*) preoperatively, normalized postoperatively. *AC* Air conduction, *BC* Bone conduction, *ABG* Air-Bone-Gap

a vibrating sounder placed on the region of the mastoid behind the ear, thereby transmitting sound through the skull base to the inner ear, known as bone conduction (BC). As both stimuli are normalized to the physiological hearing threshold of healthy young adults, baseline is at 0 dB for both tests.

In pure tone audiometry, otosclerosis immobilizing the stapes footplate is characterized by a gap between the response curve from air conduction (AC), which is affected by the fixation of the stapes footplate and therefore the attenuation of sound being transferred by the ossicular chain, and bone conduction (BC), which is less affected by the disease process in early stages. This difference is known as the air-bone-gap. However, another distinct feature in audiometry for otosclerosis is known as Carhart's notch, which marks a loss in BC around 2 kHz, whereas higher and lower frequencies remain less attenuated. This is partially due to a loss in transmitting the resonance frequency of the air-filled middle ear, but mostly caused by the loss of compliance of the inner ear capsule inflicted by the sclerotic process. If, however, the inner ear is severely affected, bone conduction loss can progress to an extent that Carhart's notch becomes indistinguishable.

Outcome in stapes surgery is equally assessed by a variety of parameters, most of which rely on pure tone audiometry as well.

Generally, the closure of the aforementioned air-bone-gap resembles the restored sound transmission over the ossicular chain. As middle ear resonance is also transmitted to the inner ear and inner ear compliance is restored against the stapes footplate, Carhart's notch disappears, as bone conduction at 2 kHz is restored as well—an effect which is known as "overclosure." In addition, unwanted effects such as sensory hearing loss of the inner ear hair cells in the course of the operative procedure can be seen by a deterioration of bone conduction, mostly around 4 kHz which is supposed to represent the most vulnerable area of the human inner ear.

However, when comparing clinical trials in terms of outcome, it has to be mentioned that a wide variety in describing hearing results makes it challenging, if not impossible, to interpret study data. This applies to beneficial results following surgery as well as unwanted hearing loss. For example, in US states data from pure tone audiograms are averaged over frequencies between 0.5, 1, 2 and 3 kHz, while in European countries, octave steps 0.5, 1, 2, and 4 kHz are preferred. However, apart from this one example, many more parameter settings have been used, which is why recommendations from the American Academy of Otolaryngology have been issued to overcome this inconsistency in the future for the US. As for now, hearing outcomes may only be compared under defined circumstances and doing so requires a certain amount of critical judgment.

Operative Procedure, Instrumentation, and Laser Application Techniques

During surgery, the outer ear canal is visualized, as the eardrum is folded anteriorly. Thus the middle ear with the ossicles is exposed (Fig. 2a). The chorda tympani, which carries sensory taste fibers for the tongue, is mobilized, and the rear wall of the outer ear canal near the eardrum, the so-called scutum, is dissected back until the stapes footplate is fully visible. Next the stapes footplate is perforated with the laser or, in more traditional fashion, mechanically with a microdissector instrument to a size of about 0.5–0.8 mm, which can accommodate the prosthesis piston with a diameter of 0.4 mm comfortably (Fig. 2b). Then the stapes suprastructure is detached from the long incus process, the stapedius tendon cut, and the suprastructure removed. A prosthesis is then introduced into the middle ear, its piston gently advanced through the perforation hole and its shaft fixed to the long incus process, either by crimping (Fig. 2c), clipping or laser fixation of a shape-memory NiTiNOL-prosthesis, which is described in another chapter of this book. Then the perforation site at the footplate and the fixation point on the long incus process is covered with little bits of connective tissue in order to facilitate firm attachment by connective tissue incorporation and to seal the inner ear, respectively [12].

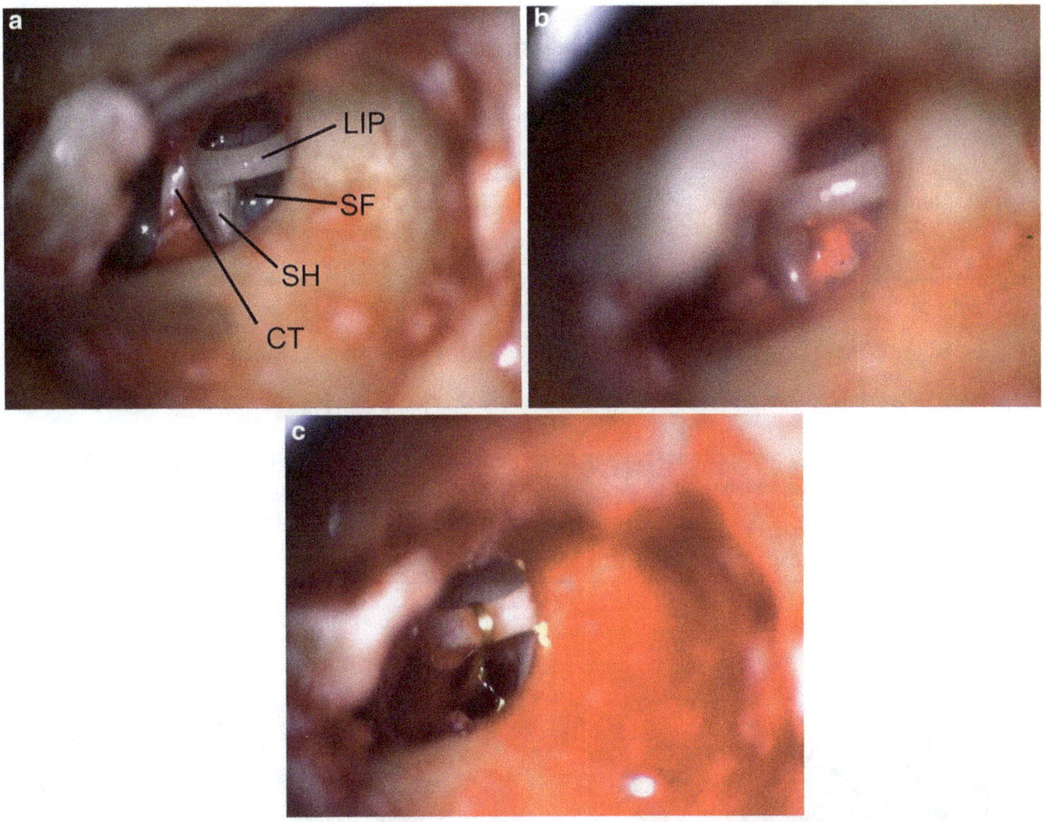

Fig. 2 (**a**) Intraoperative view of the tympanic cavity, *left ear*: the tympanic membrane is flipped to the *left*. *CT* chorda tympani, *SH* stapes head with musculus stapedius tendon, *SF* stapes footplate, *LIP* long incus process. (**b**) The same view as in (**a**), He:Ne aiming beam of an Er:YAG laser directed by a micromanipulator on the stapes footplate. (**c**) The same view as in (**a**) and (**b**), with a stapes prosthesis in situ, crimped over the long incus process

There have been many variations of this procedure, from total footplate removal to partial removal only of fixed sclerotic areas, even to the extent of leaving the suprastructure partially intact, thereby avoiding the need for prosthesis.

The use of lasers requires application techniques that are compatible to microsurgical manipulation of the stapes footplate [13], i.e., an operative field with the dimension of about 1.5 in 3 mm. Therefore, laser systems both within the range of visible light and in mid and far infrared have seen widespread use in stapes surgery. Generally, it can be said that Argon and KTP laser systems soon became popular due to their energy transmission by silica fibers of 0.2 mm diameter or less. By the use of thin laser fibers, handheld instruments of dimensions compatible with microsurgery allow direct application of laser energy to the stapes footplate over a short distance. Surgeons advocating the use of handheld instruments see the following advantages outweighing the disadvantages (Table 1, Fig. 3):

Table 1
Pro and con arguments for the use of handheld instruments concerning laser application via silica glass fibers

Pro	Con
Direct visibility of the laser beam	Obstruction of the operative field by the applicator instrument
No misalignment issues between aiming and laser beam	Manual guiding of the laser beam prone to human-related imprecisions
No direct line of sight necessary	Time consuming footplate perforation by a multitude of shots—the so-called "rosette technique" (Fig. 3)
Free angulation of the application instrument, e.g., for removal of stapes suprastructure	Imprecision in directing the laser beam can lead to unwanted irradiation of the labyrinth
Rapid defocusing of the laser beam beyond the fiber tip, therefore less damage to inner ear structures	

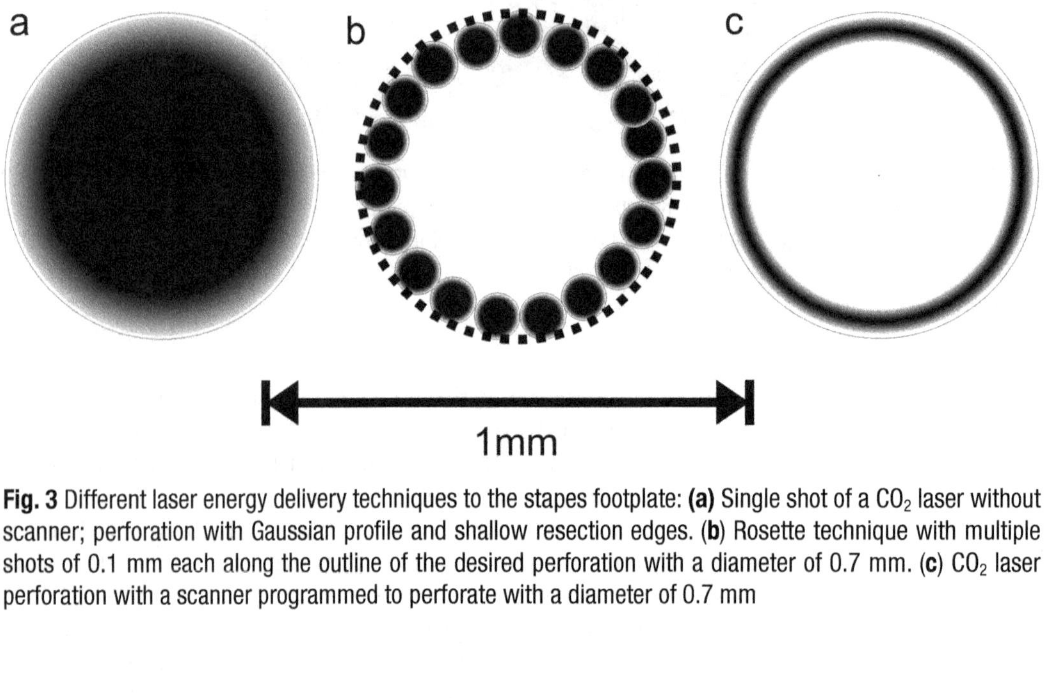

Fig. 3 Different laser energy delivery techniques to the stapes footplate: **(a)** Single shot of a CO_2 laser without scanner; perforation with Gaussian profile and shallow resection edges. (**b**) Rosette technique with multiple shots of 0.1 mm each along the outline of the desired perforation with a diameter of 0.7 mm. (**c**) CO_2 laser perforation with a scanner programmed to perforate with a diameter of 0.7 mm

Alternatively, the use of collimated and highly focused laser beam allows the transmission of laser energy over a long distance—in this case about 250–300 mm from the front lens—in free air. Therefore, micromanipulators as add-on to the operating microscope have proven useful for any kind of laser system, although they are mostly used for systems emitting in mid and far infrared,

Table 2
Pro and con arguments for the use of laser application by use of a micromanipulator

Pro	Con
Works with any type of laser system, from UV over visible light range to far infrared	Laser use only in direct line of sight. Structures occluded from view cannot be targeted
Limited expense and setup time before surgery, as an operating microscope is used anyway	Laser beam remains focused beyond the plane of the footplate, possible hazards to inner ear structures, particularly for wavelengths poorly absorbed by peri- and endolymph
The operative field is not obstructed by the laser applicator	Possible misalignment between aiming beam and surgical laser beam
Use of a laser beam scanner, allowing rapid and precise perforation of the stapes footplate (Fig. 3)	Complex mechanics of micromanipulators in comparison to handheld applicators
	Artifacts in the microscopic image by mirror coating and micromanipulator frame

whose laser beam cannot be transmitted through silica glass fibers. Pro and Con arguments for the use of micromanipulators are listed in Table 2 (see also Fig. 3).

In addition, recent advances in waveguide design have made CO_2 laser energy transmission via small diameter hollow waveguides possible. Although first trials in stapes surgery have been published, their specific benefit in this context remains to be seen.

Literature Data for Different Laser Systems Used in Stapes Surgery

Argon and KTP Laser

These two laser systems are probably the most intensively studied—in postmortem temporal bones, animal models, as well as in everyday clinical use [14–65]. Both systems display very similar properties, as it seems fair to discuss both lasers under one subheading [65]. The Argon laser has two main wavelength peaks at $\lambda = 488$ and 514 nm, while the KTP laser emits at $\lambda = 532$ nm, thus both systems produce visible green light. Laser energy is therefore well absorbed by hemoglobin, although in stapes surgery bleeding has to be strictly avoided in order to keep a clear view of the operative field. However, at this wavelength laser energy is very little absorbed by inner ear fluids, i.e., perilymph and endolymph, as these fluids are mostly clear. Laser systems operate either in continuous wave (cw) or Q-switched mode, thus phases of energy delivery are defined as "on" and "off" intervals. As it has been pointed out before, laser energy is mostly transmitted via a silica glass fiber of 50–200 μm in diameter.

Usually the stapes suprastructure is vaporized with 1.5–2 W output power at an "on" time of 0.1–0.2 s in several intervals. For the stapes footplate, the laser output power is usually reduced to 1–1.5 W, with laser "on" time of 0.1–0.2 s. The surgeon applies as many shots as needed to create a stapedotomy perforation of 0.6–0.8 mm, which accommodates a stapes piston of 0.4 mm in diameter in a way it can move freely in the stapes perforation. Modifications of the surgical technique such as preservation of the stapedius tendon [14] or partial removal of the anterior crus and the anterior third of the footplate [44] did not yield different outcomes.

Earlier studies of Vollrath and coworkers [60–62] looked at the preservation of cochlear microphonics as a functional parameter in animal experiments. They found that cochlear microphonics would be temporarily diminished following laser "on" times of 0.1 and 0.2 s, whereas at 0.5 s they would disappear. In case of perilymph leakage, cochlear microphonics would be diminished after 15 min and would recover incompletely after two hours.

In 1989, experiments on a cochlear model performed by Lesinski and coworkers [29] rendered data of temperature rise following KTP laser irradiation of 4.3–6.3 °C after one and two shots, while Argon laser would lead to an alarming temperature rise of 22.5 °C from a 0.6 mm spot up to 175 °C from a 0.05 mm spot size. Reducing the laser spot size in KTP laser, a 0.5 mm spot would lead to a temperature rise of 21 °C and a 0.05 mm spot size of 52 °C, respectively. Bartels and Gherini [15, 21] criticized these experiments for flaws in methodology, arguing that a large black thermocouple was used 2 mm behind the footplate model in clear fluids, which does not resemble the actual anatomical situation in the human vestibule. In contrast, Häusler found a temperature rise following Argon laser stapedotomy of 1.0 °C after 10 shots and 2.5 °C after 38 shots [22]. Similar data were found by Szymanski, who recorded a temperature rise of 0.2–2.47 °C, with a maximum of 2.6 °C [51]. While the temperature rise on the stapes footplate surface exceeds 100 °C [62, 64], the amount of perilymph and the surrounding temporal bone seem to act as a heat sink, which is probably why clinical results differ from experimental results mentioned before. The advantage of using a hand piece, as proposed by Causse, Garin, and Hodgson [17, 19, 24], is that the laser beam rapidly defocuses after leaving the laser fiber tip, thereby protecting the perilymph from heat spots. Nonetheless, various authors mention that using the rosette technique, only nonperforated areas should be irradiated and direct irradiation of the perilymph should be avoided [16]. However, the facial nerve canal running adjacent to the stapes footplate should be protected as well, as its temperature may equally rise between 1.4 and 15.2 °C [35], which in another study resulted in two cases of delayed facial paresis, but resolved without surgical intervention [36]. On the positive side, however, KTP and Argon lasers displayed the lowest value of pressure transients delivered to the human cochlea in clinical use, ranging between 49 and 81 dB(A) [27, 34, 42]. Consequently, there is no compelling evidence of cochlear damage following noise trauma from an argon or KTP laser while used within safe parameters.

Carbon Dioxide (CO_2) Laser

The carbon dioxide laser operates at a wavelength of $\lambda = 10{,}600$ nm, which therefore requires laser energy delivery via micromanipulator attached to the front lens of an operating microscope. Only recently, hollow waveguides for CO_2 lasers have become available in a way that their use in otologic surgery seems practicable [66]. However, it has been noted that the transmission loss of the waveguide in otosurgery is considerable, being about 66 % [59]. In any case, the CO_2 laser has been the workhorse of many otolaryngology departments worldwide, mainly in tumor surgery of the pharyngeal levels and the larynx. Thus it is hardly surprising that this laser system is available in many departments and there is an extensive body of literature on its use for stapes surgery, given the fact that laser parameters have been adapted to otologic purposes from many animal experiments and clinical data [16, 18, 26, 27, 29, 31, 34, 55, 56, 58, 59, 64, 66–96].

In the early days of CO_2 laser surgery, a single spot with varying diameter (180–500 μm) was used to produce a stapes footplate perforation in one or more shots, either in rosette technique or as a single shot, which in some cases needed widening with mechanical instruments. Extensive animal experiments performed by the workgroup of Jovanovic [26, 77–83] could show that detrimental effects on the inner ear, measured by compound action potentials (CAPs) of the auditory nerve, were avoidable. CAPs were diminished under 15 W cw laser energy for 100 and 200 ms, while animals exposed for 500 ms turned out deaf. With lower pulse durations and lower power settings, compound action potentials remained unchanged from normal.

Concerning temperature elevation, readings at 2 mm behind the stapes footplate were 8.8 °C for up to 100 ms at 4–18 W of power, while after accumulation of 10 pulses in a row, temperature could rise up to 23.8 °C at the same distance behind the stapes footplate [26, 81]. Recently, Just and coworkers set up an in vitro experiment in which they recorded temperature changes in a capillary tube under thermography, while irradiating the stapes footplate with a CO_2 laser in line with the capillary. As a result, they recorded a temperature rise of 32 K at 2 mm distance and 21 K at 3 mm distance while directly irradiating the model perilymph space [84]. However, in clinical settings, temperature rise does not seem to be as dramatic, as other workgroups found a maximum of 4.4 °C, 5.2–6.3 °C and 0.5 °C, respectively [29, 71, 89]. Gardner noted that temperature rise was up to 1 °C before opening the footplate and +12– 19 °C when directly irradiating the perilymph at two pulses per second with 0.05 s pulse duration each at 2– 4 W power and 450 μm spot size [75].

As for pressure changes induced by laser irradiation, the group of Michaelides [34] found pressure transients of 71 dB at 35 ms and a peak pressure of 89 dB over 50 μs. Kamalski [27] noted pressure of 68 dB(A) in 1 cm distance under the stapes footplate in an in vitro model, while Gardner noted no harmful acoustic effects 2 mm distant to the stapes footplate if the CO_2 laser power was 6 W cw or less. If the laser power exceeded 6 W, sound pressure transients could rise up to 92 or 106 dB.

In order to reduce the temperature rise by heat deposition to the perilymph, some authors suggest the use of superpulse mode, which is frequently used in laser surgery for the larynx and pharyngeal spaces, in order to increase the nonlaser intervals between laser pulses—thus allowing the irradiated tissue to cool down. However, in superpulse mode each pulse carries a power of up to 320 W, resulting in less perilymph heating but increased pressure deposition, [18, 74] which is why superpulse mode is generally not recommended for stapes surgery.

Recent developments employ a scanner to precisely produce a stapes perforation with sharply delineated margins. These CO_2 laser systems operate at continuous wave mode; power settings are usually 20 W for duration of about 0.05 s, which do not result in any harmful effects on the inner ear. Furthermore, the surgeon only has to set the desired perforation size, thereby avoiding the need for calculating power settings and on time duration [92, 95].

Erbium:YAG Laser

Since the mid-1990s, the Er:YAG laser became clinically available for otologic procedures. The Er:YAG laser emits at $\lambda = 2940$ nm, which is in the mid-infrared range and hits a distinct peak of absorption in water. In addition, the pulse generating characteristics of this laser are such that a sharp rise in pulse energy occurs during the first milliseconds after triggering. Pulse duration is quoted at 78 ms throughout the literature, although variations are possible [23, 50, 74, 81, 82, 92, 97–109]. Given the energy delivery over a very short time, the Er:YAG laser shows effects of nonlinear ablation, resulting in very little heating of tissue while effectively ablating bone. However, as its efficacy is best achieved on a moist surface, the stapes footplate must be kept moist at all times. Consequently, heat deposition to the perilymph is not reported as being critical with this laser system. On the contrary, pressure transients are indeed an issue, as the laser produces and audible "snap" with each pulse. While Lippert and coworkers used a fluence of 0.1–10 J/cm^2 operating the laser with favorable result [104], e.g., an ABG closure of an average of 8.1 dB, the workgroup of Häusler et al. noted pressure transients of 140– 160 dB calculated in vivo [23], which was confirmed by Gardner and coworkers estimating pressure transients of 167 dB in vitro and

110 dB in vivo [74]. Häusler and coworkers confirmed their theoretical results by sending stapedotomy patients for pure tone audiometry after 2 h and 6 h following surgery. They noted a 75 dB sensory hearing loss 2 h postoperatively in the mid- and high-frequency range, which recovered after 6 h. However, it has to be mentioned that in clinical practice pure tone audiometry is rarely performed at this early stage, while some surgeons even recommend bed rest for the patient during the first 24 h following surgery. Thus it is likely that with other laser systems and conventional surgery, a significant drop in bone conduction might be noticeable 2 h postoperatively, too. Keck and coworkers reported postoperative adverse effects over a longer period [101–103] and saw protracted cases of sensory hearing loss in 7 % of patients up to 4 kHz and in 3 % up to 3 kHz, respectively. Three of 117 patients complained of persistent tinnitus. To avoid inner ear complications, the administration of steroids intravenously 30 min before starting the operation is common practice in stapes surgery, although its evidence is still under debate [109].

In the author's institution, pulse energy was generally kept at 10–15 mJ, as under these parameters, persistent bone conduction loss or tinnitus was not seen. However, it has to be mentioned that the use of Erbium:YAG laser in stapes surgery depended particularly on one model, the Zeiss ORL E (Zeiss Meditec, Oberkochen, Germany), which consisted of an operating microscope equipped with an add-on laser that was specifically built for this purpose but mostly unsuitable for other procedures. As this model would only fulfill one task, it was discontinued from production around 2003; thus, long-term data or newer results are largely unavailable.

Other Laser Systems

Other laser systems than the aforementioned have mostly been used under conditions limited to laboratory experiments, animal models, or small series of patients. Of note is the use of diode lasers operating in between $\lambda = 808$ and 980 nm, thus in the near infrared range [2, 110–113]. In this range, absorption of laser energy and water is low, which is why this laser system, similar to the Nd:YAG laser, may not be the ideal choice for stapes surgery [112]. Instead, this laser has been used for other procedures in the middle ear, e.g., soldering of tissues [110] or cholesteatoma removal. Seven studies presented the Ho:YAG laser emitting at $\lambda = 2100$ nm [80–82, 97, 106, 114, 115], whose bone-ablating properties are well known, though this occurs with marked thermal side effects including extensive carbonization of bony margins. Although the wavelength can be propagated through glass fibers, it is probably due to the ablation characteristics, why this laser system was never used in ear surgery to a greater extent. The use of the Th:YAG laser was only mentioned in one study [27], while five further investigations presented the Er:YSSG laser in comparison with other laser systems. In conclusion, the Er:YSSG laser seems to be an interesting alternative for the Er:YAG laser as its laser–tissue interaction characteristic seemed to be less "aggressive," although also less effective on the stapes footplate [80–82, 108, 114]. The excimer laser emits in the ultraviolet range and has been investigated in four studies although its use is not recommended in mucosal tissues or the outer skin, as there is generally said to be a risk of malignant transformation of epithelial tissue by high energy UV light deposition [81, 82, 97, 106].

Finally, a new promising development is the introduction of femtosecond lasers, usually operating in the near infrared at $\lambda = 780$ or 1053 nm [97, 106, 116–118]. As laser pulses are of extremely short duration, nonlinear oblation occurs, resulting in very little thermal effects. At the same time, the extremely short duration of pulses makes pressured transients that could be harmful to the inner ear equally unlikely, thereby providing an ideal solution for the use in otology. Femtosecond lasers have demonstrated to be effective in ophthalmology, dentistry [116], and other applications on the human skin [106]. Current drawbacks are the limited number of systems available, entailing considerable costs in setting up and maintaining the laser system and the limited ablation speed resulting in long operating times. Currently, such systems are under investigation in experimental settings only, but might be entering clinical practice with the availability of smaller units with better ablation speed and lower costs.

Own Experience

To overcome the dilemma between thermal load to the inner ear and pressure transients inflicted by laser use, we investigated the ablation properties of pulsed laser systems working in the nanosecond to femtosecond range. The rationale was that extremely short-pulsed lasers would cause little heating of the perilymph due to extremely short "on" time duration, while at the same time pressure transients would be too short as to cause damage to inner ear and vestibular hair cells. In the first experiment, a nanosecond-pulsed, frequency-tripled Nd:YAG laser (Lambda Physik "Starline", Göttingen, Germany) operating at a wavelength of $\lambda = 355$ nm, pulse duration 10 ns FWHM, repetition rate 2 kHz, pulse energy 0.125 mJ, and output power 250 mW, was used to evaluate single spot ablation craters in human mallei harvested from postmortem individuals and fixed in 3.5 % formaldehyde solution. Exposure time for each spot was 0.5 s and the fluence neared 320 J/cm^2. With a beam diameter of 10 μm, crater width following 0.5 s exposure time showed about the same width as the laser beam, yet with a thermal damage zone of less than 10 μm adjacent to the crater edge (Fig. 4). As the exposure time was increased in a stepwise fashion up to 10 s, the crater width increased to 30 and 60 μm, as

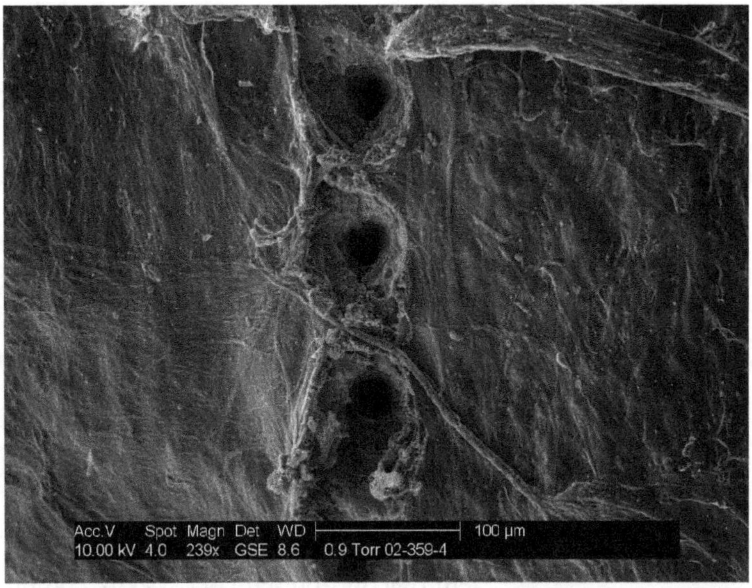

Fig. 4 Single laser spot series using a nanosecond-pulsed, frequency-tripled Nd:YAG laser at $\lambda = 355$ nm, pulse duration 10 ns FWHM, repetition rate 2 kHz, pulse energy 0.125 mJ, output power 250 mW, exposure time 0.5 s each. Note the intact connective tissue fiber between two spots

did the carbonization margin to a maximum width of 30 μm. At 10 s exposure time, however, the laser beam had cut through the long malleus process of 800 μm in diameter. The experiment showed that the results were not free of thermal side effects, however, no precautions in terms of cooling had been taken, which would have reduced the thermal damage zone considerably.

For the second experiment, a similar laser system was used, although with fourfold pulse duration of 40 ns, repetition rate of 10 kHz, and higher output power (model 210S-355-5000, ILX Lightwave, Bozeman, MT, USA). This system was coupled to a scanner and set to ablate bone material from a human malleus surface in areas of 1×1 mm^2 each within 8 s per 28 courses over the whole area. Laser parameters were a frequency-tripled Nd:YAG laser emitting at $\lambda = 355$ nm, pulse duration 40 ns FWHM, repetition rate 10 kHz, pulse energy 0.15 mJ, output power 1.5 W, fluence 95.4 J/cm^2, beam diameter 20 μm, and scan velocity 500 mm/s. This setup, as well as the laser system mentioned first in this section, emitted in TEM_{00} mode ($M^2 < 1.2$) with Gaussian intensity distribution. Under these parameters, we could observe some carbonization effects at the bottom of the ablation crater. There was also a debris zone of less than 100 μm width adjacent to the crater although this zone was not consistently present over all margins. Beyond the debris zone, there was no indication of further thermal damage, e.g., protein denaturation. As in this third experiment, the output power of the system was reduced to one-fifth of the aforementioned setting, the resection edges were delineated with sharp edges and no debris zone at all, although resection depth would be limited as expected and the crater floor showed an uneven surface. Again, no cooling was applied to the specimen during the experiment.

In a variant to the first and second experiment, we then applied 0.9 % saline solution to the malleus handle before applying laser energy under the same parameters as in the second experiment, while scan time was extended to 20 s. This resulted in no visible sign of thermal damage, although a layer of connective tissue detached and rolled back from the surface of the malleus handle over a distance of 50 μm from the resection edge. Most notably though was the fact that the scan time resulted in a full thickness cut of the malleus handle without any indication of mechanical or thermal stress, showing open Haversian (nutritional) ducts within the bone (Fig. 5).

For the fifth and sixth experiment, we then switched to a femtosecond-pulsed laser system, comprising a CrLiSAF oscillator with Colquerite amplifier, whose wavelength was set at $\lambda = 850$ nm with a bandwidth of ±26 nm FWHM. The laser spot size was 36 μm, pulse duration 100 fs at a repetition rate of 1 kHz, and a pulse energy of 40 μJ. The laser system was coupled to a scanner, ablating bone in parallel tracks with a distance of 10 μm over an area of 400×400 μm at a scan velocity of 2 mm/s. One course over the full area required a time of 40 s, while ablation depth was about 40

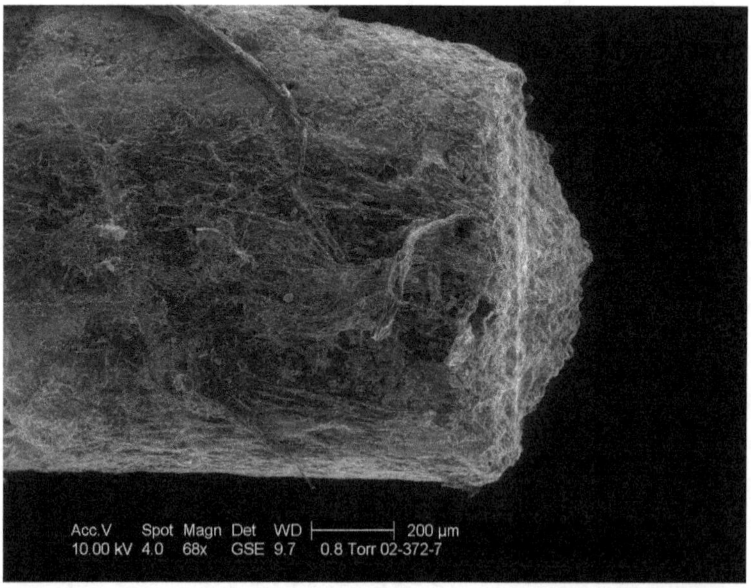

Fig. 5 Ablation of the long incus process using a nanosecond-pulsed, frequency-tripled Nd:YAG laser at $\lambda = 355$ nm, pulse duration 40 ns FWHM, repetition rate 10 kHz, pulse energy 0.15 mJ, output power 1.5 W, fluence 95.4 J/cm^2, beam diameter 20 μm, scan velocity 500 mm/s, scan time 8 s

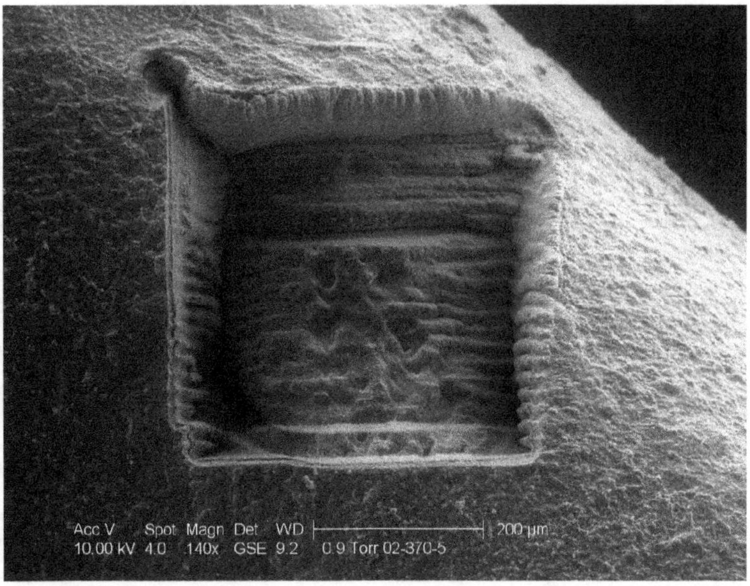

Fig. 6 Ablation zone of the long incus process, laser system as in Fig. 5, but with pulse energy 0.016 mJ, output power 0.16 W, fluence 10.2 J/cm^2, beam diameter 20 μm, scan velocity 200 mm/s, scan time 20 s. No debris on the ablation zone edges

μm per scan. The shallow excavation of one course is shown in Fig. 6 with little debris on the upper and right side edge, but sharp resection margins. Following three scanning courses with the same parameters, the debris zone was more prominent (Fig. 7) and visible on all edges, although the amount of debris is still less than expected with regard to the ablation depth. Moreover, when performing 10 courses in one area (not shown), the debris zone does not increase, suggesting that nonlinear ablation plays a relatively greater role in this setup compared to thermally ablating lasers, in which a linear increase of the amount of debris would be expected. Again, the last two ablation experiments were performed without cooling the specimen.

Finally, we investigated the ablation properties of a commercially available Er:YAG laser designed for otologic procedures, which is incorporated in an operating microscope (Zeiss Opmi ORL E, Zeiss Meditec, Oberkochen, Germany). The system operates at a wavelength of $\lambda = 2940$ nm with spot size 380 μm at a fixed focal length of 300 mm. Pulse duration varies between 50 and 500 μs, depending on pulse energy which can be set between 10 μJ and 100 μJ. As expected with the large spot size, ablation of bone resulted in very shallow craters, although with the oligothermic ablation characteristics under cooling with 0.9 % saline solution, no debris could be seen on the stapes footplate (Fig. 8). Single pulses of 10 and 25 mJ could not perforate the footplate alone, thus a rosette technique of 49 pulses with 15 μJ each was

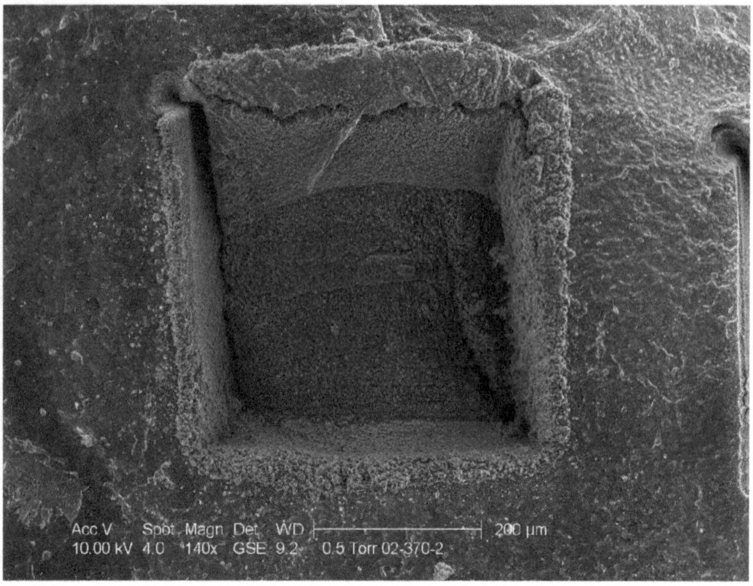

Fig. 7 Ablation zone of the long incus process, laser system as in Fig. 6, but with pulse energy 0.08 mJ, output power 0.8 W, fluence 51 J/cm^2, beam diameter 20 µm, scan velocity 200 mm/s, scan time 20 s. Marked debris on the ablation zone edges, about 100 µm wide

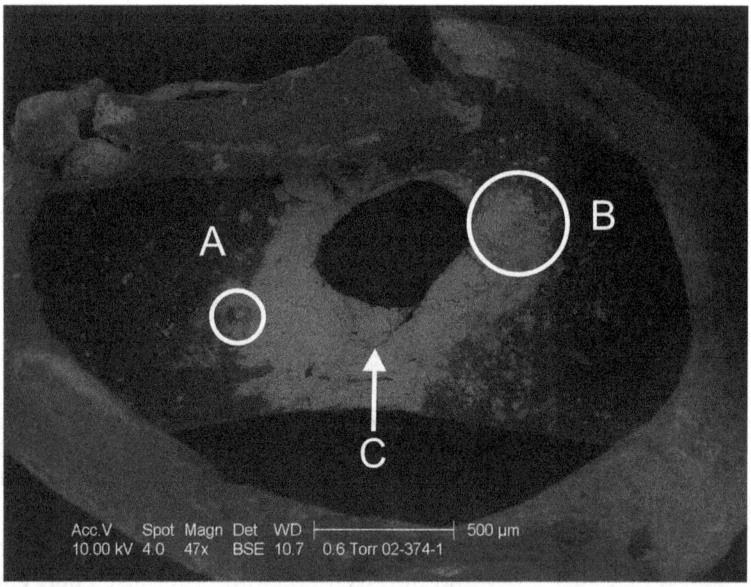

Fig. 8 Ablation on the stapes footplate by Er:YAG laser pulses of 10 mJ (A), 25 mJ (B) and a series of 49 pulses of 15 mJ each required to produce a perforation of 400 µm width in diameter (C)

required to create a perforation large enough to accommodate a stapes prosthesis piston 400 μm wide with a comfortable margin. Yet it can be seen that the zone of bone denaturation or thinning zone is somewhat larger than the actual perforation, bearing a risk of transverse stapes footplate fracture exactly halfway.

Conclusion

Given the extensive body of literature rendering a considerable amount of worldwide experience with laser use in stapes surgery, it seems fair to say that laser-assisted stapedotomy is one application in which lasers seem indispensible as they have advanced surgery for the benefit of the patient. Multiple studies confirm better outcomes for hearing in terms of air-bone-gap reduction than mechanical perforation of the footplate, particularly in revision surgery, whilst the risk of inner ear hearing loss or vestibular function loss is manageable [119, 120]. After initial concerns about damage inflicted by laser use next to the inner ear, facial nerve, and vestibular organ, there is a set of safe parameters known for every laser system applicable in this field, which, if observed and adhered to, leads to replicable and beneficial results. Moreover, meta-analysis shows that the hearing results in hearing are largely independent of the laser system used. Kamalski mentioned that there is only one study according to which a slight but significant better outcome has been achieved with the use of CO_2 laser in comparison to other laser systems [121]. However, other studies showed no significant differences in outcome depending on which laser system has been used. Thus, it is justified to say that, while none of the current laser systems displays ideal properties for middle and inner ear use, those which have been widely studied (CO_2, Argon, Er:YAG, KTP) are safe to use as long as parameter settings that have been tested and proven to be safe for a specified laser system are observed.

As for the future, challenging new developments are on the horizon, as ultrashort pulsed laser systems are able to dissect bone in a nonthermal way by photodisruption creating little pressure side effects and debris. Main obstacles to overcome are system size, usability for the surgeon, cost, and ablation speed. However, as femtosecond lasers are already an everyday tool in ophthalmology, clinical progress may help to foster their spread in otology as well.

Acknowledgements

Histological examination and electron microscopy were performed by the Institute of Pathology, RWTH Aachen University, Director: Univ.-Prof. Dr. med. R. Knüchel-Clarke

References

1. Helms J, Hoppe F. Otosklerose. In: Naumann HH, Helms J, Herberhold C, Kastenbauer E, editors. Otorhinolaryngologie in Klinik und Praxis, Band 1: Ohr. Stuttgart, New York: Georg Thieme; 1994. p. 726–41.
2. Poe DS. Laser-assisted endoscopic stapedectomy: a prospective study. Laryngoscope. 2000;110:1–37.
3. Richard C, Doherty JK, Fayad JN, Cordero A, Linthicum Jr FH. Identification of target proteins involved in cochlear otosclerosis. Otol Neurotol. 2015;36:923–31.
4. Shea Jr J. Fenestration of the oval window. Ann Otol Rhinol Laryngol. 1958;67:932–51.
5. Schuknecht HF, Oleksiuk S. The metal prosthesis for stapes ankylosis. Arch Otolaryngol. 1960;71:287–95.
6. Fisch U. Stapedotomy versus stapedectomy. Otol Neurotol. 2009;30:1160–5.
7. Fisch U. Stapedotomy versus stapedectomy (comment). Otol Neurotol. 2009;30:1166–7.
8. Sataloff J. Experimental use of laser in otosclerotic stapes. Arch Otolaryngol. 1967;86: 21–2.
9. Palva T. Argon laser in otosclerosis surgery. Acta Otolaryngol. 1979;104:153–7.
10. Perkins RC. Laser stapedotomy for otosclerosis. Laryngoscope. 1980;90:228–40.
11. Lehnhardt H. Praxis der Audiometrie. 7th ed. Stuttgart, New York: Georg Thieme; 1996.
12. Perkins R, Curto FS. Laser stapedotomy: a comparative study of prostheses and seals. Laryngoscope. 1992;102:1321–7.
13. Goldenberg RA, Brown M, Cunningham S. Laser stapedotomy. AORN J. 1992;55: 759–72.
14. Arnold A, Blaser B, Häusler R. Audiological long-term results following stapedotomy with stapedial tendon preservation. Adv Otorhinolaryngol. 2007;65:210–4.
15. Bartels LJ. KTP laser stapedotomy: is it safe? Otolaryngol Head Neck Surg. 1990;103: 685–92.
16. Buchman CA, Fucci MJ, Roberson JB, De La Cruz A. Comparison of Argon and CO_2 laser stapedotomy in primary otosclerosis surgery. Am J Otolaryngol. 2000;21:227–30.
17. Causse JB, Gherini S, Horn KL. Surgical treatment of stapes fixation by fiberoptic Argon laser stapedotomy with reconstruction of the annular ligament. Otolaryngol Clin North Am. 1993;26:395–415.
18. Garin P, van Prooyen-Keyser S, Jamart J. Hearing outcome following laser-assisted stapes surgery. J Otolaryngol. 2002;31:31–4.
19. Gherini S, Horn KL. Comment on: Small fenestra stapedotomies with and without KTP laser (Silverstein). Laryngoscope. 1990;100: 209–11.
20. Gherini SG, Horn KL, Bowman CA, Griffin G. Small fenestra stapedotomy using a fiberoptic hand-held Argon laser in obliterative otosclerosis. Laryngoscope. 1990;100:1276–82.
21. Gherini SG, Horn KL, Causse JB, McArthur GR. Fiberoptic Argon laser stapedotomy: is it safe? Am J Otol. 1993;14:283–9.
22. Häusler R, Messerli A, Romano V, Burkhalter R, Weber HP, Altermatt HJ. Experimental and clinical results of fiberoptic Argon laser stapedotomy. Eur Arch Otorhinolaryngol. 1996;253:193–200.
23. Häusler R, Schär PJ, Pratisto H, Weber HP, Frenz M. Advantages and dangers of Erbium laser application in stapedotomy. Acta Otolaryngol. 1999;119:207–13.
24. Hodgson RS, Wilson DF. Argon laser stapedotomy. Laryngoscope. 1991;101:230–3.
25. Horn KL, Gherini S, Griffin G. Argon laser stapedotomy using an endo-otoprobe system. Otolaryngol Head Neck Surg. 1990;102: 193–8.
26. Jovanovic S, Schönfeld U, Fischer R, Döring M, Prapavat V, Müller G, Scherer H. Thermische Belastung des Innenohres bei der Laserstapedotomie. Teil I: Kontinuierlich strahlende Laser. HNO. 1995;43:702–9.
27. Kamalski DM, Verdaasdonk RM, de Boorder T, Vincent R, Versnel H, Grolman W. Comparing mechanical effects and sound production of KTP, Thulium, and CO_2 laser in stapedotomy. Otol Neurotol. 2014;35: 1156–62.
28. Kisilevsky VE, Bailie NA, Hailie JJ. Modified laser-assisted stapedotomy. Laryngoscope. 2010;120:276–9.
29. Lesinski SG, Palmer A. Lasers for otosclerosis: CO_2 vs. Argon and KTP-532. Laryngoscope. 1989;99:1–8.
30. Lippy WH, Battista RA, Berenholtz L, Schuring AG, Burkey JM. Twenty-year review of revision stapedotomy. Otol Neurotol. 2003;24:560–6.
31. Lundy L. The effect of CO_2- and KTP laser on the cat saccule and utricle. Laryngoscope. 2009;119:1594–605.
32. McGee TM. The argon laser in surgery for chronic ear disease and otosclerosis. Laryngoscope. 1983;93:1177–82.
33. McGee TM, Kartush JM. Comment on: lasers for otosclerosis: CO_2 vs. Argon and KTP-532. Laryngoscope. 1990;100:106–8.

34. Michaelides EM, Kartush JM. Implications of sound levels generated by otologic devices. Otolaryngol Head Neck Surg. 2001;125: 361–3.
35. Mills M, Szymanski M, Abel E. Delayed facial palsy following laser stapedectomy: in vitro study of facial nerve temperature. Clin Otolaryngol. 2003;28:211–4.
36. Ng M, Maceri DR. Delayed facial palsy after stapedotomy using KTP laser. Am J Otol. 1999;20:421–4.
37. Nishizaki K, Kariya S, Fukushima K, Orita Y, Okano M, Maeta M. A novel laser-assisted stapedotomy technique for congenital stapes fixation. Int J Pediatr Otorhinolaryngol. 2004;68:341–5.
38. Pritchett CV, Spector ME, Kileny PR, Heidenreich KD, El-Kashlan HK. Surgical treatment of hearing loss when otosclerosis coexists with superior semicircular canal syndrome. Otol Neurotol. 2014;35: 1163–7.
39. Rauch SD, Bartley ML. Argon laser stapedectomy: comparison to traditional fenestration techniques. Am J Otol. 1992;13:556–60.
40. Schmid P, Häusler R. Revision stapedectomy: an analysis of 201 operations. Otol Neurotol. 2009;30:1092–100.
41. Schreiner C, Vollrath M. Effect of Argon laser stapedotomy on cochlear potentials. Acta Otolaryngol. 1983;95:47–53.
42. Silverstein H, Hester TO, Deems D, Rosenberg S, Crosby N, Kwiatkowski T. Outcomes after laser stapedotomy with and without preservation of the stapedius tendon. Ear Nose Throat J. 1999;78:923–8.
43. Silverstein H, Hoffmann KK, Thompson JH, Sosenberg SI, Sleeper JP. Hearing outcomes of laser stapedotomy minus prosthesis (STAMP) versus conventional laser stapedotomy. Otol Neurotol. 2004;25:106–11.
44. Silverstein H, Jackson LE, Conlon S, Rosenberg SI, Thompson JH. Laser stapedotomy minus prosthesis (Laser STAMP): absence of refixation. Otol Neurotol. 2002; 23:152–7.
45. Silverstein H, Rosenberg S, Jones R. Small fenestra stapedotomies with and without KTP laser: a comparison. Laryngoscope. 1989;99: 485–8.
46. Silverstein H, Van Ess MJ, Aalameda YA. Laser stapedotomy minus prosthesis: long-term follow-up. Otolaryngol Head Neck Surg. 2011;144:753–7.
47. Somers T, Vercruysse JP, Zarowski A, Verstreken M, Schatteman I, Offeciers FE. Transient depression of inner ear function after stapedotomy: skeeter versus CO_2 laser technique. Adv Otorhinolaryngol. 2007;65: 267–72.
48. Strunk CL, Quinn FB. Stapedectomy surgery in residency: KTP-532 laser versus argon laser. Am J Otol. 1993;14:113–7.
49. Stucken EZ, Brown KD, Selesnick SH. The use of KTP Laser in revision stapedotomy. Otol Neurotol. 2012;33:1297–9.
50. Szyfter W, Mielcarek-Kuchta D, Mietkiewska-Lezniewska D, Mlodkowska A, Laczkowska-Przybylska J. Comparison between 2 laser systems, Er-YAG and CO_2, in stapes surgery. Otol Neurotol. 2012;34:29–35.
51. Szymanski M, Mills R, Abel E. Transmission of heat to the vestibule during revision stapes surgery using a KTP laser: an in vitro study. J Laryngol Otol. 2003;117:349–52.
52. Szymanski M, Morshed K, Mills RP. The use of CO_2 laser in revision stapes surgery. Adv Otorhinolaryngol. 2007;65:250–4.
53. Thedinger BS. Applications of the KTP laser in chronic ear surgery. Am J Otol. 1990;11: 79–84.
54. Thoma J, Unger V, Kastenbauer E. Temperatur- und Druckmessungen im Innenohr bei der Anwendung des Argon-Laser. Laryngo-Rhino-Otol. 1981;60:587–90.
55. Timoshenko AP, Oletski A, Prades JM, Asanau A, Martin C, Bertholon P, Martin CH. A comparison of the hearing results of KTP and Erbium YAG laser stapedotomy. Acta Otolaryngol. 2009;129:217–9.
56. Vernick DM. A comparison of the results of KTP and CO_2 laser stapedotomy. Am J Otol. 1996;17:221–4.
57. Vernick DM. Comment on: Lasers for otosclerosis: CO_2 vs. Argon and KTP-532. Laryngoscope. 1990;100:108–9.
58. Vincent R, Bittermann AJ, Oates J, Sperling N, Grolman W. KTP versus CO_2 laser fiber stapedotomy for primary otosclerosis: results of a new comparative series with the otology-neurotology database. Otol Neurotol. 2012; 33:928–33.
59. Vincent R, Grolman W, Oates J, Sperling N, Rovers M. A nonrandomized comparison of potassium titanyl phosphate and CO2 laser fiber stapedotomy for primary otosclerosis with the otology-neurotology database. Laryngoscope. 2010;120:570–5.
60. Vollrath M, Schreiner C. Influence of Argon laser stapedotomy on cochlear potentials—I: alteration of cochlear microphonics (CM). Acta Otolaryngol Suppl. 1982;385:1–31.
61. Vollrath M, Schreiner C. Influence of Argon laser stapedotomy on inner ear function and temperature. Otolaryngol Head Neck Surg. 1983;91:521–6.

62. Vollrath M, Schreiner C. The effects of the Argon laser on temperature within the cochlea. Acta Otolaryngol. 1982;93:341–8.
63. Wiet RJ, Kubek DC, Lemberg P, Byskosh AT. A meta-analysis review of revision stapes surgery with Argon laser: effectiveness and safety. Am J Otol. 1997;18:166–71.
64. Wong BJ, Neev J, van Gemert MJ. Surface temperature distributions in Carbon Dioxide, Argon and KTP (Nd:YAG) laser ablated otic capsule and calvarial bone. Am J Otol. 1997;18:766–72.
65. Yung MW. A study of the intra-operative effect of the Argon and KTP laser in stapes surgery. Clin Otolaryngol. 2002;27:279–82.
66. Brase C, Schwitulla J, Künzel J, Meusel T, Iro H, Hornung J. First experience with the fiber-enabled CO_2 laser in stapes surgery and a comparison with the "One-Shot" technique. Otol Neurotol. 2013;34:1581–5.
67. Albers AE, Schönfeld U, Kandilakis K, Jovanovic S. CO_2 laser revision stapedotomy. Laryngoscope. 2013;123:1519–26.
68. Albers B, Wagner W, Stölzel K, Schönfeld U, Jovanovic S. Laserstapedotomie. HNO. 2011;59:1093–102.
69. Brase C, Keil I, Schwitulla J, Künzel J, Mantsopoulos K, Schmid M, Iro H, Hornung J. Bone conduction after stapes surgery: comparison of CO_2 laser and manual perforation. Otol Neurotol. 2013;34:821–6.
70. Coker NJ, Ator GA, Jenkins HA, Neblett CR, Morris JR. Carbon dioxide laser stapedotomy. Arch Otolaryngol. 1985;111:601–5.
71. Coker NJ, Ator GA, Jenkins HA, Neblett CR. Carbon dioxide laser stapedotomy: a histopathologic study. Am J Otolaryngol. 1986; 7:253–7.
72. Cuda D, Murri A, Mochi P, Solenghi T, Tinelli N. Microdrill, CO_2-laser and piezoelectric stapedotomy: a comparative study. Otol Neurotol. 2009;30:1111–5.
73. Forton GE, Wuyts FL, Delsupehe KG, Verfaillie J, Loncke R. CO_2 laser-assisted stapedotomy combined with àWengen titanium clip stapes prosthesis: Superior short-term results. Otol Neurotol. 2009;30: 1071–8.
74. Gardner EK, Dornhoffer J, Ferguson S. Photoacoustic effects of carbon dioxide lasers in stapes surgery: quantification in a temporal bone model. Otol Neurotol. 2002;23: 862–5.
75. Gardner G, Robertson JH, Tomoda K, Clark WC. CO_2 laser stapedotomy: is it practical? Am J Otolaryngol. 1984;5:108–17.
76. Haberkamp TJ, Harvey SA, Khafagy Y. Revision stapedotomy with and without the CO_2 laser: an analysis of results. Am J Otol. 1996;17:225–9.
77. Jovanovic S. Technical and clinical aspects of "one-shot" CO_2 laser stapedotomy. Adv Otorhinolaryngol. 2007;65:255–66.
78. Jovanovic S, Anft D, Schönfeld U, Berghaus A, Scherer H. Tierexperimentelle Untersuchungen zur CO_2-Laser-Stapedotomie. Laryngo-Rhino-Otol. 1995;74:36–2.
79. Jovanovic S, Anft D, Schönfeld U, Berghaus A, Scherer H. Influence of CO_2 laser application to the guinea-pig cochlea on compound action potentials. Am J Otol. 1999;20: 166–73.
80. Jovanovic S, Jamali Y, Anft D, Schönfeld U, Scherer H, Müller G. Influence of pulsed laser irradiation on the morphology and function of the guinea pig cochlea. Hear Res. 2000; 144:97–108.
81. Jovanovic S, Schönfeld U, Fischer R, Döring M, Prapavat V, Müller G, Scherer H. Thermische Belastung des Innenohres bei der Laserstapedotomie. Teil II: Gepulste Laser. HNO. 1996;44:6–13.
82. Jovanovic S, Schönfeld U, Prapavat V, Berghaus A, Fischer R, Scherer H, Müller G. Effects of pulsed laser systems on stapes footplate. Lasers Surg Med. 1997;21:341–50.
83. Jovanovic S, Schönfeld U, Scherer H. "Ein-Schuss"-CO_2-Laser-Stapedotomie. HNO. 2006;54:842–50.
84. Just T, Guder E, Pau HW. Effect of the stapedotomy technique on early post-operative hearing results—preliminary results. Auris Nasus Larynx. 2012;39:383–6.
85. Just T, Specht O, Ovatri A, Langnau E, Schmidt W, Pau HW. Themografische Untersuchung während der CO_2-Laserstapedotomie. Laryngo-Rhino-Otol. 2010;89:549–55.
86. Lescanne E, Moriniere S, Gohler C, Manceau A, Beutter P, Robier A. Retrospective case study of carbon dioxide laser stapedotomy with lens-based and mirror-based micromanipulators. J Laryngol Otol. 2003;117: 256–60.
87. Lesinski SG. Revision stapedectomy. Curr Opin Otolaryngol Head Neck Surg. 2003;11:347–54.
88. Lesinski SG, Newrock R. Carbon Dioxide lasers for otosclerosis. Otolaryngol Clin North Am. 1993;26:417–41.
89. Lesinski SG, Palmer A. CO_2 laser for otosclerosis: safe energy parameters. Laryngoscope. 1989;99:9–12.
90. Lesinski SG, Palmer A. Lasers for otosclerosis—which one if any and why. Lasers Surg Med. 1990;10:448–57.

91. Lesinski SG, Palmer A. Stapedectomy revision with the CO_2 laser. Laryngoscope. 1989;99: 13–24.
92. Marchese MR, Scorpecci A, Cianfrone F, Paludetti G. "One-shot" CO_2 versus Er:YAG laser stapedotomy: is the outcome the same? Eur Arch Otorhinolaryngol. 2011;268: 351–6.
93. Molony TB. CO_2 laser stapedotomy. J La State Med Soc. 1993;145:405–8.
94. Motta G, Moscillo L. Functional results in stapedotomy with and without CO_2 laser. ORL. 2002;64:307–10.
95. Sergi B, Scorpecci A, Parrilla C, Paludetti G. Early hearing assessment after "one shot" CO2 laser stapedotomy: is it helpful to predict inner ear damage and functional outcome? Otol Neurotol. 2010;31:1376–80.
96. Shabana YK, Allam H, Pedersen B. Laser stapedotomy. J Laryngol Otol. 1999;113: 413–6.
97. Armstrong WB, Neev JA, DaSilva LB, Rubenchik AM, Stuart BC. Ultrashort pulse laser ossicular bone ablation and stapedotomy in cadaveric bone. Lasers Surg Med. 2002;30:216–20.
98. Arnoldner C, Schwab B, Lenarz T. Clinical results after stapedotomy: a comparison between the Erbium:Yttrium-Aluminium-Garnet laser and the conventional technique. Otol Neurotol. 2006;27:458–65.
99. Frenz M. Physical characteristics of various lasers used in stapes surgery. Adv Otorhinolaryngol. 2007;65:237–49.
100. Galli J, Parrilla C, Fiorita A, Marchese MR, Paludetti G. Erbium:Yttrium-Aluminium-Garnet laser application in stapedotomy. Otolaryngol Head Neck Surg. 2005; 133:923–8.
101. Keck T, Bürner H, Rettinger G. Prospective clinical study on cochlear function after Erbium:Yttrium-Aluminium-Garnet laser stapedotomy. Laryngoscope. 2005;115:1627–31.
102. Keck T, Wiebe M, Rettinger G, Riechelmann H. Safety of the Erbium:Yttrium-Aluminium-Garnet laser in stapes surgery in otosclerosis. Otol Neurotol. 2002;23:21–4.
103. Keck T, Wiebe M, Riechelmann H, Rettinger G. Ergebnisse nach Stapedotomie mit dem Erbium:YAG-Laser. Laryngo-Rhino-Otol. 2003;82:157–61.
104. Lippert BM, Gottschlich S, Külkens C, Folz BJ, Rudert H, Werner JA. Experimental and clinical results of Er:YAG laser stapedotomy. Lasers Surg Med. 2001;28:11–7.
105. Maier W, Lohnstein PU, Klenzner T, Schipper J. Cochleaprotektion und chirurgische Präzision bei der Er:YAG-laserchirurgischen Stapedotomie. Laryngo-Rhino-Otol. 2006; 85:333–7.
106. Neev J, Nelson JS, Critelli M, McCullough JL, Cheung E, Carrasco WA, Rubenchik AM, DaSilva LB, Perry MD, Stuart BC. Ablation of human nail by pulsed lasers. Lasers Surg Med. 1997;21:186–92.
107. Parrilla C, Galli J, Fetoni AR, Rigante M, Paludetti G. Erbium:Yttrium-Aluminium-Garnet laser stapedotomy—a safe technique. Otolaryngol Head Neck Surg. 2008; 138:507–12.
108. Pratisto H, Frenz M, Ith M, Romano V, Felix D, Grossenbacher R, Altermatt HJ, Weber HP. Temperature and pressure effects during Erbium laser stapedotomy. Lasers Surg Med. 1996;18:100–8.
109. Riechelmann H, Tholen M, Keck T, Rettinger G. Perioperative Glucocorticoid treatment does not influence early post-laser stapedotomy hearing thresholds. Am J Otol. 2000;21:809–12.
110. Ditkoff M, Blevins NH, Perrault D, Shapshay SM. Potential use of Diode laser soldering in middle ear reconstruction. Lasers Surg Med. 2002;31:242–6.
111. Djalilian HR, Lee AD. Stapedotomy using continuous wave Diode laser (comment). Otol Neurotol. 2008;29:1215.
112. Gerard JM, Serry P, Gersdorff MC. Outcome and lack of prognostic factors in stapes surgery. Otol Neurotol. 2008;29:290–4.
113. Kamalski DM, de Boorder T, Bittermann AJ, Wegner I, Vincent R, Grolman W. Capturing thermal, mechanical and acoustic effects of the Diode (980 nm) laser in stapedotomy. Otol Neurotol. 2014;35:1070–6.
114. Jamali Y, Jovanovic S, Schönfeld U, Anft D, Ertl T, Scherer H, Berghaus A, Müller G. Wirkung des gepulsten Er:YSSG und Ho:YAG-Lasers auf das Corti-Organ der Meerschweinchen-Cochlea—eine rasterelektronenmikroskopische Studie. Laryngo-Rhino-Otol. 1998;77:689–94.
115. Kautzky M, Trödhan A, Susani M, Schenk P. Infrared laser stapedotomy. Eur Arch Otorhinolaryngol. 1991;248:449–51.
116. Kasenbacher A, Leitner M, Weigl P. Mit Laserpulsen gegen Karies. Der Femtosekundenlaser als Werkzeug in der Zahnmedizin. LTJ. 2005;4:57–62.
117. McCaughey RG, Sun H, Rothholtz VS, Juhasz T, Wong BJ. Femtosecond laser

ablation of the stapes. J Biomed Opt. 2009;14:024040.

118. Schwab B, Hagner D, Müller W, Lubatschowski H, Lenarz T, Heermann R. Knochenablation mittels ultrakurzer Laserpulse. Eine neue Idee für die Mittelohrchirurgie. Laryngo-Rhino-Otol. 2004;83:219–25.

119. Ilgner J, Wehner M, Lorenzen J, Bovi M, Westhofen M. Morphological effects of nano-second- and femtosecond-pulsed laser ablation on human middle ear ossicles. J Biomed Opt. 2006;11(1):014004.

120. Fang L, Lin H, Zhang TY, Tan J. Laser versus non-laser stapedotomy in otosclerosis: a systematic review and meta-analysis. Auris Nasus Larynx. 2014;41:337–42.

121. Somers T, Vercruysse JP, Zarowski A, Verstreken M, Offeciers FE. Stapedotomy with microdrill or Carbon Dioxide laser: influence on inner ear function. Ann Otol Rhinol Laryngol. 2006;115:880–5.

Chapter 8

Laser-Assisted Implantation of Nitinol Stapes Prosthesis

Ronald Sroka, Joachim Müller, and Florian Schrötzlmair

Introduction

Since the introduction of stapesplasty in the 1950s [1], many innovative approaches have been undertaken in order to improve safety, surgical manageability, and postoperative hearing improvement of otosclerosis surgery [2]. New materials had been established in clinical routine (e.g., gold, titanium, teflon, metallic, and metalloplastic alloys) and some disappeared after a while [3]. Also new prosthesis designs have been developed (e.g., wire, band, and clip prostheses) [3]. Nevertheless, a delicate detail problem of stapesplasty still remains the fixation of the prosthesis on the long process of the incus, a clinical procedure called "crimping." On the one hand, tight prosthesis fixation prevents lateralization of the piston [4] and secures long-time hearing improvement [5]. On the other hand, too strong attachment can lead to incus necrosis and consequently to a loss of initially restored hearing [6]. Using a prosthesis which has to be crimped manually requires the surgeon to have a good feeling for the force which is applied. However, even experienced surgeons may apply forces that could damage the incus, disarticulate the malleoincudal joint, or damage the inner ear [7]. To address this problem, "self-crimping" prostheses have been developed. These implants are mainly produced of nitinol, a nickel–titanium shape-memory alloy, delivered in an open form which can be put onto the long process of the incus. Heating of the prosthesis loop above a certain temperature by applying energy (e.g., laser, radiofrequency) leads to closure of the prosthesis around the long process and thereby to tight fixation [8]. As the forces of

Brian J.-F. Wong and Justus Ilgner (eds.), *Biomedical Optics in Otorhinolaryngology: Head and Neck Surgery*, DOI 10.1007/978-1-4939-1758-7_8, © Springer Science+Business Media New York 2016

this memory shaping are minimal, pressure necrosis of the incus tissue should be avoided. With regard to acoustic properties, a recent meta-analysis of stapesplasty with nitinol prostheses has documented that use of this alloy is not inferior to established prostheses [9].

Until recently, there have been only nitinol prostheses with circular closure around the incus in clinical use. In 2010, a novel prosthesis called NiTiBOND® consisting of a piston of pure titanium and a nitinol attachment loop was designed. As shown in Fig. 1, the loop resembles a shamrock composed of four distinct contact zones and three contact-free zones which are thermally active areas. This design should prevent thermal damage during application of energy for closure. Between these zones are the elastic spring regions for deformation of the prosthesis during surgeon individual modeling around the incus. The prosthesis is delivered with a so-called "thermo-dummy" with the same properties as the prosthesis itself allowing extracorporal testing of energy parameters individually for each energy delivery and application system and each patient [7]. To avoid thermal damages and side effects, preclinical studies were performed followed by a clinical feasibility and retrospective comparison study including the experience of the physician also.

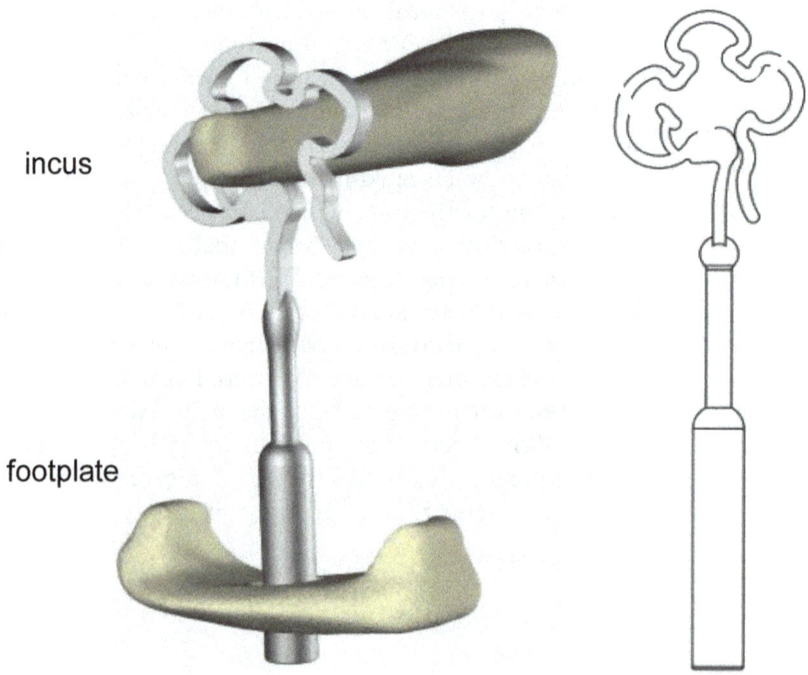

Fig. 1 Scheme of closure and fixation of NitiBond® stapes implant to the incus (courtesy of KURZ)

Preclinical Investigations

The preclinical investigation included the laser related closure of the nitinol prosthesis like fiber diameter and distance between fiber tip and target, energy per pulse, and the combination of the factor pulse duration and intensity, wavelength, furthermore investigation on the material–laser interaction, and finally safety and destruction aspects.

Experiments were performed on stapes nitinol implants available under the trade name NiTiBond® (Heinz Kurz GmbH, Dusslingen, Germany). As sketched in Fig. 2, the samples were fixed to a mount at the piston, thus allowing the thermoactive areas to be irradiated by fiber maneuvers in all directions; thus perpendicular irradiation could be performed. Irradiation was performed using mainly a 200-µm fiber transmitting the energy of a diode laser which emits at 940 nm (Medilas D OPAL, Dornier MedTech GmbH, Weßling, Germany). Thus, a variety of laser parameters could be varied. Reproducible positioning and changes in prosthesis form and closure were documented by means of a camera (Telecam® Endoscopic Camera, Karl Storz GmbH, Tuttlingen, Germany) attached to an endoscope (Cystoscope 0°, Karl Storz GmbH, Tuttlingen, Germany). Evaluation was performed by comparison of the images using conventional image processing software. In this way, the closure of the shamrock was measured after laser energy application. For statistical analysis,

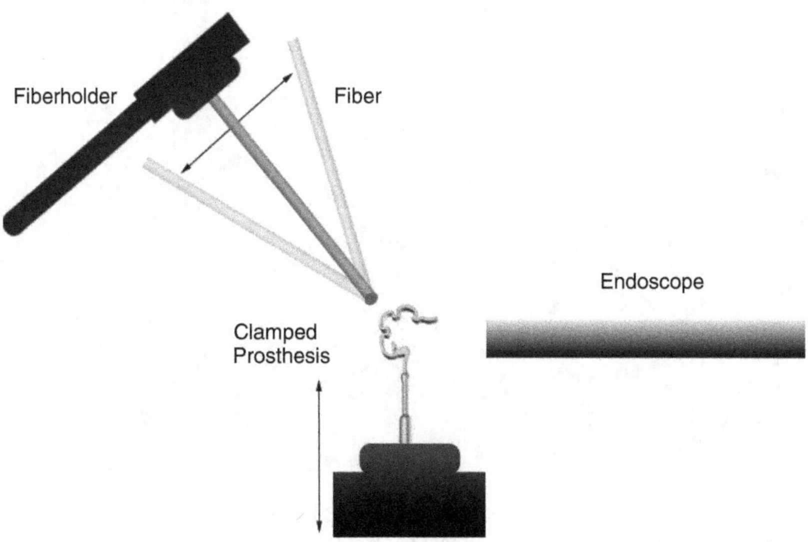

Fig. 2 Experimental set-up

mean and standard deviations were calculated. Student's t-test (SigmaPlot 11.0; Jandel Scientific, San Rafael, USA) was applied for comparison; a p-value <0.05 was considered as statistically significant.

In a first iterative experimental approach with the 940 nm-wavelength emitting diode laser and at a fiber tip distance of approximately 0.5 mm to the nitinol target, the application of a laser pulse energy of 40 mJ/pulse resulted in a suitable closure of the loop. Specific investigations on the influence by the distance between laser fiber tip and target surface on the bending process showed that in near contact mode a closure of almost 30° could be obtained, while at a distance of 1 mm the induced shaping was just 5°, which is illustrated in Fig. 3. In a similar manner, varying fiber diameters at constant laser parameters showed an increase in closure angle for a 200 μm-fiber compared to a 400 μm-fiber. These observations could be explained as the area size which is under illumination changes with respect to distance between fiber tip and target, or the diameter of the fiber core. Calculations taking the divergency (numerical aperture of a fiber) into account showed a reduction of the irradiation and the irradiance by a factor of 10 in case of the 200 μm fiber and by a factor of 4.5 in case of the 400 μm fiber, as listed in Table 1.

Additionally, in a set of single pulse experiments the dependency on the pulse duration was investigated while holding the applied energy per pulse constant at 40 mJ/pulse. Therefore, varying the pulse duration between t(pulse) = 80, 40, 20, 10, and 5 ms the laser power was increased from P = 0.5, 1, 2, 4, and 8 W accordingly, to obtain constant energy per pulse, simply by multiplication using the formula $E(\text{pulse}) = t(\text{pulse}) \times P$. Using the 940

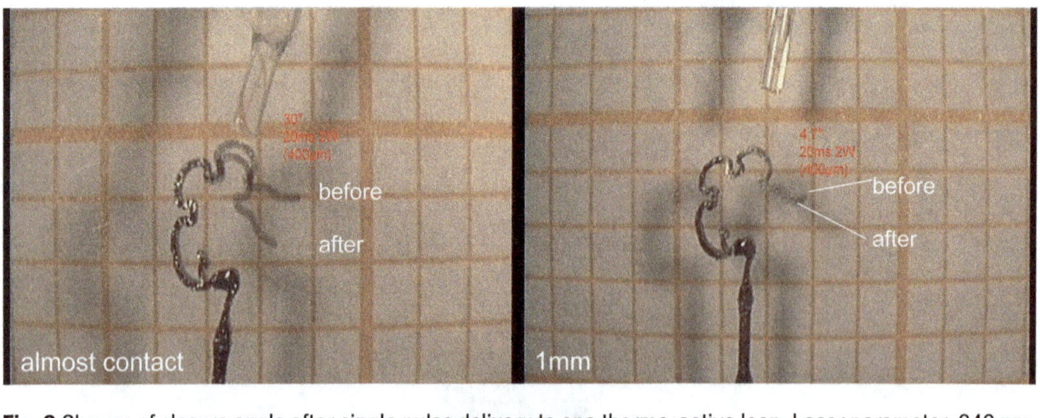

Fig. 3 Change of closure angle after single pulse delivery to one thermo-active loop. Laser parameter: 940 nm; 400 μm fiber; 2 W; 20 ms; 40 mJ/pulse). *Left*: Almost contact mode application results in closure angle of 30°. *Right*: 1 mm distance between fiber results in closure of 5°

Table 1
Change of irradiation and irradiance on the target by varying the distance between almost contact and 1 mm distance between fiber tip and target surface

	Irradiation (J/cm²) for 40 mJ		Irradiance (W/cm²) for 2 W	
Distance (mm)	200 μm	400 μm	200 μm	400 μm
0	127.3	31.8	6366.2	1591.5
1	12.4	7.2	621.7	360.9

E(pulse) = 40 mJ

Table 2
Variation of closure angle (mean ± std.dev.) with respect to applying a constant energy/pulse while changing the pulse duration *t*(pulse)

Energy	0.5 W 80 ms	1 W 40 ms	2 W 20 ms	4 W 10 ms	8 W 5 ms
mean	57.0°	57.7°	61.2°	69.5°	63.7°
std. dev.	±18.1°	11.3°	17.4°	4.7°	4.1°

nm-laser emission transported by a 200 μm-fiber positioned almost in contact to single thermoactive loop and applying a single pulse, the resulting closure values (mean and standard deviation) were listed in Table 2. From this, it could be clearly derived that a mean maximum closure angle of 69.5° ±4.7° could be obtained at 4 W and 10 ms. Longer and shorter pulse duration showed reduced closure potential.

Experiments concerning the wavelength dependency of clinically available laser systems emitting in the NIR spectral region and with potential of fiber-assisted energy application showed no obviously significant differences in closure behavior. Experiments on the laser-induced temperatures using thermal camera imaging showed an intense temperature increase within the thermoactive zone of the loop, while in the tissue contact zones only a minimal temperature increase could be observed.

Finally, potential risk factors from the technical point of view were investigated. Even when applying high amount of laser energy (in clinical terms) to the nitinol target, a real destruction could not be observed. With regard to the potential tissue side effects, it must be pointed out that the width of the target loop on the incus is about 250 μm in diameter. Laser application in a defocused mode or with large spot size may result in uncontrolled irradiation of the underlying and surrounding tissue structures, as sketched in

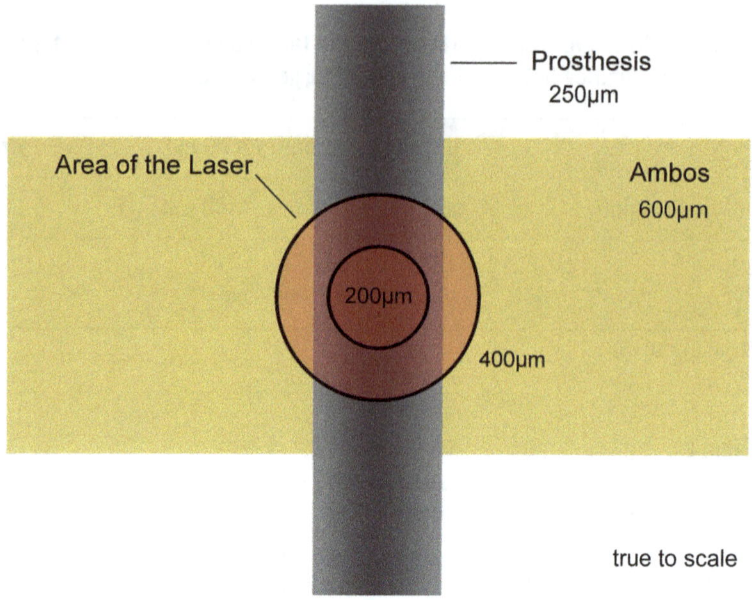

Fig. 4 True scale sketch to show the possible of irradiation of surrounding tissue if not proper targeting

Fig. 4. Theoretical simulations showed that an application of laser pulse energy of 40 mJ/pulse (10 ms; 4 W; wavelength > 1500 nm) to soft and hard tissues can induce temperature of more than 120 °C. To prevent undesired tissue temperature increase, precise targeting, laser spot size adapted to target size, and distance control (no movement in the axial direction) should be mandatory for safe treatment.

Clinical Study

In a small cohort clinical study, patients ($n = 15$) underwent stapes surgery after giving informed consent [15]. According to the technique described by Helms [14], a posterior partial stapedectomy was performed. Using a perforator of 0.6 mm in diameter, a hole was drilled in the stapes footplate and its posterior third was removed. For closure of NiTiBOND® prosthesis, a diode laser (Medilas D Multibeam, Dornier MedTech GmbH, Weßling, Germany) emitting at 940 nm and using a 400-µm laser fiber was used to apply the energy on the prosthesis in order to induce its closure around the incus. Pre-operative testing was performed by means of the delivered test prosthesis immediately before implantation as shown in Fig. 5. In this study, laser parameters were set to 2 W at a pulse duration of 20 ms, thus applying 40 mJ/pulse.

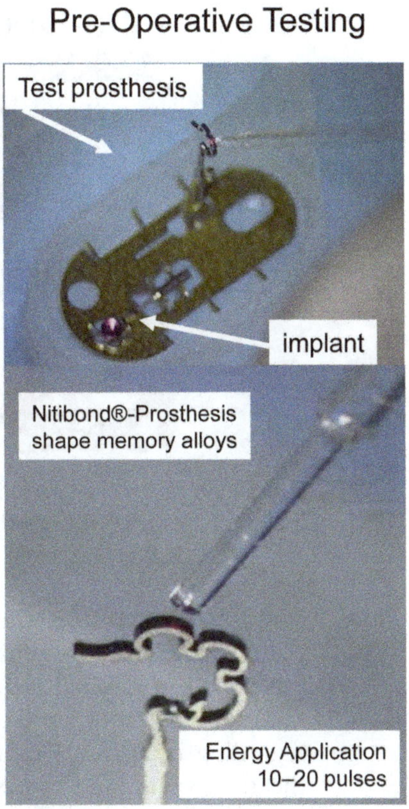

Fig. 5 Unpacked NitiBond®-Prosthesis showing test prosthesis and implant (*top*) and during test application of laser pulses to the test prosthesis (*bottom*) (courtesy of KURZ)

The number of applied laser pulses depends on the manual testing by the surgeon for a reliable fixation. The intraoperative procedure is shown in Fig. 6 with the fiber tip targeting to the loop of the nitinol implant. Following this procedure, a total of 10–25 laser pulses were applied in a stepwise fashion to the three thermo-active loops to induce loop closure and stepwise adaptation to the incus. In this way a maximum of 1 J laser energy in total was applied. Evaluation of the clinical outcome was performed by pure-tone audiometry according to ISO 8253-1 standard. Mean remaining air-bone gap (ABG) and mean ABG reduction were determined.

The result of this study showed that the clinical use of NiTiBOND® prosthesis combined with laser-assisted fixation led to an overall postoperative hearing improvement. Patients benefited from this operation over the full hearing frequency spectrum. An ABG reduction of 17 ± 4 dB could be observed, while the remaining mean postoperative ABG was reduced to 11 ± 2 dB. For all hearing frequencies, stapesplasty with NiTiBOND® prosthesis led to less remaining ABG after stapes surgery. Furthermore, it

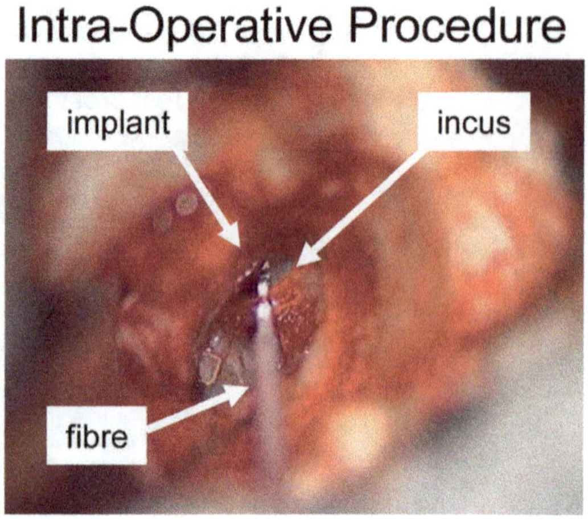

Fig. 6 Intraoperative setting during laser assisted application of laser energy for fixation of the NiTiBOND® prosthesis to the incus

could be derived from the surgeons that NiTiBOND® prosthesis was suitable for experienced stapes surgeons, as well as for ear surgeons with limited experience in stapes surgery. Normally, the experienced stapes surgeon achieved better audiometric results regarding mean ABG reduction and mean remaining ABG than the nonexperienced stapes surgeons. Remarkably, when the less experienced stapes surgeons used NiTiBOND® prosthesis, they achieved a similarly mean ABG reduction as the experienced stapes surgeon using this prosthesis type.

Discussion

Laser energy application for fixation of stapes implants seems to be a promising and easy-to-train technique. As a diversity of lasers and wavelengths are available in clinical use in the area of otorhinolaryngology, it must be mentioned that there are a variety of parameters which should be tested separately to find the suitable set of parameters, e.g., wavelength, irradiation, irradiance, application angle, etc. Thus, this study could be seen as the basic of necessary test procedures for clinical application. Additional investigations on the laser–material interaction should be performed to identify optimized parameter settings, handling procedures, and risks for side effects [12, 13].

The preclinical study investigated the use of the 940-nm wavelength in combination with a 200-μm bare fiber with flat cut-polished fiber tip and the application of a constant pulse energy of 40 mJ/pulse. A combination of 4 W in 10 ms and a fiber-to-target distance of nearly contact looks favorable for secure and safe closure of the implant. For safety reasons and to protect the incus tissue from laser-induced thermal necrosis, high laser powers should be avoided. As the width of the nitinol-target-loop is about 250 μm the use of a suitable focus or spot size is mandatory. This could be achieved by using the 200 μm-fiber and in near contact mode.

In the preclinical experiments, only single pulses were applied to each of the three thermoactive loops. Due to the complex geometric clinical *in situ* situation during the operation the number of laser pulses and thus the amount of laser energy is higher when compared to the experiment. From the technical point of view, a perpendicular laser energy application could be achieved only on one single loop, as the others were angled in different degrees up to about tangential. Furthermore, the distance between fiber tip and loop surface may change in the millimeter range during laser application, be it due to remaining tremor of the physician's hand or by the patient's breathing and vascular pulse. For safety reasons, laser energy should only be applied when the reflex of the laser pilot beam can be identified on the loop surface. Supported by those observations, the clinical potential of laser energy-assisted fixation of NiTiBOND® prosthesis was proven by using a 400-μm fiber coupled to the clinically available laser system at that time. Careful laser energy application was performed to avoid laser–tissue interaction with the incus.

Improving the laser energy application with a fiber bendable at the very end to achieve a more perpendicular energy application could be of clinical interest. Nevertheless, this clinical test clearly demonstrated the simple application of laser energy to model the NiTiBOND® prosthesis precisely to the incus. The 4-week post-operation audiogram showed improved hearing over the complete hearing frequency range. Comparing the audiometric results of the laser-assisted fixation of NiTiBOND® implants with other piston-prosthesis techniques, e.g., K-piston or CliP® piston [10, 11], the mean remaining ABG is reduced and the mean ABG reduction is increased [15]. Additionally, due to precise handling and reproducible maneuvers, it looks like the learning curve of a proper and safe use of laser-assisted NiTiBOND® prosthesis implantation could be improved.

Conclusion

Fiber-assisted diode laser energy application allows controlled and precise closure of NiTiBOND® prosthesis while modeling to the incus. Clinically, the promising audiometric results encourage further clinical use of laser assistance during nitinol-prosthesis fixation for experienced, as well as nonexperienced stapes surgeons. Given the positive results, prospects are that this novel prosthesis fixation technique will continue to allow good functional outcome and overcome implantation problems of historical prosthesis types.

Acknowledgement

F. Suchan, T. Pongratz, D. Saal, D. Rust for technical assistance during experiments. The companies Heinz Kurz GmbH, Dusslingen, Germany and Dornier MedTech GmbH, Wessling, Germany are acknowledged for device support. The pre-clinical investigation was supported by an Innovation grant of the Ministry of Baden-Wuertemberg, Germany.

References

1. Shea JJ. Symposium: the operation for the mobilization of the stapes in otosclerotic deafness. Laryngoscope. 1956;66:729–84.
2. Häusler R. General history of stapedectomy. Adv Otorhinolaryngol. 2007;65:1–5.
3. Fritsch MH, Naumann IC. Phylogeny of the stapes prosthesis. Otol Neurotol. 2008;29: 407–15.
4. Lagleyre S, Calmels MN, Escude B, Deguine O, Fraysse B. Revision stapes surgery: the "lateralized piston syndrome". Otol Neurotol. 2009;30:1138–44.
5. Huber AM, Veraguth D, Schmid S, Roth T, Eiber A. Tight stapes prosthesis fixation leads to better functional results in otoslerosis surgery. Otol Neurotol. 2008;29:893–9.
6. Gerlinger I, Tóth M, Lujber L, Szanyi I, Móricz P, Somogyvári K, Németh A, Ráth G, Pytel J, Mann W. Necrosis of the long process of the incus following stapes surgery: new anatomical observations. Laryngoscope. 2009; 119:721–6.
7. Huber AM, Schrepfer T, Eiber A. Clinical evaluation of the NiTiBOND stapes prothesis, an optimized shape memory alloy design. Otol Neurotol. 2012;33:132–6.
8. Know GW, Reitan H. Shape-memory stapes prosthesis for otosclerosis surgery. Laryngoscope. 2005;115:1340–6.
9. Van Rompaey V, Claes G, Potvin J, Wouters K, Van de Heyning PH. Systematic review of the literature on nitinol prosthesis in surgery for otosclerosis: assessment of the adequacy of statistical power. Otol Neurotol. 2011;32: 357–66.
10. Zuur CL, De Bruijn AJ, Lindeboom R, Tange RA. Retrospective analysis of early postoperative hearing results obtained after stapedotomy with implantation of a new titanium stapes prosthesis. Otol Neurotol. 2003;24:863–7.
11. Wengen DF. A new self-retaining titanium clip stapes prosthesis. Adv Otorhinolaryngol. 2007;65:184–9.
12. Sroka R, Rühm A, Suchan F, Pongratz T, Russ D, Saal D, Schroetzlmair F, Müller J. Physical investigation of the laser induced NitiBond© stapesprosthesis—Preliminary result. Presentation: EAONO—6th International Workshop and Consensus in Auditory Implants, Bratislava, Slovak Republic, 30.08.2012–02.09.2012
13. Sroka R, Pongratz T, Suchan F, Schroetzlmair F, Müller J, Saal D, Russ D. Laser assisted fixation of NiTiBond prosthesis. Presentation at 4th Symposium on Topical Problems of Biophotonics, Nishni Novgorod, Russia, 21.–27.07.2013.
14. Helms J. Sanierende und rekonstruktive Operationen an Gehörgang, Mittelohr und Felsenbein. In: Naumann HH, editor. Kopf- und Halschirurgie, vol. 2. Stuttgart: Thieme; 1996.
15. Schroetzlmair F, Suchan F, Kisser U, Hempel JM, Sroka R, Müller J. Promising clinical results of an innovative self-crimping stapesprosthesis in otosclerosis surgery. Otol Neurotol. 2013;34(9):1571–5.

Chapter 9

Endonasal Laser Ablation of Soft Tissue

Justus Ilgner and Martin Westhofen

Introduction

Starting in the late 1970s, lasers have been widely used for endonasal applications in order to resect, vaporize, or ablate soft tissue and even bone. The objective is to alleviate nasal breathing, resolve obstruction, enable mucosal drainage, and modulate inflammatory response. While benign and malignant neoplasms are less frequently the cause of endonasal obstruction, most of air flow impairment is caused by hyperplastic turbinates as in allergic rhinitis and by polyp formation in the course of chronic rhinosinusitis. Laser turbinate reduction is subject to a separate chapter in this book.

Chronic rhinosinusitis (CRS), on the other hand, is a widespread condition which affects about 11 % of the general population. In its variety, the annual burden on the U.S. health care system has been estimated at 4.3 billion US$. The disease comes in a form without nasal polyps (CRS-NP) or with nasal polyps (CRS + NP). A variety of factors associated with CRS has been addressed in the past. Bronchial asthma, in general, is associated with CRS in 19–46 % of cases, as is allergic rhinitis with 22 %. 10 to 64 % of CRS patients also suffer from a variety of allergies, while an allergic disposition, in turn, does not seem to trigger CRS [1–3]. There is, however, an established link between intolerance for acetyl salicylic acid (ASS), nonallergic bronchial asthma, and CRS, known as Samter's or Widal's triad. ASS intolerance can be found in 7–22 % of patients [3–6].

Apart from associated factors, the cause of chronic rhinosinusitis is still largely unknown. In recent years, CRS has been related to infectious triggers—either *Staphylococcus aureus*, whose superantigens are able to trigger up to 25 % of the native population of T lymphocytes [7, 8] or to an eosinophilic reaction to fungi [9, 10]. As for bacterial infection, the role of biofilm has been highlighted

Brian J.-F. Wong and Justus Ilgner (eds.), *Biomedical Optics in Otorhinolaryngology: Head and Neck Surgery*, DOI 10.1007/978-1-4939-1758-7_9, © Springer Science+Business Media New York 2016

in the recent years [11, 12]. It was shown that bacteria, whose colonial growth has exceeded a certain threshold, can form a mass of mucopolysaccharides which is impenetrable for antibodies as well as cells from the human immune system. Confocal laser scanning microscopy for biofilm in the paranasal sinuses is a growing research area in order to characterize the formation and the components of biofilm. Understanding its mechanisms will potentially result in new therapeutic approaches which can be more pertinent and cost-effective.

Following this research, it is now generally understood that CRS is a disease that cannot be addressed by surgery alone. While up to the 1970s it was an accepted concept to exenterate the mucosa from diseased areas of the paranasal sinuses as widely as possible, the work of Messerklinger and Stammberger radically changed the surgical approach to CRS [13, 14]. They could show that once ventilation and mucosal drainage from diseased sinuses were re-established in certain key areas, opening the natural pathways in a minimally invasive fashion, even large areas of dependent inflamed mucosa could functionally be restored. Thus, the approach of functional endoscopic sinus surgery (FESS) using an endoscope or microscope became the gold standard in sinus surgery since the 1980s. However, in any case, given the complex inflammatory process, patients have to undergo an extensive follow-up under medical treatment with, e.g., topical steroids in order to prevent symptomatic recurrence [3, 15, 16]. According to Kennedy, 10–27 % of patients suffer from recurrent events of symptoms during postoperative follow-up even after many years, which in many cases result in revision surgery [1]. Consequently, the role of laser surgery in primary cases as well as in recurrent disease has been evaluated since the 1990s as it can be minimally invasive and highly directional, addressing diseased areas while leaving healthy mucosa intact.

Overview of Literature

In 1977, Lenz [17] performed first experiments on nine human postmortem individuals in order to enlarge the bony medial wall of the maxillary sinus. In 14 procedures, bone with a thickness of 0.4–1.8 mm was cut with a beam diameter of 0.5–1.5 mm by an Argon laser, with power rates between 0.1 and 100 W. One of the first clinical endonasal applications of lasers in humans was reported by Strong. He employed a CO_2 laser in order to obliterate septum vessels in hereditary teleangiectasia and to remove solitary papillomas. However, as the CO_2 laser beam cannot be transmitted by glass fibers, this circumstance prevented its use in deeper areas, i.e., the posterior nasal cavity as well as off-axis, i.e., the paranasal sinuses. However, despite these limitations, the CO_2 laser has been used in a variety of clinical settings for endonasal surgery, given its ability to operate in continuous wave (cw) mode, as well as in pulsed mode [18–21]. Shapshay compared tissue effects of the CO_2 laser with those of a Holmium:YAG laser [22, 23]. While used in cw mode at 6 W and fired in single intervals of 0.1–0.5 s, the CO_2 laser produced more carbonization than the Holmium:YAG laser with a pulse energy of 1.0–1.2 J at 3–5 Hz repetition rate. However, carbonization effects were less for the CO_2 laser than for the Holmium:YAG when the CO_2 laser was set to superpulse mode at 6 W average power and 90–110 pulses per second. Selkin reported 250 endonasal CO_2 laser operations, whose cases consisted largely of hyperplastic inferior turbinates (61 cases) and 31 bilateral and 19 unilateral excisions of endonasal polyps [24]. Complications were endonasal obstruction in 4 cases, intra and postoperative hemorrhage in 11 cases, 2 septal perforations, and one Rhinitis sicca. In various studies, Sato combined the use of CO_2 laser with deflective hand pieces in order to reach areas within the nasal cavity that are off axis or situated in the paranasal sinuses. Deflection angles were 45°, 90°, and 135°. With these, he was able to ablate antrochoanal polyps in seven children and three adults. As for endonasal polyps, these were removed with a CO_2 laser alone (4 cases), in conjunction with a microdebrider (4 cases), or with a microdebrider alone (17 cases) [19–21]. Bone removal, however, was achieved with conventional resecting instruments. The 135° reflective handheld device was used in another study for maxillary sinus surgery by Sato [19]. The rationale is that in endonasal sinus surgery, the ostium to the maxillary sinus is enlarged by opening its medial wall, while the anterior wall is still difficult to reach. It can only be seen by using optical devices and reached by instruments with a bending angle of greater than 90°, unless the medial wall of the maxillary sinus is not resected completely, as in medial maxillectomy. Sato resected 10 inflammatory polyps and benign neoplasms with this deflective device. Laser parameters were not noted.

In recent years, a number of hollow waveguides have been developed in order to widen the operative range for CO_2 lasers. While their potential is only at the beginning of being exploited, waveguides could become a useful adjunct for endonasal application of CO_2 lasers in the future. Agarwal et al. reported a series of 12 patients treated endonasally with a CO_2 laser using a handheld hollow waveguide between the years 2007 and 2009 [18]. Three patients suffered from adhesions following primary radiotherapy for malignant disease, while in nine patients the laser was used to excise or reduce a variety of malignant and nonmalignant neoplasms in the nose (6), nasopharynx (3), or in both regions (2), as well as in the sphenoid sinus and adjacent sella region (1). Power was set at 6–12 W cw, however, further parameters were not indicated.

As for fiber-based laser systems, mostly Yttrium–Aluminum–Garnet (YAG) systems have been under review, including the frequency-doubled (KTP) Neodymium:YAG laser. In the recent years, particularly the Neodymium:YAG laser has been complemented by a variety of diode lasers, whose wavelength is similarly localized in the near-infrared range. While the Neodymium:YAG laser has been used extensively in laser turbinate reduction, its use in CRS with polyps and particularly with recurrent disease is limited [25–28]. Scherer and Hopf described a procedure to resect polyps from their base in the middle meatus in contact mode at 3–5 W cw [28]. Resection was performed with a combination of an endoscope with a laser fiber guiding instrument, deflecting the tip of the laser fiber by means of an Albarran lever as used in Urology. Ohyama reported a series of 21 patients in which he vaporized polyps or resected those from their stalk [29]. In follow-up, a longer duration of crust formation was noted compared to conventional surgery, while blood loss was less. Also, the procedure took longer to perform than in the conventional fashion. Laser parameters were not reported. In an early study with the Neodymium:YAG laser, Zhang described its use to superficially coagulate the mucosa along the sinus walls from which the polyps had been resected by conventional instrumentation. In noncontact mode, laser settings were 25 W cw. In comparison to 48 patients without laser treatment, 54 patients with laser coagulation were reported to run a smaller risk of polyp recurrence (46.6 % versus 66.6 %) [30].

More extensively than Neodymium:YAG laser systems, Holmium:YAG laser systems were evaluated for endonasal sinus surgery [31, 32]. Gleich et al. reported of 37 endonasal operations, while 29 had been performed for treating chronic rhinosinusitis [31]. Of note is the fact that he also used the laser to incise or ablate bone in addition to soft tissue. This was less the case in 10 revision cases, who had been primarily operated via a transantral window (Caldwell–Luc technique). Bone was cut at an energy of 1 J with a pulse rate of 3 Hz, while polyps were resected at 0.8 J with 3 Hz repetition rate. During follow-up, 24 of 29 patients were reported as symptom free, while wound healing was comparable to FESS. One patient had another polyp recurrence and another suffered postoperative hemorrhage. As for bone resection, Kautzky et al. also used the Holmium:YAG Laser at 0.9 J pulse energy and 5 Hz repetition rate in order to incise bone to access paranasal sinuses intraoperatively [32]. The bone itself was removed with conventional instruments following laser incision. Of note was a marked zone of bone necrosis (370–520 μm width), while carbonization was not seen. Some impairment was noted by the authors as bony debris often contaminated the endoscope lens which required frequent cleaning, thereby attenuating the benefits of bloodless resection with a laser. After a feasibility study with animals, Shapshay resected the uncinate process, opened the ethmoid bulla and the maxillary sinus ostium in 17 patients with a

Holmium:YAG laser, set at 0.5–1.2 J at a pulse rate of 3–10 Hz [22, 23]. The ethmoid cells, however, were resected conventionally. The total laser power applied ranged between 380 and 5048 J. 10 patients were described as having an excellent result, while 4 noted partial reobstruction and 3 patients returned with a recurrence of polyps in a range between 6 and 8 months. The average duration of the procedure was 1 h 50 min. As for Holmium:YAG laser resection of endonasal soft tissue, Metson published a randomized controlled prospective trial of 32 patients who were operated with conventional FESS technique on one side and with a laser technique on the other [33]. Laser energy was delivered via a 400 μm glass fiber, while the laser parameters were set to a pulse energy between 0.5 and 2 J at a pulse rate between 5 and 220 Hz which resulted in a power range between 2.5 and 15 W. The ablation depth ranged between 1.2 and 1.7 mm. Noteworthy was a thermal necrosis zone 0.5–1.0 mm adjacent to the ablated region. In fact, a prolonged crust formation was noted on the laser operated side after 6 weeks, although crust formation was more prevalent on the conventionally operated side after 1 week. Moreover, postoperative edema was more pronounced on the laser operated side. The laser procedure took an average of 121 min, which was significantly longer than on the FESS side.

A similar study was performed by Gerlinger using a KTP laser with 24 patients whose laser procedure on one side was compared to conventional FESS procedure on the contralateral side [34]. Different power settings were used for a variety of subtasks, i.e., 20–30 W for bone ablation, 5–8 W for polyp resection, and 3–5 W for coagulating vessels. Moreover, the laser was set to cw mode for soft tissue resection and to pulsed mode of 20–50 ms pulse duration for bone ablation. As with Metson, Gerlinger noted marked edema on the laser operated side after 1 week, while at the same time crust formation was more prevalent on the FESS side. Generally, there were no great differences in wound healing. The total energy applied ranged between 484 and 1788 J. Blood loss was diminished greatly on the laser operated side, while the laser process was more time consuming and required single use instruments that were more expensive. Two more studies addressed KTP laser procedures during follow up or in revision surgery following FESS. Wang reported of 13 patients undergoing endonasal laser revision surgery following recurrence of polyps after FESS [35]. The laser was set at 15–20 W cw while the energy was output through a laser fiber of 0.4 mm diameter, resulting in a spot size of 0.4 mm in contact or 0.8 mm in near-contact mode. The technique was to cut polyps off the stalk or to vaporize the contents. During an average follow-up of 24.7 months, two of 13 patients had another recurrence, while no complications were seen by the procedure itself. In postoperative follow-up, Levine used the KTP laser to resect synechiae at 8–12 W laser power with 0.1 s "on" and

0.1 s "off" intervals [36]. Single polyps were resected in the same way at 6–10 W laser power. During a 24-month follow-up period, which included concomitant medical treatment for CRS, 22 patients were free of symptoms, 18 improved, 4 unchanged, and 2 were worse.

In order to avoid extensive opening of the paranasal sinuses as in midfacial degloving, Kaluskar and coworkers (2009) evaluated the use of a fiber-based KTP laser to remove inverted papilloma, which is a benign lesion with a potential for malignant transformation [37]. Over 6 years, nine cases were resected endonasally. Mucosa close to the lesion was incised as the lesion itself was lifted off the bony surface by vaporization and/or coagulation of the underlying soft tissue. Using this technique, the group recorded one case of recurrence 12 months following laser surgery.

In 2011, Hesham and coworkers suggested the use of a diode laser emitting infrared light at a wavelength of 980 nm with a power rating at 20 W cw through a 0.4 mm fiber in contact or near-contact mode, which resulted in a spot size of 0.4–0.8 mm [38]. Their objective was to treat 25 patients in whom synechiae, i.e., transverse scar formation between the turbinates and the septum, had occurred following functional endoscopic sinus surgery with conventional instruments. However, their laser procedure was combined with local application of Mitomycin C, an antiproliferative drug, in a concentration of 0.4 mg/ml for 5 min. While 32 synechiae in 20 patients had been resected with this procedure, three patients had a recurrence with 4 synechiae (1 bilaterally).

In order to apply lasers endonasally not only for resection purposes, but also for tissue repair, Bleier et al. performed an animal experiment in 20 white rabbits in order to weld endonasal sinus mucosa, which was simultaneously tested for bond strength under water pressure [39]. His group used a diode laser of 808 nm set at 1.0 W, applying a power density of 31.8 W/cm^2 with intervals of 0.5 s "on" and 0.1 s "off" duration. As for the bonding agent, a mixture of albumin, hyaluronic acid and indiocyanine green (used as a color indicator) was employed. The group noticed a significant increase of bond strengths over conventional wound healing at days 0 and 5, while this difference leveled to non-significance from day 15.

Own Experience

Starting in 1997, we developed a clinical algorithm in which the use of laser procedures is embedded in our follow-up of patients who have undergone one or more FESS procedure(s) for CRS with polyps (Fig. 1). It has to be stated that, in the light of aforementioned studies, we regard the use of laser in primary FESS as feasible, but comparatively time-consuming. Although even hard

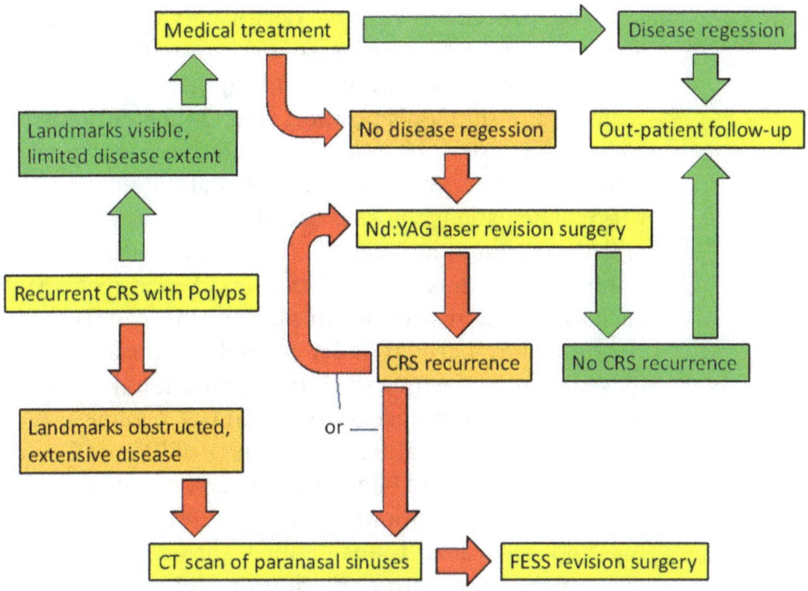

Fig. 1 Algorithm for the indication of Neodymium:YAG laser intervention for recurrent CRS with polyps

tissue ablation is possible with a laser during FESS, the benefits of laser use are limited compared to conventionally instrumented FESS surgery. However, in postoperative follow-up, particularly in cases with limited extent of recurrent disease which do not respond to medical treatment, laser procedures can be very useful to limit recurrence and re-establish mucosal function before the extent of recurrence makes another full FESS revision inevitable.

Generally, the use of topical steroids is widely accepted as the treatment of choice during wound healing as well as for polyp recurrence. Evidence is less extensive for the use of systemic steroids, leukotriene antagonists, and antihistamines in CRS with polyps. However, medical treatment is generally given priority over surgical steps unless severe complications require immediate intervention. If, after three weeks of medical treatment, local recurrence of disease is not controlled, laser surgery is considered as the next step. Typical landmarks, e.g., the periorbit, the middle meatus, or the superior area of the inferior turbinate, must remain visible in order to maintain orientation in the operative field. For practical reasons and time considerations, three regions out of five on one side of the septum (anterior ethmoid, posterior ethmoid, maxillary sinus ostium, frontal sinus recess, sphenoid sinus ostium) can be treated in one session, otherwise the procedure should be split into two. Contraindications are former dehiscence of the Dura with CSF leak, dehiscence of the orbital wall with prolapse of orbital fat, and excessive bleeding during previous surgeries. Arterial hypertension should be medically controlled before laser intervention is started.

The procedure can be performed under local or general anesthesia. In any case, the patient is rested on the operating table in a supine position with his head slightly rotated to the right side, which is the surgeon's position (Fig. 2). Laser safety protocols are followed as usual. If under local anesthesia, the patient wears the same protective goggles as all the staff present in the operating room. The patient's nose is anesthetized with 10 % lidocaine spray and decongested and anesthetized again with cotton swabs containing a 50 % mixture of lidocaine 2 % and oxymetazoline 0,1 % each. These swabs remain in place for at least 10 minutes before the procedure starts. If under general anesthesia, the patient's goggles are replaced with a sheet of aluminum foil wrapped in a 10 cm wide strip of cotton gauze soaked in 0.9 % saline.

The instrumental setup consists of a 30° and 70° Hopkins rod endoscope, a suitable light source, a conventional suction device for fluids and—additionally—a smoke evacuator. Video monitoring and recording is maintained throughout the procedure—either with a standard definition or high definition CCD camera attached to the endoscope, allowing all staff to follow the procedure and to maintain ergonomically optimal working conditions for the surgeon.

The Neodymium:YAG laser system which is used (Dornier MediLas 5060 N, Dornier GmbH, Germering, Germany) allows, besides power settings, the application of feedback power control,

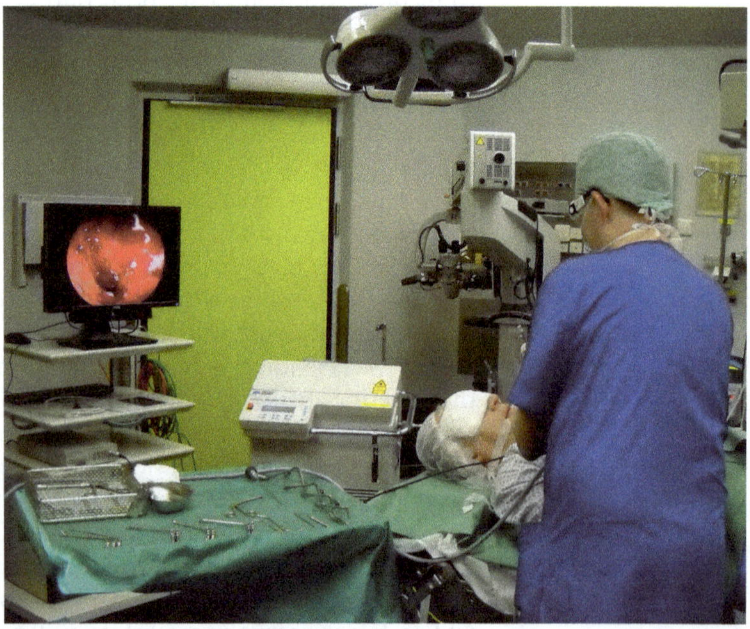

Fig. 2 Setup during endonasal Neodymium:YAG laser tissue excision. From **left** to *right*: video recording and monitoring facility, Neodymium:YAG laser unit, patient under general anesthesia, surgeon

which can be applied when working in contact mode: With feedback power control (Fibertom C (R)) turned on, the infrared to visible light which is emitted by the tissue under thermal ablation is picked up by the laser fiber simultaneously while emitting energy. This feedback information is uncoupled from the laser fiber inside the laser system and used as a parameter to reduce the laser power accordingly, should the temperature inside the tissue rise too high. The "tightness" of feedback loop can be set to three different levels, independently from the laser power that is chosen. In most cases, 10 W cw from a Neodymium:YAG laser are sufficient to ablate soft tissue inside the nasal cavity and sinuses swiftly without causing collateral damage. The latter is particularly important, as with the laser's main emission line at 1064 nm, absorption in water is particularly low. This is why the initial use of the Neodymium:YAG laser in non-contact mode, as first used by Lesserson [40], Lenz and Eichler [17], as well as Metson [33] resulted in good coagulation of tissue, but with risks to adjacent structures as the dura or the periorbit. Werner reported a zone of thermal damage of 10 mm maximum from the center of irradiation and later postulated the risk of atrophying ostitis of the underlying bone [27]. Likewise, Rathfoot reported a damage zone of 4 mm in soft tissue [41] as did Ossoff [42] with a combined zone of coagulation and necrosis up to 4 mm. However, despite the warnings that concerned the use of a Neodymium:YAG laser in particular it has to be mentioned that the laser parameters used are not always available in detail from these reports. This applies in particular to the laser energy delivery in non-contact versus contact mode. In the latter, the tip of the laser fiber is deliberately contaminated with debris, either from resected tissue or from burning a wooden spatula before application, so that all laser energy is absorbed at the fiber tip and not propagated into depth of tissue. Consequently, when limiting laser output power to 3–5 W as done by Scherer and Hopf [28], they as well as Shapshay [22, 23] could not detect any collateral damage to the tissue. In our department, contact mode in combination with feedback power control is a standard procedure when ablating soft tissue endonasally. It is worth mentioning, that feedback power control often limits the output laser power to less than the power setting, e.g., 10 W, so that the total laser energy applied at the end of the procedure is far less than the power setting multiplied with "laser on"-time.

As with all lasers emitting in the near infrared or visible light range, conventional glass silica fibers can be used to deliver laser light into tissue. However, as the paranasal sinuses require bending the fiber to a very small radius at times, fibers with small diameters are preferable. Fibers with a core diameter of 60 μm have a limited working range to areas that are close to the direct line if sight, which is the nasal cavity itself, the ethmoid and the sphenoid sinus. For the frontal sinus recess and the maxillary sinus, fibers with

400 μm or even 200 μm diameter are preferable. As energy density rises inversely with the square of cross sectional fiber radius, 200 μm fibers usually carry a maximum of 10 W cw from a Neodymium:YAG laser. However, energy loss due to bending the fiber to an, e.g., 10 mm radius is negligible compared to 400 μm or even 600 μm diameter fibers bent to the same radius. As stated above, 10 W cw is generally sufficient for ablating soft tissue in the nasal cavity. Sometimes re-cutting the fiber is necessary during the procedure when the tip breaks, e.g., when hitting bone. In these cases, the shape of the re-cut fiber should be checked for sharp edges and/or beam deviation and if necessary cut again. Beam scattering, however, is not a too big problem when working in contact mode.

Coming to laser application devices, it should be kept in mind that space inside the nasal cavity is limited. The operative field has to accommodate an endoscope, usually 4.0 mm in diameter, the laser fiber with a guide and suction instruments to evacuate smoke or fluids. Generally, endonasal laser procedures can be performed two-handed or single-handed. In a two-handed procedure, the right hand usually carries the laser fiber applicator, which, in our case, is a rigid irrigation tube with a tip bent in various angles from 30° over 45° to 90° and a lateral tap, to which the smoke evacuation tube can be attached (Fig. 3). The laser fiber port is sealed

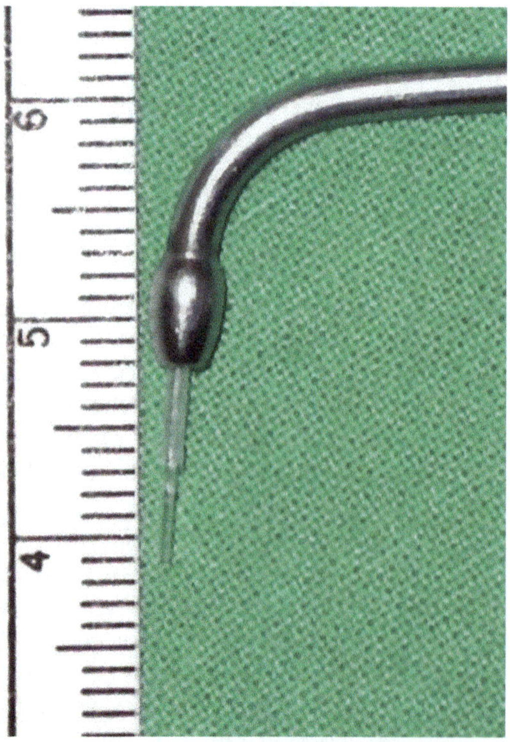

Fig. 3 Rigid 90° angled applicator as guide for 600 μm (core diameter) laser fiber

airtight in order to prevent vacuum leaks. The left hand carries the endoscope with the CCD camera attached to it. This arrangement has the advantage of flexibly guiding both devices, which can be useful whenever the laser fiber should be retracted inside the guide for greater rigidity in close tissue contact, while the endoscope stays further away to maintain the overview and become less susceptible to lens contamination. The disadvantage is that handling two devices independently inside the nasal cavity can be difficult. For a single-handed procedure, we have developed and used a semi rigid applicator (PolyDiagnost GmbH, Pfaffenhofen, Germany) with a flexible tip of 25 mm in length which can be bent to a 180° angle unloaded, which is reduced to 120° accommodating a 20 μm core fiber (Fig. 4). This device has an outer diameter of 4 mm, giving maximum flexibility inside the operative field. The inner lining of the device contains two ducts of 300 μm diameter each and further two ducts with an inner diameter of 1200 μm each. Usually one of the smaller ducts accommodates the laser fiber of 200 μm in diameter while the larger ducts are used for smoke evacuation and, if available, a thin flexible endoscope. However, as the ducts are very limited in size, smoke evacuation capacity and image quality from the endoscope is limited.

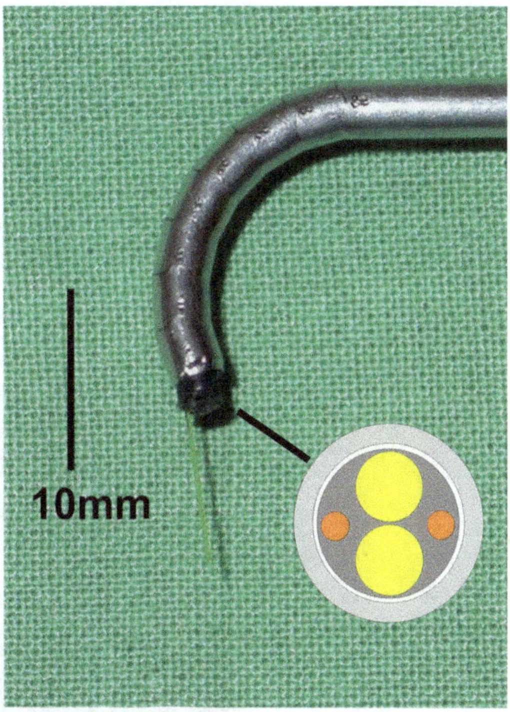

Fig. 4 Adjustable tip of flexible applicator with a 200 μm laser fiber and (*insert*) cross-sectional sketch of four channels contained in the inner sleeve (two channels with an inner diameter of 300 μm, accommodating a 200 μm laser fiber, and two channels of 1200 μm diameter for, e.g., irrigation, smoke suction, and flexible miniature endoscopes)

Techniques for Treating Different Types of Tissue

Endonasal polyps are soft, flabby structures with a grayish looking color representing a high water content with little vascularization. They can be pedunculated, differentiating them from mucosal edema, which is broad-based and more generalized over the mucosal area. Polyps can be shrunk in near-contact mode by evaporating their contents, although the temperature of irradiated tissue can rise exponentially as soon as its water content is used up. Therefore, in our experience it is preferable to cut polyps from the stalk in contact mode in a brush-like fashion. If the polyp is resected, it usually sticks to the laser fiber, making harvesting easy. This procedure is usually swift and has the advantage of leaving the polyp intact, which is therefore available for histological examination. It is useful to subcategorize polyps for their content with either neutrophil or eosinophil granulocyte content, in order to adapt medication and postoperative care to the underlying pathology.

Mucoceles are retention cysts that occur when previous surgery or trauma with fracture across the paranasal sinuses leads to scar tissue formation, which blocks the drainage of mucous from mucosal glands. Due to considerable internal pressure building up from the inside, mucoceles can destroy adjacent bone which can lead to penetration of the anterior skull base or the periorbit. As in these cases the dura of the frontal brain or the orbit is exposed, care should be taken to avoid irradiation in contact mode. However, the fluid inside the mucocele usually prevents the underlying tissue from overheating, so "uncapping" the cystic wall in contact mode is feasible with a Neodymium:YAG laser (Fig. 5). In postoperative follow-up, however, care should be taken to remove crusts and mucus across the resection margins, which may lead to reformation of mucoceles.

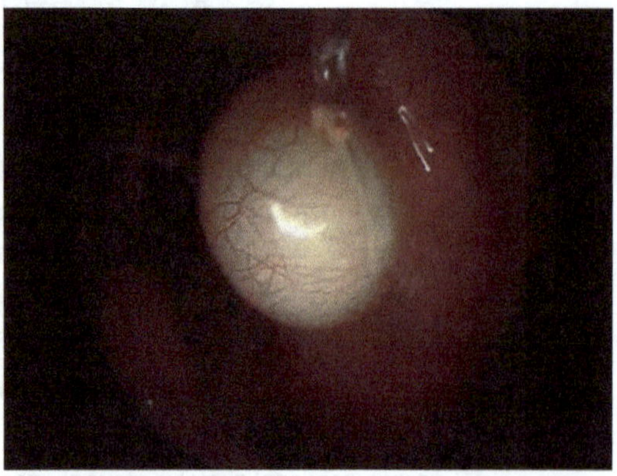

Fig. 5 600 μm laser fiber in contact with a retention cyst of the left maxillary sinus ostium. View through 30° angled Hopkins endoscope (Karl Storz, Tuttlingen)

Synechiae, as mentioned before, are transverse formations of scar tissue that usually occur between the septal wall and one of the three nasal turbinates attached to the lateral wall of the nasal cavity. They usually occur during wound healing following surgery or trauma in nasal cavities that are narrow, whenever mucus or crusts form a bridge between the two wound areas. Fibroblasts can grow over the mucus and turn temporary adhesions into permanent scars. By means of a fiber-guided laser, transverse scars can be cut at either end, therefore making reformation of synechiae less likely. In some cases as in narrow endonasal cavities, however, it is necessary to place silicone sheets in between wound areas until the first phases of wound healing have passed, which is usually accomplished after 14 days.

Granulating tissue is a part of normal wound healing following FESS and therefore should be primarily addressed with topical steroids, systemic leukotriene antagonists, etc. However, granulating tissue sometimes overgrows the endonasal wound during the healing process following FESS, so that, when granulating tissue is populated with fibroblasts, there is a risk of scar formation across paranasal sinus ostia inflicting mucocele formation and synechiae. Thus, in selected cases, removal of excessive granulating tissue can be helpful in order to guide local wound healing and prevent scar formation in unwanted areas [43, 44]. Normally granulating tissue is quite flat and adherent to the base of wound. Thus it is difficult to excise, harvesting it for histological examination. However, thermal injury should be avoided as far as possible, using small fiber diameters, working in contact mode and limiting laser power settings to 10 W maximum.

In summary, we compared 175 Neodymium:YAG laser revision procedures with 268 FESS revision surgeries for the recurrence of CRS. As for histological features of wound healing, the only difference between laser procedures and FESS surgery was that there was a prolonged appearance of tissue edema following laser surgery. This effect was also seen by Metson and Gerlinger as mentioned earlier. However, this observation did not show any impact on wound healing at all, as in both modalities, the distinct histological stages of healing process, i.e., the appearance of fibrin coating after the operation, the prevalence of granulocytes, lymphocytes, collagen, as well as epithelialization with squamous cell epithelium versus respiratory epithelium were comparable.

Histology showed that from Neodymium:YAG laser application in edematous endonasal tissue in contact mode at 10 W cw under feedback power control, no carbonization could be observed, while the coagulation zone extended about 50 μm into the resection margins (Fig. 6). At 30 W, there was a carbonization zone of about 2 μm width, as coagulation zone extended 50–100 μm into the lateral resection margins (Fig. 7).

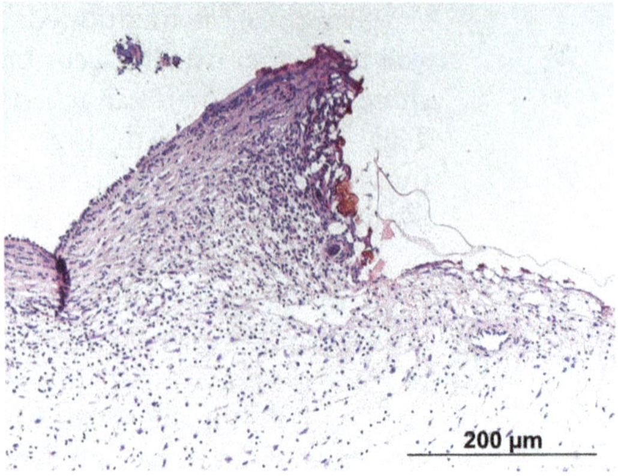

Fig. 6 Histological image of laser–tissue interaction from Neodymium:YAG laser in contact mode, 10 W, cw, under negative feedback temperature control: no visible carbonization, coagulation zone extending about 50 μm into resection margin (source: Institute of Pathology, RWTH Aachen University, Director: Univ.-Prof. Dr. med. R. Knüchel-Clarke)

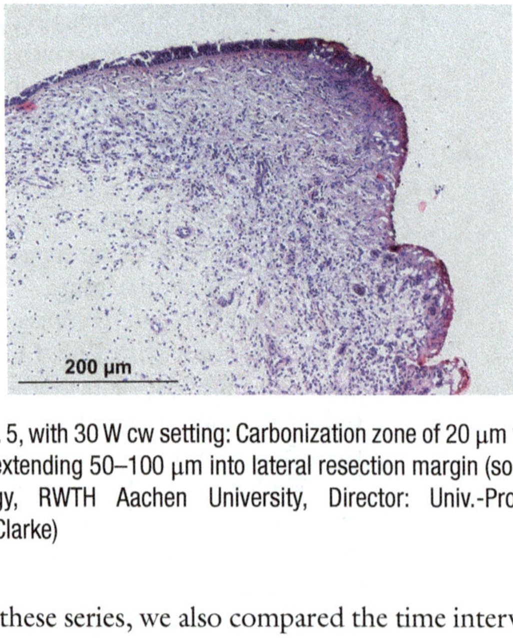

Fig. 7 As Fig. 5, with 30 W cw setting: Carbonization zone of 20 μm width, coagulation zone extending 50–100 μm into lateral resection margin (source: Institute of Pathology, RWTH Aachen University, Director: Univ.-Prof. Dr. med. R. Knüchel-Clarke)

From these series, we also compared the time intervals starting from the point of intervention to the next, when symptomatic reappearance of polyps, restenosis of paranasal sinus ostia, etc. in chronic rhinosinusitis required yet another surgical intervention—either another laser procedure or a full FESS revision. As a result, patients who had one revision by laser versus one FESS reintervention did not have a different risk to undergo a second revision ($P = 0.1529$).

In conclusion, lasers in endonasal surgery provide a useful addition to the repertoire of surgical tools [45–48] for a variety of procedures. Mainly the benefit for the patient, besides cost and time effectiveness, should be the guide for indicating laser interventions in contrast to conservative treatment or conventional surgery. The proximity of vital structures, in particular the contents of the orbit, the frontal dura and the internal carotid artery requires judicious choice of suitable laser systems, laser parameters and instrumentation. With these considerations in mind, the use of lasers in the nose and paranasal sinuses is a safe and reliable treatment option for suitable indications.

Acknowledgments

Histological examination was performed by the Institute of Pathology, RWTH Aachen University, Director: Univ.-Prof. Dr. med. R. Knüchel-Clarke

References

1. Kennedy DW. Prognostic factors, outcomes, and staging in ethmoid sinus surgery. Laryngoscope. 1992;102(Suppl57):1–18.
2. Rosenfeld RM, et al. Clinical practice guideline: Adult sinusitis. Otolaryngol Head Neck Surg. 2007;137:S1–S31.
3. Fokkens W, Lund V, Mullol J et al.. EPOS 2012: European Position Paper on Rhinosinusitis and Nasal Polyps 2012. *Rhinology* 2012;Suppl. 23:1–298
4. Ragab S, Scadding GK, Lund VJ, Saleh H. Treatment of chronic rhinosinusitis and its effects on asthma. Eur Respir J. 2006;28:68–74.
5. Seybt MW, McMains KC, Kountakis SE. The prevalence and effect of asthma on adults with chronic rhinosinusitis. Ear Nose Throat J. 2007;86:409–11.
6. Batra PS, Kern RC, Tripathi A, Conley DB, Ditto AM, Haines III GK, et al. Outcome analysis of endoscopic sinus surgery in patients with nasal polyps and asthma. Laryngoscope. 2003;113:1703–6.
7. Bachert C, Gevaert P, Holtappels G, van Cauwenberge P. Mediators in nasal polyposis. Curr Allergy Asthma Rep. 2002;2:481–7.
8. Bachert C, Gevaert P, van Cauwenberge P. Staphylococcus aureus enterotoxins: a key in airway disease? Allergy. 2002;57:480–7.
9. Ponikau JU, Sherris DA, Kephart GM, Adolphson C, Kita H. The role of ubiquitous airborne fungi in chronic rhinosinusitis. Curr Allergy Asthma Rep. 2005;5:472–6.
10. Ponikau JU, Sherris DA, Kita H, Kern EB. Intranasal antifungal treatment in 51 patients with chronic rhinosinusitis. J Allergy Clin Immunol. 2002;110:862–6.
11. Hochstim CJ, Masood R, Rice DH. Biofilm and persistent inflammation in endoscopic sinus surgery. Otolaryngol Head Neck Surg. 2010;143:697–8.
12. Singhal D, Foreman A, Jervis-Bardy J, Wormald PJ. Staphylococcus aureus biofilms: Nemesis of endoscopic sinus surgery. Laryngoscope. 2011;121:1578–83.
13. Stammberger H. Endoscopic endonasal surgery. Concepts in treatment of recurrent sinusitis. Part 1: Anatomic and pathophysiologic considerations. Otolaryngol Head Neck Surg. 1986;94:143–7.
14. Stammberger H. Endoscopic endonasal surgery. Concepts in treatment of recurrent sinusitis. Part 2: Surgical technique. Otolaryngol Head Neck Surg. 1986;94:147–56.
15. Mehanna H, Mills J, Kelly B, McGarry GW. Benefit from endoscopic sinus surgery. Clin Otolaryngol. 2002;27:464–71.
16. Larsen K, Tos M. A long-term follow-up study of nasal polyp patients after simple polypectomies. Eur Arch Otorhinolaryngol. 1997;254(Suppl1):S85–8.
17. Lenz H, Eichler J. Endonasal surgical technique with the argon laser. Laryngo-Rhino-Otologie. 1984;63:534–40.
18. Agarwal G, Kupferman ME, Holsinger FC, Hanna EY. Sinonasal and nasopharyngeal

applications of the hand-held CO2 laser fiber. Int Forum Allergy Rhinol. 2011;1:109–12.

19. Sato K. Endoscopic sinus surgery for the anterior maxillary sinus, using a 135 degrees reflective CO2 laser. J Laryngol Otol. 2008;122: 918–20.
20. Sato K, Nakashima T. Endoscopic sinus surgery for antrochoanal polyp using CO_2 laser and / or microresektor: a long-term result. J Laryngol Otol. 2005;119:362–5.
21. Sato K, Nakashima T. Endoscopic sinus surgery for chronic sinusitis with antrochoanal polyp. Laryngoscope. 2000;110:1581–3.
22. Shapshay SM, Rebeiz EE, Pankratov MM. Holmium:yttrium aluminium garnet laser-assisted endoscopic sinus surgery: clinical experience. Laryngoscope. 1992;102:1177–80.
23. Shapshay SM, Rebeiz EE, Bohigian K, Hybels RL, Aretz HT, Pankratov MM. Holmium: yttrium aluminium garnet laser-assisted endoscopic sinus surgery: laboratory experience. Laryngoscope. 1991;101:142–9.
24. Selkin SG. Pitfalls in intranasal laser surgery and how to avoid them. Arch Otolaryngol Head Neck Surg. 1986;112:285–9.
25. Lippert BM, Werner JA. Nd:YAG laser light-induced reduction of the nasal turbinates. Laryngo-Rhino-Otologie. 1996;75:523–8.
26. Jovanovic S, Dokic D. Nd:YAG laser surgery in treatment of allergic rhinitis. Laryngo-Rhino-Otologie. 1995;74:419–22.
27. Werner JA, Rudert H. Use of the Nd:YAG laser in otorhinolaryngology. HNO. 1992;40: 248–58.
28. Scherer H, Reichert K, Schildhauer S. Laser surgery of the middle nasal meatus in recurrent sinusitis. Laryngo-Rhino-Otologie. 1999;78: 50–3.
29. Ohyama M. Laser polypectomy. *Rhinology* 1989;Suppl.8:35-43
30. Zhang BQ. Comparison of results of laser and routine surgery therapy in treatment of nasal polyps. Chin Med J. 1993;106:707–8.
31. Gleich LL, Rebeiz EE, Pankratov MM, Shapshay SM. The Holmium:YAG laser assisted otolaryngologic procedures. Arch Otolaryngol Head Neck Surg. 1995;121:1162–6.
32. Kautzky M, Bigenzahn W, Steurer M, Susani M, Schenk P. Holmium:YAG laser surgery: possibilities for use in inflammatory paranasal sinus diseases. HNO. 1992;40:468–71.
33. Metson R. Holmium:YAG laser endoscopic sinus surgery. Laryngoscope. 1996;106:1–18.
34. Gerlinger I, Lujber L, Jarai T, Pytel J. KTP-532 laser-assisted endoscopic nasal sinus surgery. Clin Otolaryngol. 2003;28:67–71.
35. Wang HK, Wang PC, Tsai YH, Huang TC, Hsu SY. Endoscope-assisted KTP laser sinus clear-out procedure for recurrent ethmoid polyps. J Clin Laser Med Surg. 2003;21:93–8.
36. Levine HL. Lasers in endonasal surgery. Otolaryngol Clin N Am. 1997;30:451–5.
37. Kaluskar SK, Mehta R, Farnan TB, Basha SI. Endoscopic 532-nm KTP laser excision of inverted papilloma of the nose and paranasal sinuses: a series of 9 patients. Ear Nose Throat J. 2009;88:880–7.
38. Hesham A, Fathi A, Attia M, Safwat S, Hesham A. Laser and topical mitomycin C for management of nasal synechia after FESS: a preliminary report. Eur Arch Otorhinolaryngol. 2011;268:1289–92.
39. Bleier BS, Palmer JN, Gratton MA, Cohen NA. In vivo laser tissue welding in the rabbit maxillary sinus. Am J Rhinol. 2008;22:625–8.
40. Lesserson LA, Schaefer SD. Instrumentation for endoscopic sinus surgery. Ear Nose Throat J. 1984;73:522–31.
41. Rathfoot CJ, Duncavage J, Shapshay SM. Laser use in the paranasal sinuses. Otolaryngol Clin N Am. 1996;29:943–8.
42. Ossoff RH, Coleman JA, Courey MS, Duncavage JA, Werkhaven JA, Reinisch L. Clinical applications of lasers in otolaryngology—head and neck surgery. Lasers Surg Med. 1994;15:217–48.
43. Mori K, Tamura M, Kawamoto M, Shikina T, Asada H, Itami S, Kurane I, Kubo T. Modulation of T-cell functions by laser surgery in patients with allergic rhinitis. Acta Otolaryngol. 2003;123:704–8.
44. Kass EG, Massaro BM, Komorowski RA, Toohill RJ. Wound healing of KTP and argon laser lesions in the canine nasal cavity. Otolaryngol Head Neck Surg. 1993;108: 283–92.
45. Grevers G. A new surgical system for endoscopic paranasal sinus surgery. Laryngo-Rhino-Otologie. 1995;74:266–8.
46. Selivanova O, Kuehnemund M, Mann WJ, Amedee RG. Comparison of conventional instruments and mechanical debriders for surgery of patients with chronic rhinosinusitis. Am J Rhinol. 2003;17(4):197–202.
47. Slatkine M, Krespi YP. Instrumentation for office laser surgery. Operative techniques in otolaryngology. Head Neck Surg. 1994;5: 211–7.
48. Vauterin T, van der Poorten V, Jorissen M. Long term effects of cutting forceps in endoscopic sinus surgery. Rhinology. 2006;44: 123–7.

Chapter 10

Current Concepts in Laser Surgery: Endonasal Laser Turbinate Reduction

Miriam Havel and Andreas Leunig

Introduction

Inferior turbinate hypertrophy is a common cause of nasal airway obstruction. Whilst the initial mainstay of treatment for this condition is with the use of pharmacologic therapy such as steroids and antihistamines, there remains a considerable cohort of patients that are refractory to this treatment and require surgery. Numerous surgical techniques for inferior turbinate hypertrophy have been employed over the years, including total or partial turbinectomy, turbinoplasty (submucous resection, microdebrider, conchopexy, outfracture), laser surgery, and thermal techniques (electrocautery, cryosurgery, radiofrequency ablation) [1]. Techniques aiming at removal of most of the turbinate tissue including bony structures seem to provide the most distinct and long-lasting effects, but are also accompanied by higher morbidity [2]. Besides intra- and postoperative bleeding, adverse side effects observed include synechiae, nasal dryness and crusting, osteitis, foetor, atrophic rhinitis, etc. There is a general trend in the last decades leading toward mucosal sparing/tissue sparing techniques and steering away from extensive mucosal destruction (e.g., turbinectomy) as the latter modes of turbinate reduction are thought to be most associated with the mentioned secondary effects including empty nose syndrome [3–5]. Since the introduction of laser technology in the field, it has been demonstrated in numerous clinical studies that endonasal laser treatments cause

Brian J.-F. Wong and Justus Ilgner (eds.), *Biomedical Optics in Otorhinolaryngology: Head and Neck Surgery*,
DOI 10.1007/978-1-4939-1758-7_10, © Springer Science+Business Media New York 2016

limited tissue trauma with little or no bleeding and reach a high patient acceptance as they can be usually performed without nasal packing and under outpatient conditions [6].

Nasal Airway Obstruction and Inferior Turbinate

The inferior turbinate represents the main decongestant-responsive structure of the nasal cavity. Decongestion of the nasal mucosa is supposed to increase the volume of the nasal cavity by 35 % [7]. Surgical procedures for the treatment of hyperplastic inferior turbinates aim at reducing the volume of the inferior turbinate tissue, particularly its head or anterior portion, which is a component of the nasal valve representing the most resistive region in the nasal airway. The important physiological functions of inferior turbinate including warming, humidifying and filtering, as well as directing of the inspired air indicate that the nasal airflow improvement has to occur without affecting the nasal physiology. The mechanism of airflow perception is not fully understood. Nasal obstruction is commonly associated with an increased resistance in the nasal airway. However, objective measurements of nasal airway resistance often do not correlate with subjective extent of nasal obstruction. Damaged or resected trigeminal nerve endings can create the sensation of nasal obstruction without an objective increase in nasal airway resistance [2]. Thus, the preferred turbinate reduction procedure should aim at reducing the turbinate volume, preserving the airflow perception and turbinate shape responsible for directing the air stream, preserving physiological function while minimizing iatrogenic complications. Any technique resulting in extensive destruction of the turbinate mucosa runs a risk of a loss of physiological function leading to crusting and synechiae [8].

Laser Systems for Inferior Turbinate Surgery

Since the early 1980s, laser systems of various types have been employed for surgical endonasal applications including carbon dioxide (CO_2, λ[lambda] = 10.600 nm), Argon-ion (λ[lambda] = 488/514 nm), potassium titanyl phosphate (KTP, λ[lambda] = 532 nm), neodymium:yttrium–aluminium–garnet (Nd:YAG, λ[lambda] = 1.064 nm), holmium:yttrium–aluminium–garnet (Ho:YAG, λ[lambda] = 2.080 nm), and diode (λ[lambda] = 805/810/940/980/1470 nm) laser. Systems most frequently involved in inferior turbinate reduction include CO_2- and Nd:YAG lasers in the 1980s and 1990s, whereas in the course of 2000s clinical trials investigating the use of Ho:YAG, KTP, diode of different wavelengths, and argon ion lasers emerge [1, 6].

The basic difference between these medical laser systems is the wavelength of the emitted light, leading to altering light–tissue interactions due to optical parameters of the tissue. Besides the emitted wavelength, laser settings such as output power, operating mode (pulsed or continuous wave), and application mode (contact or non-contact application) fundamentally influence the induced tissue effects (see Table 1). Apart from the CO_2 laser, which has to be delivered via rigid hand piece/waveguide in clinical routine, all listed laser types can be delivered via a flexible quartz fibre providing precise and well-controlled application of the laser light toward the treated tissue in the narrow anatomical landscape of the nasal cavity. Recently, delivery mode for CO_2 laser by means of a hollow optical fibre also has been reported [9].

Regarding the laser light–tissue interaction, some laser type specific differences have to be taken into account. CO_2 laser is highly absorbed by water and provides superficial vaporization of turbinate tissue with a broad thermal coagulation zone of the surrounding tissue. In contrast, diode and Nd:YAG laser are poorly absorbed by water, tissue proteins, and blood and penetrate deeply into the tissue. In "noncontact" application, a large zone of coagulation results, whereas the "contact mode" offers effective tissue cutting with a small zone of coagulation. The pulsed Ho:YAG laser is also highly absorbed by water and combines bone and tissue vaporization abilities with good hemostasis in "contact" as well as "noncontact" mode. Due to the high absorbance by endogenous chromophores such as melanin and hemoglobin, light of Argon ion and KTP lasers shows good coagulative effects on venous

Table 1
Laser systems for inferior turbinate surgery (from Janda et al. [6], modified)

Laser	Wavelength (nm)	Mode	Delivery
Argon	488/514	cw	SiO_2-quartz
KTP	532	Pulsed	SiO_2-quartz
Diode	Various	cw	SiO_2-quartz
Nd:YAG	1064	cw/pulsed	SiO_2-quartz
Ho:YAG	2080	Pulsed	SiO_2-quartz
CO_2	10,600	cw/pulsed	Halide fibre Hollow waveguide

plexus of the lower turbinate providing an effective reduction of the cavernous body with preservation of the surrounding tissue [6, 10] and are also suitable for therapy of vascular malformations (e.g., hemangioma and hereditary hemorrhagic telangiectasia). In general, the optical penetration depth of the laser light applied to the turbinate tissue during the laser treatment depends on the optical properties of the tissue, described by the absorption and scattering coefficients.

Clinical Note

Careful patient selection, patient information, and indication prior to surgical decision-making are crucial for a favorable and patient-centered outcome. Preoperative workup including detailed history taking and endoscopic, as well as laboratory examination where appropriate, considering potential etiologic factors for nasal obstruction such as grossly deviated nasal septum, acute rhinitis/sinusitis, chronic rhinosinusitis, nasal polyps, or allergy are mandatory and should be addressed specifically. The cause and degree of the inferior turbinate enlargement is to be assessed and documented. The underlying pathology may require pre- and postoperative medical management to prevent recurrences of turbinate hypertrophy.

Besides the implementation of laser safety measures, an adequate preoperative preparation of the patient includes decongestion and anesthesia of the nasal cavity. For this purpose insertion of cotton pads soaked with, e.g., 4 % tetracaine and 0.5 % xylometazoline solution (1:1) applied for 10–15 min are effective.

Laser light application itself is facilitated by endoscopes (except for CO_2 laser, where a microscope and a micromanipulator is commonly used) and can be carried out via guiding the fibre from the posterior to the anterior free edge of the inferior turbinate under endoscopic control producing controlled tissue effects in linear or punctiform application mode (Fig. 1a, b). The induced tissue effect of laser light results in visible blanching of the tissue. Visually controlled and targeted application of laser light is mandatory to prevent lesions of surrounding tissue with intraoperative bleeding and/or subsequent synechiae in case of corresponding lesions.

In cases where the head of inferior turbinate seems especially prominent, some single laser spots can be directed additionally onto the head of the turbinate. Postoperatively, nasal cavities can be treated with an antibiotic and steroid-containing ointment and patient may receive prescriptions for nasal ointments and topical

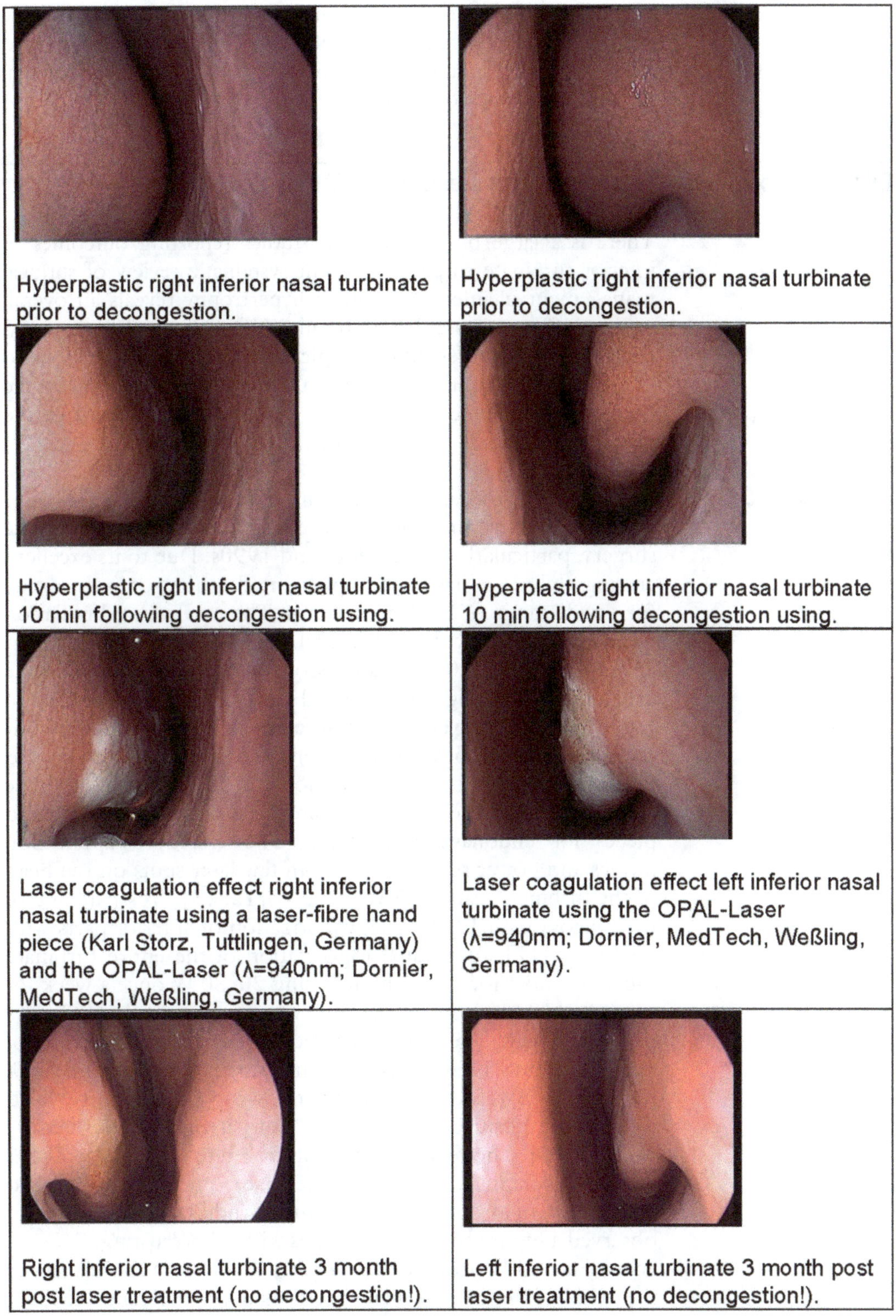

Fig. 1 (a, b). Application of laser light (*left panel* punctiform, *right panel* linear application mode); in this example performed in a "non-contact" mode using a flexible silica fibre (600 μm core diameter) fixed onto a custom-designed device for precise endonasal fibre guidance (ENT-Fibre Guidance System, Karl Storz, Tuttlingen, Germany)

decongestants. Postoperative care visits including endoscopic examination and documentation allow for the assessment of wound healing condition and evaluation, as well as for treatment of possibly occurring complications.

Clinical Outcomes of Laser Surgery for Treatment of Turbinate Hypertrophy

There is a large body of clinical studies reporting outcomes of inferior turbinate surgery. A recent systematic review of surgical management of inferior turbinate hypertrophy reveals an overall positive effect on nasal breathing in 97 % of almost 100 reviewed clinical trials regardless of the surgical technique used [1]. Around one-third (32 %) of the reviewed studies consists of reports on the use of laser technology for inferior turbinate reduction, with the oldest being published in 1982 [11].

Carbon dioxide Laser

Regarding the to date published literature, carbon dioxide laser seems to be the most widely used laser system for turbinate surgery, particularly in the 1980s and 1990s. Due to its excellent cutting abilities is has been implemented in the surgical routine for a wide range of ENT procedures. The mid infrared radiation of CO_2 laser is effectively absorbed by water with a limited penetration depth of 0.01 mm and poor coagulation and hemostatic capabilities. Laser light is delivered via a mirror beam guide system with hollow waveguides of different shapes. Microscope controlled application of waveguide delivered beam might be limited by the narrow anatomical conditions of the nasal cavity. Some authors describe the use of custom made or self-designed hand pieces for endonasal procedures. The employed application modes and power settings vary from few laser spots on the head of the turbinate using 1–5 W or 10 W [12, 13], crosshatching of the mucosa with 12 W [14], vaporization of anterior parts with 15 W [15–17], to gradual vaporization of the entire turbinate mucosa (under local anesthesia) using 20–30 W once a week for 5 weeks [18, 19]. Nasal packing was often used for 1–2 days postoperatively. The degree of the subjective improvement of nasal breathing 12 months following surgery varied from 57 % [14] to 93 % [15], a long-term follow up of 5 years revealed long-lasting positive effects in 77 % of patients as described by Lippert [13]. The reported complication rate amounts to 3–4 % with postoperative bleeding, synechiae, mucosa dryness and around 1 % of atrophic rhinitis in most studies. However, Passali observed a higher complication rates with 74 % crusting, 7 % synechiae, and 11 % atrophic rhinitis [20]. CO_2-laser vaporization of the whole inferior turbinate performed in local anesthesia in pediatric patient cohort (age 9–15 years) under microscopic control using 5–10 W defocused laser beam as compared to Nd:YAG laser treatment was reported by Araki et al. with 86 % of beneficiary outcome 2 weeks postoperatively regardless of the laser system used. Adverse effects were not observed, a long-term follow up was not provided [21].

Argon-Ion Laser

In one of the first reports published on laser reduction of hyperplastic inferior nasal turbinates more than 2000 patients with nasal obstruction due to vasomotor rhinitis were treated with a continuous wave argon laser in noncontact mode by laser strip carbonization with 8 W. A group of 96 patients was followed up for 2 years with 80 % reporting improved nasal breathing. Besides an extensive crusting for 4–6 weeks, tissue necrosis on the nasal septum in six cases and bony sequestra of the turbinate bone in two cases were observed [10]. No adverse effects in smaller patient groups treated with this laser type were reported decades later [22, 23]. High purchase cost, as well as power supply and cooling requirements are mentioned as drawbacks of this laser system.

KTP Laser

Also absorbed by chromophores, the pulsed KTP laser was applied at 6–8 W on anterior part of the inferior turbinate by crosshatching the mucosa with islands of healthy nasal mucosa left between the vaporizations in noncontact mode in 29 patients suffering from allergic or vasomotor rhinitis. After a follow-up period of 6–12 months, 81 % of the patients described a subjective improvement of the nasal airway passage, as well as less nasal congestion and rhinorrhea. No side effects and complications were reported [24]. A retrospective assessment of 124 patients treated with KTP laser at 7 W revealed an improved nasal airway in 87 % after 1 year [25].

Ho:YAG Laser

Some studies investigated the value of the Ho:YAG laser in the reduction of hyperplastic inferior nasal turbinates. Leunig et al. treated 85 patients with nasal obstruction due to allergic or vasomotor rhinitis with a pulsed Ho:YAG laser in contact mode at a repetition rate of 4 ± 8Hz and an energy of 0.8 ± 1.2 J per pulse. A follow up period of 12 months was completed by 52 patients showing subjective improvement of the nasal airflow in 77 %. Minor bleedings and postoperative pain in two cases, as well as nasal dryness in one case, were observed [26]. Serrano et al. used a Ho:YAG laser of 0.8 J per pulse in a contact mode at a repetition rate of 5 Hz for treatment of 46 patients. Improvement in nasal obstruction was noted in 52 % of patients 16 months after the laser treatment and prolonged crusting in three cases, one synechia and dysaesthesia of the nose in some cases were described [27]. In a small patient group of children

($n = 8$, age 8–16 years) Ho:YAG laser application efficacy was assessed retrospectively as compared to a group treated with surface diathermy and showed lower morbidity in the laser treated patients. However, both treatment modalities had a poor long-term outcome [28].

Nd:YAG Laser

Several clinicians evaluated Nd:YAG laser in the 1990s era with its excellent coagulation capabilities due to the deep tissue penetration. A noncontact application of Nd:YAG laser at 5–10 W under endoscopic control in a group of 89 patients with 40 eligible for a follow-up reporting improvement of nasal breathing in 73 % after 1 year and 65 % after 2 years of surgery was presented. Concerning postoperative healing, extensive nasal crusting in 24 % of patients was observed [29]. Olthoff et al. used a continuous wave Nd:YAG laser for turbinate surgery in contact mode in 117 patients at a power of 8 W. Forty patients were followed up for a period of 22 months, of which 80 % described a subjective improvement of the nasal airflow. In 15 % of the cases, pain during the treatment and postoperative nasal dryness after the surgery was observed [30]. A combination of interstitial and contact approaches using Nd:YAG laser photocoagulation for treatment of inferior turbinate hypertrophy under local anesthesia yielded improved results in terms of postoperative nasal patency at 1-year follow-up of 86 % in a group of 121 patients with very low complication rate. The relapse rate was approximately 14 %, predominantly in patients with allergic rhinitis. Thus, the authors concluded an accurate preoperative evaluation of the cause of the turbinate hypertrophy to be fundamental to achieve better results after laser turbinectomy and reduce the risk of recurrences [31].

Diode Laser

Similar to the Nd:YAG laser, diode laser systems also provide good coagulation capabilities. The tissue penetration depth is not as deep as in Nd:YAG laser, thus some authors regard diode lasers to produce deep but controllable tissue coagulation with a little risk of periostal damage of the turbinate bone and a favorable postoperative outcome in terms of improved postoperative healing due to reduced tissue swelling period [32]. These observations yielded from a clinical study with continuous wave diode laser light (940 nm) applied in noncontact mode at 8 ± 10 W on 76 patients. Fifty patients were followed up for 1 year. Six months following surgery 86 % of the patients described a subjective improvement of the nasal airflow, while 1 year after the laser treatment the number decreased to 76 %. Minor bleeding was observed in 6 % of the cases but did not require nasal packing. Concerning complications, 8 % of the patients reported about nasal dryness and 6 % about pain shortly after the operation [32].

Min et al. reported about the value of contact turbinate surgery in 53 patients using a diode laser (810 nm). The laser light was applied in continuous wave at a power of 15 W, photocoagulating the turbinate surface by crosshatching the mucosa. No postoperative packing was used. Six months after the treatment the authors observed a significant improvement of the nasal airway objectively documented by rhinomanometry. There were no complications or side effects described and the mucociliary function was postoperatively restored as assessed by saccharine transit time [33].

In a prospective clinical investigation, the therapeutic effect of diode laser (830 nm) inferior turbinate reduction on nasal obstruction and decongestant abuse in 42 patients was evaluated. Treatment efficiency was assessed 1 and 6 weeks, as well as 6 and 12 months following surgery. Subjective pre and posttherapeutic nasal airflow and patient satisfaction were rated on visual analogue scales. Assessment of the long-term objective clinical effectiveness was based on rhinomanometry, photodocumentation, and the need for decongestants. No perioperative complications occurred. Postoperative edema disappeared within the first week and crusting within 6 weeks after surgery. A total of 88 % of patients managed to successfully stop decongestant abuse after 6 months, 74 % after 1 year [34].

In summary, most of the commonly available diode laser systems provide light at wavelengths of $\lambda = 800–1000$ nm, mainly causing coagulative tissue effects when applied in noncontact mode. Diode lasers also have lower acquisition and maintenance costs than the CO_2 or Nd-YAG devices. Due to their smaller size, transportability, and power supply requirements they are also more versatile in the clinical setting. Reflecting these advantages, diode laser systems of various wavelengths were increasingly employed in inferior turbinate surgery in the last years as indicated in the recent literature [35–39].

Comparative Studies

A comparative evaluation of three laser systems: CO_2, Nd:YAG, and diode (805 nm) lasers for inferior turbinate reduction surgery under endoscopic control was conducted in a total of 46 patients, who were randomized into three treatment groups and followed for more than 1 year. The laser application was endoscopically guided using a hollow waveguide in the case of the CO_2 laser and a flexible fibres for the diode and Nd:YAG laser. In the latter cases, a continuous wave laser beam of a power of 8 W was applied in contact mode in a crosshatched way onto the entire turbinate. Subjective and objective data were collected. Subjective improvement of nasal airway was achieved in 41 % (diode), 47 % (Nd:YAG), and 57 % (CO_2) of patients The difference between the groups was not statistically significant. There was more postoperative bleeding in the CO_2 laser group with three patients requiring nasal packing. The CO_2 laser procedure also took longer to perform [14].

A large group of patients ($n=533$) with hyperplastic inferior turbinates was treated CO_2 and Nd:YAG laser techniques. The therapeutic results of both types of laser turbinectomy were reported and compared with those of submucosal diathermy. The CO_2 laser treatment was conducted under operating microscope by the application of laser spots to the head of the turbinate, whereas in the Nd:YAG laser procedure, diffuse, low-power irradiation of the entire concha was performed under endoscopic control. The authors observed positive effect only already few days following the CO_2 laser procedure and state that no follow-up treatment was required in this group of patients. By contrast, positive effects of Nd:YAG laser treatment only became evident within weeks or months and was attributed to the slow scarring process. Compared to submucosal diathermy, both laser methods produced better long-term results. Two years postoperatively, the overall success rate as defined by patient satisfaction was 80 % for the CO_2 laser, 68 % for the Nd:YAG laser, and 36 % for submucosal diathermy [13].

Another comparative evaluation of long-term effects of the Ho:YAG laser with diode laser (940 nm) for turbinate surgery showed a significant subjective and objective (rhinomanometry) improvement of nasal airflow within a follow-up of 6 months and 3 years as compared to the preoperative data in 68 % (Ho:YAG, $n=80$) and 74 % (diode, $n=113$) of patients. Adverse effects (nasal dryness and pain) were rare (<5 %) and occurred solely during the first weeks after the intervention. A wound healing period of 3–4 weeks (diode) and of 1–2 weeks (Ho:YAG) was observed. No significant long-term differences between the two investigated groups were detected [40].

Current Concepts in Turbinate Surgery

In recently published investigations the authors direct their attention more toward patient-centered issues that are beyond feasibility examination of the involved laser systems. Evaluation of postoperative patients' comfort (day surgery, no nasal packing), quality of life, and patient satisfaction, as well as assessment of wound healing during the postoperative period seems to come to the fore.

From the technical point of view also the needs of the user seem to be adequately met in the last years, considering the compact design of the laser system devices enhancing their transportability, as well as the moderate costs increasing their clinical availability.

Conclusion

Since the beginning of the 1980s, increasing involvement of laser-based techniques for the treatment of inferior turbinate hypertrophy as well as other endonasal application aside from conventional surgical procedures has been reported. Generally, the aims of surgery are to reduce the size of the turbinate to increase airflow, avoid complication and preserve nasal physiology (humidifying, warming, and directing of inhaled air). Moreover, further general considerations for technique selection include clinical setting (in-office versus operating room), cost of the device used, efficacy of the procedure, and extent of possible postoperative complications such as bleeding, adhesion formation, and crusting potentially compromising patient's safety and comfort.

The treatment of hyperplastic inferior nasal turbinates by means of different laser systems represents an effective alternative to conventional therapeutic procedures and has been established in the rhinological routine since several decades. The cost-effective and timesaving application can be performed as an outpatient procedure under local anesthesia in a short operation time without nasal packing providing high patient acceptance. Currently, various laser systems are in clinical use for the reduction of hyperplastic inferior nasal turbinates. Along with the variety of possible laser settings and application modes, it is comprehensible that there is no single technique which is effective in all patients or which represents a gold standard. Depending on the chosen parameters and the clinical experience and expertise of the surgeon, it is possible to induce very similar tissue effects with laser emissions of different wavelengths rendering good patient-centered results in terms of satisfactory symptom relieve and reasonable long-term outcome. However, to determine the exact value of laser treatment in comparison to other surgical techniques, prospective controlled trials implementing different methods for the reduction of hyperplastic inferior nasal turbinates are needed.

Laser treatment of hyperplastic inferior turbinates can be considered as a useful, cost effective, time-saving procedure that can frequently be performed as an outpatient procedure under local anesthesia, providing satisfactory symptom relieve and high patient comfort. The choice of laser device is dependent on personal preference, training curve of the surgeon and personal experience in treatment and postoperative clinical results, revealing advantages and drawbacks of the specific laser device used.

References

1. Batra PS, Seiden AM, Smith TL. Surgical management of adult inferior turbinate hypertrophy: a systematic review of the evidence. Laryngoscope. 2009;119(9):1819–27.
2. Willatt D. The evidence for reducing inferior turbinates. Rhinology. 2009;47(3):227–36.
3. Moore GF, Freeman TJ, Ogren FP, Yonkers AJ. Extended follow-up of total inferior turbinate resection for relief of chronic nasal obstruction. Laryngoscope. 1985;95(9 Pt 1):1095–9.
4. Warwick-Brown NP, Marks NJ. Turbinate surgery: how effective is it? A long-term assessment. ORL J Otorhinolaryngol Relat Spec. 1987;49(6):314–20.
5. Chhabra N, Houser SM. The diagnosis and management of empty nose syndrome. Otolaryngol Clin North Am. 2009;42(2):311–30.
6. Janda P, Sroka R, Baumgartner R, Grevers G, Leunig A. Laser treatment of hyperplastic inferior nasal turbinates: a review. Lasers Surg Med. 2001;28(5):404–13.
7. Grymer LF, Hilberg O, Pedersen OF, Rasmussen TR. Acoustic rhinometry: values from adults with subjective normal nasal patency. Rhinology. 1991;29(1):35–47.
8. Hol MK, Huizing EH. Treatment of inferior turbinate pathology: a review and critical evaluation of the different techniques. Rhinology. 2000;38(4):157–66.
9. Temelkuran B, Hart SD, Benoit G, Joannopoulos JD, Fink Y. Wavelength-scalable hollow optical fibres with large photonic bandgaps for CO2 laser transmission. Nature. 2002;420(6916):650–3.
10. Lenz H. 8 years' laser surgery of the inferior turbinates in vasomotor rhinopathy in the form of laser strip carbonization. HNO. 1985; 33(9):422–5.
11. Mittelman H. CO2 laser turbinectomies for chronic, obstructive rhinitis. Lasers Surg Med. 1982;2(1):29–36.
12. Mladina R, Risavi R, Subaric M. CO2 laser anterior turbinectomy in the treatment of nonallergic vasomotor rhinopathia. A prospective study upon 78 patients. Rhinology. 1991; 29(4):267–71.
13. Lippert BM, Werner JA. CO2 laser surgery of hypertrophied inferior turbinates. Rhinology. 1997;35(1):33–6.
14. DeRowe A, Landsberg R, Leonov Y, Katzir A, Ophir D. Subjective comparison of Nd:YAG, diode, and CO2 lasers for endoscopically guided inferior turbinate reduction surgery. Am J Rhinol. 1998;12(3):209–12.
15. Englender M. Nasal laser mucotomy (L-mucotomy) of the interior turbinates. J Laryngol Otol. 1995;109(4):296–9.
16. Elwany S, Abdel-Moneim MH. Carbon dioxide laser turbinectomy. An electron microscopic study. J Laryngol Otol. 1997;111(10): 931–4.
17. Lagerholm S, Harsten G, Emgård P, Olsson B. Laser-turbinectomy: long-term results. J Laryngol Otol. 1999;113(6):529–31.
18. Fukutake T, Yamashita T, Tomoda K, Kumazawa T. Laser surgery for allergic rhinitis. Arch Otolaryngol Head Neck Surg. 1986;112(12):1280–2.
19. Kawamura S, Fukutake T, Kubo N, Yamashita T, Kumazawa T. Subjective results of laser surgery for allergic rhinitis. Acta Otolaryngol Suppl. 1993;500:109–12.
20. Passàli D, Lauriello M, Anselmi M, Bellussi L. Treatment of hypertrophy of the inferior turbinate: long-term results in 382 patients randomly assigned to therapy. Ann Otol Rhinol Laryngol. 1999;108(6):569–75.
21. Araki S, Suzuki N, Sato H, Yamaguchi T, Fujita H, Umezawa Y, Suzuki M. Endoscopic laser treatment for pediatric nasal allergy. Diagn Ther Endosc. 2000;6(4):189–92.
22. Ferri E, Armato E, Cavaleri S, Capuzzo P, Ianniello F. Argon plasma surgery for treatment of inferior turbinate hypertrophy: a long-term follow-up in 157 patients. ORL J Otorhinolaryngol Relat Spec. 2003;65(4):206–10.
23. Ottaviani F, Capaccio P, Cesana BM, Manzo R, Peri A. Argon plasma coagulation in the treatment of nonallergic hypertrophic inferior nasal turbinates. Am J Otolaryngol. 2003;24(5): 306–10.
24. Levine HL. The potassium--titanyl phosphate laser for treatment of turbinate dysfunction. Otolaryngol Head Neck Surg. 1991;104(2): 247–51.
25. Wang HK, Tsai YH, Wu YY, Wang PC. Endoscopic potassium-titanyl-phosphate laser treatment for the reduction of hypertrophic inferior nasal turbinate. Photomed Laser Surg. 2004;22(3):173–6.
26. Leunig A, Janda P, Sroka R, Baumgartner R, Grevers G. Ho:YAG laser treatment of hyperplastic inferior nasal turbinates. Laryngoscope. 1999;109(10):1690–5.
27. Serrano E, Percodani J, Yardeni E, Lombard L, Laffitte F, Pessey JJ. The holmium:YAG laser for treatment of inferior turbinate hypertrophy. Rhinology. 1998;36(2):77–80.

28. Rejali SD, Upile T, McLellan D, Bingham BJ. Inferior turbinate reduction in children using Holmium YAG laser-a clinical and histological study. Lasers Surg Med. 2004;34(4):310–4.
29. Lippert BM, Werner JA. Comparison of carbon dioxide and neodymium: yttrium-aluminum-garnet lasers in surgery of the inferior turbinate. Ann Otol Rhinol Laryngol. 1997;106(12): 1036–42.
30. Olthoff A, Martin A, Liebmann F. Nd:YAG laser treatment of the lower turbinates with contact in hyperreflexic and allergic rhinopathy. Laryngorhinootologie. 1999;78(5):240–3.
31. Vagnetti A, Gobbi E, Algieri GM, D'Ambrosio L. Wedge turbinectomy: a new combined photocoagulative Nd:YAG laser technique. Laryngoscope. 2000;110(6):1034–6.
32. Janda P, Sroka R, Tauber S, Baumgartner R, Grevers G, Leunig A. Diode laser treatment of hyperplastic inferior nasal turbinates. Lasers Surg Med. 2000;27(2):129–39.
33. Caffier PP, Frieler K, Scherer H, Sedlmaier B, Göktas O. Rhinitis medicamentosa: therapeutic effect of diode laser inferior turbinate reduction on nasal obstruction and decongestant abuse. Am J Rhinol. 2008;22(4): 433–9.
34. Min YG, Kim HS, Yun YS, Kim CS, Jang YJ, Jung TG. Contact laser turbinate surgery for the treatment of idiopathic rhinitis. Clin Otolaryngol Allied Sci. 1996;21(6):533–6.
35. Parida PK, Surianarayanan G, Alexander A, Saxena SK, Santhosh K. Diode laser turbinate reduction in the treatment of symptomatic inferior turbinate hypertrophy. Indian J Otolaryngol Head Neck Surg. 2013;65 Suppl 2:350–5.
36. Kassab AN, Rifaat M, Madian Y. Comparative study of management of inferior turbinate hypertrophy using turbinoplasty assisted by microdebrider or 980 nm diode laser. J Laryngol Otol. 2012;126(12):1231–7.
37. Cakli H, Cingi C, Güven E, Gurbuz MK, Kaya E. Diode laser treatment of hypertrophic inferior turbinates and evaluation of the results with acoustic rhinometry. Eur Arch Otorhinolaryngol. 2012;269(12):2511–7.
38. Caffier PP, Scherer H, Neumann K, Lück S, Enzmann H, Haisch A. Diode laser treatment in therapy-resistant allergic rhinitis: impact on nasal obstruction and associated symptoms. Lasers Med Sci. 2011;26(1):57–67.
39. Havel M, Sroka R, Leunig A, Patel P, Betz CS. A double-blind, randomized, intra-individual controlled feasibility trial comparing the use of 1,470 and 940 nm diode laser for the treatment of hyperplastic inferior nasal turbinates. Lasers Surg Med. 2011;43(9):881–6.
40. Sroka R, Janda P, Killian T, Vaz F, Betz CS, Leunig A. Comparison of long term results after Ho:YAG and diode laser treatment of hyperplastic inferior nasal turbinates. Lasers Surg Med. 2007;39(4):324–31.

Chapter 11

Laser-Lithotripsy of Salivary Stones

Ronald Sroka, Vanessa von Holzschuher, Pamela Zengel, and Florian Schrötzlmair

Introduction

The risk of developing salivary calculi during lifetime is approximately 1–2 % [1], while the incidence of symptomatic sialolithiasis was estimated to be 56/1,000,000 inhabitants in England [2]. Sialoliths originate within the submandibular (83 %), parotid (10 %), or sublingual gland (7 %). They are located either within the glandular tissue or in the salivary ducts [1]. Depending on the size and location of the stone, salivary duct obstruction occurs, causing pain, swelling, and sometimes infection, which may lead to the development of abscess, phlegmonous inflammation, and fistula. In order to remove stones from the salivary system, different methods are in clinical use.

Patients suffering from sialoliths of less than 2 mm in diameter without any acute symptoms underwent conservative treatment, such as stimulation of salivary production, dilatation of the orifice, or "wait and see" strategy as first treatment options [3]. In case of larger, intraductal sialoliths, enoral slitting of the duct is one of the most effective and safe methods for stone removal from the submandibular duct if the sialoliths are located near to the papilla, though it carries several risks if the stone is positioned beyond the knee of Wharton's duct [4]. Enoral slitting is not recommended for the removal of parotideal duct sialoliths. Extracorporeal shock wave lithotripsy is preferred for intraglandular stones and is effective in more than 50 %. However, this treatment holds several disadvantages like the risk of bleed-

Brian J.-F. Wong and Justus Ilgner (eds.), *Biomedical Optics in Otorhinolaryngology: Head and Neck Surgery*,
DOI 10.1007/978-1-4939-1758-7_11,

ing, hematoma, infection (<1 %), abscess formation, hearing impairment, tinnitus, or damage to teeth. Additionally, it is a time-consuming procedure as 4–8 sessions of about 30 min each are needed [4–6]. Over the last decades interventional sialendoscopy has been developed, which allows removal of stones up to a size of 5 mm by suction, basket, balloon, grasper, or miniforceps with and without fragmentation [7–13]. External removal by small incisions is rarely indicated and holds the risk of facial nerve palsy, bleeding, reduced skin sensitivity, or scar formation. Surgical removal of the affected gland is indicated for intraglandular stones that are refractory to other methods. Furthermore, this method holds the risk of a permanent damage to the marginal mandibular branch of the facial nerve (submandibular gland) or the facial nerve (parotid gland) [14, 15]. Both, intracorporeal electrohydraulic and piezoelectric lithotripsy have shown to have fairly good fragmentation capability. However, there is a high percentage of ductal perforations [16, 17]. Endoscopic laser lithotripsy of salivary stones has rarely been published so far and thus there is a lack of experience [5, 8, 18–23], while for urolithiasis, several laser types are in clinical use and have been intensively investigated. Possible reason is the small diameter of the salivary ducts and thus the sialendoscopes need to have reduced diameter in comparison to the ureteroscopes used in the urinary tract. Though first reports on laser lithotripsy of salivary stones using the excimer- [19, 22], the pulsed-dye laser [8, 20], and the CO_2 laser [18] date back to the early 1990s, only some single case studies have been published since then [5, 24]. Newer laser systems such as the Ho:YAG laser and the Er:YAG laser, both with low risk of tissue damage and good fragmentation rates of uroliths [25, 26], have only recently been investigated in sialolithiasis [23, 27, 28]. Another development in laser lithotripters is the FREDDY laser, which is expected to carry an extremely low risk of tissue damage due to the low absorption of the laser pulses by the tissue at this wavelength [29–32].

With respect to the insufficient information about the laser impact on salivary stones and its possible interaction with tissue, this manuscript summarizes experiences using clinically available laser systems, e.g., FREDDY laser and the Ho:YAG laser. In addition to that, it became of interest whether the composition of the salivary stone may have any impact on laser type or laser parameter chosen by the physician. Thus, different optical techniques were used to identify the components of sialoliths, as these data were correlated to their fragmentation properties.

Optical Techniques to Characterize Salivary Stones

Photonic techniques to distinguish the components of salivary stones are fluorescence, FTIR spectroscopy, Raman spectroscopy, and dual energy computer tomography (DECT). Salivary stones extracted from patients with clinical symptoms of sialolithiasis were examined in vitro. After extraction, the stones were kept in Ringer solution until experiments were started.

By means of fluorescence techniques, the macroscopic stone was illuminated using filtered light of a xenon-arc lamp to emit in the spectral range of $\lambda = 355–425$ nm. The fluorescence was documented by means of a digital camera equipped with a long pass filter; $\lambda < 440$ nm. Thereafter, excitation–emission matrices (EEM) were obtained by using a spectrometer (FluoroMax-2, HORIBA Jobin Yvon GmbH) equipped with a specific measurement compartment coupled to a bifurcated fiber probe. Excitation was performed in the range of $\lambda = 400–450$ nm with increments of 5 nm, while emission was detected in the spectral range between $\lambda = 480$ nm and $\lambda = 750$ nm. Evaluating the fluorescence, green and red-green fluorescing salivary stones could be distinguished as shown in Figs. 1 and 2. The associated EEM also shows the dependencies of the emission spectra on the excitation wavelength. Unfortunately, a direct correlation to a fluorescing composite of the stone could not be done so far.

Standard analysis procedure of stone composites is FTIR spectrometry. Salivary stones were investigated by means of FTIR spectrometry in the range from 4000 to 400 cm^{-1} (Nicolet 380 FTIR-Spectrometer, Thermo Electron Corporation). The results from FTIR spectrometric analysis showed that most sample content of 75–95 % from carbonate apatite ($Ca_{10}(PO_4)(CO_3OH)6(OH)_2$) and minor samples were from complete organic compound. Weddellit ($CaC_2O_4 \cdot 2H_2O$) and Struvit ($(NH_4)Mg[PO_4] \cdot 6H_2O$) could be identified.

Raman spectrometry analysis procedure was performed in the range of 200–3500 cm^{-1} after excitation with $\lambda = 1064$ nm of the Nd:YAG laser of the Raman spectrometer device (FT-Raman-Spectrometer IFS66 and Raman Modul FRA106, Bruker Corporation). Evaluation was performed using the data base HaveItAll Raman and software KnowItAll Raman (Bio-Rad Laboratories) for qualitative comparison. The evaluation by means of the database results in identifying keratin and carbonate apatite in different ratios as the two major components in the salivary stone samples. In Fig. 3, the overlay of the two components and a typical salivary stone Raman spectrum is shown.

Dual energy computer tomography (DECT) analysis is based upon the linear decay of X-ray energy within a stone sample. The

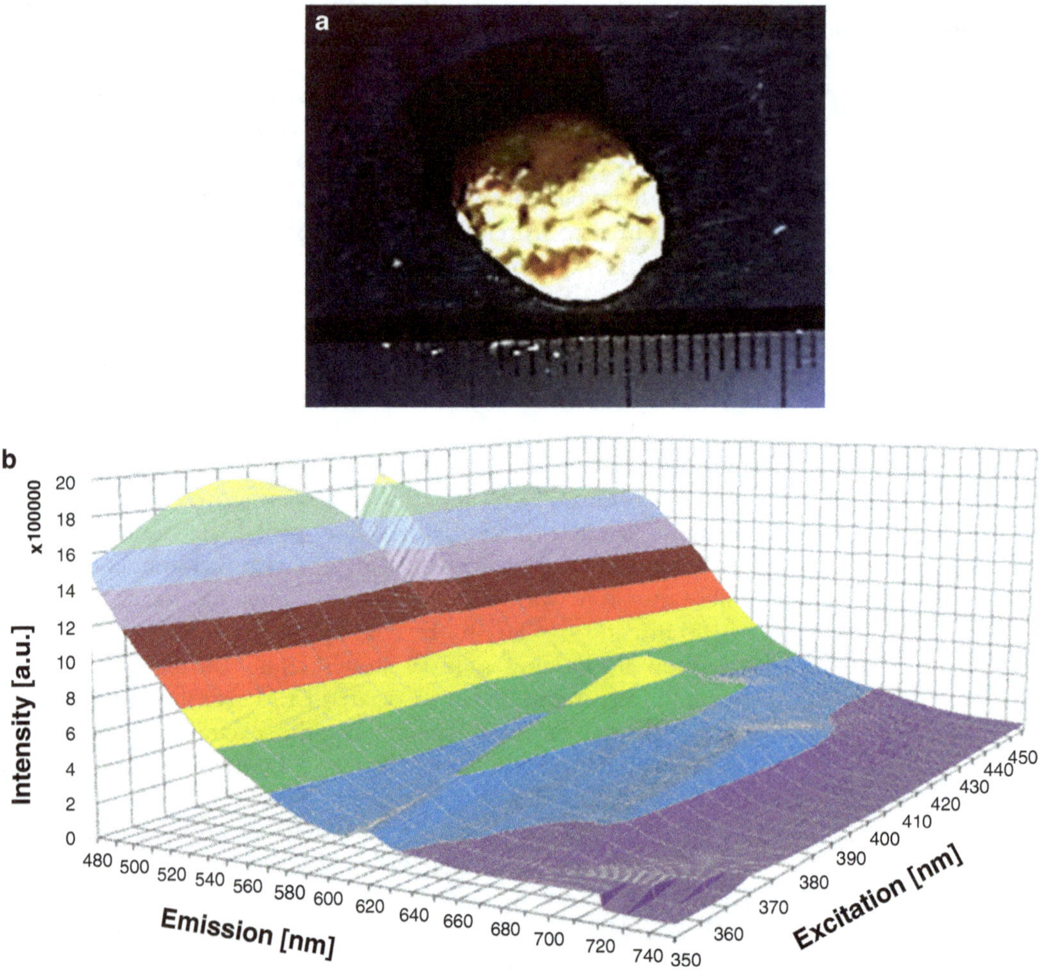

Fig. 1 (**a**) *Green* and *red* fluorescent salivary stones viewed under blue light excitation (**b**, mm-scale). The associated EEM shows prominent *blue*/*green* fluorescence, while especially red fluorescence emission ($\lambda = 600$–680 nm) could be observed when excitation wavelength is at around $\lambda = 400$ nm

dependency on the X-ray energy correlates with the order number of the main composites [33, 34]. Collected stone samples embedded in Ringer solution were investigated by means of the clinically available DECT system (Somatom Definition Flash, Siemens Medical Solutions) applying two different energies of 80 and 140 kV in a perpendicular setup. Evaluation was performed by characterization of the sample density in a region of interest ($x80$, $x140$) and calculation of the dual energy (DE) index according to the following equation: DE index $= (x80 - x140)/(x80 - x140 + 2000)$. According to this evaluation, it had been

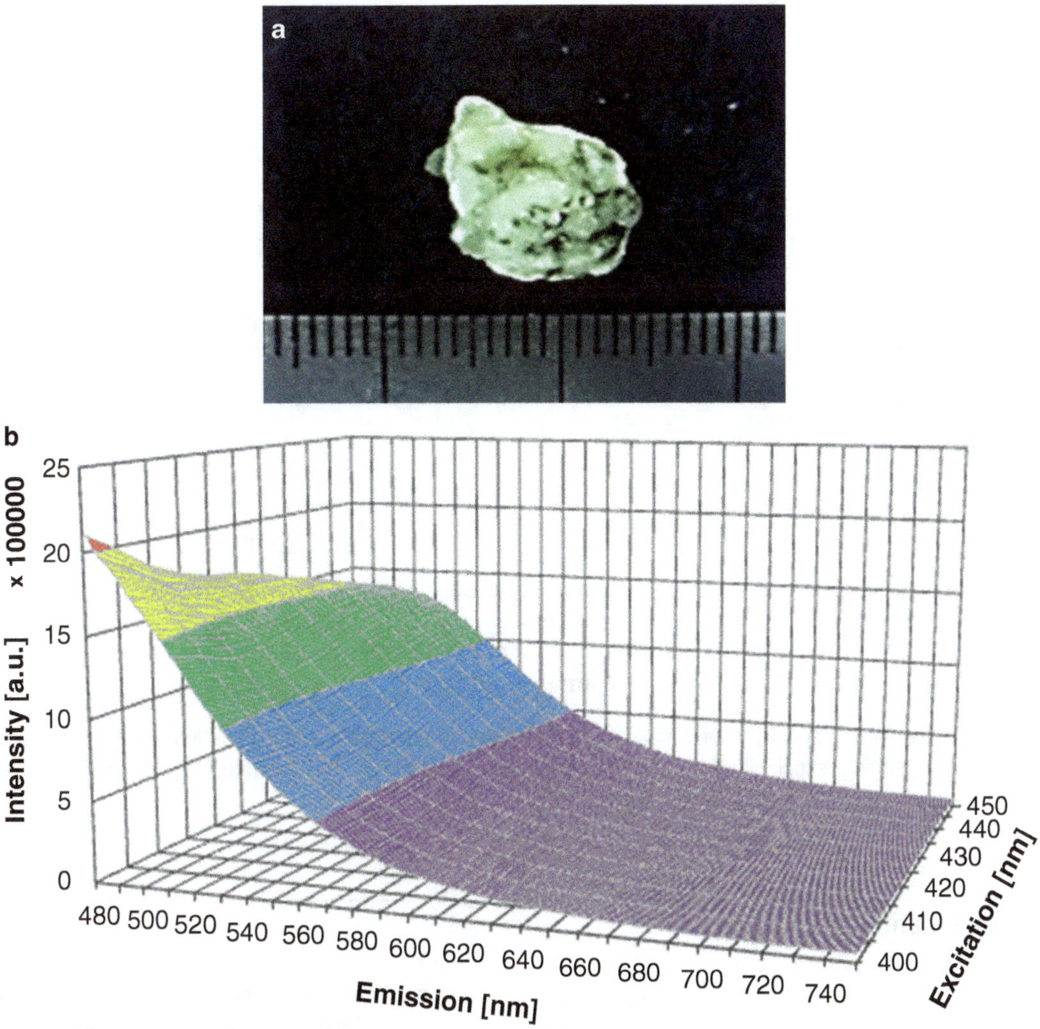

Fig. 2 (**a**) Pure *green* fluorescent salivary stone viewed under *blue light* excitation (**b**, mm-scale) and associated EEM without any spectral differentiation

shown that the DE index of pure water is DE(H_2O) = 0 and for bone DE(bone) = 0.1148 [35]. DECT evaluation results in density values for the tested sialoliths in the mean of $x80 = (1643 \pm 478)$ HU in case of the lower X-ray energy and $x140 = (851 \pm 267)$HU for the higher X-ray energy. The calculated DE index was 0.1726 ± 0.022 which is in the range of calcified urea stones. Thus, especially the calcification could be derived though a differentiation between carbonate apatite and weddellite seems not possible.

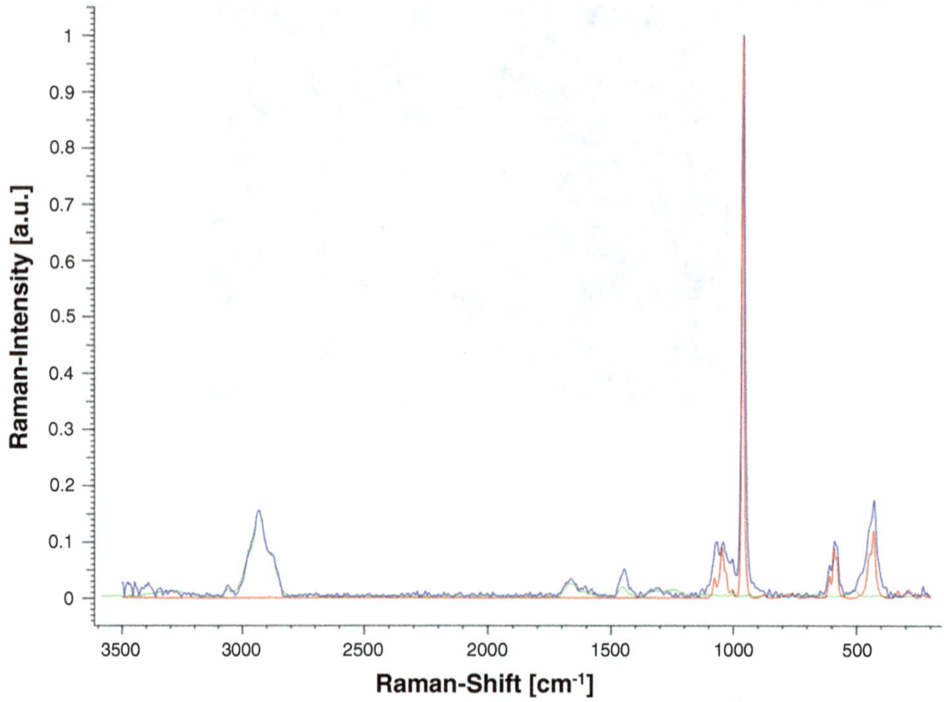

Fig. 3 Typical Raman spectrum of a salivary stone (*blue*) superimposed with identified keratin spectrum (*green*) representing, especially the band nearby 2900 cm^{-1} and carbonate apatite (*red*) representing the bands ranging from 1100 to 400 cm^{-1}

Fragmentation

In vitro fragmentation experiments were performed in a standard aquarium setup [36, 37] using a lattice with 1.5 mm mesh size through which small fragments could escape. Laser energy sources for fragmentation served two clinically established Ho:YAG lasers (Medilas H20, Dornier MedTech, Germany; Auriga, StarMedTec GmbH, Starnberg, Germany) emitting at $\lambda = 2100$ nm with pulse durations of less than 400 μs. With respect to the clinical goal of sialolith fragmentation, use of the 200 μm-fiber was mandatory. The repetition rate was set to the lowest parameter of 3 Hz, and the energy per pulse values were varied: 0.5, 1.0, and 1.5 J/pulse. Additional experiments were performed by means of the FREDDY laser system (FREquency Doubled Q-switched-Double-pulse Nd:YAG Laser) (U100plus, WOM World of Medicine AG, Berlin, Germany), which is a short-pulse (pulse duration < 5 μs) solid state laser emitting the two wavelengths of 532 and 1064 nm simultaneously [35]. In these experiments, a certain number of salivary stones per group were randomly selected to perform experimental fragmentation.

For evaluation purposes, the salivary stones were weighed before and their residuals after fragmentation, additionally the number of pulses and the total applied energy were documented. Thus, the fragmentation rate related to time (FT [mg/min]) and to energy (FE [mg/J]) could be calculated. Statistical analysis included evaluation of mean, standard deviation, and significance (one-way ANOVA) with $p<0.05$.

As for the results, Ho:YAG laser fragmentation of sialoliths proved successful with every laser parameter setting. Even the lowest laser parameter setting available confirmed that as little as 400 mJ/pulse at a repetition rate of 3 Hz is far above the potential ablation threshold for salivary stones. The fragmentation rate related to the duration time of the experiment showed an increase from 36.6 ± 29.3 mg/min to 74.4 ± 59.3 mg/min and 87.0 ± 72.5 mg/min without any significance for the group of 0.5 J/pulse, 1 J/pulse, and 1.5 J/pulse, respectively. The fragmentation rate related to the energy setting showed nearly no difference, figures reading 0.41 ± 0.33 mg/J to 0.41 ± 0.33 mg/J and 0.32 ± 0.27 mg/J without any significance for the group of 0.5 J/pulse, 1 J/pulse, and 1.5 J/pulse, respectively. In case of the FREDDY laser, stone fragmentation failed in some stones. Stone fragmentation into pieces smaller than 0.3 mm in diameter with the Ho:YAG laser required more total applied energy than in the FREDDY laser group. Comparing the mean fragmentation rates of salivary stones, the FREDDY laser is significantly more effective than the Ho:YAG laser.

Soft Tissue Effects

Harvested salivary gland tissue was exposed to single pulses of laser energy while keeping the fiber in direct smooth contact to the tissue surface. Tissues were histologically prepared and transversal sections were performed to get the depth of the induced effects (HE-stain, 5 μm slide).

Superficially, all impacts, independent of the laser system under investigation, could be observed. Histology showed no sign of impact by FREDDY and Ho:YAG energy of 0.5 J/pulse at tissue depth of 30–50 μm, while the higher Ho:YAG laser energy parameter resulted in holes within this layer. As shown in Fig. 4, operating at 1 J/pulse tissue effects could be observed up to a depth of 50–70 μm, while the 1.5 J/pulse induced effects more deeply.

Discussion

Endoscopic laser lithotripsy has been commonly used as a treatment for urinary calculi since the 1980s [38–40]. Its quick development into a routine clinical procedure worldwide is mainly due to the fact that the Ho:YAG laser became widely available for clinical use

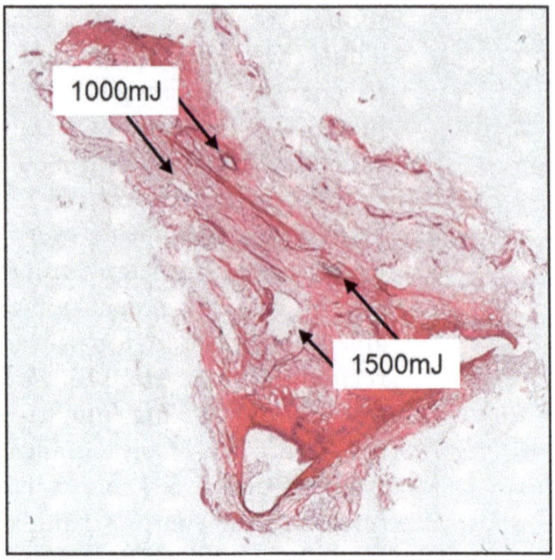

Fig. 4 Tissue slice of layer depth 50–70 μm showing the impacts of single laser pulses given at energy levels of 1 and 1.5 J/pulse. At this depth impacts of laser pulses of 0.5 J are not visible

within this time span. This laser system has several advantages: its ability to fragment all stones regardless of composition and size, its ability to deliver higher energies even through small diameter fibers that are easily deflected, and minimal retrograde propulsion as well as minimal fragment migration when low power settings are used [41–43].

So far laser lithotripsy of salivary stones has not evolved into a routine procedure. First attempts and experiences in laser-assisted destruction of sialoliths during the last century [8, 19, 20, 22] used pulsed-dye lasers and excimer lasers. Minor experiments have been published since the millennium [5, 21, 24]. Following urologic experiments [41–43], the in vitro study comparing the Ho:YAG and the Er:YAG lasers in fragmentation of salivary stones showed good fragmentation rates [23]. The main drawback of using Er:YAG laser irradiation clinically was to develop a specific biocompatible laser energy application system, which in contrast is already available for Ho:YAG laser application [43].

Experiments show that compared to the short-pulse duration FREDDY laser, the Ho:YAG laser was able to disintegrate all stones in a rather slow, but efficient soft milling process to powder, while the type of fragmentation caused by the FREDDY laser looked more like cracking stones and was not successful in all cases. The aim of lithotripsy in sialolithiasis is the fragmentation of the calculus into pieces of optimally less than 0.3 mm, to be washed out during manipulation or at least less than 2 mm, as these fragments could then easily be eliminated from the duct by endoscopy. These aims could be achieved with both laser systems.

The mechanism of the FREDDY laser is based upon plasma-induced shockwave generation, which results in high pressure for cracking the stone. This also serves for increased acceleration of stone fragments, which then may be impacted into the surrounding tissue. Furthermore, increased acceleration results also in effective repulsion of the stone, away from the laser fiber, which is an energy per pulse dependent effect [44]. Those effects also increase the potential of fiber burn back. Otherwise the FREDDY technique is equipped with a passive soft tissue detection unit to guard soft tissue from accidental laser impacts. In detail, the green 532 nm pulse is used to induce the formation of plasma between the fiber and the stones, while the IR energy is deployed to pump the plasma, amplifying bubble formation. Its collapse generates a mechanical shock wave, which leads to fragmentation of the stone. It is supposed that the energy of the green pulse is not high enough for any soft tissue interaction in front of the fiber tip. Instead it penetrates into the soft tissue and gets absorbed without major thermal effects and without any plasma formation. The IR light then also penetrates into the soft tissue causing only a slight increase of temperature. Therefore, this technique is thought to provide a "passive" safety for soft tissues.

The mechanism of the Ho:YAG laser system is related to the thermoablation of the stone composites by vaporizing the water molecules within the stone, thus being independent from the stone composites. Furthermore, between Ho:YAG laser fiber and target stone, a channel (Moses effect) is created by vaporizing the water in between; thus a free transmission of the Ho:YAG laser energy through the channel onto the target becomes possible. As there is no shockwave, the induced pressure waves are reduced compared to the FREDDY laser. In addition, the fibers burn back as well as the repulsion effects are also reduced. Unfortunately, there is no tissue identification technique comparable to the FREDDY laser; thus, the full Ho:YAG laser energy can be delivered to the surrounding tissue resulting in unwanted soft tissue effects.

The optical techniques to identify different composites within the salivary stones showed some correlation. Although fluorescence correlates with the results of the Raman Spectra, it does neither correlates to FTIR spectroscopy nor to DECT. Otherwise DECT measurements do correlate with Raman- as well as with FTIR spectroscopy. Finally, FTIR spectroscopy showed correlation to Raman spectroscopy. Fragmentation and ablation showed no correlation to any of the optical diagnostic techniques and thus to salivary stone compositions. Fragmentation using Ho:YAG laser seems to be independent from stone composition.

The analysis of salivary stones due to their components by different photonic techniques showed that each optical technique has potential for differentiating the stone components. However, the absolute composites could not be identified. Clinical and in situ

X-ray techniques are only available. FTIR—as well as Raman—spectroscopy can only be performed on harvested sialolith samples. Fluorescence is not available but could be adapted to endoscopes compared to fluorescence-assisted cystoscopy developed to improve clinical diagnosis in bladder cancer [45, 46]. Although fluorescence is not itself suited to improve diagnostic information, it could be helpful in discovering the stone as there is an improved differentiation to the surrounding tissue. Fragmentation using Ho:YAG laser seems to be independent of stone composition. Thus a specific differentiation for setting up effective laser parameters seems unnecessary. With respect to prevent adjacent tissue from injury and the endoscope from potential destruction lowest possible energy per pulse values above the ablation threshold of sialoliths should be applied.

Conclusion

Although several optical techniques could be used to identify salivary stone compositions, there is no correlation to the fragmentation properties using the Ho:YAG laser. Thus, differential diagnostic considerations and decision making for specific laser parameters by the operating surgeon seem to be unnecessary. Optical techniques could be easily adapted and may support the physician, e.g., by means of intraoperative fluorescence guidance through the submandibular channel to target salivary stones. Furthermore, during laser light application fluorescence techniques may help to differentiate the target stone from surrounding tissue to prevent soft tissue from unwanted laser impact. For the treatment of sialoliths by means of laser-assisted lithotripsy by Ho:YAG laser, a suitable endoscope with working channel to guide the laser fiber is essential. Ho:YAG induced fragmentation rates in terms of mg/J did not differ significantly, as shown in the presentedexperiments. Thus low energy per pulse and repetition rates, e.g., 0.5 J/pulse and 3 Hz can be recommended and side effects to soft tissue can be reduced. Adhering to these principles, beneficial clinical outcome while maintaining the patient's safety can be achieved.

Acknowledgements

M. Domes, G. Scheib, L. Bienert, M. Heide, and T. Pongratz for technical assistance during experiments. The companies Dornier MedTech GmbH, StarMedtec GmbH, and WOM GmbH for support of equipment.

References

1. Rauch S, Gorlin RJ. Diseases of the salivary glands. In: Gorlin RJ, Goldman HM, editors. Thoma's oral pathology, vol. 2. 6th ed. St. Louis: Mosby; 1970. p. 997–1003.
2. Escudier MP, McGurk M. Symptomatik sialadenitis and sialolithiasis in the English population, an estimate of the cost of hospital treatment. Br Dent J. 1999;187(4):180.
3. Iro H, Zenk J. Konzepte zur Diagnostik und Therapie des Speichelsteinleidens. Deutsches Ärzteblatt. 2003;100(9):A-556/B-457/C-448.
4. McGurk M, Escudier MP, Brown JE. Modern management of salivary calculi. Br J Surg. 2005;92:107–12.
5. Katz P. New techniques for the treatment of salivary lithiasis: sialendoscopy and extracorporeal lithotropsy: 1773 cases. Ann Otolaryngol Chir Cervicofac. 2004;121(3):123–32.
6. Zenk J, Gottwald F, Bozzato A, Iro H. Speichelsteine der Glandula submandibularis. Steinentfernung mit Organerhalt. HNO. 2005;53:243–9.
7. Harold DB. Submandibular salivary stones: current management modalities. J Oral Maxillofac Surg. 2004;62:369–78.
8. Iro H, Zenk J, Waldfahrer F, Benzel W. Current status of minimally invasive treatment methods in sialolithiasis. HNO. 1996;44(2):78–84.
9. Katz P, Fritsch MH. Salivary stones: innovative techniques in diagnosis and treatment. Curr Opin Otolaryngol Head Neck Surg. 2003;11(3):173–8.
10. Marchal F, Dulguerov P, Becker M, Barki G, Disant F, Lehmann W. Submandibular diagnostic and interventional sialendoscopy: new procedure for ductal disorders. Ann Otol Rhinol Laryngol. 2002;111:27–35.
11. Marchal F, Dulguerov P, Guyot JP, Lehmann W. Sialendoscopie et lithotripsie intracanalaire. Otorhinolaryngol Nova. 1998;8:262–4.
12. Nahlieli O, Nakar LH, Nazarian Y, Turner MD. Sialoendoscopy: a new approach to salivary gland obstructive pathology. J Am Dent Assoc. 2006;137(10):1394–400.
13. Ziegler CM, Steveling H, Seubert M, Muhling J. Endoscopy: a minimally invasive procedure for diagnosis and treatment of diseases of the salivary glands. Six years of practical experience. Br J Oral Maxillofac Surg. 2004;42(1):1–7.
14. Berini-Aytes L, Gay-Escoda C. Morbidity associated with removal of the submandibular gland. J Craniomaxillofac Surg. 1992;20:216–9.
15. Lyall JB, Fleet J. Morbidity study of submandibular gland excision. Ann R Coll Surg Engl. 1986;68:327.
16. Iro H, Zenk J, Hosemann WG, Benzel W. Electrohydraulic intracorporeal lithothripsy of salivary calculi. In vitro and animal experiment studies. HNO. 1993;41(8):389–95.
17. Königsberger T, Feyh J, Goetz A, Kastenbauer E. Endoscopically controlled electrohydraulic intracorporeal shock wave lithotripsy (EISL) of salivary stones. J Otolaryngol. 1993;22(1):12–3.
18. Arzoz E, Santiago A, Esnal F, Palomero R. Endoscopic intracorporeal lithotripsy for sialolithiasis. J Oral Maxillofac Surg. 1996;54(7):847–50.
19. Gundlach P, Scherer H, Hopf J, Leege N, Muller G, Hirst L, Scholz C. Endoscopic-controlled laser lithotripsy of salivary calculi: in vitro studies and initial clinical use. HNO. 1990;38(7):247–50.
20. Ito H, Baba S. Pulsed dye laser lithotripsy of submandibular gland salivary calculus. J Laryngol Otol. 1996;110(10):942–6.
21. Kerr PD, Krahn H, Brodovsky D. Endoscopic laser lithotripsy of a proximal parotid duct calculus. J Otolarynol. 2001;30(2):129–30.
22. Königsberger R, Feyh J, Goetz A, Schilling V, Kastenbauer E. Endoscopic controlled laser lithotripsy in the treatment of sialolithiasis. Laryngorhinootologie. 1990;69(6):322–3.
23. Raif J, Vardi M, Nahlieli O, Gannot I. An Er:YAG laser endoscopic fiber delivery system for lithotripsy of salivary stones. Lasers Surg Med. 2006;38(6):580–7.
24. McGurk M, Prince MJ, Jiang ZX, King TA. Laser lithotripsy: a preliminary study on its application for sialolithiasis. Br J Oral Maxillofac Surg. 1994;32(4):218–21.
25. Chan KF, Lee H, Teichman JM, Kamerer A, McGuff HS, Vargas G, Welch AJ. Erbium:YAG laser lithotripsy mechanism. J Urol. 2002;168(2):436–41.
26. Teichmann JMH, Kang HW, Glickman RD, Welsh AJ. Update on erbium:YAG lithotripsy. AIP Conf Proc. 2007;900:216–27. Print ISSN 0094-243X.
27. Grases F, Santiago C, Simonet BM, Costa-Bauza A. Sialolithiasis: mechanism of calculi formation and etiologic factors. Clin Chim Acta. 2003;334(1–2):131–6.
28. Sterenborg HJCM, Van Den Akker HP, Van Der Meulen FW, Van Swol CFP, Van Leeuwen AGJM, Van Gemert MJC. Laserlithotripsy of salivary stones: a comparison between the

pulsed dye laser and the Ho-YSGG laser. Lasers Med Sci. 1990;5(4):357–63.

29. Zörcher T, Hochberger J, Schrott KM, Kuhn R, Schafhauser W. In vitro study concerning the efficiency of the frequency doubled double-pulse Neodymium:YAG laser (FREDDY) for lithotripsy of calculi in the urinary tract. Lasers Surg Med. 1999;25(1):38–42.
30. Fried NM. Potential applications of the erbium:YAG laser in endourology. J Endourol. 2001;15(9):889–94.
31. Delvecchio FC, Auge BK, Brizuela RM, Weizer AZ, Zhomg P, Preminger GM. In vitro analysis of stone fragmentation ability of the FREDDY laser. J Endourol. 2003;17(3):177–9.
32. Yates JK, Pareek G, Zabbo A. Comparison of the FREDDY and holmium lasers for laser lithotripsy of ureteral calculi. In: 75th annual meeting of the American Urological Association; 2006.
33. Primak AN, Giraldo JCR, Eusemann CD, Schmidt B, Kantor B, Fletcher JG, McCollough CH. Dual-source dual-energy CT with additional tin filtration: dose and image quality evaluation in phantoms and in-vivo. AJR Am J Roentgenol. 2010;195(5):1164–74. doi:10.2214/AJR.09.3956.
34. Johnson TR. Dual-energy CT: general principles. AJR Am J Roentgenol. 2012;199(5 Suppl):S3–8. doi:10.2214/AJR.12.9116.
35. Graser A, Johnson TR, Bader M, Staehler M, Haseke N, Nikolaou K, Reiser MF, Stief CG, Becker CR. Dual energy CT characterization of urinary calculi: initial in vitro and clinical experience. Invest Radiol. 2008;43(2):112–9. doi:10.1097/RLI.0b013e318157a144.
36. Siedek V, Betz C, Hecht V, Blagova R, Vogeser M, Zengel P, Berghaus A, Leunig A, Sroka R. Laser induced fragmentation of salivary stones: an in vitro comparison of two different, clinically approved laser systems. Lasers Surg Med. 2008;40:257–64.
37. Sroka R, Haseke N, Pongratz T, Hecht V, Tilki D, Stief CG, Bader MJ. In vitro investigations of repulsion during laser lithotripsy using a pendulum set-up. Lasers Med Sci. 2012;27(3):637–43. doi:10.1007/s10103-011-0992-0. Epub 2011 Oct 20.
38. Grasso M. Laser as an endoscopic lithotrite. Urology. 1996;48(2):199–206.
39. Hofstetter AG. Laser lithotripsy in the treatment of ureteral lithiasis. Arch Esp Urol. 1992;45:227–9.
40. Hofstetter AG. Laser qualities and areas of application, current status and perspectives. Langenbecks Arch Chir Suppl II Verh Dtsch Ges Chir. 1989;315–8.
41. Teichman JM, Chan KF, Cecconi PP, Corbin NS, Kamerer AD, Glickman RD, Welch AJ. Erbium:YAG versus holmium:YAG lithotripsy. J Urol. 2001;165(3):876–9.
42. Varkarakis IM, Inagaki T, Allaf ME, Chan TY, Rogers CG, Wright EJ, Fried NM. Comparison of erbium:yttrium aluminium garnet and holmium:yttrium-aluminium-garnet lasers for incision of urethra and bladder neck in an in vivo porcine model. Urology. 2005;65(1):191–5.
43. Fried NM, Tesfaye Z, Ong AM, Rha KH, Hejazu P. Optimization of the erbium:YAG laser for precise incision of ureteral and urethral tissues: in vitro and in vivo results. Lasers Surg Med. 2003;33(2):108–14.
44. Marguet CG, Sung JC, Springhart WP, L'Esperance JO, Zhou S, Zhong P, Albala DM, Preminger GM. In vitro comparison of stone retropulsion and fragmentation of the frequency doubled, double pulse nd:yag laser and the holmium:yag laser. J Urol. 2005;173(5):1797–800.
45. Kriegmair M, Stepp H, Steinbach P, Lumper W, Ehsan A, Stepp HG, Rick K, Knüchel R, Baumgartner R, Hofstetter A. Fluorescence cystoscopy Fluorescence cystoscopy following intravesical instillation of 5-aminolevulinic acid: a new procedure with high sensitivity for detection of hardly visible urothelial neoplasias. Urol Int. 1995;55(4):190–6.
46. Zaak D, Kriegmair M, Stepp H, Stepp H, Baumgartner R, Oberneder R, Schneede P, Corvin S, Frimberger D, Knüchel R, Hofstetter A. Endoscopic detection of transitional cell carcinoma with 5-aminolevulinic acid: results of 1012 fluorescence endoscopies. Urology. 2001;57(4):690–4.

Chapter 12

Laser Treatment for Vascular Malformations and Hemangiomas in the Head and Neck

Tara L. Rosenberg, James D. Phillips, and Gresham T. Richter

Background

In the 1960s, continuous wave argon and carbon dioxide (CO_2) lasers were used in the treatment of port-wine stains (PWS) and hemangiomas. However, these lasers resulted in skin changes and scarring, thus limiting their use in the treatment of cutaneous vascular lesions. Since the early attempts at therapeutic usage, laser technology and laser use in vascular anomalies have significantly improved. In particular, the work of Anderson and Parrish in the 1980s revolutionized laser treatment for skin and vascular lesions [1].

The International Society for the Study of Vascular Anomalies (ISSVA), an organization founded in 1992, established a commonly used classification system for vascular anomalies. This was based upon the 1982 work of Mulliken and Glowacki [2, 3] and has been updated in 2014. Vascular tumors and vascular malformations comprise the two main types of vascular anomalies. Infantile hemangioma is the most common vascular tumor. Vascular malformations are divided into slow flow, fast flow, and combined vascular malformations, with each specific malformation's classification based upon the type(s) of vessels involved [4].

Lesions with the following features respond best to laser treatment: superficial, small caliber vessels that are slow flow. Such lesions include capillary malformations (i.e., port-wine stains), superficial hemangiomas, and venous malformations (VMs). Patients with fast-flow lesions (e.g., arteriovenous malformations) currently have no established treatment options with

Brian J.-F. Wong and Justus Ilgner (eds.), *Biomedical Optics in Otorhinolaryngology: Head and Neck Surgery*,
DOI 10.1007/978-1-4939-1758-7_12, © Springer Science+Business Media New York 2016

laser therapy. Clinical work is underway, however, to identify effective laser therapy options for these patients. This chapter will focus on the most common vascular anomalies managed with laser therapy, how to identify them, and the ideal laser options for each lesion.

Introduction to Vascular Anomalies

Port-Wine Stains

Approximately, 75 % of port-wine stains (PWSs) (i.e., capillary malformations of the dermis) are located in the head and neck regions [5]. They occur in approximately 0.1–0.3 % of infants and are the most common congenital vascular malformation [6]. PWSs are red to purple in color and have a flat, macular appearance. They are composed of ectatic and superficial small vessels that gradually increase in diameter over time. The natural progression of the affected areas involves darkening and hypertrophy of the lesions, resulting in nodular, thick plaques that may cause disfigurement and resultant psychological disturbance [7, 8].

Sturge–Weber syndrome [7] is a sporadic congenital neuro-oculo-cutaneous disorder that classically involves the following: PWS of the ophthalmic branch of the trigeminal nerve (V_1) skin distribution, leptomeninges of the brain, and eye(s). Clinical manifestations may include stroke, seizures, glaucoma, and intellectual disability [9]. Ocular and/or neurologic findings are more likely to be found in patients with a PWS involving the entire V_1 distribution [10].

Venous Malformations

Venous malformations (VMs) frequently occur in the head and neck, especially in muscle, skin, subcutaneous tissue, and mucous membranes. They may be focal, multifocal, or diffuse, and their location and size may vary [11–14]. VMs are comprised of tortuous, thin-walled veins with a single endothelial lining [15]. Gradual vascular expansion makes these congenital lesions more noticeable with age. Rapid expansion may occur during fluctuations in hormones (e.g., puberty or oral contraceptive use), after trauma, or with acute thrombosis. With episodes of acute thrombosis, VMs demonstrate local intravascular coagulation (LIC), which is thought to lead to acute or chronic pain, a phenomenon unique to VM patients when compared to other vascular anomalies. VMs produce a characteristic blue hue when near the surface of skin/mucosa. Also, they are soft and compressible and expand when in a dependent position, during exercise, or with Valsalva [14].

Lymphatic Malformations

Lymphatic malformations (LMs), previously known as lymphangiomas or cystic hygromas, are comprised of ectatic lymph vessels that convalesce into a neoplastic lesion. Defined by the caliber of the vessels involved, LMs may be macrocystic (>2 cm^3), microcystic (<2 cm^3), or contain mixed components of each [16]. As slow-flow lesions, LMs lack pulsation and warmth. They are noncompressible and do not engorge when in a gravity-dependent position (as do venous malformations). LMs vacillate in size according to the relative production of lymph from local inflammation. Microcystic LMs can be infiltrative into tissue and represent a very difficult entity to address. At times, VMs and LMs will occur together to create a venous lymphatic malformation. This is common in microcystic or mixed LMs.

Hemangiomas

Hemangiomas, the most common vascular tumors [4], are divided into two main types: infantile hemangiomas (IHs) and congenital hemangiomas (CHs). Approximately 5 % of children are born with IHs. These lesions have a unique growth curve that begins with a rapid growth phase (proliferating phase) that occurs in the first few weeks to months of life. The second phase is a quiescent period of several months, which is then followed by the third phase of involution. The process of involution involves slow regression of the hemangioma until around the age of 5–6 years. After completion of this natural course, a fully involuted hemangioma may result in normal-appearing skin, atrophic skin, scattered superficial red vascular staining, a fibro-fatty residuum, or a combination of these findings. IHs may be defined by their depth of involvement: superficial, compound (involving the skin and subcutaneous structures) and deep. They may also be classified as focal or segmental. Segmental lesions have a more aggressive nature and tend to be diffuse, larger, and plaque-like [17]. Each growth phase in segmental disease is prolonged. Glucose transporter-1 protein (GLUT-1) is a marker for the endothelium of IHs, since they are positive for this immunostain [4].

Infantile hemangiomas may also occur in the subglottis. Though rare, they can be life threatening if airway obstruction occurs. Patients with subglottic hemangiomas present with biphasic stridor, usually during the proliferative phase at 6–12 weeks of age. It is important to be cognizant of the potential presence of subglottic hemangiomas in patients with cutaneous IHs in a beard distribution as they are at increased risk (>50 %) of having these lesions compared to other patients with focal disease. Patients with hemangiomas in the beard distribution should also be evaluated for PHACES syndrome (posterior fossa malformation, hemangiomas, arterial anomalies, cardiac defects, eye abnormalities, and sternal defects). Subglottic hemangiomas have been effectively treated with a number of therapies including oral propranolol, systemic steroids, intralesional steroid injection, open excision, and endoscopic laser ablation [18, 19].

Basic Laser Concepts

Hemoglobin (either oxygenated or deoxygenated) is the target chromophore during the laser treatment of vascular lesions. Superficial lesions are treated by lasers with short wavelengths because they have more shallow depth of penetration. The pulse duration of each laser determines in part the vessel diameter that can be treated. Less time (i.e., shorter pulse duration) is needed to cause destruction of smaller vessels. Early PWSs and proliferating hemangiomas are examples of small vessel lesions (vessels ≤100 μm in diameter). The flashlamp-pumped dye laser (i.e., pulsed dye laser or PDL) has a pulse duration of 500–1500 μs and is used to treat small vessel lesions. Intermediate to advanced PWSs and involuting hemangiomas are examples of medium vessel lesions (vessels 100–400 μm in diameter). These lesions require a pulse duration between 10 and 100 ms for an appropriate response, and the potassium titanyl phosphate (KTP) laser may also be used. Advanced PWSs and VMs are examples of large vessel lesions (vessels >400 μm in width). These lesions require a longer pulse duration (e.g., around 0.1–1 s) for treatment. Neodymium:yttrium–aluminum–garnet (Nd:YAG) lasers may be used for some large vessel lesions, such as VMs, partly because they are able to deliver a longer pulse duration [1]. Laser wavelengths and settings for the most commonly used lasers in the treatment of vascular anomalies are listed in Table 1.

Laser Use in Vascular Anomalies

Port-Wine Stains

The standard treatment for PWS is PDL therapy. This treatment may begin as early as infancy. Early treatment has proven to be safe and effective with or without anesthesia. PDL therapy has been shown by some to be more effective in the pediatric population when compared to adults [20]. Ashinoff et al. reported that after an average 2.9 treatment sessions for their PWSs, 83 % of the infants demonstrated greater than 50 % lightening of the lesions. After an average 3.8 sessions, 45 % of patients experienced 75 % lightening. These results were obtained without skin complications [21].

Lighter, circular spots may be seen after PDL treatment from the focused area of laser application. The dark areas in between are treated with repeat therapy, and continued therapy is required for

Table 1
Laser wavelengths, settings, and additional information for the most commonly treated vascular anomalies

Laser	Main indications in vascular anomalies	Typical settings	Additional information
PDL 595 nm	Hemangiomas, port-wine stains, and others	Two main options: 1. Joules: 8–15 J Duration: 1.5 ms Spot size: 7 mm 2. Joules: 10 J max Duration: 1.5 ms Spot size: 10 mm	Place coolant on maximum level. Joules vary on response. 7 mm spot is most frequently used with average treatment range between 8 and 15 J. With 10 mm spot size, maximum Joule range is 10 because of the spot size. The smaller the spot size, the higher the Joule maximum level
Alexandrite 755 nm	Hemangiomas, port-wine stains, and others (Often used on lesions that are resistant to PDL treatment and lesions with more purple coloration)	Joules: 60–100 J Duration: 3 ms Spot size: 8 mm Hertz: 1 Hz Coolant settings: pre 90/delay 80/post OFF	Joule level varies with response. Not recommended for use on dark skin. It will be absorbed by melanin and results in hypopigmentation
GentleYAG® 1064 nm	Various vascular anomalies, usually venous malformations	Two main options: 1. Joules: 180–220 J Duration: 20 ms Spot size: 3 mm 2. Joules: 80–100 J Duration: 20 ms Spot size: 8 mm Constant settings: Hertz: 1 Hz Coolant settings: pre 40/delay 30/post OFF	Consider this laser on darkly pigmented skin. 8 mm spot size maxes out at 120 J. Referred to as "gentle" due to the coolant spray. Same wavelength as Nd:YAG laser. Joules vary with response

(continued)

Table 1 (continued)

Laser	Main indications in vascular anomalies	Typical settings	Additional information
Nd:YAG 1064 nm	Venous malformations (Airway, intraoral and interstitial treatments)	Most settings are standard Watts: 15–25 W Duration: 1–2 ms	Various hand pieces and fibers exist for use in the head and neck region. SFE 0.6 fiber is used for interstitial cases along with a 14-gauge 1¼″ needle
CO_2 10,600 nm	Mucosal aerodigestive lymphatic malformations	Settings for surface ablation: Watts: 18 W Mode: scanning Settings for removing bulky disease: Watts: 4–5 W Mode: cutting	

This table was borrowed and altered with permission from Springer from another chapter overall long-term control. Serial PDL treatments are typically scheduled every 4–6 weeks. However, some advocate for better results with shorter intervals [22]. Intervals of every 2–3 months may be selected for younger patients who require general anesthesia. When a plateau is reached (no improvement in appearance), treatment should be discontinued.

About 20 % of PWSs are PDL-resistant, and complete resolution with PDL as a single modality therapy only occurs in less than 10 % [23]. There are multiple factors that have been postulated to contribute to PWS laser resistance: lesion size, patient age, skin thickness, anatomical location, number of prior treatments, and vessel characteristics [24]. Poor responders may include midfacial lesions and those in the trigeminal distribution. At 5 years after the completion of PDL treatments, 16–50 % of patients experience darkening of their lesions [25, 26], thought to be due to vessel regeneration and lesion revascularization [27].

Other laser therapies have been used with some benefit in PDL-resistant PWSs such as the Alexandrite laser. The Alexandrite laser has a longer wavelength and thus a greater depth of penetration than the PDL at a 755 nm wavelength. It also has greater affinity for deoxyhemoglobin, which is present in higher concentrations in large capillary, venular, and venous channels [28]. The GentleYAG® laser may also be applied to PDL-resistant PWSs [24] as well as intense pulsed light (IPL) therapy [29]. The latter treatment modality has a rectangular treatment spot with a broad base, which may be advantageous. PDL, however, seems to remain the preferred initial treatment by some patients [7].

Therapeutic adjuncts exist for laser treatment in PWSs. There are reported studies in site-specific pharmaco-laser therapy and PWS lesion hemodynamic changes in the perioperative period [24, 29]. Rapamycin (antiangiogenic agent) applied topically has been combined with PDL treatment, which shows some promising results in animal models to decrease lesion regeneration/revasularization. This may increase the overall efficacy and duration of PDL treatment effects in PWS [27, 29–32]. Compared to PDL therapy, Klein et al. reported patient subjective improved outcomes with indocyanine green-augmented diode laser (ICG+DL) therapy in PWS. However, there was no objective difference in outcomes between the two therapies. Furthermore, patient-reported pain levels were higher for ICG+DL treatment when compared to standard PDL therapy [33]. Klein et al. reported later that ICG+DL therapy benefits only a minor portion of PWS patients [34].

Venous Malformations

Treatment of head and neck venous malformations usually requires multimodality treatment: sclerotherapy, surgical excision, laser therapy, or a combination of these treatments. In 2012, Richter and Braswell summarized the treatment modalities for head and neck VMs, which included laser therapy. Some deep VMs of the

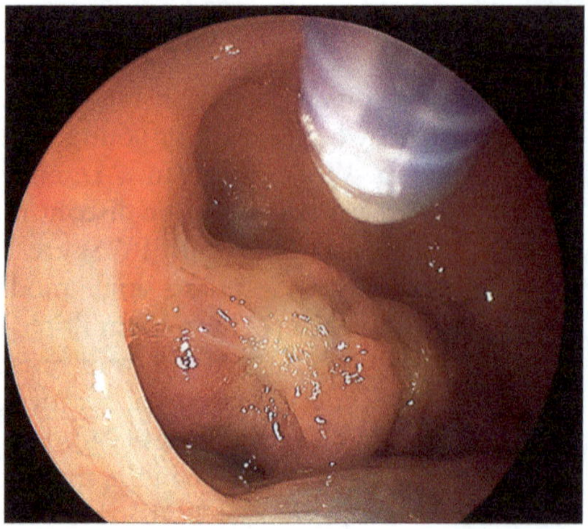

Fig. 1 Nd:YAG laser therapy of mucosal venous malformation of the nasopharynx. Immediate shrinkage at laser site with pinpoint mucosal thermal injury

parotid, muscle, or tongue may respond to laser intervention. Other VMs that may be treated with laser therapy include superficial and deep mucosal lesions and superficial cutaneous lesions [14]. Nd:YAG (1064 nm) and Alexandrite (755 nm) lasers are often used due to their affinity for deoxyhemoglobin and their longer wavelengths [29].

The GentleYAG® laser and Alexandrite laser are used to treat cutaneous VMs. The benefit of the GentleYAG® laser is the emission of a cryogen burst immediately before and/or after the laser pulse in order to decrease thermal damage to the skin [14, 35]. Venous telangiectasias are better treated by the Alexandrite laser, and larger superficial veins respond better to the GentleYAG® laser [14]. Laser therapy may be used in the management of complex cervicofacial VMs to treat mucocutaneous disease and to thicken the tissue at the sites of the lesions to allow for better response and fewer complications when subsequent sclerotherapy and/or surgery are employed [35].

Mucosal VMs respond well to the Nd:YAG laser. Aerodigestive lesions of the lips, gingiva, buccal mucosa, tongue, tongue base, pharynx, nasopharynx, hypopharynx, larynx, and trachea may all be treated with this laser via direct visualization or endoscopic application (Fig. 1). Distal lesions, may require the use of the Nd:YAG laser fiber attached to a Hopkins telescope to allow for simultaneous visualization and treatment of the lesions. There is instant decrease in size of the treated mucosal VMs after the laser pulse as the ectatic venous channels shrink. Initially, treatment sessions are performed about every 3 months until lesion control is reached. Patients with a low burden of disease may require only 1–2 treatments for disease control, but for many patients, an average of four treatments is necessary [13]. A short course of

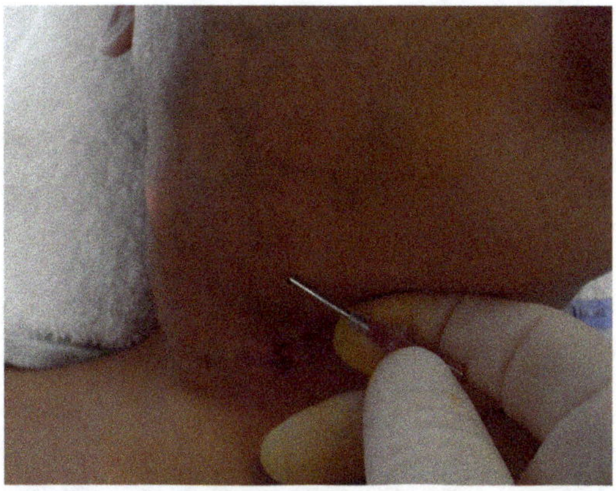

Fig. 2 Interstitial Nd:YAG laser therapy of right neck venous malformation

postoperative steroids may help alleviate edema and pain. Rare complications include bleeding, scarring, and mucosal sloughing [11, 13, 14, 35].

Interstitial laser therapy using the Nd:YAG laser is an alternative treatment to surgical excision for deep, large vessel VMs located in the masseter muscle, deep parotid, tongue, and neck (Fig. 2). Often with ultrasound guidance, a 14-gauge needle is inserted directly into the VM, and a Nd:YAG glass laser fiber is passed through the needle. This permits ablation of the VM within the vessels, while the needle and laser fiber are slowly withdrawn from the lesion [11, 36]. During treatment, one may experience an audible pop of the vessels responding to the laser, and instant lesion shrinking may be seen [14].

Lymphatic Malformations

Depending on the location and caliber of an individual LM, surgical excision and aspiration with sclerotherapy represent the mainstays of treatment, with both modalities achieving comparable rates of success [37]. However, for lesions near the surface of the mucosa in the head and neck, laser therapy has proven to be a useful adjunct for treatment.

As space-occupying lesions, LMs of the upper aerodigestive tract may cause dysphagia, dysarthria, or airway obstruction. Lesions of the tongue can ulcerate, leading to halitosis or bleeding [38]. Complete surgical resection is often not an option for infiltrative lesions of the upper aerodigestive tract due to the associated risks to tongue mobility, swallow function, glottic impairment, etc. Laser debulking or resurfacing thus becomes an effective measure for the temporization of symptoms. Both CO_2 and Nd:YAG lasers have been effectively applied to lesions of the oral tongue [39, 40], tongue base [41, 42], and larynx [43] (Fig. 3). Glade and Buckmiller reported a 10-year experience using CO_2 laser resurfacing of oral LMs, indicating both the efficacy and safety of this technique [39]. In the study, patients underwent an average of three laser procedures.

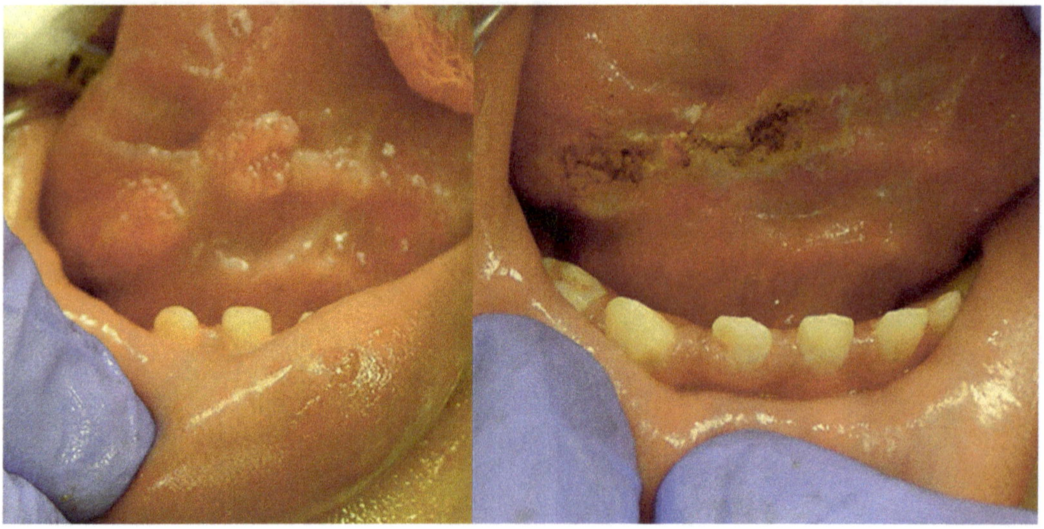

Fig. 3 Floor of mouth and tongue microcystic lymphatic malformation before and after CO_2 laser therapy

Though a small sample size due to the rarity of the disease, all patients reported improvement of symptoms including swelling, bleeding, and pain. Combined with suspension of the airway and microscopic or endoscopic techniques, serial intervention is often required as lesions wax and wane.

Hemangiomas

Not all hemangiomas are candidates for laser therapy. The main lesions that may be treated effectively with laser therapy include the following: (1) cutaneous precursor lesions, (2) early proliferating superficial lesions (particularly in cosmetically concerning areas), (3) hemangiomas (superficial or compound) with skin ulceration/bleeding [44], (4) superficial hemangiomas with extremely fast growth, and (5) involuting hemangiomas with residual telangiectasias [45]. There are several possible risks of laser treatment to IHs: pain, swelling, hypo/hyperpigmentation, temporary purpura, ulceration/blistering, and scarring [46–48].

The pulsed-dye laser (PDL) is the most commonly used laser for the treatment of hemangiomas (Fig. 4). Treatment of superficial IHs in the proliferative phase by PDL results in decreased overall growth of the lesion [44]. PDL therapy is not as effective on lesions greater than 3 mm in thickness, deep lesions, or compound disease due to limited depth of tissue penetration by this laser [49, 50].

Involuted IHs may require various interventions depending on the residual changes that are present. For overlying telangiectasias, PDL therapy is indicated [45]. The fractionated CO_2 laser may be used for skin resurfacing of involuted IHs that have atrophic skin or scarring [51]. Involuted IHs with substantial volume may result in residual fibrofatty tissue. This bulky, nonpigmented tissue does not respond to laser therapy, and surgical excision is usually necessary to give a good cosmetic outcome.

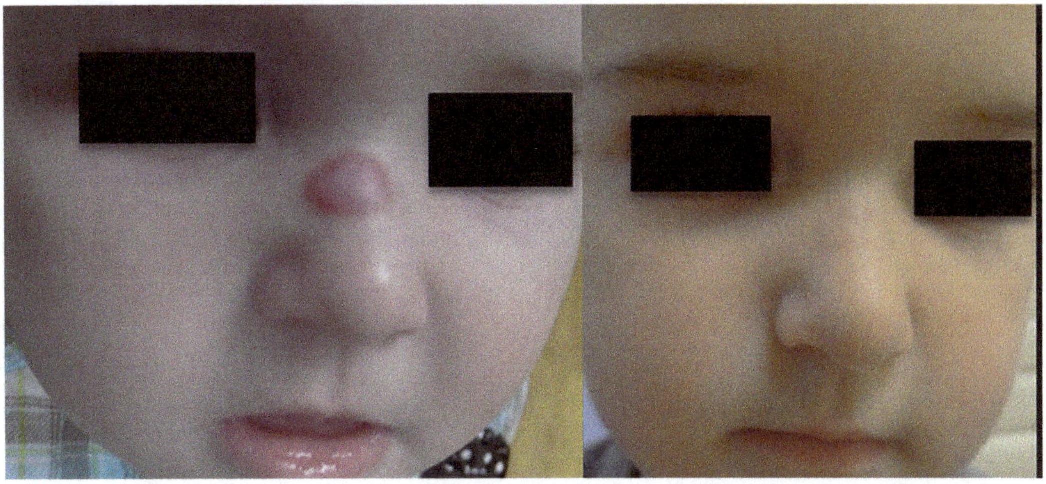

Fig. 4 Nasal superficial infantile hemangioma before and 6 months after three pulsed-dye laser (PDL) treatments

The CO_2 laser is the most commonly used laser in the treatment of subglottic hemangiomas. This laser is effective (~89 % success rate) in reducing the lesion size and decreasing symptoms. However, subglottic stenosis may occur if multiple or overly aggressive laser treatments are performed and sparing the underlying perichondrium from laser damage is paramount [18]. With the advent of propranolol therapy in the treatment of IHs (including those in the subglottis), CO_2 laser use may not be needed. Instead, combination therapy with oral administration of propranolol and intralesional injection of steroids (kenalog/celestone) for subglottic hemangiomas may be sufficient.

Propranolol is now the first-line medical therapy for large, multiple, or complicated IHs. Given the good response rates to this therapy, surgery or other intervention may not be necessary in many patients [52, 53]. However, in many patients the PDL is required to assist in final control of superficial vascular staining from IH.

Conclusion

The treatment of head and neck vascular anomalies using laser therapy has steadily advanced since the 1980s. Capillary malformations, venous malformations, lymphatic malformations, and infantile hemangiomas are good candidates in select cases for laser therapy of superficial cutaneous or mucosal disease. The PDL, Nd:YAG, Alexandrite, and CO_2 lasers are most commonly used for vascular anomalies. Significant complications are rare, and good patient outcomes/satisfaction support the continued use of laser therapy for these lesions. Further research in this area is imperative to continue progress and innovation in the field.

References

1. Keller GS, Toft KM. Lasers in aesthetic surgery. New York: Thieme; 2001. xvi, 368 p.
2. Mulliken JB, Glowacki J. Hemangiomas and vascular malformations in infants and children: a classification based on endothelial characteristics. Plast Reconstr Surg. 1982;69(3): 412–22.
3. Mulliken JB, Glowacki J. Classification of pediatric vascular lesions. Plast Reconstr Surg. 1982;70(1):120–1.
4. Enjolras O, Wassef M, Chapot R. Color atlas of vascular tumors and vascular malformations. Cambridge: Cambridge University Press; 2007. x, 299 p.
5. Frigerio A, Bhama PK, Tan OT. Quantitative three-dimensional assessment of port-wine stain clearance after laser treatments. Lasers Surg Med. 2013;45(10):633–8.
6. Habif TP. Clinical dermatology: a color guide to diagnosis and therapy. 4th ed. Edinburgh: Mosby; 2004. xv, 1004 p.
7. Faurschou A, et al. Lasers or light sources for treating port-wine stains. Cochrane Database Syst Rev. 2011;(11):CD007152.
8. Malm M, Carlberg M. Port-wine stain—a surgical and psychological problem. Ann Plast Surg. 1988;20(6):512–6.
9. Shirley MD, et al. Sturge-Weber syndrome and port-wine stains caused by somatic mutation in GNAQ. N Engl J Med. 2013;368(21):1971–9.
10. Ch'ng S, Tan ST. Facial port-wine stains—clinical stratification and risks of neuro-ocular involvement. J Plast Reconstr Aesthet Surg. 2008;61(8):889–93.
11. Glade RS, et al. Diagnosis and management of pediatric cervicofacial venous malformations: retrospective review from a vascular anomalies center. Laryngoscope. 2010;120(2):229–35.
12. Koncz O, Burrows PE, Mulliken JB. Cervicofacial venous malformations. MRI features and interventional strategies. Interv Neuroradiol. 2002;8(3):227–34.
13. Eivazi B, et al. Laser treatment of mucosal venous malformations of the upper aerodigestive tract in 50 patients. Lasers Med Sci. 2010;25(4):571–6.
14. Richter GT, Braswell L. Management of venous malformations. Facial Plast Surg. 2012; 28(6):603–10.
15. North PE, Mihm Jr MC. Histopathological diagnosis of infantile hemangiomas and vascular malformations. Facial Plast Surg Clin North Am. 2001;9(4):505–24.
16. Colletti G, et al. Contemporary management of vascular malformations. J Oral Maxillofac Surg. 2014;72(3):510–28.
17. Craig LM, Alster TS. Vascular skin lesions in children: a review of laser surgical and medical treatments. Dermatol Surg. 2013;39(8):1137–46.
18. Bitar MA, Moukarbel RV, Zalzal GH. Management of congenital subglottic hemangioma: trends and success over the past 17 years. Otolaryngol Head Neck Surg. 2005; 132(2):226–31.
19. Raol N, et al. Propranolol for the treatment of subglottic hemangiomas. Int J Pediatr Otorhinolaryngol. 2011;75(12):1510–4.
20. Stier MF, Glick SA, Hirsch RJ. Laser treatment of pediatric vascular lesions: port wine stains and hemangiomas. J Am Acad Dermatol. 2008;58(2):261–85.
21. Ashinoff R, Geronemus RG. Flashlamp-pumped pulsed dye laser for port-wine stains in infancy: earlier versus later treatment. J Am Acad Dermatol. 1991;24(3):467–72.
22. Tomson N, et al. The treatment of port-wine stains with the pulsed-dye laser at 2-week and 6-week intervals: a comparative study. Br J Dermatol. 2006;154(4):676–9.
23. Lanigan SW. Port-wine stains unresponsive to pulsed dye laser: explanations and solutions. Br J Dermatol. 1998;139(2):173–7.
24. Savas JA, et al. Pulsed dye laser-resistant port-wine stains: mechanisms of resistance and implications for treatment. Br J Dermatol. 2013;168(5):941–53.
25. Michel S, Landthaler M, Hohenleutner U. Recurrence of port-wine stains after treatment with the flashlamp-pumped pulsed dye laser. Br J Dermatol. 2000;143(6):1230–4.
26. Orten SS, et al. Port-wine stains. An assessment of 5 years of treatment. Arch Otolaryngol Head Neck Surg. 1996;122(11):1174–9.
27. Tan W, et al. Topical rapamycin suppresses the angiogenesis pathways induced by pulsed dye laser: molecular mechanisms of inhibition of regeneration and revascularization of photocoagulated cutaneous blood vessels. Lasers Surg Med. 2012;44(10):796–804.
28. Izikson L, Anderson RR. Treatment endpoints for resistant port wine stains with a 755 nm laser. J Cosmet Laser Ther. 2009;11(1):52–5.
29. Chen JK, et al. An overview of clinical and experimental treatment modalities for port wine stains. J Am Acad Dermatol. 2012; 67(2):289–304.

30. Jia W, et al. Long-term blood vessel removal with combined laser and topical rapamycin antiangiogenic therapy: implications for effective port wine stain treatment. Lasers Surg Med. 2010;42(2):105–12.
31. Loewe R, et al. Stem cell marker upregulation in normal cutaneous vessels following pulsed-dye laser exposure and its abrogation by concurrent rapamycin administration: implications for treatment of port-wine stain birthmarks. J Cutan Pathol. 2010;37 Suppl 1:76–82.
32. Phung TL, et al. Can the wound healing response of human skin be modulated after laser treatment and the effects of exposure extended? Implications on the combined use of the pulsed dye laser and a topical angiogenesis inhibitor for treatment of port wine stain birthmarks. Lasers Surg Med. 2008;40(1):1–5.
33. Klein A, et al. Indocyanine green-augmented diode laser treatment of port-wine stains: clinical and histological evidence for a new treatment option from a randomized controlled trial. Br J Dermatol. 2012;167(2):333–42.
34. Klein A, et al. A randomized controlled trial to optimize indocyanine green-augmented diode laser therapy of capillary malformations. Lasers Surg Med. 2013;45(4):216–24.
35. Scherer K, Waner M. Nd:YAG lasers (1,064 nm) in the treatment of venous malformations of the face and neck: challenges and benefits. Lasers Med Sci. 2007;22(2):119–26.
36. Chang CJ, Fisher DM, Chen YR. Intralesional photocoagulation of vascular anomalies of the tongue. Br J Plast Surg. 1999;52(3):178–81.
37. Adams MT, Saltzman B, Perkins JA. Head and neck lymphatic malformation treatment: a systematic review. Otolaryngol Head Neck Surg. 2012;147(4):627–39.
38. April MM, et al. Laser therapy for lymphatic malformations of the upper aerodigestive tract. An evolving experience. Arch Otolaryngol Head Neck Surg. 1992;118(2):205–8.
39. Glade RS, Buckmiller LM. CO2 laser resurfacing of intraoral lymphatic malformations: a 10-year experience. Int J Pediatr Otorhinolaryngol. 2009;73(10):1358–61.
40. Suen JY, Waner M. Treatment of oral cavity vascular malformations using the neodymium: YAG laser. Arch Otolaryngol Head Neck Surg. 1989;115(11):1329–33.
41. Edwards PD, et al. Lymphatic malformation of the lingual base and oral floor. Plast Reconstr Surg. 2005;115(7):1906–15.
42. Shapshay SM, David LM, Zeitels S. Neodymium-YAG laser photocoagulation of hemangiomas of the head and neck. Laryngoscope. 1987;97(3 Pt 1):323–30.
43. Cohen SR, Thompson JW. Lymphangiomas of the larynx in infants and children. A survey of pediatric lymphangioma. Ann Otol Rhinol Laryngol Suppl. 1986;127:1–20.
44. Bencini PL, et al. Laser use for cutaneous vascular alterations of cosmetic interest. Dermatol Ther. 2012;25(4):340–51.
45. Franca K, et al. Lasers for cutaneous congenital vascular lesions: a comprehensive overview and update. Lasers Med Sci. 2013;28(4):1197–204.
46. Batta K, et al. Randomised controlled study of early pulsed dye laser treatment of uncomplicated childhood haemangiomas: results of a 1-year analysis. Lancet. 2002;360(9332):521–7.
47. Kono T, et al. Comparison study of a traditional pulsed dye laser versus a long-pulsed dye laser in the treatment of early childhood hemangiomas. Lasers Surg Med. 2006;38(2):112–5.
48. Witman PM, et al. Complications following pulsed dye laser treatment of superficial hemangiomas. Lasers Surg Med. 2006;38(2):116–23.
49. Garden JM, Bakus AD, Paller AS. Treatment of cutaneous hemangiomas by the flashlamp-pumped pulsed dye laser: prospective analysis. J Pediatr. 1992;120(4 Pt 1):555–60.
50. Poetke M, Philipp C, Berlien HP. Flashlamp-pumped pulsed dye laser for hemangiomas in infancy: treatment of superficial vs mixed hemangiomas. Arch Dermatol. 2000;136(5):628–32.
51. Brightman LA, et al. Ablative fractional resurfacing for involuted hemangioma residuum. Arch Dermatol. 2012;148(11):1294–8.
52. Marqueling AL, et al. Propranolol and infantile hemangiomas four years later: a systematic review. Pediatr Dermatol. 2013;30(2):182–91.
53. Menezes MD, et al. Status of propranolol for treatment of infantile hemangioma and description of a randomized clinical trial. Ann Otol Rhinol Laryngol. 2011;120(10):686–95.

Part II

Advanced Therapeutic Concepts of Light Therapy

Introduction

Light interacts with tissue through photothermal, photoacoustic, and photochemical mechanisms. Essentially, the tissue effect of these interactions is related to the characteristics of the light and the resulting distribution of photons within the tissue. Accordingly, the properties of light can be selected to modify tissue in a highly specific way. In clinical applications within the head and neck, the importance of using an optical technique is that light can be precisely delivered to alter tissue using minimally invasive technologies.

There are innumerable areas where light can be used to alter tissue structure and behavior. As such, optical therapeutics and diagnostics are appearing in many advanced applications. The topics selected in this subsection focus on emerging areas where clinical efficacy is beginning to be established within the head and neck. These selected applications are associated with optimistic results and are continuing to be developed through translational research.

An important emerging application within optical therapeutics is the use of lasers as applied to transoral robotic surgery (TORS). Tumors can be resected from within the upper airway using this minimally invasive technique, while reducing the cosmetic and functional morbidity associated with more radical surgical maneuvers. The robotic approach improves visualization and access to constrained spaces and aims to increase precision and stability.

Although robotic surgery was initially designed to use electrocautery as a method to cut and coagulate, the implementation of laser systems for performing similar functions has been gaining popularity. Compared to electrocautery, lasers have been shown to decrease collateral thermal tissue damage and increase precision during tumor resection. Both carbon dioxide (CO_2) and thalium-doped yttrium-aluminum-garnet (Th:YAG) lasers have been demonstrated with positive results. The well-fitting union between TORS and lasers will continue to strengthen with improved integration of flexible laser light carriers and optimization of laser parameters.

Optical therapeutics also play a significant a role in minimally invasive cartilage reshaping, such as for correcting deformities of the ear and nasal septum. This novel technique treats cartilage tissue similar to a thermoplastic material by using heat to alter the biophysical properties of the cartilage and producing shape change. The significant advantage of this technique is that it does not rely on making incisions through the skin or mucosa. The process of laser cartilage reshaping simply involves deforming the tissue into the required shape, irradiating the deformed region with laser energy, and splinting the tissue for a period after the procedure. Laser cartilage reshaping has not been widely adopted; however, several large case series have demonstrated successful results with nasal septal straightening auricular reshaping.

In contrast to the various high-powered laser applications that rely on the generation heat, low level laser therapy (LLLT) uses low energy to alter tissue without a significant increase in temperature. This therapeutic modality, which relies on photochemical effects, has been investigated for the treatment of several head and neck conditions that otherwise have limited treatment options. In hearing-related studies performed on animal models, LLLT demonstrates strong evidence for improving acute noise-induced hearing loss and ototoxic hearing loss, likely as a result of recovery of cochlear hair cells. Furthermore, there is encouraging evidence for the use of this technology for the treatment of vestibular dysfunction. Several clinical studies have been performed using transcanal LLLT for the treatment of tinnitus, but with mixed results, which may be due to differences in dosing. Clinical studies have also been performed for the use of LLLT for the treatment of allergic rhinitis, oral mucositis, and neck pain with promising findings.

A wide range of advanced optical therapeutic applications within the head and neck are gaining clinical acceptance through translational research. The subsequent chapters will provide a detailed description, operating principles, and recent progress of these emerging application technologies.

Chapter 13

Transoral Robotic Surgery and Lasers

James Attra and Niels Kokot

Introduction to Transoral Robotic Surgery

The concept of automata devised to replace or enhance human function dates back millennia. Scattered throughout the writings of the earliest great civilizations, one can find myriad examples of constructs devised to mimic humans in form and performance [1]. Among the most intriguing and anatomic of these early robot designs were the creations of the great Renaissance polymath Leonardo da Vinci, which included plans for a mechanical knight complete with an articulating neck and mandible [2]. Although medical robotics was initially pioneered in the 1980s, the intersection of robotics and otolaryngology began in 1995 with robot-automated microdrill stapedotomy and over the past decade has progressed to more sophisticated applications in head and neck surgery [3].

The aptly named da Vinci Surgical System (Intuitive Surgical, Sunnyvale, California, USA) has been approved for use in general surgery since 1997 and has been predominantly utilized in urologic and cardiac procedures [4–6]. It remains the only robot currently approved for clinical use in head and neck surgery, and in December of 2009, the Food and Drug Administration approved the system for use in transoral resection of benign and malignant tumors of the upper aerodigestive tract relegated to T1 and T2 status.

Engineered to improve visualization, precision and stability, the system consists of four components: a surgeon's console, patient sidecart, vision system, and Endowrist instruments (Fig. 1). The operating surgeon is seated at the console and manipulates glove-like master controls, which direct instruments in the

Brian J.-F. Wong and Justus Ilgner (eds.), *Biomedical Optics in Otorhinolaryngology: Head and Neck Surgery*,
DOI 10.1007/978-1-4939-1758-7_13,

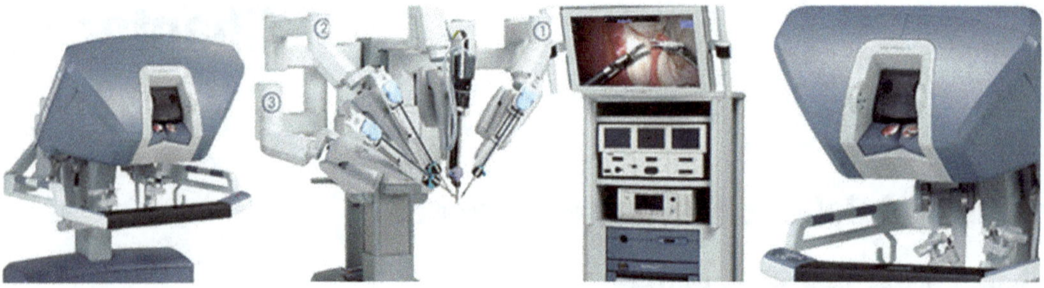

Fig. 1 Schematic demonstrating components of the da Vinci Surgical System, including operator console, Endowrist instruments, and video tower

operative field (Fig. 2). Each instrument arm has seven degrees of freedom: three translational (up and down, left and right, forward and backward), three rotational (roll, yaw, and pitch), and one grip (cutting, grasping, etc.). The system provides for precise motion-scaling of the operators hands to a microlevel and adds tremor reduction. The vision system utilizes a dual-lens endoscope to provide a high-definition stereoscopic 3D view of the operative field. The endoscope is available in 0 and 30° orientations, enabling nonlinear exposure if necessary, such as in surgery of the tongue base or larynx. The patient side cart supports four robotics arms which accommodate an array of surgical instruments including various dissectors, graspers, monopolar and bipolar cautery, as well as the endoscope (Fig. 2). While costly, the system has been embraced in the fields of urology, general surgery, cardiac surgery, and gynecology based on demonstrated benefits in reducing blood loss and complication rates while ameliorating the learning curve for novice surgeons [7, 8]. Increased cost (approximately US$1.5 million coupled with US$100,000 yearly maintenance fee) and operating room setup time as well as a lack of tactile sensory feedback have been commonly cited as general drawbacks of the system and of robotic surgery in general.

Rationale for TORS

The head and neck is a sensitive anatomic region that associates the critical functions of respiration, phonation, and deglutition, while the cosmetic form of the head and neck is of obvious societal and psychological importance. Thus, preservation of function and avoidance of deforming, radical maneuvers are paramount principles well-served by minimally invasive surgery through the oral aperture. Traditionally, most malignant lesions of the oropharynx are accessed via lip-splitting mandibulotomy, allowing for direct visualization and direct manual access to the tumor to

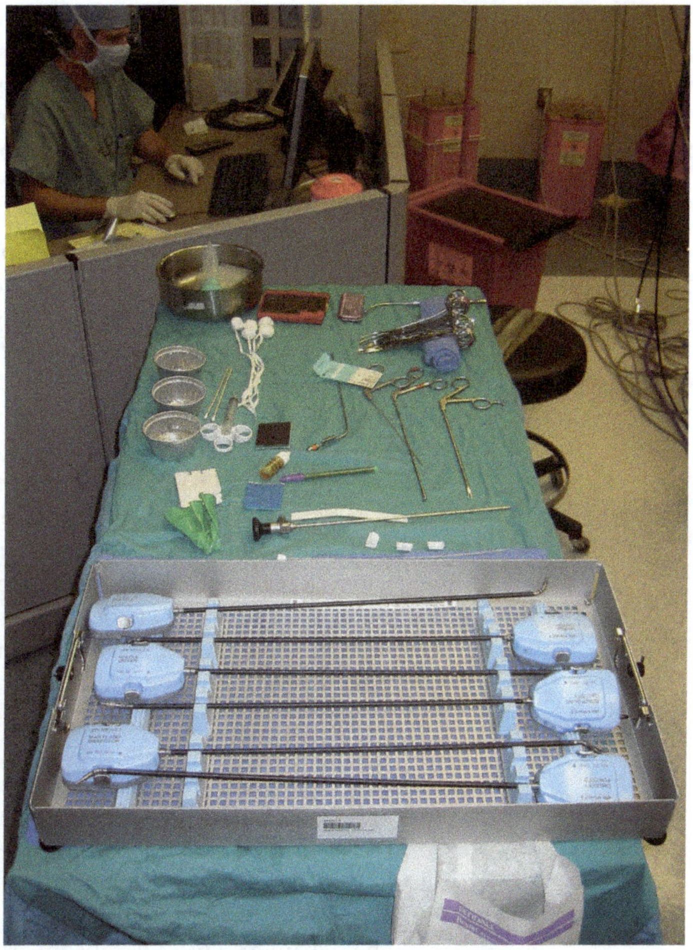

Fig. 2 Array of different Endowrist instruments used in TORS

achieve adequate surgical margins, as well as control of the great vessels in the neck. Immediate surgical morbidity includes the need for either regional or free flap reconstruction, requisite long operative times, and increased blood loss. In general, the natural orifices in the head and neck are inviting to minimally invasive endoscopic techniques. Additionally, most patients undergoing these procedures require a tracheotomy and feeding tube placement. Patients undergo prolonged rehabilitation with variable recovery of speech and swallowing function that may be further impaired by adjuvant radiation or chemoradiation.

In an effort to curtail the morbidity associated with open approaches, investigators in the 1980s and 1990s led landmark trials of organ-preserving combined therapy for head and neck squamous cell carcinoma. The Veterans' Affairs Laryngeal Cancer study and RTOG 91-11 demonstrated equivalent survival with laryngeal preservation in patients treated with primary combined chemoradiation compared to total laryngectomy followed by adjuvant radiation [9, 10]. Similar survival outcomes were seen when these treatment schema were applied to oropharyngeal carcinomas [11]. Increased sensitivity of human papillomavirus-induced carcinomas to primary chemoradiation seems to also have expanded the role for nonsurgical protocols [12]. Given the results of these organ preservation trials, primary treatment for head and neck squamous cell carcinoma has undergone a paradigm shift whereby chemoradiation is viewed as a viable organ-preserving first-line therapy at many institutions.

Despite this evolution, there continues to be an impetus to develop a therapy that avoids the morbidity of radical surgery while mitigating the long-term functional sequelae of primary chemoradiation. The development of transoral laser microsurgery (TLM) in the 1970s heralded the possibility of equivalent locoregional control of disease through a minimally invasive approach, but technical challenges have hindered its widespread use among head and neck cancer surgeons [13]. Necessitating single-handed surgery performed through a rigid laryngoscope and utilizing a "line-of-sight" microscope-mounted CO_2 laser, TLM presents many equipment-related compromises that are elegantly obviated by robotic technology. Offering nonlinear endoscopy and wristed instrumentation, the da Vinci system grants the operator a much wider view of the surgical field and allows more natural multiplanar tissue dissection than transoral surgery using a microscope.

The acronym TORS (transoral robotic surgery) was coined by investigators at the University of Pennsylvania, whose systematic and pioneering work in cadaver laboratory feasibility studies and later in animal and human series helped to establish a definitive role and safety profile for robotics in head and neck surgical oncology [14–17]. Through their efforts, operating room setup of the da Vinci robot for TORS was made systematic and reproducible and the importance of utilizing a suitable mouth gag for introducing the instrument arms into the surgical field was elucidated (Figs. 3, 4, and 5). The investigators found that TORS offered the benefits of avoiding the negative functional and cosmetic sequelae of lip-splitting mandibulotomy while providing for decreased operative time, blood loss, and increased visualization for tumors of the oropharynx and larynx [17–19]. Wristed instrumentation rendered possible various "open" surgical maneuvers unable to be performed with more restrictive traditional techniques, including dissection in an axial plane and caudal-to-cranial vector. Patients treated with TORS also enjoy more rapid recovery and decreased rates of tracheotomy and feeding

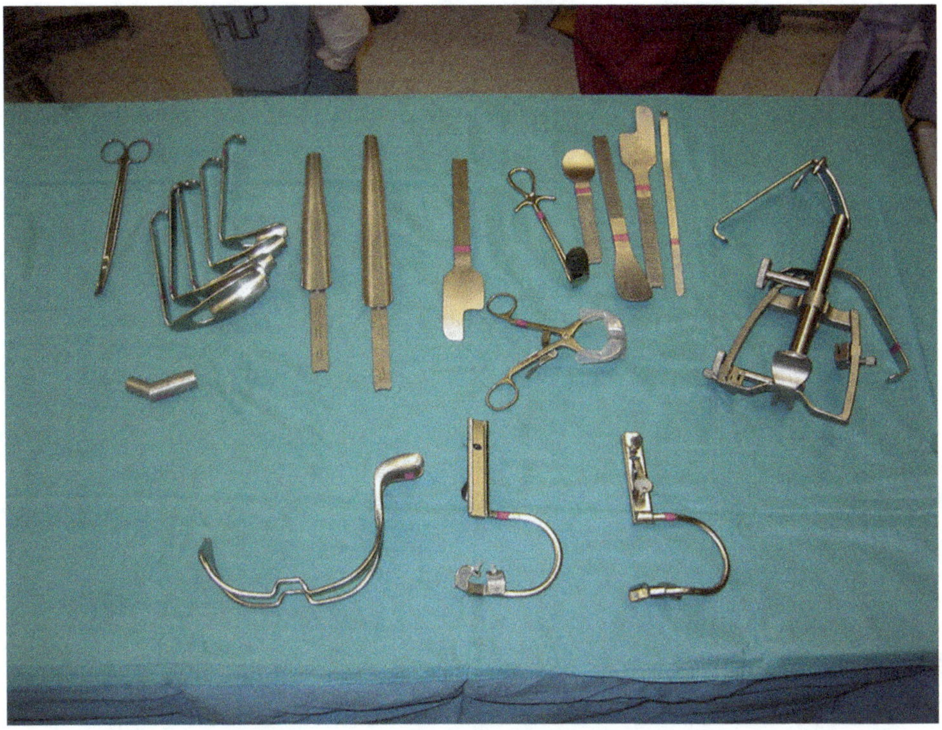

Fig. 3 Operating room side table with mouth gags commonly employed in TORS

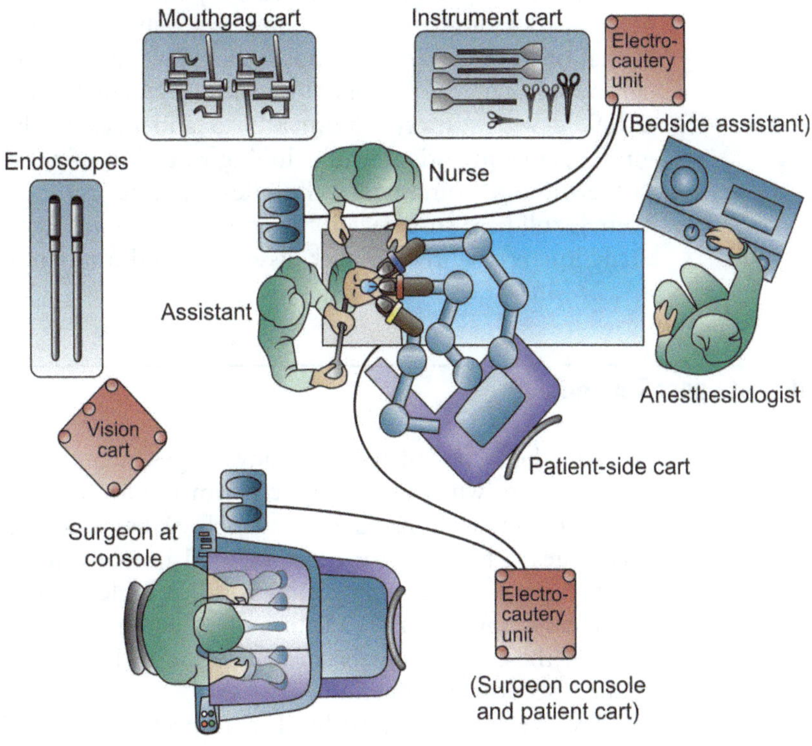

Fig. 4 Standard operating room layout using the da Vinci Surgical System for TORS

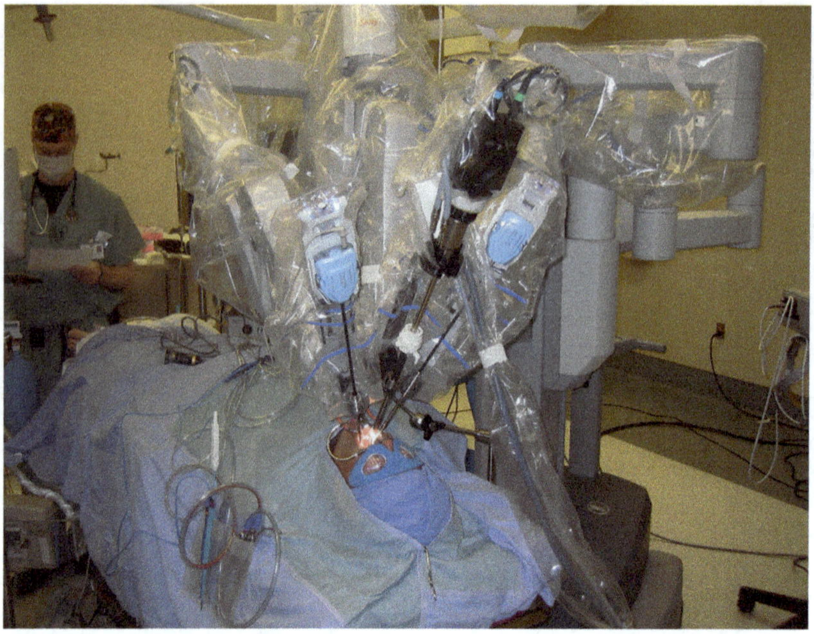

Fig. 5 Patient sidecart orientation for TORS, with instruments arms oriented at the head of bed

tube placement, all while experiencing equivalent oncologic outcomes [19–26]. Thus, robotic surgery through the oral aperture developed widespread applicability as a viable alternative to traditional open and transoral approaches for definitive treatment of laryngopharyngeal tumors. Following FDA approval of TORS in 2009, a wide variety of other head and neck applications are under active investigation, including resection of parapharyngeal space tumors, combined techniques for transoral total laryngectomy, skull base surgery, glottic surgery, intraoral free flap reconstruction, retroauricular neck dissection, and submandibulectomy [4, 27–35].

Incorporation of Laser Technology

Despite the litany of technical advantages, adaptation of the da Vinci system, which was designed primarily for abdominal procedures, to applications in otolaryngology has not been without challenges. The need for more tailored instrumentation, smaller robotic arms and a more acute working angle continue to spur technical innovation in the field of head and neck robotic surgery. Among these has been the incorporation of laser technology for tissue resection and ablation.

Proven and celebrated by their respective bodies of literature in otolaryngology, TORS and laser technology seem an ideal marriage for the treatment of head and neck malignancies, particularly of the supraglottic and glottic larynx. Since its introduction to transoral surgery in the 1970s, transoral CO_2 laser resection of laryngopharyngeal tumors has been recognized as advantageous in reducing collateral thermal damage and offering improved precision and hemostasis when compared to conventional monopolar electrocautery, properties ideal for laryngopharyngeal surgery [13, 36]. However, as alluded to previously, the protocol for TLM utilizes an instrument setup with a fixed single axis of resection via the line-of-sight of the mounted laser through a rigid laryngoscope, placing the surgeon a good distance from the operative field and necessitating sometimes awkward and constrained surgical maneuvers. Difficulty in mastering the subtleties of this technique has limited its use in earnest to a handful of major centers [37].

TORS has traditionally relied upon the proprietary monopolar and bipolar electrocautery instruments manufactured by Intuitive Surgical for cutting and hemostasis, raising concerns over unnecessary collateral tissue carbonization, increased postoperative crusting and edema, and histologic distortion of the specimen. Studies of mucosal incisions in animal models have suggested superiority of laser tissue ablation compared to conventional electrocautery in this regard [38, 39]. This consideration is particularly relevant to laryngeal and hypopharyngeal surgery, where precision and minimization of edema are of added importance [40, 43]. It would seem that the convention of TLM offers an ideal resecting and ablating tool in the CO_2 laser but with a nuanced and sometimes difficult delivery of the instrument, while conventional TORS presents a more capable delivery platform but suffers from the drawbacks of electrocautery. Therefore, it was no long before surgeons began searching for ways to adapt laser technology to the robot to reap the potential benefits of both.

CO_2 Laser

The carbon dioxide laser uses a gaseous state active medium to deliver energy at 0.1–100 W with a wavelength of 10,600 nm. It generally ablates to a depth of 200 μm and its chromophore is water. The benefits of the CO_2 laser for resection of laryngeal lesions are well-described, particularly within the context of TLM. With the advent of the first hollow-tube flexible carrier for the CO_2 laser (OmniGuide company, Cambridge, MA, USA) it became possible to channel laser energy distally to the tip of the da Vinci instrument arms, empowering the laser with a range of motion unprecedented in previous transoral surgery techniques. Pilot studies emerged in the late 2000s documenting feasible use of the CO_2 laser in resection of supraglottic and oropharyngeal tumors. Early mechanics for introducing the hollow fiber into the operative field included a side channel manually welded to an instrument arm, which proved to be unsatisfactory, an Endo-Sheath (Vision Sciences, Natick, MA, USA), and fastening the fiber to the tip of the monopolar cautery [41, 42]. Currently, Omniguide manufactures a metallic flexible coil (Flexguide ULTRA, Omniguide company, Cambridge, MA, USA) that attaches to the proprietary da Vinci needle driver and accommodates a CO_2 laser fiber. Pictured is the instrument setup and use in performing a robotic supraglottic laryngectomy (Figs. 6, 7, 8, 9, 10, 11, 12, and 13). In 2007, Solares et al. presented use of a flexible hollow-core fiber to conduct a CO_2 laser for cadaveric, animal, and human trials of robot-assisted supraglottic partial laryngectomy [41]. An Endo-Sheath system was used to couple the laser to the robotic arm. Laser energy was delivered in continuous wave mode at 7.2–10 W. Proof-of-concept and feasibility were demonstrated in human cadaver and living canine models and the authors were able to successfully perform the procedure on a single patient, for the first time combining laser technology with a TORS approach to treat a living human subject. Inadequate exposure prevented surgery in the remaining two patients in the series. Later in 2008, Desai et al. conducted a prospective trial of laser-assisted TORS on eight patients using the CO_2 laser fiber

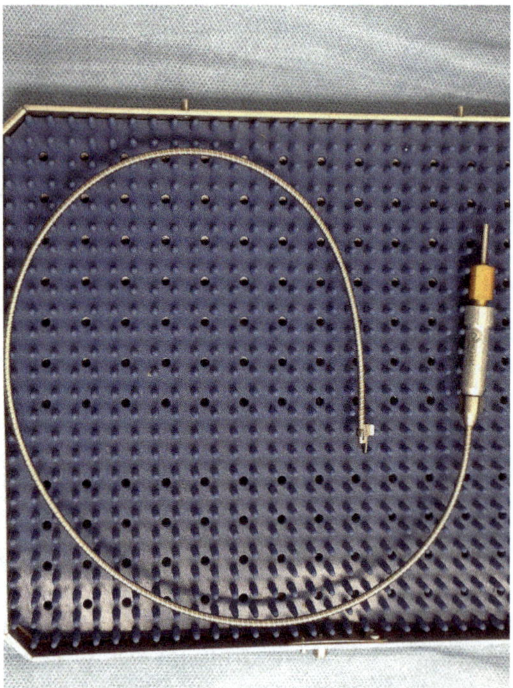

Fig. 6 Omiguide Flexguide ULTRA coil used to accommodate a CO_2 laser fiber in TORS

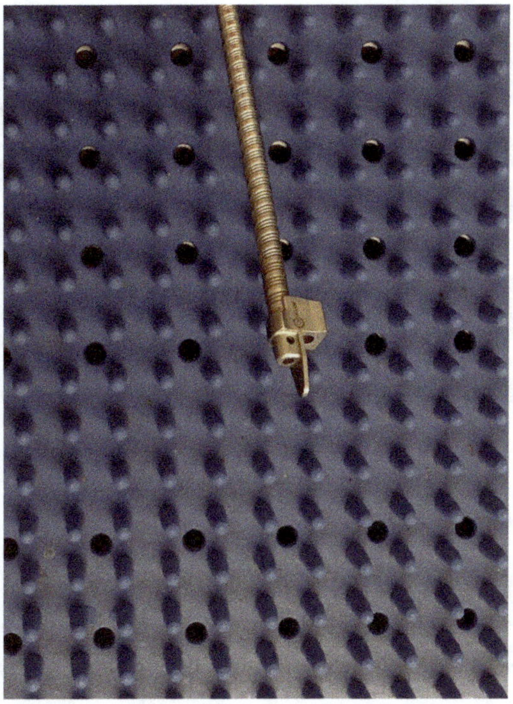

Fig. 7 Flexguide ULTRA tip detail

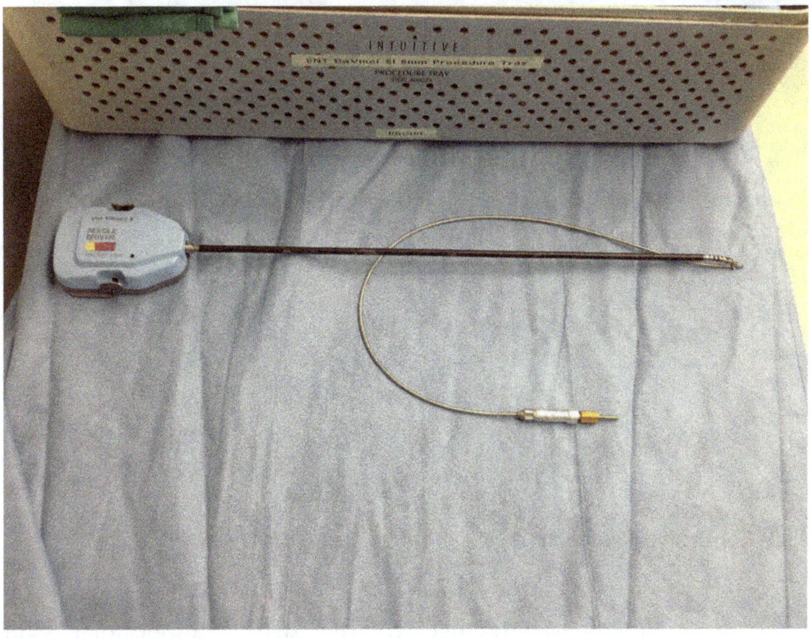

Fig. 8 Flexguide ULTRA articulates with da Vinci propriety needle driver

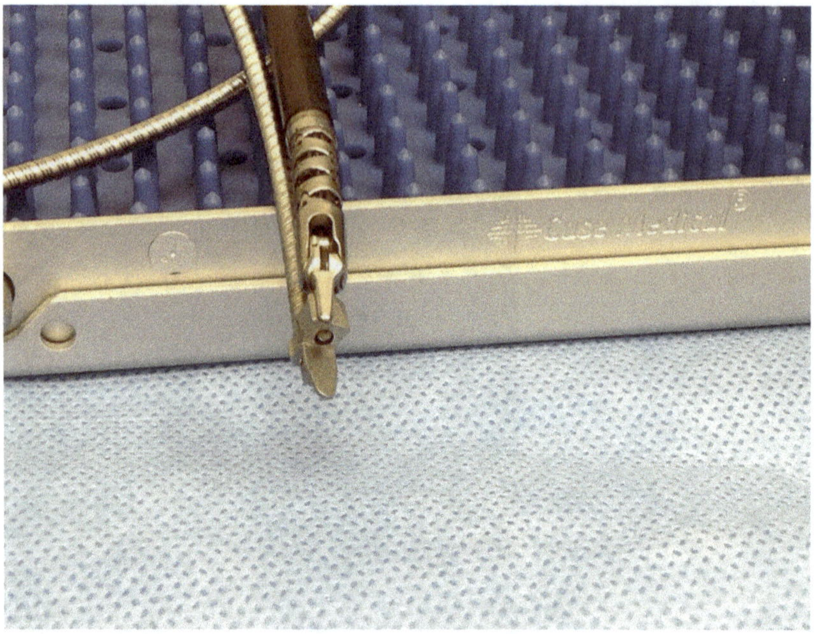

Fig. 9 Flexguide ULTRA articulates with da Vinci propriety needle driver (detail)

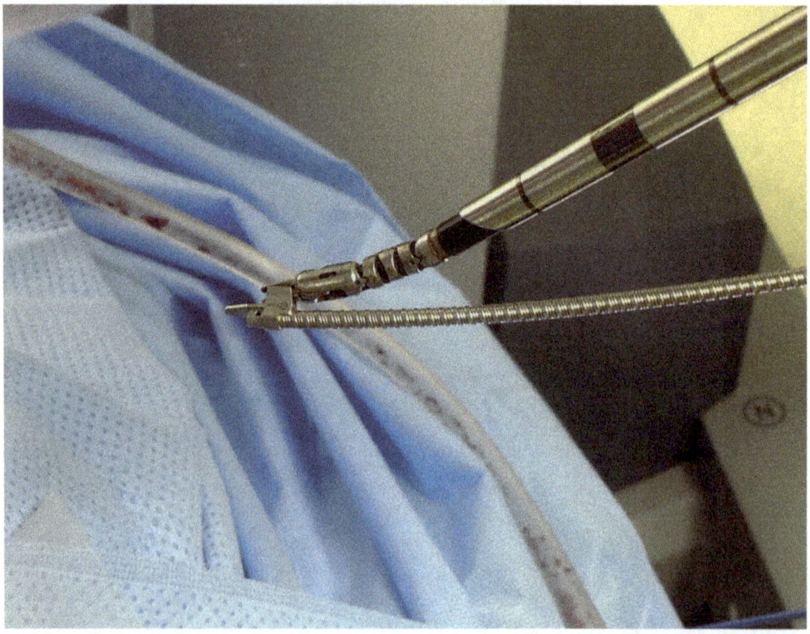

Fig. 10 Flexguide ULTRA articulates with da Vinci propriety needle driver (detail)

manually attached to the spatula monopolar cautery [42]. Pathology included six oropharyngeal and one supraglottic malignancy. Laser energy was delivered in a continuous wave between 7 and 14 W with a 200 μm spot size. The approach proved feasible

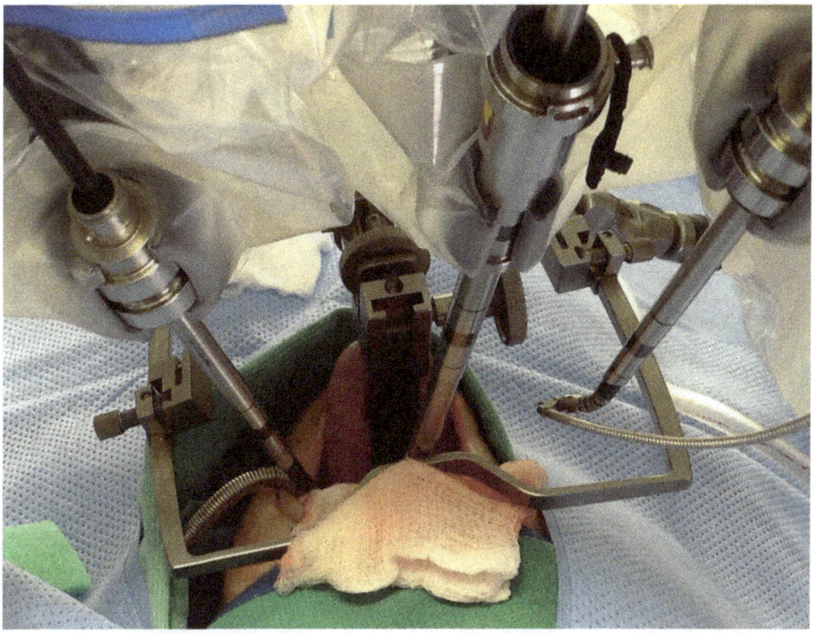

Fig. 11 CO_2 laser fiber employed in TORS

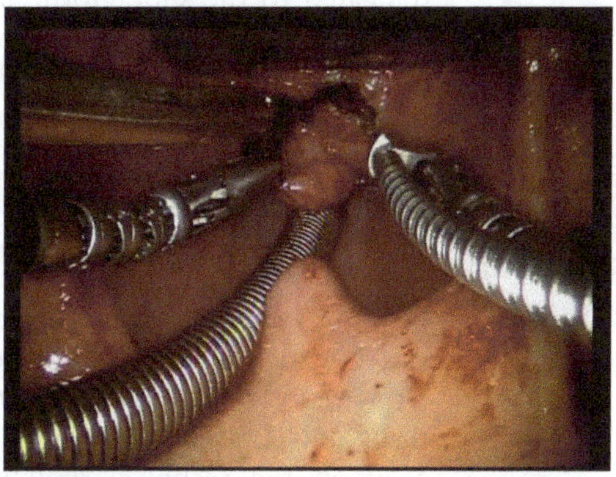

Fig. 12 Endoscopic view of CO_2 laser fiber used in TORS supraglottic laryngectomy

in seven of the eight patients, with insufficient exposure of the supraglottis preventing surgery in one patient. One patient with a supraglottic tumor underwent a precautionary tracheotomy but this was avoided in the remaining six patients. All six patients with oropharyngeal tumors began tolerating an oral diet on the first postoperative day, while the patient with a supraglottic carcinoma began an oral diet 3 days following the procedure. There were no postoperative complications and no evidence of disease recurrence at an average follow-up time of 4 months. The authors conducting both of these early series recognized the superior visualization

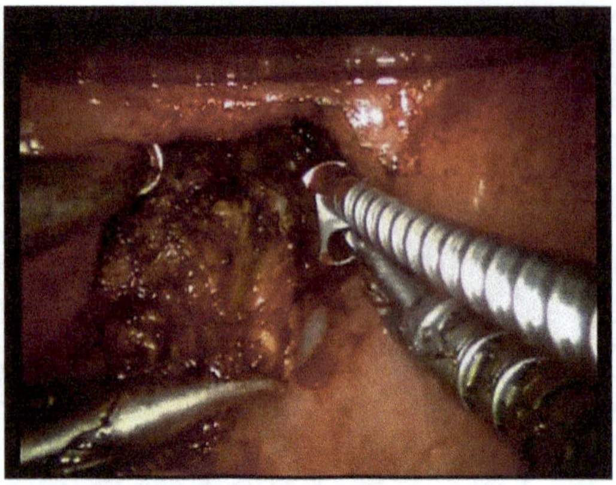

Fig. 13 Endoscopic view of CO_2 laser fiber used in TORS supraglottic laryngectomy

and instrument dexterity afforded by TORS combined with the precise cutting properties of the laser, but were significantly restrained by instrument arm size and a lack of sophisticated integration of the laser into the robot mechanism and cited a serious need for technological improvement in these areas.

Laryngeal applications of TORS, as in TLM, have mostly been relegated to the supraglottic larynx, as access to the level of the glottis has proven difficult with the current instrumentation. However, recently in 2013 Lallement et al. reported a retrospective study on a series of patients with early staged (T1 and T2) laryngeal tumors treated with TORS, with more than half of the lesions being glottic in origin (13 out of 23 patients) [43]. He was largely successful and able to demonstrate feasibility of the technique, with only three patients requiring tracheotomy and 11 needing a nasogastric tube postoperatively. At 12 months of follow-up patients enjoyed oncologic outcomes commensurate with TLM reports, with 10 % recurrence rate, 95 % laryngeal preservation, and 100 % global survival. The authors commented specifically on the technical drawbacks of monopolar cautery when utilized in laryngeal surgery, including inadvertent collateral tissue damage and pathologic distortion of the tumor specimen. In one case, intraoperative breach of the cricothyroid membrane while resecting an anterior commissure lesion was ascribed to the imprecision of the electrocautery as a cutting tool. Use of maximum motion scaling when using cautery was recommended and the potential benefits of laser technology in this context were cited, although no lasers were utilized in the series.

Similar concerns over tissue carbonization and crusting when using electrocautery were reported in a similarly sized series of 24 patients reported by Lawson et al. in 2011 [44]. His patients underwent TORS for various early staged tumors of the supraglottic larynx, oropharynx and oral cavity. All tumors in the study were safely and satisfactorily removed, but the lack of available laser technology at the time was plainly cited as a drawback of TORS.

Application of laser-assisted TORS to the glottic larynx advanced in 2011 when Blanco et al. reported successful excision of a T1a glottic squamous cell carcinoma using TORS [45]. He used a CO_2 fiber fastened to an effector arm with a 16Fr red rubber catheter. The tumor was removed with oncologically sound 2 mm margins and tracheotomy was not required. This marked the first use of laser-assisted TORS for glottic surgery in a human patient.

Across these reports, investigators reported several advantages when using the laser with TORS. Specifically, the finer tissue cutting of the CO_2 laser aided in more controlled tumor resection and also in construction of pharyngeal reconstructive flaps. Authors reported reduced burn artifact on histologic analysis of the specimen as well as the depth and width of acute burn injury. Additionally, the multidirectional and tangential capabilities of the instrument arm as a point of origin for the laser allowed for more intuitive tissue handling when compared to using a "line-of-sight" laser mounted well away from the operative field. This obviated time required for repositioning the microscope and laryngoscope as in TLM. Obstacles encountered in these early trials were related to bulkiness of the instrument arms and proved prohibitive in some scenarios as described previously [41, 42]. Authors cited better integration of the laser delivery fiber into the system and reduction of instrument arm size as particular areas of future improvement.

In 2011, Remacle et al. completed a small prospective trial to establish the safety and feasibility of a new hollow-core glass wave guide (Lumenis, Santa Clara, CA) to channel a CO_2 laser in TORS [46]. Unlike previous trials combining TORS with the CO_2 laser, the authors were able to utilize the 5Fr proprietary fiber introducer designed by Intuitive Surgical for use with the da Vinci system. They presented four patients with early-stage (T1 and T2) tumors of the oropharynx and supraglottis. Average setup time was 30 min and average operative time was 94 min. Patients experienced an average inpatient stay of 6 days. Complete tumor resection with negative pathological margins was accomplished in all cases and no patient required tracheotomy. At 9 months' follow-up, there were no reported complications. Intraoperative settings for the laser were 7–15 W, continuous delivery.

Thulium-Doped YAG Laser

A technical step forward was made in 2008 when the FDA approved the Intuitive Surgical 5Fr fiber introducer for use with validated surgical lasers, including the CO_2 and Thulium-doped yttrium–

aluminum–garnet (Th:YAG) lasers. The Th:YAG laser is a diode-pumped solid-state laser generated in a continuous-wave beam with a wavelength of 2013 nm (about 2 μm) [47]. Like the CO_2 laser, its target chromophore is water. While less widely utilized than the CO_2 laser in otolaryngology, it has been employed to treat airway pathology in both adult and pediatric populations and has also been used in conjunction with surgical robotics in both urologic and neurosurgical applications [47–50]. Additionally, it has been used for the endoscopic treatment of sialolithiasis [51]. The laser boasts ideal qualities for use in mucosal surgery, including a soft tissue penetration depth of <1 mm, closed water absorption peak, and shorter wavelength than the CO_2 laser [52].

In 2012, Benazzo et al. completed a series of operations utilizing the da Vinci 5Fr introducer coupled with a Thulium-doped YAG laser fiber to remove early (T1-staged) supraglottic and oropharyngeal carcinomas [53]. The investigators demonstrated feasibility, with all six patients in the series undergoing successful extirpation of their tumors with clear pathologic margins and excellent functional outcomes. A 2 μm continuous wave Thulium laser was carried with a 273 μm fiber at powers ranging from 5 to 8.5 W. Open neck dissection was completed at the time of excision of the primary tumor when indicated. Patients underwent prophylactic tracheotomy but were decannulated at a mean of 7.5 days. Average length of inpatient stay was 10.7 days, and patients tolerated an oral diet at a mean of 5.0 days.

In the same year, Van Abel et al. submitted a prospective cohort trial of 15 patients undergoing removal of upper aerodigestive tract malignancies with the TORS using the Th:YAG laser matched with 30 controls treated with TORS coupled with conventional electrocautery [52]. A 70-W 2 μm continuous wave Th-YAG laser was used. They assessed safety, feasibility, and 30-day functional outcome, demonstrating comparable safety thulium laser-assisted TORS. All tumors were excised completely with negative surgical margins in both arms of the study and open neck dissection was done at the time of TORS when feasible. They achieved statistical significance in reducing the percentage of intraoperative pharyngotomies (8 % vs. 42 % in the control group), as well as less postoperative pain and need for analgesia. Intraoperative blood loss and postoperative complications were comparable to patients treated with electrocautery, with no statistically significant differences noted. The investigators postulated that the finer cutting action and potentially improved hemostasis seen with the Th:YAG laser led to better visualization and subsequently better preservation of the buccopharyngeal fascia tissue plane. Lessened postoperative pain in the investigative arm was attributed to the deeper and wider thermal damage zone associated with electrocautery as well as the finer tissue ablation granted by the laser.

As the availability of lasers for use in TORS has increased, investigators have begun to compare their properties alongside those of other cutting tools used with the da Vinci system. In 2013, Mattheis et al. reported a prospective series of six patients who underwent CO_2 laser-assisted TORS for T1–T2 oropharyngeal tumors and compared technical feasibility, cutting properties, operative time, and hemostasis with a series of 17 patients undergoing TORS using the Th:YAG laser and electrocautery [54]. Using the CO_2 laser at 15 W energy level, they reported smaller vaporization and coagulation zones than those associated with the other cutting modalities. Based on their results, the CO_2 laser was recommended over the Th:YAG laser as a more precise cutting tool for use in TORS.

Also in 2013, Hoffman et al. demonstrated the various physical cutting properties and subjective intraoperative performance scores of an array of resection tools suited for TORS, including the CO_2 and Th:YAG lasers, radiofrequency (RF) needle, and conventional electrocautery [55]. Evaluation was carried out on porcine tongue specimens as well as on human TORS patients. Histopathologic analysis of both the cut and coagulation zone width was completed for cuts made along the porcine base of tongue (corresponding to lymphoid tissue), lateral tongue (corresponding to muscular tissue with thin mucosa), and tongue tip (representing thick mucosa) at varying energy levels for each instrument. A second component to the study compiled subjective performance grades given independently by the two authors evaluating use of each of the instruments when performing TORS on human patients (the exception being the radiofrequency needle, which currently lacks approval for use in TORS and therefore was evaluated during nonrobotic surgery only). These subjective scales were a modification of that proposed by Sinha et al, and included qualities such as hemostasis, user friendliness, tissue sticking, coagulation, and speed [38]. The third component of the report was a cost evaluation for each instrument system, considering list price and cost to replace disposable components over a range of 5–60 cases. On histopathologic evaluation of the specimens, the CO_2 laser and monopolar cautery had the largest incision width in all three tongue tissue zones, while the RF needle resulted in the narrowest. In all three zones, the largest coagulation zone was produced by the monopolar electrocautery, while the narrowest was produced by the RF needle. The monopolar cautery collected the worst performance scores for bleeding, tissue sticking and user friendliness, with both lasers and the RF needle performing superiorly in those categories, partially owing to the noncontact nature of the lasers. The RF needle and cautery prevailed on cost analysis, with both lasers touting a higher initial acquisition expense as well as high replacement costs for laser fibers. Overall, the study confirmed previously demonstrated superiority of laser fibers in achieving hemostasis and minimizing the zone of coagulation, while also bolstering the case for approving radiofrequency technology for use in TORS.

In this author's experience, the physicality of the laser as a "noncontact" instrument confers both advantages and drawbacks when considering tissue handling and access to deeper structures. The spatula tip of the monopolar electrocautery allows use as a blunt dissector as well as a tissue-cutting instrument, a valuable convenience with limited availability among current laser delivery systems. Conversely, the ability of the laser to ablate tissue at a distance gives the instrument greater "reach" than electrocautery and other instruments which require tissue contact, rendering lasers invaluable when operating on areas of the larynx and hypopharynx that are difficult to contact with the instrument arms.

Conclusion

The application of surgical robotics to otolaryngology has led to a minimally invasive, oncologically effective approach to head and neck tumors that has yielded impressive oncologic and functional outcomes and expanded visualization and bimanual, multiplanar access to the surgical field. However, robotic technology as related to transoral surgery is still completely nascent, nonspecialized, and ripe for innovation. Coupling the laser, a proven superior resecting tool, with the unprecedented access and visualization capable via TORS has been largely successful when pioneered and holds promise for becoming the standard of care for surgical treatment of early-stage laryngopharyngeal tumors. As head and neck surgeons continue to adapt robotic technology to meet their specific needs, the successful integration of evidence-supported tools, such as the CO_2 and Th:YAG lasers, provides an encouraging precedent for enterprising practitioners aiming to advance the capabilities of TORS through the use of proven otolaryngic techniques.

References

1. Robotics Research Group. University of Texas at Austin. Robotics: history. http://www.robotics.utexas.edu/rrg/learn_more/history. Accessed 8 Oct 2010.
2. Rosheim ME. Leonardo's lost robots. Heidelberg: Springer; 2006. p. 69.
3. Brett PN, Baker DA, Reyes L, et al. An automatic technique for microdrilling a stapedotomy in the flexible stapes footplate. Proc Inst Mech Eng. 1995;209:255–62.
4. Maan ZN, et al. The use of robotics in otolaryngology-head and neck surgery: a systematic review. Am J Otolaryngol. 2012;33(1):137–46.
5. Modi P, Rodriguez E, Chitwood Jr WR. Robot-assisted cardiac surgery. Interact Cardiovasc Thorac Surg. 2010;9:500–5.
6. Carpentier A, Loulmet D, Aupecle B, Kieffer JP, Tournay D, Guibourt P, et al. [Computer assisted open heart surgery. First case operated

on with success]. C R Acad Sci III. 1998;321(5):437–42.

7. Woods ME, Wiklund P, Castle EP. Robot-assisted radical cystectomy: recent advances and review of the literature. Curr Opin Urol. 2010;20:125–9.
8. Poffo R, Toschi AP, Pope RB. Robotic surgery in cardiology: a safe and effective procedure. Einstein (Sao Paulo). 2013;11(3):296–302.
9. Induction chemotherapy plus radiation compared with surgery plus radiation in patients with advanced laryngeal cancer. The Department of Veterans Affairs Laryngeal Cancer Study Group. N Engl J Med. 1991;324(24):1685–90.
10. Forastiere AA, Goepfert H, Maor M, Pajak TF, Weber R, Morrison W, et al. Concurrent chemotherapy and radiotherapy for organ preservation in advanced laryngeal cancer. N Engl J Med. 2003;349(22):2091–8.
11. Calais G, Alfonsi M, Bardet E, Sire C, Germain T, Bergerot P, et al. Randomized trial of radiation therapy versus concomitant chemotherapy and radiation therapy for advanced-stage oropharynx carcinoma. J Natl Cancer Inst. 1999;91(24):2081–6.
12. Ang KK, Harris J, Wheeler R, Weber R, Rosenthal DI, Nguyen-Tan PF, et al. Human papillomavirus and survival of patients with oropharyngeal cancer. N Engl J Med. 2010;363(1):24–35.
13. Steiner W, Ambrosch P. Endoscopic laser surgery of the upper aerodigestive tract: with special emphasis on cancer surgery. Stuttgart: Thieme; 2000.
14. Hockstein NG, Nolan JP, O'Malley Jr BW, Woo YJ. Robotic microlaryngeal surgery: a technical feasibility study using the daVinci surgical robot and an airway mannequin. Laryngoscope. 2005;115(5):780–5.
15. Hockstein NG, Nolan JP, O'Malley Jr BW, Woo YJ. Robot-assisted pharyngeal and laryngeal microsurgery: results of robotic cadaver dissections. Laryngoscope. 2005;115(6):1003–8.
16. Weinstein GS, O'Malley Jr BW, Hockstein NG. Transoral robotic surgery: supraglottic laryngectomy in a canine model. Laryngoscope. 2005;115(7):1315–9.
17. Hockstein NG, Weinstein GS, O'Malley Jr BW. Maintenance of hemostasis in transoral robotic surgery. ORL J Otorhinolaryngol Relat Spec. 2005;67(4):220–4.
18. Hockstein NG, O'Malley Jr BW, Weinstein GS. Assessment of intraoperative safety in transoral robotic surgery. Laryngoscope. 2006;116(2):165–8.
19. Weinstein GS, O'Malley Jr BW, Snyder W, Sherman E, Quon H. Transoral robotic surgery: radical tonsillectomy. Arch Otolaryngol Head Neck Surg. 2007;133(12):1220–6.
20. Weinstein GS, O'Malley Jr BW, Cohen MA, Quon H. Transoral robotic surgery for advanced oropharyngeal carcinoma. Arch Otolaryngol Head Neck Surg. 2010; 136(11):1079–85.
21. de Arruda FF, Puri DR, Zhung J, Narayana A, Wolden S, Hunt M, et al. Intensity-modulated radiation therapy for the treatment of oropharyngeal carcinoma: the Memorial Sloan-Kettering Cancer Center experience. Int J Radiat Oncol Biol Phys. 2006;64(2): 363–73.
22. Lawson JD, Otto K, Chen A, Shin DM, Davis L, Johnstone PA. Concurrent platinum-based chemotherapy and simultaneous modulated accelerated radiation therapy for locally advanced squamous cell carcinoma of the tongue base. Head Neck. 2008;30(3): 327–35.
23. Cohen MA, Weinstein GS, O'Malley Jr BW, Feldman M, Quon H. Transoral robotic surgery and human papillomavirus status: oncologic results. Head Neck. 2011;33(4):573–80.
24. Weinstein GS, Quon H, O'Malley Jr BW, Kim GG, Cohen MA. Selective neck dissection and deintensified postoperative radiation and chemotherapy for oropharyngeal cancer: a subset analysis of the University of Pennsylvania transoral robotic surgery trial. Laryngoscope. 2010;120(9):1749–55.
25. White HN, Moore EJ, Rosenthal EL, Carroll WR, Olsen KD, Desmond RA, et al. Transoral robotic-assisted surgery for head and neck squamous cell carcinoma: one- and 2-year survival analysis. Arch Otolaryngol Head Neck Surg. 2010;136(12):1248–52.
26. Genden EM, Kotz T, Tong CC, Smith C, Sikora AG, Teng MS, et al. Transoral robotic resection and reconstruction for head and neck cancer. Laryngoscope. 2011;121(8):1668–74.
27. O'Malley Jr BW, Weinstein GS. Robotic skull base surgery: preclinical investigations to human clinical application. Arch Otolaryngol Head Neck Surg. 2007;133(12):1215–9.
28. Hanna EY, Holsinger C, DeMonte F, Kupferman M. Robotic endoscopic surgery of the skull base: a novel surgical approach. Arch Otolaryngol Head Neck Surg. 2007;133(12):1209–14.
29. McCool RR, Warren FM, Wiggins 3rd RH, Hunt JP. Robotic surgery of the infratemporal fossa utilizing novel suprahyoid port. Laryngoscope. 2010;120(9):1738–43.

30. O'Malley Jr BW, Quon H, Leonhardt FD, Chalian AA, Weinstein GS. Transoral robotic surgery for parapharyngeal space tumors. ORL J Otorhinolaryngol Relat Spec. 2010;72(6):332–6.
31. Wei WI, Ho WK. Transoral robotic resection of recurrent nasopharyngeal carcinoma. Laryngoscope. 2010;120(10):2011–4.
32. Mukhija VK, Sung CK, Desai SC, Wanna G, Genden EM. Transoral robotic assisted free flap reconstruction. Otolaryngol Head Neck Surg. 2009;140(1):124–5.
33. Haus BM, Kambham N, Le D, Moll FM, Gourin C, Terris DJ. Surgical robotic applications in otolaryngology. Laryngoscope. 2003;113(7):1139–44.
34. Terris DJ, Haus BM, Gourin CG. Endoscopic neck surgery: resection of the submandibular gland in a cadaver model. Laryngoscope. 2004;114(3):407–10.
35. Smith RV, Schiff BA, Sarta C, Hans S, Brasnu D. Transoral robotic total laryngectomy. Laryngoscope. 2013;123(3):678–82.
36. Steiner W, Fierek O, Ambrosch P, Hommerich CP, Kron M. Transoral laser microsurgery for squamous cell carcinoma of the base of the tongue. Arch Otolaryngol Head Neck Surg. 2003;129(1):36–43.
37. Haughey BH, Hinni ML, Salassa JR, Hayden RE, Grant DG, Rich JT, et al. Transoral laser microsurgery as primary treatment for advanced-stage oropharyngeal cancer: a united states multicenter study. Head Neck. 2011;33(12):1683–94.
38. Sinha UK, Gallagher LA. Effects of steel scalpel, ultrasonic scalpel, CO2 laser, and monopolar and bipolar electrosurgery on wound healing in guinea pig oral mucosa. Laryngoscope. 2003;113(2):228–36.
39. Liboon J, Funkhouser W, Terris DJ. A comparison of mucosal incisions made by scalpel, CO2 laser, electrocautery, and constant-voltage electrocautery. Otolaryngol Head Neck Surg. 1997;116(3):379–85.
40. Yan Y, Olszewski AE, Hoffman MR, Zhuang P, Ford CN, Dailey SH, et al. Use of lasers in laryngeal surgery. J Voice. 2010;24(1):102–9.
41. Solares CA, Strome M. Transoral robot-assisted CO2 laser supraglottic laryngectomy: experimental and clinical data. Laryngoscope. 2007;117(5):817–20.
42. Desai SC, Sung CK, Jang DW, Genden EM. Transoral robotic surgery using a carbon dioxide flexible laser for tumors of the upper aerodigestive tract. Laryngoscope. 2008;118(12):2187–9.
43. Lallemant B, Chambon G, Garrel R, Kacha S, Rupp D, Galy-Bernadoy C, Chapuis H, et al. Transoral robotic surgery for the treatment of T1-T2 carcinoma of the larynx: preliminary study. Laryngoscope. 2013;123(10):2485–90.
44. Lawson G, Matar N, Remacle M, Jamart J, Bachy V. Transoral robotic surgery for the management of head and neck tumors: learning curve. Eur Arch Otorhinolaryngol. 2011;268(12):1795–801.
45. Blanco RG, Ha PK, Califano JA, Saunders JM. Transoral robotic surgery of the vocal cord. J Laparoendosc Adv Surg Tech A. 2011;21(2):157–9.
46. Remacle M, Matar N, Lawson G, Bachy V, Delos M, Nollevaux MC, et al. Combining a new CO2 laser wave guide with transoral robotic surgery: a feasibility study on four patients with malignant tumors. Eur Arch Otorhinolaryngol. 2012;269(7):1833–7.
47. Zeitels SM, Burns JA, Akst LM, Hillman RE, Broadhurst MS, Anderson RR. Office-based and microlaryngeal applications of a fiber-based thulium laser. Ann Otol Rhinol Laryngol. 2006;115(12):891–6.
48. Ayari-Khalfallah S, Fuchsmann C, Froehlich P. Thulium laser in airway diseases in children. Curr Opin Otolaryngol Head Neck Surg. 2008;16(1):55–9.
49. Tang K, Xu Z, Xia D, Ma X, Guo X, Guan W, et al. Early outcomes of thulium laser versus transurethral resection of the prostate for managing benign prostatic hyperplasia: a systematic review and meta-analysis of comparative studies. J Endourol. 2014;28(1):65–72.
50. Passacantilli E, Antonelli M, D'Amico A, Delfinis CP, Anichini G, Lenzi J, et al. Neurosurgical applications of the 2-mm thulium laser: histological evaluation of meningiomas in comparison to bipolar forceps and an ultrasonic aspirator. Photomed Laser Surg. 2012;30(5):286–92.
51. Durbec M, Dinkel E, Vigier S, Disant F, Marchal F, Faure F. Thulium-YAG laser sialendoscopy for parotid and submandibular sialolithiasis. Lasers Surg Med. 2012;44(10):783–6.
52. Van Abel KM, Moore EJ, Carlson ML, Davidson JA, Garcia JJ, Olsen SM, et al. Transoral robotic surgery using the thulium:YAG laser: a prospective study. Arch Otolaryngol Head Neck Surg. 2012; 138(2):158–66.
53. Benazzo M, Canzi P, Occhini A. Transoral robotic surgery with laser for head and neck cancers: a feasibility study. ORL J Otorhinolaryngol Relat Spec. 2012;74(3): 124–8.

54. Mattheis S, Hoffmann TK, Schuler PJ, Dominas N, Bankfalvi A, Lang S. The use of a flexible CO2-laser fiber in transoral robotic surgery (TORS). Laryngorhinootologie. 2014;93(2):95–9.

55. Hoffmann TK, Schuler PJ, Bankfalvi A, Greve J, Heusgen L, Lang S, et al. Comparative analysis of resection tools suited for transoral robot-assisted surgery. Eur Arch Otorhinolaryngol. 2014;271(5):1207–13.

Chapter 14

1540 nm-Er/Glass Laser-Assisted Cartilage Reshaping For Protruding Ears (LACR)

Franck Marie Leclère, Serge Mordon, and Mario A. Trelles

Introduction

Approximately, one in 5000 children are born with auricular malformations [1]. The most common deformity, the protruding ears, or "bat ears,", can be a subject of much teasing from schoolmates. In the girls, the bat ears become even more prominent if they tie their hair above the head, say for ballet practice.

Prominent ears like other deformational auricular anomalies are best treated nonsurgically [2] by molding within the first 3 months of life, as the cartilage is malleable during this early period because of the influence of maternal estrogens. After this period, the deformity is fixed and a surgical therapy is usually necessary. Since the pioneer work of Dieffenbach [3] in 1845, over 170 surgical techniques have been described for the correction of protruding ears and each method has been reported to produce acceptable results. Classic open surgery, however, requires incisions to expose cartilage tissue and alter its shape. It is a technically challenging operation that produces variable results depending on the preferences, experience, and skill of the surgeon.

Since the first work of Sobol in 1993 [4, 5], laser-assisted cartilage reshaping has generated increasing clinical interest. In 2004, we reported a new technique using a 1540 nm laser to reshape protruding ears [6]. This wavelength allowed for cartilage reshaping with neither skin nor cartilage incision, without cartilage scoring and with no anesthesia. In this chapter, we present the surgical technique of LACR and we discuss our results. Apart from

Brian J.-F. Wong and Justus Ilgner (eds.), *Biomedical Optics in Otorhinolaryngology: Head and Neck Surgery*,
DOI 10.1007/978-1-4939-1758-7_14, © Springer Science+Business Media New York 2016

deviation from normality, congenital deformity of pinna also exists in a variety of forms, but their management is not relevant in the context of this work and will not be covered.

The Animal Model

Since the preliminary work of Sobol et al. [4], cartilage reshaping has gained an interest, particularly in the field of nasal and plastic surgery. Historically, laser-assisted cartilage reshaping was first developed for septoplasty. In 2004, Mordon et al. [6] proposed the possibility to adopt this technique for protruding ears. The animal model chosen was the rabbit as it was easily accessible to the laboratory and has large ears. However, as compared to the human ear, the rabbit ear has powerful auricular muscles, thus limiting its suitability. In the laboratory, LACR treatment (laser-assisted cartilage reshaping) was performed in vivo using a 1540 nm Er:Glass laser connected to a hand piece with an integrated cooling system (Fig. 2). The treatment consisted of 15 contiguous spots (3 ms, 7 pulses, 12 J/cm^2, 2 Hz, cumulative fluence 84 J/cm^2) applied in eight parallel rows along the ear. An aluminum preformed splint was then placed for a period of 1 week. For Helidonis et al., the reshaping is obtained through increased cartilage malleability at temperatures between 65 and 75 °C. For Mordon et al., proliferation and regeneration of cartilaginous cells have been observed and are considered as the main contributor to the stability of long-term shape change [6–8].

From Laboratory to Bedside

The difficulties associated with the transition from animal to the clinic were of three types. (1) The risk of skin burns and cartilage denaturation were directly related to the nature of the technique. Sobol et al. [4, 5] had initially claimed that the cartilage remodeling could be stable if the temperature delivered to the cartilage was close to 70 °C. Further studies by Diaz-Valdes et al. [7] have shown that, however, at this temperature the viability of chondrocytes was compromised. Meanwhile, Chae et al. [8] determined that the temperature associated with cartilage remodeling was between 50 and 65 °C. If biopsies on irradiated ears have shown no burning of the skin and the viability of chondrocytes, the temperature range appears reduced. Considering the variable thickness of the human ear and skin sensitivity, particular attention should be paid to the cooling system of surface to achieve an optimal temperature within the cartilage without skin alteration (Fig. 1). (2) With the rise in temperature, pain related to LACR treatment should be prevented. We had at our disposal an integrated cooling system and systematic anti-inflammatory prescription was the rule. (3) Finally, the success of this new technique was significantly associated with the presence of a mold in the immediate postoperative phase. The latter should be able to maintain the desired shape in its position. The challenge then was to impose this constraint to young patients and obtain their cooperation.

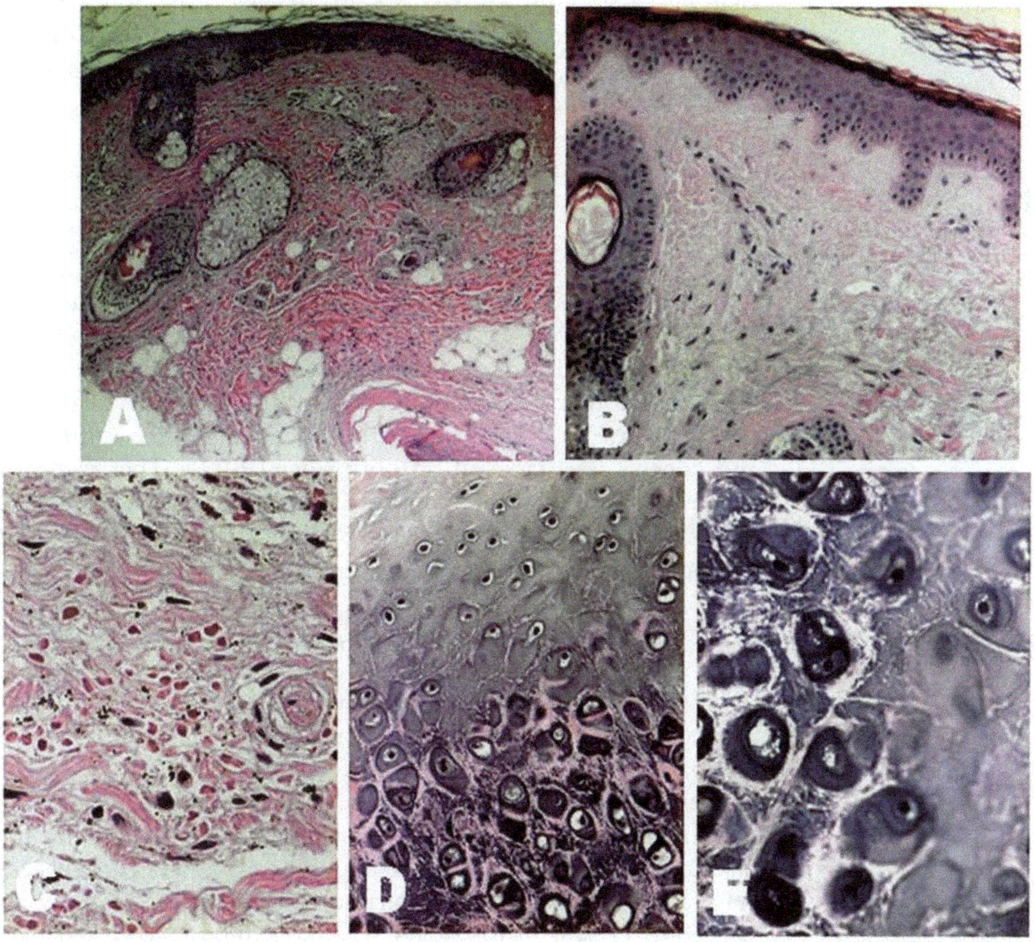

Fig. 1 (**a**) Skin ×125 HE/EO before treatment. Skin is of normal appearance with epidermis, dermis, and cartilage of normal aspect. (**b**) Skin and cartilage ×200 HE/EO immediately after treatment. Epidermis shows no damage and there is an inflammatory reaction in the dermis with coagulation phenomenon. (**c**) Skin and cartilage ×200 HE/EO 7 days after laser irradiation. Important inflammatory infiltration will cell proliferation. Polymorphonuclear cells are seen with cartilage hyalinization and traces of coagulation. (**d**) Cartilage ×400 HE/EO 15 days after irradiation. Cartilage cell formation is noticed in the areas which correspond to laser irradiation. There is a chondroblastic proliferation around a contracted cartilage. (**e**) Cartilage ×400 HE/EO 30 days after, cartilage is in the phase of getting thicker showing chondroblastic proliferation. Cells are observed in clusters formed by several cell divisions

The Clinical Examination

The surgeon should assess and record the three major pathological characteristics of the protruding ear deformity.

1. Poorly defined or absent antihelical fold
2. Conchoscaphal angle >90°
3. Exaggerated concha

The skin should be carefully examined in order to exclude discharging ears, otitis externa, or scars. To assess the postoperative improvement, cephaloauricular distances should be carefully measured before and after LACR. Skin sensation should also be carefully evaluated before and after the procedure.

The Surgical Technique

The 1540 nm Er/Glass laser (Aramis, Quantel Derma GmbH, Erlangen, Germany) is set at 12 J/cm^2 per pulse [9–11]. The treatment requires seven stacked pulses (3 ms, 2 Hz, 84 J/cm^2 cumulative fluence) applied using a 4-mm spot hand piece with integrated cooling (Koolburst, Quantel Derma GmbH, Erlangen, Germany) on both sides of the entire helix and concha so that the entire helix and concha are irradiated on both sides [9–11]. The treatment requires at least 50 (x7) pulses on each side to be effective. Contact cooling makes the treatment very tolerable, eliminating the need for topical anesthesia (Fig. 2).

The Silicone Elastomer

After irradiation, a silicone elastomer (Hydro-C, Detax, Ettlingen, Germany) is inserted inside the helix to give it the desired shape. Three minutes later the elastomer hardens and a solid mold is obtained. Patients are asked to wear this mold at all times for the first 2 weeks and then only at night for an additional 4 weeks (Fig. 3). A nonsteroidal anti-inflammatory drug (NSAID) is prescribed to all patients for 3 days. The mold appears to be the main limitation of the technique. It should be precisely adapted and carefully controlled after the operation.

Clinical Studies

The French National Institute of Health and Medical Research (INSERM) U703 (nom U 1189) has been working in cooperation with two centers and since its first report in 2004 on the

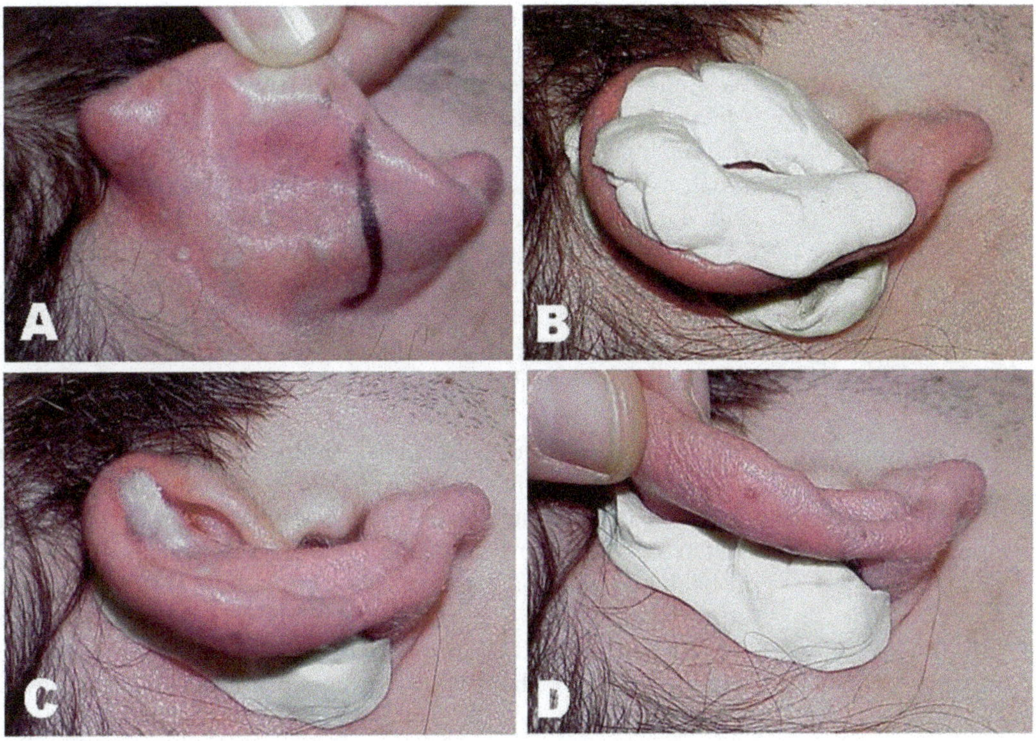

Fig. 2 (**a**) Behind the ear, the *line* defines de limit of laser irradiation. (**b**) The elastometer is in place on the external side of the ear. (**c, d**) Show the elastometer placed behind to force the helix to bend and to adopt its new position

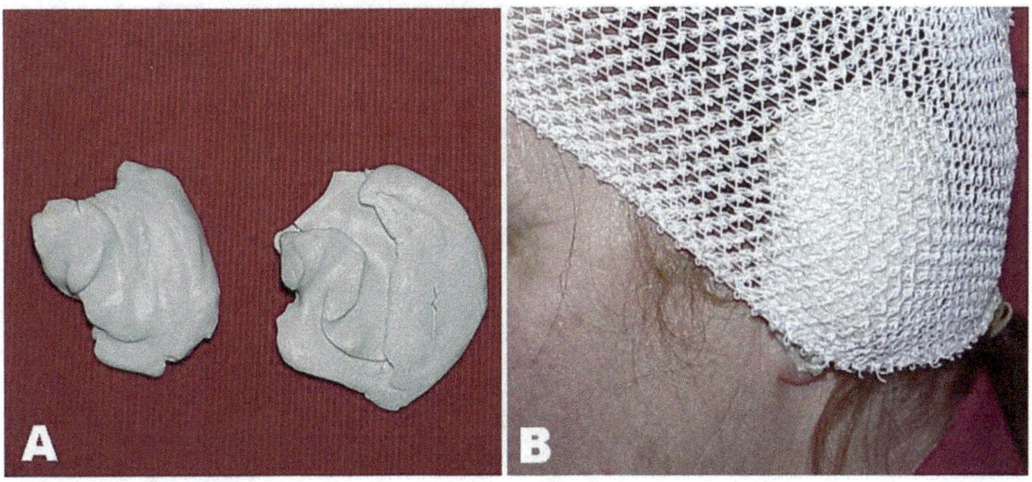

Fig. 3 (**a**) Elastometers, which mimic the shape or the external ear, are already hard as a fixed mold, to maintain the ear helix in the new position after laser cartilage reshaping. (**b**) The mold is kept in place by an elastic cap band

rabbit, three clinical trials were achieved [9–11]. Our first clinical study published by Trelles et al. on 12 ears in 8 patients showed thickening of the perichondrium and the cartilage layers at 2 weeks [9]. This thickening was confirmed at 3 weeks and 1 month with an intact matrix. The chondrocytes were viable and functional, as confirmed by the binucleation of some chondrocytes (Fig. 4). This reshaping was found to be stable 6 months post-LACR. Laser irradiation leads to an increase of temperature which could induce a coordinated expression of growth factors. Among them TGFb1 that has proved to develop when temperature increases in laser-irradiated tissue [12, 13]. Furthermore, we noticed that LACR provides a smoother and more natural curvature than conventional techniques and without any scarring (Fig. 5). In a second clinical trial published by Leclère et al. in 2006 [10], 24 patients underwent LACR of both ears using our 1540 nm laser. Postoperative follow up was uneventful for all ears, except for six on which minor contact dermatitis developed probably because of inappropriate mold design. This did not require additional therapy and those patients (four children and two adults) stopped wearing the mold leading to incomplete shape correction. There were no cases of infection, hematomas,

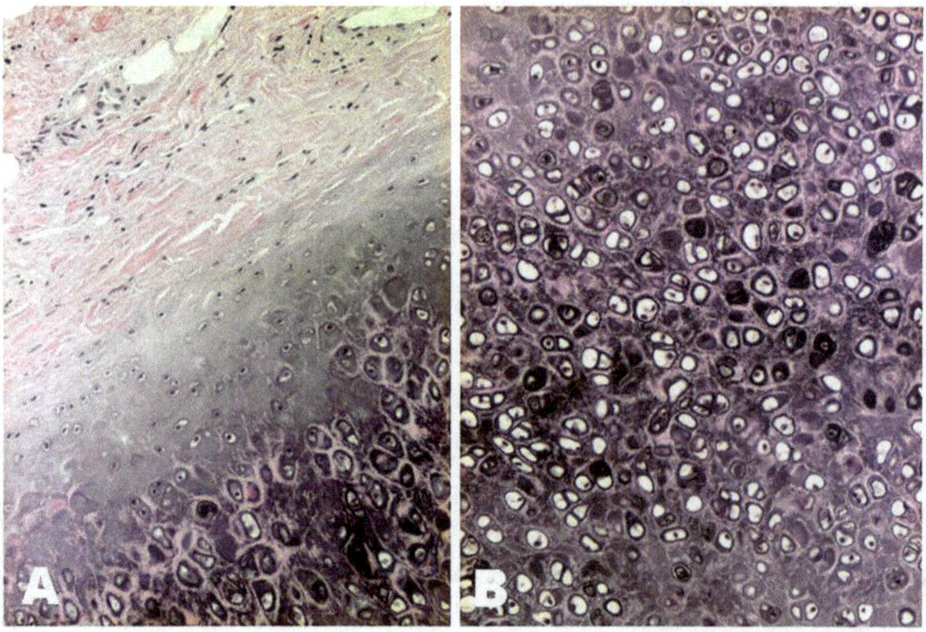

Fig. 4 (**a**) Cartilage ×200 HE/EO 6 months after laser irradiation. Cartilage appears well restructured, thicker, and a well defined margin between active chondrocytes and an area of new cartilage formation. (**b**) Abundant proliferation of chondrocytes, some of them appear binuclear in an active phase, well formed and of a standard pattern

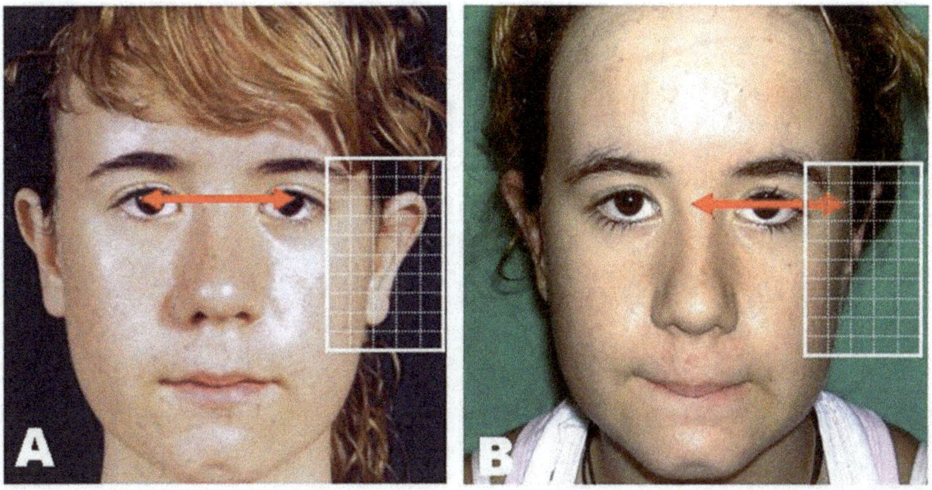

Fig. 5 (**a**) Before and (**b**) 6 months after ear remodeling by laser cartilage. *Arrows* of same length are centered at the eyes pupils to define equal proportions of both photographs. The graduated grid superimposed on both left ears permits clear detection of improvement of protruding ears after laser surgery for cartilage reshaping

or skin necrosis. For the remaining 18 patients (six children and nine adults) the expected ear reshaping was achieved (fluence = 84 J/cm^2); in three adults, partial or incomplete reshaping was observed and correlated to a lower fluence (70 J/cm^2). Those patients were retreated at 3 months at 84 J/cm^2 fluence and all achieved suitable reshaping. Again, no postoperative discomfort was reported. A third 4-year prospective evaluation of LACR for 32 protruding ears was published in 2011 by Leclère et al. [11]. There were 15 patients with bilateral ear protrusion, and the remaining two cases had unilateral protruding ears. The mean age for this series was 34.5 years, much higher than our previous study (16 years). Except for two cases of dermatitis, there were no early complications. Long term follow-up outcomes were incomplete shape correction in two patients and slight asymmetry in five patients, but there was no recurrence, no cases of keloid and no alteration in sensitivity and growth in the entire series. Moreover, the mean superior and middle cephaloauricular distances were, respectively, 12.3 ± 1.9 and 13.7 ± 1.6 mm compared to 17.8 ± 3.1 mm ($p < 0.01$) and 23.9 ± 1.9 mm ($p < 0.01$) before operation. Mean patient satisfaction was 8.6/10 with all patients reporting that they would be willing to undergo the procedure again, if required. Efficacy data from all these studies suggest that LACR is a reproducible and efficient technique irrespective of the age of the patient (Fig. 6).

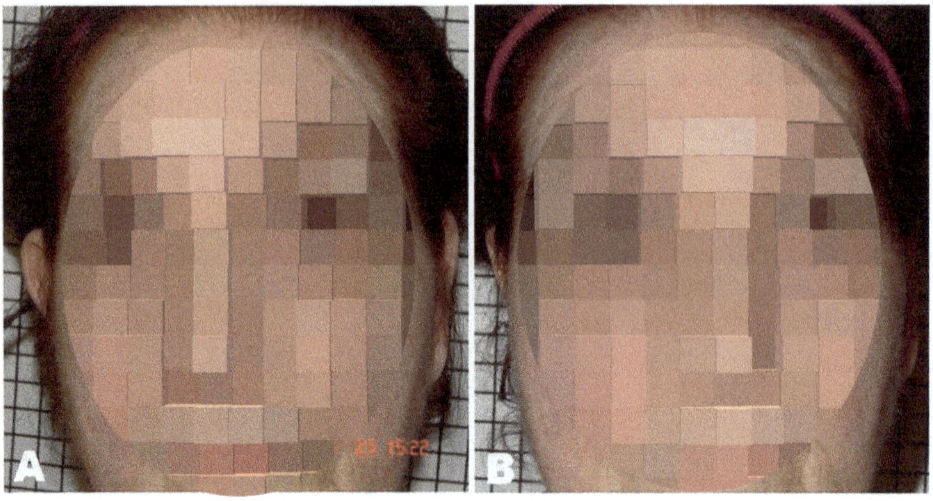

Fig. 6 (**a**) Right protruding ear, before treatment. (**b**) Six months after laser cartilage reshaping. Notice repositioning of the helix as shown by the graduated scale placed behind

Evolution of the LACR Procedure and the Other Possibilities of Cartilage Reshaping

Alternative methods have been developed to provide nonsurgical approaches to reshaping cartilage [1]. Specifically, cartilage biomechanics is temperature dependent, with temperatures between 50 and 70 °C producing stress relaxation which leads to gross shape change [1, 7, 8]. Moreover, a few months after laser irradiation cartilage thickening appears to be related to formation of apatite [14]. In our understanding, apatite plays a key role in the permanent stabilization of the changed shape of the cartilage in the treated area. Thus, thermal-based mechanisms, such as radiofrequency [15], electrical current [16–19], or lasers, have been investigated to produce shape change in cartilage in place of classic "cut and suture" methods. The main advantage afforded by these optical technologies is that cartilage reshaping may be achieved through an incision-free procedure with limited cutaneous injury and no associated risks and economic costs of surgery and anesthesia which translates to a shorter recovery time, reduced costs, and lower overall discomfort for the patient [1]. Other teams have tried to perform LACR with a similar technique [20], but are still faced with the challenge of the correct use of the mold or the difficulty in obtaining approval for clinical trials. Another approach was recently proposed by Ragab et al. [21]. Use of the CO_2 laser permitted cartilage reshaping with both vaporization and incisions. In his technique, the open approach allowed precise laser application and cartilage suturing provided great stabilization. Postoperative care involved wearing a simple headband for a week, representing a considerable advantage. However, this method uses both laser and surgery, which undermines the basis of a technique whose primary objective is simplicity to perform, elimination of need for anesthesia, and minimum complication rate. Additionally, even if their results seem attractive, larger series are required to assess risk factors arising from using sutures, i.e., hematoma, hypertrophic scars, and keloids. Finally, among all LACR applications, this technique currently stands alone in providing cartilage biopsies, long-term clinical follow up and a standardized technique. Other applications currently studied for deviated septum [22, 23], alar cartilage reshaping [24], or costal graft reshaping [25, 26] need to provide more histological and clinical evidence in order to clarify their action mechanism.

Conclusion

The LACR technique for protruding ears was developed at the INSERM institute in Lille (France), with a view to both improve patient comfort and reduce complications. Based on three clinical trials, the 1540 nm Er/Glass laser appears to be an ideal wave length for cartilage reshaping. (1) The wavelength's penetration depth matches the thickness of the cartilage, allowing for the homogenous heat generation; (2) contact cooling makes the treatment very tolerable; (3) the degree of correction appears similar to that obtained by conventional techniques. (4) Furthermore, LACR provides a smoother and more natural curvature than conventional techniques and without any scarring.

References

1. Wu EC, Sun V, Manuel CT, Protsenko DE, Jia W, Nelson JS, Wong BJ. Ex vivo investigations of laser auricular cartilage reshaping with carbon dioxide spray cooling in a rabbit model. Lasers Med Sci. 2013;28(6):1475–82.
2. Dieffenbach JF. Die operative chirurgie. Wiesbaden: Leipzi FA Brook-Haus; 1845.
3. van Wijk MP. Non-surgical correction of congenital deformities of the auricle: a systematic review of the literature. J Plast Reconstr Aesthet Surg. 2009;62:727–36.
4. Helidonis E, Sobol E, Kavvalos G, Bizakis J, Christodoulou P, et al. Laser shaping of composite cartilage grafts. Am J Otolaryngol. 1993;14:410–2.
5. Sobol E, Bagratashvili NV, Omel'chenko A, Sviridov A. Laser shaping of cartilage. In: Anderson RR, Katzir A, editors. Laser surgery: advanced characterization, therapeutics, and systems, vol. 2128. 4th ed. Bellingham, WA: SPIE; 1994. p. 43–9.
6. Mordon S, Wang T, Fleurisse L, Creusy C. Laser cartilage reshaping in an in vivo rabbit model using a 1.54 micron Er:glass laser. Lasers Surg Med. 2004;34:315–20.
7. Diaz-Valdes SH, Aguilar G, Basu R, Lavernia EJ, Wong BJ. Modeling the thermal response of porcine cartilage to laser irradiation. In: Laser–tissue interaction XIII: photochemical, photothermal, and photomechanical, San Jose, CA, USA; 2002. p. 47–56.

8. Chae Y, Aguilar G, Lavernia EJ, Wong BJ. Characterization of temperature dependent mechanical behavior of cartilage. Lasers Surg Med. 2003;32:271–8.
9. Trelles MA, Mordon S. Correction of ear malformations by laser-assisted cartilage reshaping (LACR). Lasers Surg Med. 2006;38:659–62.
10. Leclère FM, Petropoulos I, Mordon S. Laser-assisted cartilage reshaping (LACR) for treating ear protrusions: a clinical study in 24 patients. Aesthetic Plast Surg. 2010;34:141–7.
11. Leclère FM, Trelles MA, Mordon S. Laser assisted cartilage reshaping for protruding ears (LACR): a prospective Long term follow-up of 32 procedures. Lasers Surg Med. 2011; 43(9):875–80.
12. Souil E, Capon A, Moron S, Xuan ATD, Polla B, Bachelet M. Treatment with 85 nm diode laser induces long-lasting 2-kDa heat shock protein expression in normal rat skin. Br J Dermatol. 2001;144:260–6.
13. Welch WJ. Mammalian stress response: cell physiology, structure/function of stress proteins and implications for medicine and disease. Physiol Rev. 1992;72:1063–81.
14. Heger M, Mordon S, Leroy G, Fleurisse L, Creusy C. Raman microspectrometry of laser-reshaped rabbit auricular cartilage: preliminary study on laser-induced cartilage mineralization. J Biomed Opt. 2006;11(2):024003.
15. Keefe MW, Rasouli A, Telenkov SA, Karamzadeh AM, Milner TE, Crumley RL, Wong BJ. Radiofrequency cartilage reshaping: efficacy, biophysical measurements, and tissue viability. Arch Facial Plast Surg. 2003;5(1): 46–52.
16. Ho KH, Diaz Valdes SH, Protsenko DE, Aguilar G, Wong BJ. Electromechanical reshaping of septal cartilage. Laryngoscope. 2003;113(11):1916–21.
17. Protsenko DE, Ho K, Wong BJ. Stress relaxation in porcine septal cartilage during electromechanical reshaping: mechanical and electrical responses. Ann Biomed Eng. 2006; 34(3):455–64.
18. Manuel CT, Foulad A, Protsenko DE, Sepehr A, Wong BJ. Needle electrode-based electromechanical reshaping of cartilage. Ann Biomed Eng. 2010;38(11):3389–97.
19. Wu EC, Protsenko DE, Khan AZ, Dubin S, Karimi K, Wong BJ. Needle electrode-based electromechanical reshaping of rabbit septal cartilage: a systematic evaluation. IEEE Trans Biomed Eng. 2011 Aug;58(8).
20. Holden PK, Chlebicki C, Wong BJ. Minimally invasive ear reshaping with a 1450-nm diode laser using cryogen spray cooling in New Zealand white rabbits. Arch Facial Plast Surg. 2009;11:399–404.
21. Ragab A. Carbon dioxide laser-assisted cartilage reshaping otoplasty: a new technique for prominent ears. Laryngoscope. 2010;120:1312–8.
22. Bourolias C, Prokopakis E, Sobol E, Moschandreas J, Velegrakis GA, Helidonis E. Septal cartilage reshaping with the use of an Erbium doped glass fiber laser. Preliminary results. Rhinology. 2008;46(1):62–5.
23. Leclère FM, Petropoulos I, Mordon S. Laser assisted septal cartilage reshaping (LASCR): a prospective study in 12 patients. Lasers Surg Med. 2010;42:693–8.
24. Leclère FM, Wang T, Mordon S. Reshaping du cartilage alaire par laser Er:Glass 1540 nm: premiers résultats cliniques chez l'en fant. In: Congrès Soc Fran Laser Med (SFLM), Janvier 2011.
25. Sobol E, Shekhter A, Guller A, Baum O, Baskov A. Laser-induced regeneration of cartilage. J Biomed Opt. 2011;16:080902.
26. Baum OI, Soshnikova YM, Sobol EN, Korneychuk AY, Obrezkova MV, Svistushkin VM, Timofeeva OK, Lunin VV. Laser reshaping of costal cartilage for transplantation. Lasers Surg Med. 2011;43:511–5.

Chapter 15

Cartilage Reshaping of the Nose

Emil Sobol, Valery Svistushkin, and Emmanuel Helidonis

Introduction. The Problem

A patent nasal airway alters the quality of the voice, aids in maintain adequate ventilation, and heats, filters, and humidifies the air before it reaches the lung. Nasal airway obstruction can lead to subjective complaints and also impair ventilation during sleep leading to a number of sequelae associated with obstructive sleep apnea (arrhythmia, reduced mentation, cor pulmonale). In the airway, estimating flow is a complex process that depends upon anatomy and accurate calculation requires numerical modeling (e.g., computational fluid dynamics). However, it can be grossly estimated using Poiseuille's law which describes flow through a cylindrical tube; flow is proportional to the fourth power of the diameter of the tube.

Hence, a decrease in the nasal lumen size by a factor of two could reduce flow through the nasopharynx up to 16 times. Any combination of nasoseptal deformity and mucosal edema producing such an epic change may lead to nasal respiratory insufficiency. The nasal cavity and the nasal septum are complex structures. Septal deformities ("deviated septum") are readily amenable to surgical treatment and were classified by Cottle [1] by anatomic location.

Area 1. The nasal vestibule (caudal septum).

The caudal (most distal and anterior) end of the cartilaginous septum extends into one nostril distorting the airway.

Brian J.-F. Wong and Justus Ilgner (eds.), *Biomedical Optics in Otorhinolaryngology: Head and Neck Surgery*,
DOI 10.1007/978-1-4939-1758-7_15, © Springer Science+Business Media New York 2016

Area 2. The internal nasal valve area.

The internal nasal valve is the narrowest point of the airway and bounded by the septum, upper lateral cartilage, and inferior turbinate. Septal deformities here are usually along the dorsum of the septum and often C-shaped. At this locus the impact on airflow may be severe and the lateral wall of the nose may collapse with inspiration.

Area 3. The attic area (or keystone).

The cartilaginous septum, bony septum (perpendicular plate), upper lateral cartilage, and nasal bones meet at the "keystone" region, which is the key structural point for the nose. Airway obstruction may occur here due to bony and cartilaginous deformities beneath the nasal bones. Deformations of the bony septum here generally lead to deformities of cartilaginous septum as well.

Area 4. The anterior turbinate area.

Obstructions in this area cause stuffiness, headaches, cough, and sinus problems. Often, deformities in this region are a consequence of osseocartilaginous deformities at the junction of the septum and maxillary crest (vomer bone).

Area 5. The posterior turbinate area or the sphenopalatine ganglion area.

Obstruction in this region may cause facial pain, stuffiness, headaches, postnasal discharge, and eustachian tube dysfunction.

Nasal septum deviations are a common etiology of nasal obstruction and does not occur in isolation with other structural anomalies, the most common being hypertrophy of the inferior turbinates. It is estimated that 75–80 % of individuals of European origin may present with some type of anatomic deformity of the nose [2]. The treatment of choice for patients with significant deviations of the nasal septum up to now has been surgery focused on the bony and/or the cartilaginous septum.

The most common nasal operation performed is the correction of deformed or deviated septum. Nasal surgery was first performed in ancient India and Egypt, where nasal fractures and gross deformities of the septum were corrected with digital manipulation. In the Renaissance, advances in the practice of rhinoplasty and nasal reconstruction (changing the external shape of the nose) were made by Tagliacozzi and Brancas [3]. In the early nineteenth century treatises on nasal diseases were published in France and Germany. Credit for developing submucous resection (SMR) of the nasal septum (surgical removal of cartilage regions that obstruct the airway) belongs to Freer [4] and to Killian [5] and the procedures used, today, have evolved from this technique. In 1958 Cottle, Loring, and Fisher presented the intranasal maxillary–

premaxillary approach for correcting nasal septal deformities [1]. Cottle and Loring not only preserved the septal–columellar relationship, but also preserved the mobility of the cartilaginous septum. This technique is considered even today the best approach for correcting all types of nasal septal deformities and is usually done under local or general anesthesia, and it is often required for the patient to be hospitalized for a period of time. Contemporary septal surgery leads to the absence from work, a financial burden for both patient and family, etc. There are also contraindications for performing surgery, such as age, and comorbidities such as cardiac disease, stroke, etc.

The cartilaginous nasal septum is firm, semi-flexible, and is irregularly quadrangular in shape. It must be capable of movement to withstand trauma and with the shift of head position during sleep. It is attached to the upper lateral cartilages along its dorsal aspect and its caudal–ventral corner, posteriorly in articulates with the perpendicular plate of the ethmoid bone and vomer, inferoposteriorly it rests in the groove of the maxillary spine (crest). Subluxations of the caudal end as a result of injury are common as is a "C shaped" deformity along the dorsum. The relationship between the upper lateral cartilage and cartilaginous septum is very important. The normal upper lateral cartilage creates 10–15° with a straight septum and narrower angles may lead to dynamic collapse of the airway during respiration. These two structures along with the anterior aspect of the inferior turbinate define the internal nasal valve. A C-shaped deformity of the septum may compromise one or both upper lateral cartilages a significant restriction of flow. The accepted approach to the correction of septal deformities involves incisions through the mucoperichondrium, elevation of flaps, and resection or reshaping of deformed cartilage via scoring, suturing, or morselization. Changing the shape of septal cartilage can now be corrected in a much simpler and atraumatic technique using a laser. The plastic deformation of cartilage following laser radiation was first described in 1992 [6] with detailed analysis of this process performed in subsequent years.

The Laser Solution: Cartilage Reshaping with Laser Irradiation

Phenomenon of Laser Reshaping. Optical, Mechanical, and Thermal Effects in Laser Reshaping of Cartilage

When cartilage is acutely bent into a new shape, the deformation creates internal stresses that counter the imposed shape change, and these forces act to restore the tissue to its initial configuration. The idea underlying the laser reshaping of cartilage (LRC) is to first mechanically deform the tissue to the desired shape and then to irradiate the areas of maximum internal stress for a short period

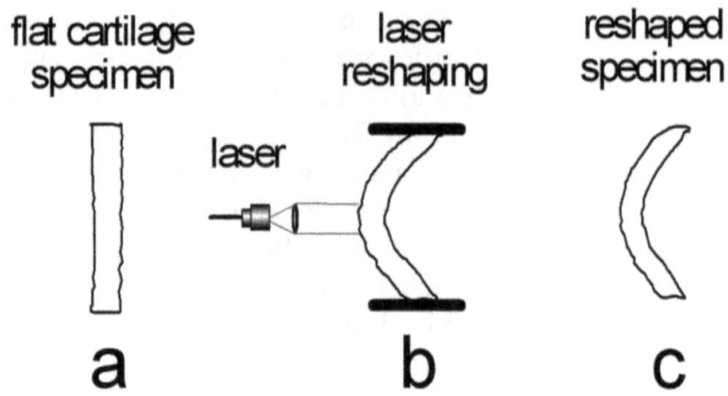

Fig. 1 Laser reshaping of cartilage: (a) initial cartilage slab, (b) deformation and laser irradiation, (c) reshaped cartilage

of time to produce stress relaxation and achieve a new stable cartilage shape (Fig. 1) [7, 8].

Stress relaxation in cartilage is a time and temperature-dependent process; alterations in tissue properties (optical and mechanical) are the functions of the temperature profile of the cartilage during heating (Fig. 2). In the early stages of the laser reshaping process, the increase in stress may be due to tissue expansion during heating where water in the tissue does not have adequate time to diffuse to the periphery of the laser spot. After a few seconds, the movement of water leads to a redistribution of stress and results in stress relaxation.

A number of thermal, optical, and mechanical effects accompany the laser-induced stress relaxation of cartilage including:

1. Laser radiation accelerates a reduction in internal stress when the tissue temperature reaches ~70 °C [7].
2. Laser-induced changes in the slope of a "stress–strain" curve which manifests as a temporal decrease in cartilage elasticity [9].
3. Light scattering kinetics in cartilage during irradiation demonstrates an increase (a change of the sign of the slope) when internal stress relaxation occurs (Fig. 2) [7, 10]. This may arise from the nucleus of a new phase (water droplets, gas bubbles, micropores) increasing the number of light-scattering centers.
4. Calorimetric measurements reveal a peak at ~70 °C which disappears when the sample is heated a second time, and reappears after immersion in a water bath for 20 min [11, 12].
5. A change of slope of the heating curve is observed at ~70 °C. When the heating rate is not very high and the laser power density is nearly constant, the time dependent temperature change becomes constant at approximately 70 °C [7].

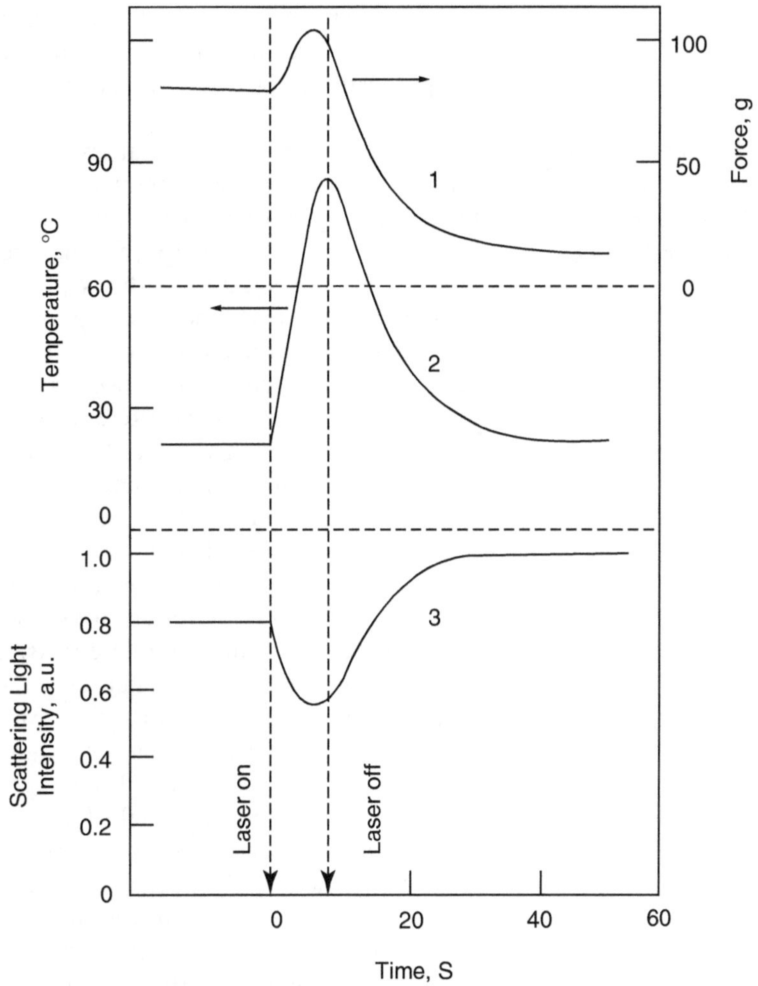

Fig. 2 Time dependences of (1) stress, (2) temperature, and (3) light scattering in cartilage in the course of laser irradiation

From the duration of this constant section in the heating curve and using calorimetric measurements, the energy consumption of this transition was estimated to be between 1200 and 1800 J/cm^3.

6. A maximum at 70 °C for the temperature dependence of the internal friction in cartilage undergoing forced oscillation [9].
7. The photo-acoustic response of cartilage during laser heating changes at 70 °C due to changes in tissue mechanical properties [13].

It can therefore be deduced from these studies that the process of laser-induced stress relaxation in cartilage has the characteristics of a type-I phase transition and that there is a strong correlation between temperature, stress and optical properties of cartilage irradiated (Fig. 2).

The Effect of Laser Radiation on Cartilage Tissue Structure and Chondrocytes

Laser-induced structural alterations in cartilage have been studied for different dosimetry parameters including laser wavelength, fluence, and types of cartilaginous tissues using conventional histological techniques [8, 14, 15], atomic force microscopy [8, 16] and optical (light scattering) methods [17]. Two types of structural alterations have been identified: primary, appearing immediately after laser irradiation and secondary that arise after some time, as a result of tissue regeneration processes [8, 18].

No dramatic structural alterations in the tissue were observed using conventional histological technique for some regimes of laser reshaping of cartilage. The structural integrity of the tissue appears to survive when the laser energy and exposure times are not too excessive [8]. Therapeutic window of laser dosimetry for cartilage reshaping has been presented in Fig. 3 (zone I). Lower fluence (zone III) does not ensure stress relaxation. High fluence (zone II) results in undesirable effects, including tissue denaturation and cell damage. Upper boundary in Fig. 3 represents denaturation of cartilage structure. Since stress relaxation may occur over a shorter time than denaturation, laser reshaping may be accomplished without visible damage or denaturation of tissue structure. A theoretical model of laser-induced structural alterations in biopolymers [19] predicts the existence of a therapeutic window (zone I) allowing stress relaxation without dramatic alterations in tissue structure. Range of laser fluences in the therapeutic window decreases with increasing exposure time. Upper and lower boundaries of the therapeutic window depend on laser wavelength, pulse characteristics, thickness of cartilage specimen, and water content.

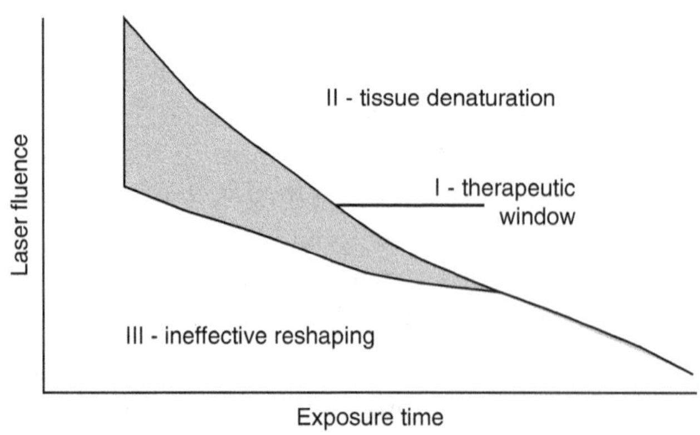

Fig. 3 Optimal laser settings for cartilage reshaping

Chondrocytes are more sensitive to damage by laser irradiation than the cartilage matrix and their alterations depend on dosimetry. Sviridov et al. [20] demonstrated that laser shaping with a holmium laser was accompanied by some alterations in chondrocyte morphology. Two types of cell alterations were distinguished: cytoplasmic focal vacuolation (FV), which may be associated with reversible cell injury, and nuclear condensation (NC), which is generally regarded as being indicative of cell death. The histological changes in chondrocytes have been quantified using a semi-quantitative rating of severity according to the proportion of cells affected. However, there are conditions (such as laser fluence of 1.7 J/cm^2, exposure time of 4 s) which allow laser shaping without nuclear condensation and only produce minor cell vacuolation [20]. Pronounced damage in the chondrocyte population was observed [21, 22] when relative higher laser fluences were applied.

The potential to reshape cartilage without significant injury to chondrocytes was established in ex-vivo experiments for porcine nasal septum cartilage [23]. The threshold laser settings are found (3 s, 0.8 W for 1560 nm fiber laser) which facilitates stable reshaping without significant alterations to chondrocytes. Exceeding these regimes may lead to substantial injury (including necrosis) of the cells. Both mechanical and thermal events may create changes in the chondrocytes, which are modest for 3 s, but increase with exposure time and laser power. However, cellular injury may activate regeneration processes resulting in new tissue formation and therefore in some future alteration of cartilage shape obtained immediately after laser procedure. A recent study [24] used a 1460 nm diode laser to reshape cartilage. The extent of chondrocytes necrosis was dependent on the laser exposure time and power. Necrotic regions produced following irradiation with lower laser powers (0.3 and 0.5 W) repopulated with chondrocytes within 4 weeks. Specimens irradiated with 1 W did not show chondrocyte repair within 4-week time interval. It must be noted that this elastic cartilage is surrounded by a dense, vascularized perichondrium laden with stem cells, and outcomes may be different in the hyaline cartilage of the nasal septum.

Mechanisms of LRC

Various mechanisms for the laser-induced stress relaxation in cartilage have been discussed in the literature [8, 18]. Laser-induced stress relaxation appears like a phase transformation of the first kind, and there are evidences that this transformation is connected with a transition in cartilaginous water from the boundto free state which may be followed by different processes: (1) Local depolymerization ("melting") of proteoglycan aggregates under short-term laser heating exceeding 70 °C followed by the formation of a new proteoglycan structure without pronounced dramatic structural changes (denaturation) of the cartilage matrix [8]. Short-lived breaking of chemical bonds between collagen and proteoglycan subsystems is also possible to reduce internal stress in cartilage by some alterations in the spatial structure of proteoglycans [18]. (2) Formation of nanopores in the cartilage matrix [25]. Pore formation is a well-known mechanism of stress relaxation in solids and was established also for biological tissues. It is discussed in the framework of spatial macroscopic heterogeneity of the structural and mechanical properties of the cartilage matrix, specifically, the existence of relatively strong regions (domains) separated by softer layers. Laser photothermolysis of these layers leads to domain mobility and induces nanopore formation that may result in stress relaxation [26]. This mechanism, when considering heterogeneity of chemical bond breaking and structural changes in biopolymers requires adequate energy consumption and can provide long-term stability of cartilage shape. (3) Local tissue mineralization (neutralization) of negative charged groups on proteoglycans by Na or Ca cations without any changes in collagen and proteoglycan structures [16]. (4) Reorganization (aligning) of spatial structure of the cells in cartilage matrix decreases stress [27]. This mechanism is similar to the polygonization in solids including aligning of the structural defects (dislocations). Since mechanical properties of the cells in cartilage are materially lower than that for cartilage matrix, the cells play a role of the structural defects similar to dislocations in crystals. Figure 4 demonstrates structural redistribution of the cells in cartilage after laser irradiation.

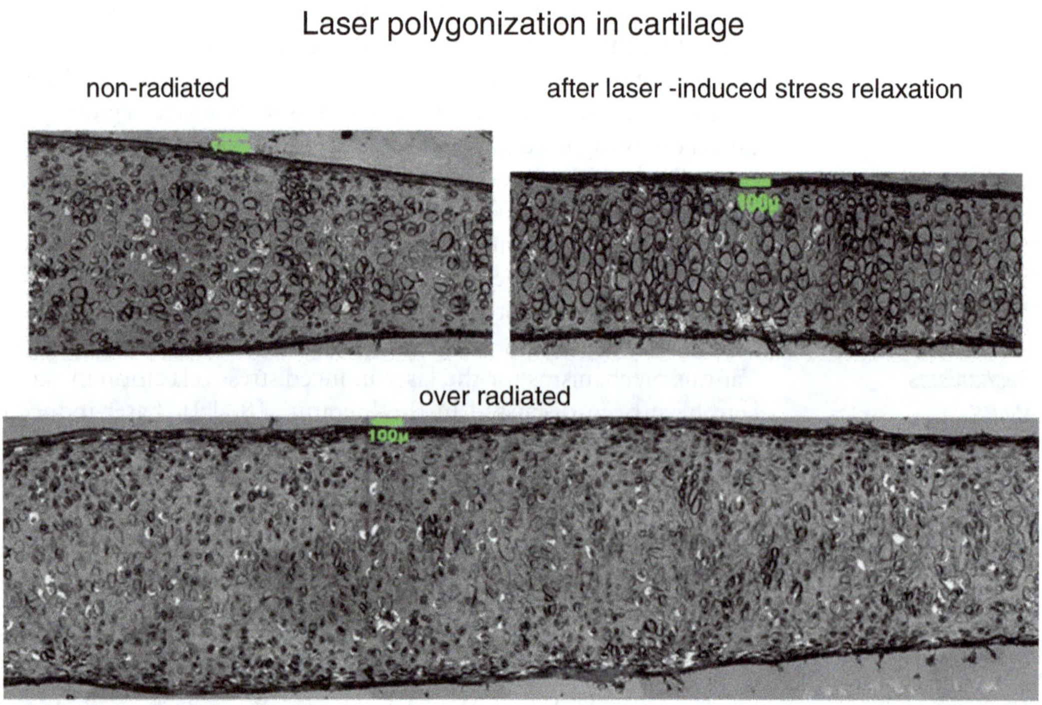

Fig. 4 Laser-induced modification of chondron structure in cartilage

Optimal and Safe Laser Settings for LRC. Choice of Laser Wavelength and Exposure Time

The appropriate conditions for laser reshaping clearly depend on the laser wavelength used, and on the optical properties and thickness of cartilage. Various lasers have been used for cartilage reshaping such as CO_2 laser, pulse-periodic Nd:YAG, Ho:YAG lasers, diode (1.45 μm), and Er-glass fiber (1.56 μm) lasers. The principal difference between these lasers is in the depth of light penetration into the tissue. Er-glass fiber laser provides a more uniform axial temperature profile than either CO_2 or Ho:YAG lasers, as it has a penetration depth of about 1 mm which is comparable to the thickness of human nasal septum (1–2 mm). It is among the most suitable tools for the shaping of nasal cartilage. The 1.56 μm radiation is mainly absorbed by tissue water. That allowed one to apply mechanical pressing of nasal septum surface to decrease water content in the superficial layers of the septum and therefore to prevent overheating and damage of the mucosa [18].

Laser power density (W) must be adequate to rapidly reach 70 °C, which is necessary to achieve stress relaxation. The selection of power density depends on thickness, laser exposure time, and (for pulse repetitive mode) pulse duration and frequency. The detailed theoretical description of the temperature field in laser treated materials is described elsewhere [28]. As stress relaxation takes usually less time than tissue denaturization, for short exposure times, there is a therapeutic window (a range of laser power density) when stress relaxation occurs without substantial changes in cartilage structure (Fig. 3). Theoretical calculation of the minimal time required for stress relaxation in cartilage matrix is about 0.3 s. This value is true when laser radiation heats cartilage samples along all its depth (when cartilage thickness is substantially less than laser light penetration depth). When the thickness of cartilage is greater than or equal to the light penetration depth, more time is required for stress relaxation. Histological examinations of porcine and human cartilages following laser reshaping did not reveal substantial alterations of the cartilage matrix structure when exposure time was less than 8 s [8]. Therefore, the exposure times for the nasal septum vary between 0.3 and 8 s. Laser spot diameter is chosen about 1.5 mm, which is approximately equal to the average thickness of nasal septum and slightly larger than the light penetration depth.

To guarantee safety of this laser procedure, a feedback control system should monitor temperature (Fig. 5). In our device, temperature is monitored using two thin thermocouples at the periphery of laser spot [29, 30]. Numerical simulations have shown that the 70 °C critical temperature required for cartilage reshaping in region of light distribution corresponds to a temperature of 41 ± 2 °C measured at the periphery. This estimate was confirmed experimentally using 64 nasal septal cartilage specimen obtained from 16 pigs.

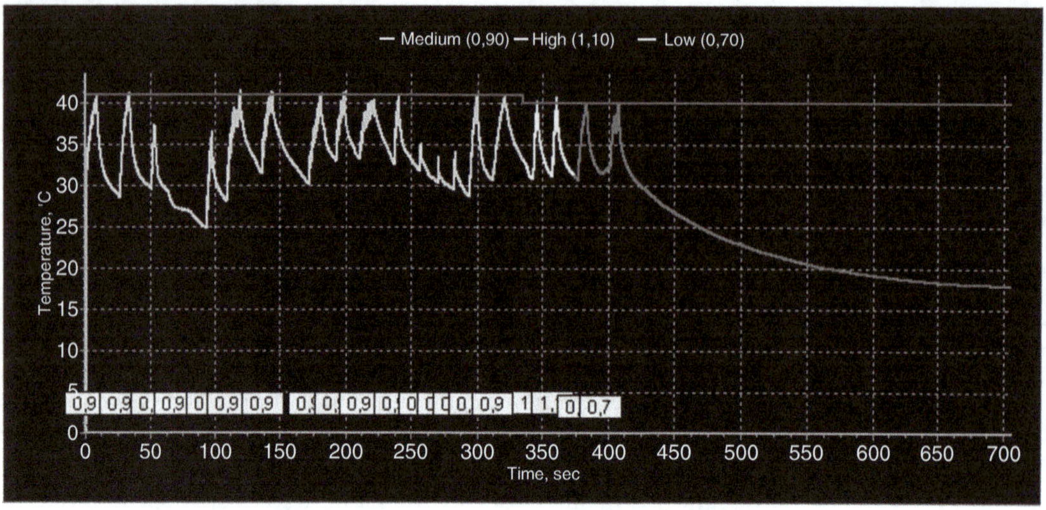

Fig. 5 Temperature measurements in the course of laser reshaping of nasal septum

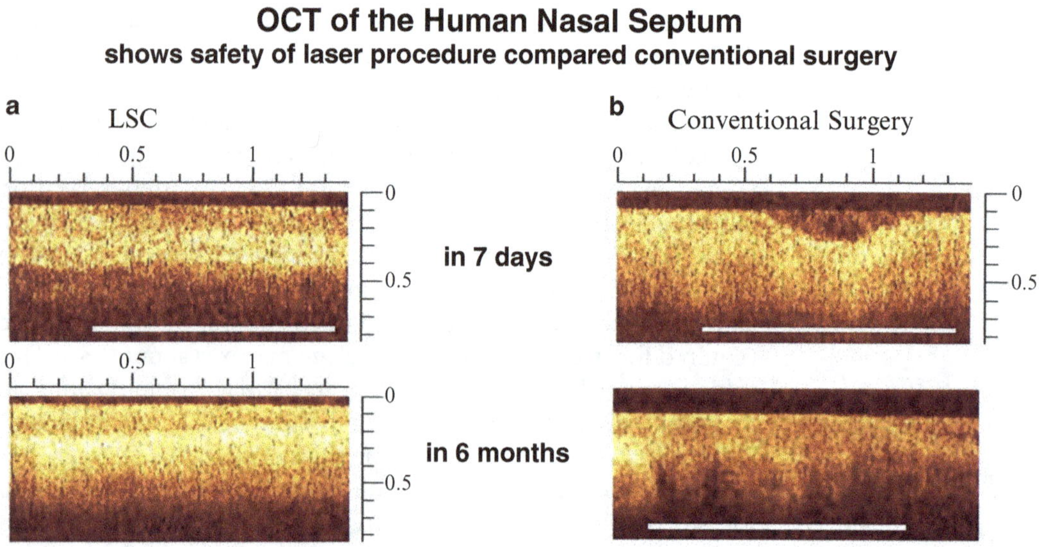

Fig. 6 OCT images of nasal septum cartilage (**a**, **b**) of a patient after laser reshaping (on the *left*) and for a patient underwent conventional surgery (on the *right*)

The feedback control system terminates laser irradiation when 41 ± 1 °C is recorded by the thermocouples.

Another noninvasive technique to monitor laser-induced structural alterations in cartilage is optical coherence tomography (OCT) [31]. OCT images of nasal septum cartilage of a patient after laser reshaping and in a patient following conventional surgery show that laser reshaping preserved initial layered structure of nasal septum since conventional surgery resulted in dramatic alterations in cartilage structure even after 6 months [26] (Fig. 6).

Clinical Applications of Laser Septochondrocorrection

Indications and Contraindications for Laser Reshaping of Nasal Septum Cartilage

Indications for laser septochondrocorrection (LSC) [26, 32, 33]

1. Nasal airway obstruction due to cartilaginous deformation of the nasal septum. Since the best shape of deformity for LSC is the C-shaped deformity, various types of deformities can be corrected (Fig. 7).
2. Nasal airway obstruction due to deformation of the cartilaginous and bony nasal septum in patients with contraindications to classical surgical approaches. The atraumatic correction with laser of the cartilaginous part anterior, usually, improves the breathing even if the bony part is deformed due to the wider space of the nasal cavity posterior. This approach can also be combined with treatment of the hypertrophy of the inferior turbinates.
3. The presence of chronic rhinosinusitis with considerable deviation of the cartilaginous septum, which is judged to be responsible for the presence, the aggravation, or the persistence of the above problems.
4. Changes in the shape of the anterior aspect of the nose due to the deformity of the cartilaginous septum.
5. Narrowing of the nasal valve area, creating difficulty in breathing due to C-shaped deformity of the septal cartilage.
6. Preventing the deformity of the hard palate and of the teeth in children having a C-shaped deformity of the cartilaginous septum.

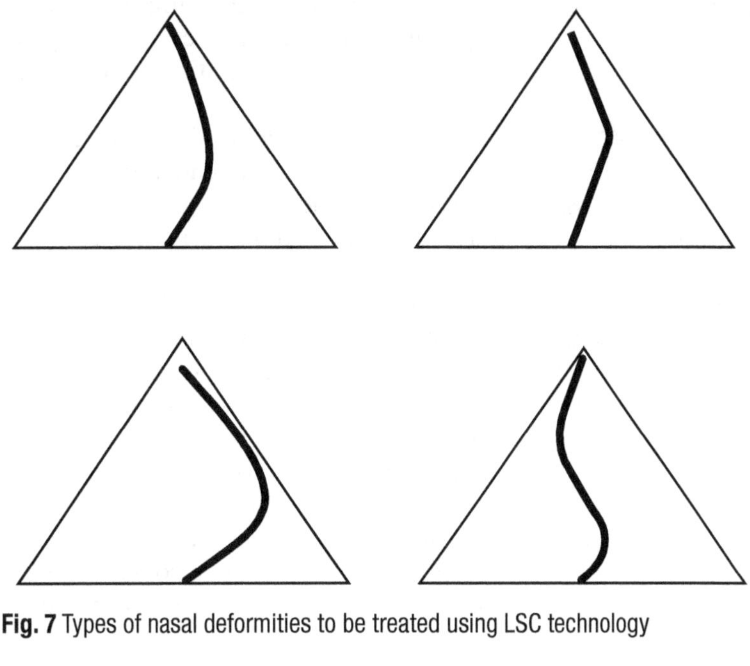

Fig. 7 Types of nasal deformities to be treated using LSC technology

7. Presence of other pathological problems, such as relapsing secretory otitis media, Eustachian tube dysfunction, and infections of the upper and/or lower respiratory system thought to be related to the presence of deformity of the nasal septum.
8. Sleep apnea and snoring related to the presence of a deformity of the septum.
9. In cases of nasal polyposis where the correction of the nasal septum can be combined with the removal of the polyps.
10. In aged people and older children, who need improvement of their nasal breathing.
11. For increasing the performance of certain groups such as workers, athletes, etc.

Contraindications [33]

1. Malignant tumors, schizophrenia, serious cardiovascular and other problems, unless it is judged otherwise by the physician, who wants to improve the patient's quality of life without endangering his life.
2. Vertical fractures of septal cartilage.
3. Horizontal septal cartilage.
4. Presence of cartilaginous spur.
5. Thickening and/or calcification of the cartilaginous nasal septum.
6. Dislocation of the quadrangular cartilaginous septum.

Technology of LSC

The technology of laser septochondrocorrection includes the (a) mechanical straightening of cartilage of nasal septum using a special instrument and the (b) delivery of laser radiation to deviated part of nasal septum **LSC** is performed as follows [26, 33].

Determination of Deviated Part of Nasal Septum and Kind of Septonasal Deformities

The nasal septal deformity is visually assessed using anterior and posterior rhinoscopy, endoscopic and/or microscopic examinations. Rigid endoscopes (0°, 30°) and also any microscopes with a focal length of 30 mm may be used.

Topical Anesthesia in the Area of Deformation

Anesthesia of nasal mucosa is necessary to reduce possible pain due to the insertion of the instrument used for the mechanical alignment of the cartilage. The patient will feel a pressure on the septum and lateral wall of nasal cavity. This sensation decrease gradually and disappears at the beginning of laser treatment as stress relaxation occurs. Local anesthetic application is used. A standard topical anesthetic with addition of 0.1 % solution of epinephrine or a similar decongestant (i.e., 0.1 % naphthizin solution) is applied. This is applied to nasal mucosa of the septum and to the lateral wall of a nasal cavity in the vicinity of the inferior turbinate. Anesthetic spray (e.g., 10 % lidocaine solution) may also be used. The anesthetic is adequate for the subsequent laser procedure that lasts collectively 10–12 min.

Straightening out of the Deviated Cartilage by Mechanical Treatment

Cartilage of nasal septum is straightened and fixed in the median position using special instrument. This instrument is a modified nasal speculum that is stabilized and secured to the patient's head using a brace. The placement of the instrument to deform the septum and general approach to laser irradiation are illustrated in Figs. 8 and 9, respectively.

Laser Radiation Delivery to Deviated Part of Nasal Septum

Laser light is delivered via a quartz fiber to an optothermomechanical handpiece with a sapphire window-indenter at the tip that is applied to the deviated part of septum. The handpiece is inserted into the nostril and positioned so that the sapphire window is in contact with the region of nasal cartilage where energy is applied.

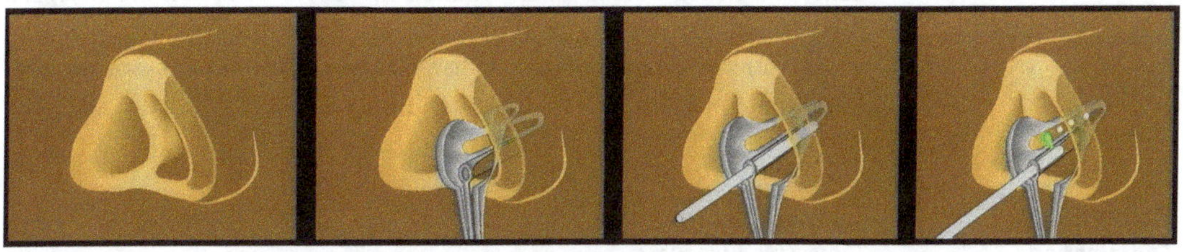

Fig. 8 Scheme of LSC. Initial deformation of septonasal cartilage; straightening out of the deviated cartilage by mechanical treatment; introduction of contactor; laser treatment

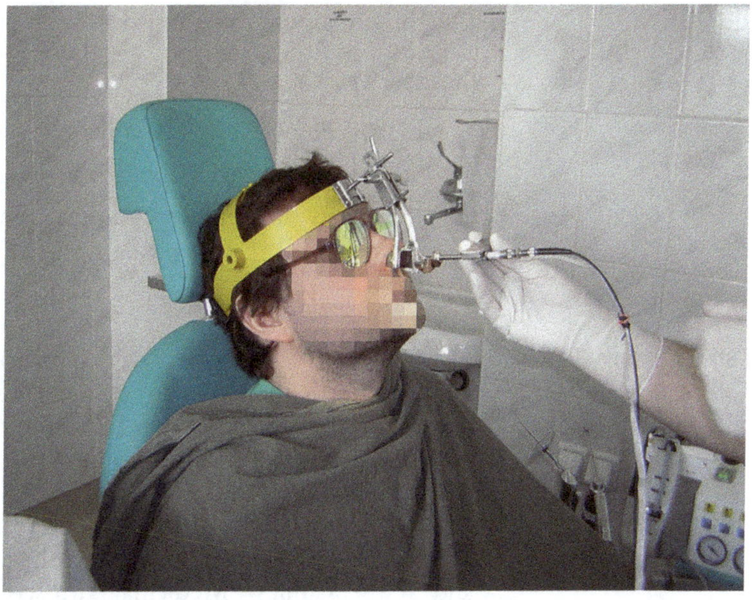

Fig. 9 LSC procedure for a patient

Laser Treatment of Deviated Cartilage

Treatment is computer controlled. Laser dosimetry is first determined by the surgeon using system software. Laser radiation is switched on by pressing of a pedal. The areas of maximum mechanical stress are treated by laser radiation. The treatment is carried out in linear direction from the inside part of the septum to the outside. The temperature is monitored and controlled by the thermocouple sensors, built into contactor, and the data are displayed on the screen of a computer. Laser radiation is automatically terminated at the attainment of a preset temperature. Then the surgeon moves the handpiece to the next point. The indenter depresses the mucosa of the septum and the laser is switched on. The size of a laser spot is of 1.5 mm. Thus 4–6 points with distance between them of 3–4 mm are processed.

After laser treatment begins, the patient experiences some relief of discomfort as there is a decrease of pressure of the instrument acting on the septum. After treatment, the device is taken out. Short-term stabilization of septal position in the midline is achieved using cotton packs soaked in Vaseline, which are inserted into the nostril where there is a convex deformity.

Laser procedure proceeds for 10–12 min, and it is not accompanied by bleeding. Usually the patients can leave 30 min after the procedure.

Postoperation Examination of Patients

Clinical examination

Objective measures

1. The use of anterior rhinoscopy demonstrates the correction of the septal deformity, which includes the reduction in C-shaped deformity and overall widening of the airway.
2. Rhinomanometric examination can be used to measure flow.

Objective signs

1. Improvement in nasal breathing.
2. Reduction and/or disappearance of snoring and sleep apnea.
3. Improvement of the psychological status of the patient.
4. Improvement in performance in various physical activities (swimming, running, etc.).

Clinical Follow Up Results

The first 250 LSC surgeries were performed in 1999–2006 at the ENT clinics of the Sechenov 1st Medical University of Moscow (Russia) using Holmium and Erbium-doped glass fiber lasers. More recently, an improved system for LSC (Arcuo Medical Inc.) was used in 830 patients (2007–present) whose age ranged between 12 and 88 years at the Vladimirsky Research and Clinical Institute of Moscow Region, Sechenov 1st Medical University of Moscow and at the Clinics "Medicina," Moscow, Russia. A prospective study was conducted between January 2007 and June 2007 at the

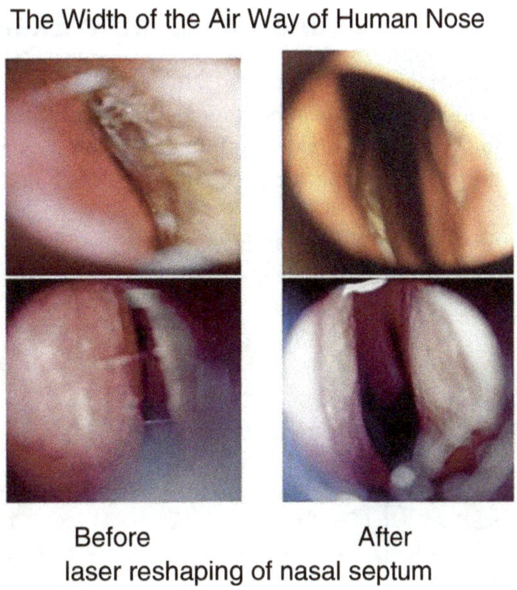

Fig. 10 Nasal way of two patients before (*left*) and after (*right*) laser irradiation

Department of Otolaryngology, School of Medicine, University of Crete, Greece on 67 patients, 49 male, and 18 female between 16 and 70 years of age [32–35].

Results Preoperatively, all patients experienced considerable difficulty in nasal breathing due to a C-shaped deviation of their cartilaginous septum. The straightening of the nasal septum and with improvement in breathing were obtained immediately after laser procedure in all the patients (Fig. 10).

This was also shown by the results of the active anterior rhinometric examination (Fig. 11) and the Nasal Obstruction Symptom Evaluation (NOSE) scale, answered by the patients. No age limitations, no complications, and no negative secondary effects were observed [33].

Equipment for Laser Reshaping of Nasal Cartilage

The Laser Septocorrector LSC-701 was developed by the Arcuo Medical Inc., USA (Fig. 12). It includes an Erbium-doped glass fiber laser, special instrument (Fig. 13), optothermomechanical contactor (Fig. 14), and feedback control system measuring temperature in the course of laser procedure and switching the laser off when preset value of temperature is achieved [29, 30]. The thermomechanical contactor has three functions: (1) deliver

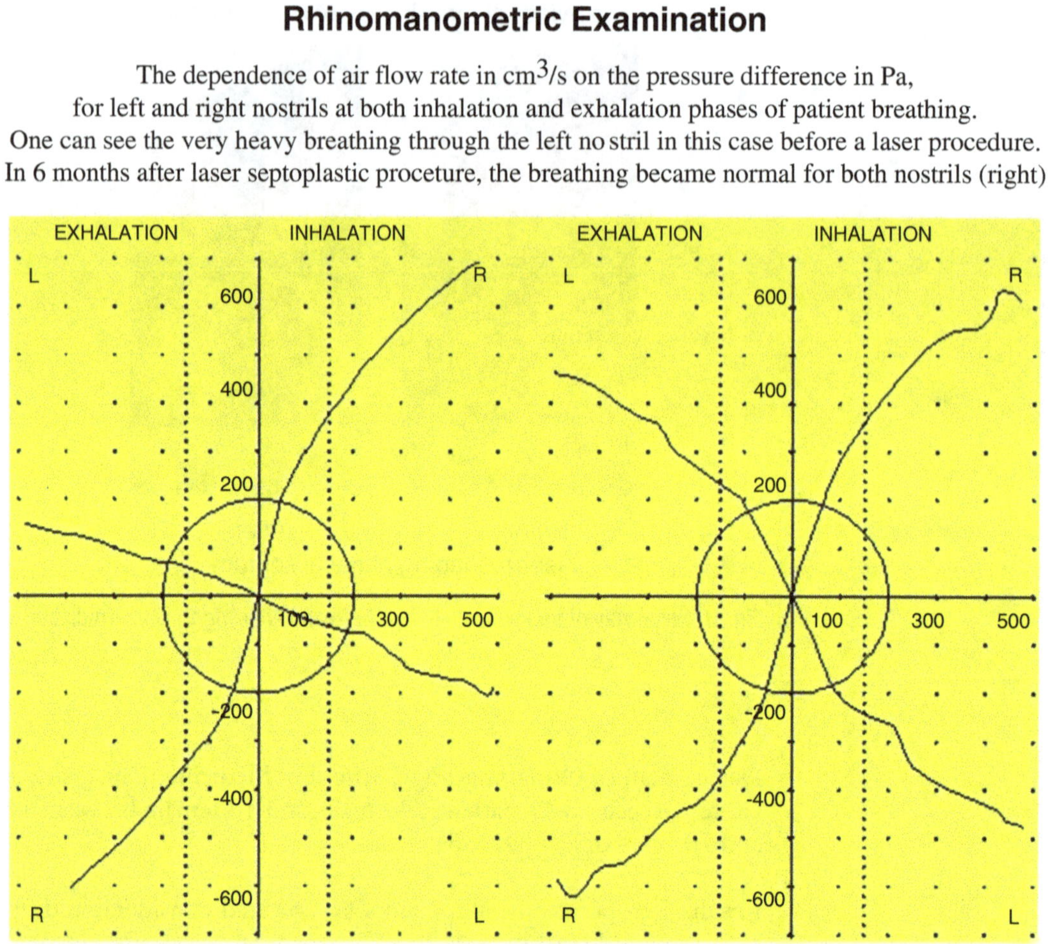

Fig. 11 Rhinomanometric measurements for a patient before (*left*) and after (*right*) laser irradiation

laser energy, (2) press nasal septum to remove water and prevent mucosa heating and damage, and (3) monitor temperature using two thin thermocouples mounted on the contactor sapphire window at the periphery of laser spot. The temperature measured in the course of LSC is presented in Fig. 5. The technical specification of LSC is presented in the Table 1.

Another device with similar technology was evaluated in 12 patients [36]. The Er-glass laser (1.54 μm) dosimetry was pulse duration of 10 ms, laser fluence of 30–50 J/cm^2. That fluence represents a laser power density of 3–5 kW/cm^2 which is much higher than the power density of 200–300 W/cm^2 used in the LSC technology in our series [34, 35]. Since contact cooling of the surface reduced potential mucosal injury, their laser settings may have led to pronounced denaturation of cartilage with chondrocytes necrosis. Hence, in theory, the final shape of nasal septum may change after laser procedure because of regeneration processes

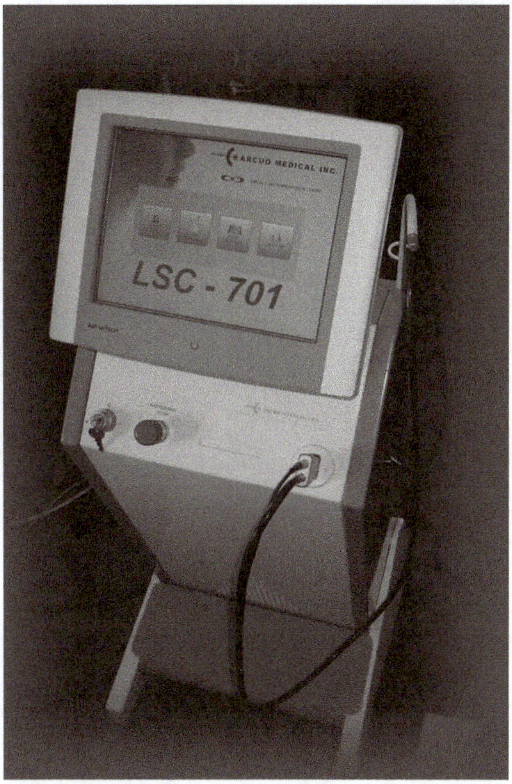

Fig. 12 Equipment for LSC [35]

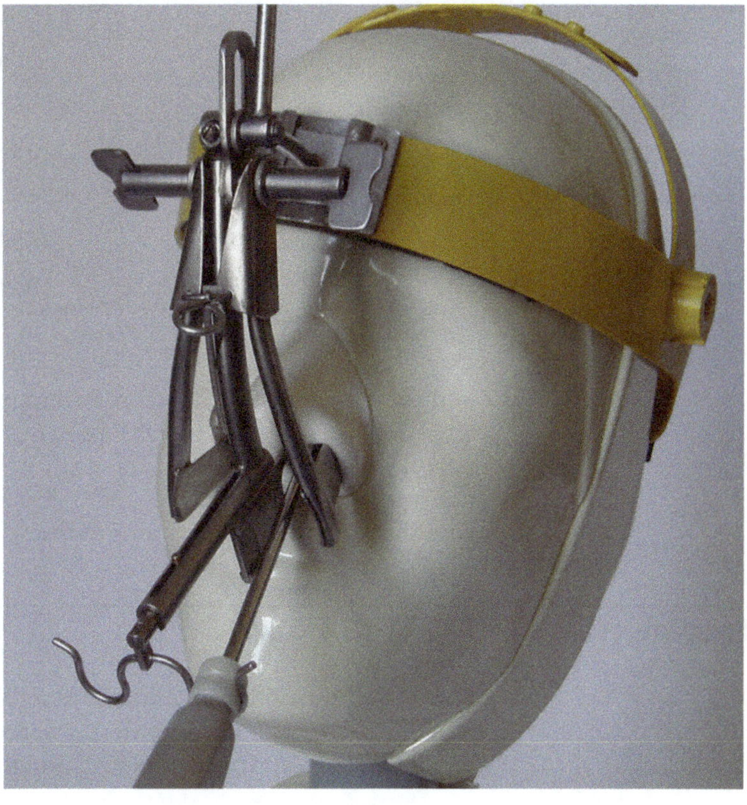

Fig. 13 A variant of the instrument for LSC [26]

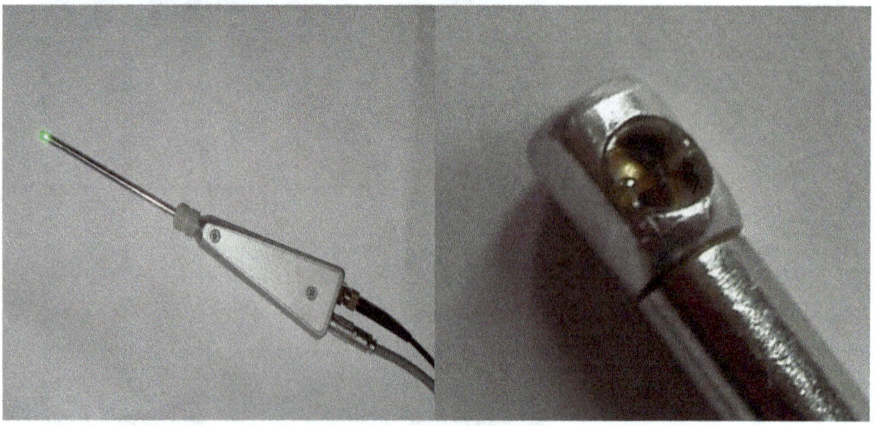

Fig. 14 Optothermomechanical contactor and indenter with two thermocouples [29]

Table 1
The technical specification LSC (Arcuo Medical Inc.)

Technical data	
Output laser power	Up to 3 W
Laser type, wavelength	Erbium-doped glass fiber laser, infrared, 1560 nm
Mode of operation	Modulated
Length of combined cable	3 m
Feedback control system	Microprocessor based
Laser spot diameter	1.5–2.0 mm
Maximum power consumption	500 W
Dimensions in mm (LWH)	500 × 450 × 1150
Weight	40 kg

in the damaged tissue. Therefore in the approach [36], immediately after the procedure, an internal septal splint was inserted into the nostril and kept for 7 days. In contrast, the LSC procedure does not lead to the tissue damage and allows to obtain stable results without the weekly applications of the splints [32–35].

Prospects of Laser Reshaping of Cartilage

For many cases, the atraumatic bloodless procedure LRC will potentially replace the conventional approach to the correction of septal deformities involves incisions through the mucoperichondrium, elevation of flaps, and resection or reshaping of deformed cartilage via scoring, suturing, or morselization.

The phenomenon of laser cartilage reshaping is compelling and innovative advancement in clinical laser research and its clinical use will extend beyond just otolaryngology. As research continues new applications appear in anatomical areas, where cartilage exists and this will prove beneficial for the patients and industry. Laser procedures can be accomplished with minimal morbidity and with considerable reduced cost. The laser technology will continue to develop and transform diagnosis and treatment. As far as the specialty of otolaryngology is concerned, the laser reshaping of the cartilage will find new possible applications in the ears, the nose, the larynx, and the trachea [37–43].

Conclusions

Heating cartilage with a laser accelerates stress relaxation. Then internal forces causing cartilage to resist shape change dissipate and a new stable geometry is achieved. Nasal septal cartilage reshaping with laser, when compared to the conventional surgery, is a straightforward, relatively painless, atraumatic, and bloodless approach. It is an office-based or outpatient procedure, not limited by age or most medical comorbid conditions. As the technology is further developed and refined, other deformities of cartilage in the head and neck may be amendable to treatment using this approach and modality.

References

1. Cottle NH, Loring RM, Fisher GC, Gaynon IE. The maxilla-premaxilla approach to extensive nasal septum surgery. Arch Otolaryngol. 1958;68:303–13.
2. Gray LP. Deviated nasal septum. Incidence and etiology. Ann Otol Rhinol Laryngol. 1978;87:1–20.
3. Rhinology. The collected writings of Maurice H. Cottle, MD. American Rhinologic Society. Editorial Board. Pat A. Barelli, Walter E.E. Loch, Eugene B. Kern, Albert Steiner; 1987. p. 35–37.
4. Freer OT. The correction of deflections of the nasal septum with minimum of traumatism. JAMA. 1902;38:636–42.
5. Killian G. The submucous window resection of the nasal septum. Ann Otol (St Louis). 1905;14:363–93.
6. Helidonis E, Sobol EN, Kavvalos G, Bizakis J, Christodoulou P, Velegrakis G, Segas J, Bagratashvili VN. Laser shaping of composite cartilage grafts. Am J Otolaryngol. 1993; 14:410–2.
7. Sobol EN, Bagratashvili VN, Sviridov AP, Ovchinnikov YM, Shechter AB, Nikiforova GN, Svistushkin VM. Cartilage shaping under laser radiation. Proc Soc Photo Opt Instrum Eng. 1994;2128:43–9.
8. Helidonis E, Sobol EN, Velegrakis G, Bizakis J. Shaping of nasal septal cartilage with the carbon dioxide laser—preliminary report of an experimental study. Lasers Med Sci. 1994; 9:51–4.
9. Sobol E, Sviridov A, Omel'chenko A, Bagratashvili V, Kitai M, Harding SE, Jones N, Jumel K, Mertig M, Pompe W, Ovchinnikov Y, Shekhter A, Svistushkin V. Laser reshaping of cartilage. Biotechnol Genet Eng Rev. 2000;17:553–78.
10. Wong B, Milner T, Anvari B, Sviridov A, Omel'chenko A, Bagratashvili V, Sobol E, Nelson JS. Thermo-optical response of cartilage during feedback-controlled laser-assisted reshaping. Proc Soc Photo Opt Instrum Eng. 1997;2970:380–91.

11. Bagratashvili VN, Sobol EN, Sviridov AP, Omel'chenko AI, Popov VK. Thermal and diffusion processes in laser-induced stress relaxation and reshaping of cartilage. J Biomech. 1997;30:813–7.
12. Wong B, Milner T, Kim H, Telenkov SA, Chew CF, Sobol E, Nelson J. Characterization of temperature-dependent biophysical properties during laser mediated cartilage reshaping. Sel Top Quant Electron. 1999;5:1095–102.
13. Omelchenko AI, Bagratashvili VN, Sobol EN, Karabutov AA. Control of tissue mechanics upon the repetitive-pulse laser heating of cartilage. Laser Phys. 2006;16(12):1681–8.
14. Helidonis EM, Volitakis I, Naumidi E, Velegrakis G, Bizakis J, Andchristodoulou P. The histology of laser thermo-chondroplasty. Am J Otolaryngol. 1995;15:423–8.
15. Sviridov AP, Sobol EN, Bagratashvili V, Omel'chenko A, Ovchinnikov YM, Shechter AB, Svistushkin VM, Nikiforova GN, Jones N. In vivo study and histological examination of laser reshaping of cartilage. Proc Soc Photo Opt Instrum Eng. 1999;3590:222–8.
16. Sobol E, Omel'chenko A, Mertig M, Pompe W. Scanning force microscopy of the fine structure of cartilage irradiated with a CO2 laser. Lasers Med Sci. 2000;15:15–23.
17. Sobol EN, Sviridov A, Kitai M, Gilligan J, Tolk NH, Edwards G. Time-resolved, light scattering measurements of cartilage and cornea denaturation due to FEL radiation. J Biomed Opt. 2003;8(2):216–22.
18. Sobol EN, Milner TE, Shekhter AB, Baum OI, Guller AE, Ignatieva NY, Omelchenko AI, Zakharkina OL. Laser reshaping and regeneration of cartilage. Laser Phys Lett. 2007;4(7):488–502.
19. Sobol EN, Kitai MS, Jones N, Sviridov AP, Milner T, Wong B. Heating and structural alterations in cartilage under laser radiation. IEEE J Quant Electron. 1999;35(4):532–9.
20. Sviridov AP, Sobol EN, Jones N, Lowe J. Effect of holmium laser radiation on stress, temperature and structure in cartilage. Lasers Med Sci. 1998;13:73–8.
21. Rasouli A, Sun CH, Basu R, Wong BJ. Quantitative assessment of chondrocyte viability after laser mediated reshaping: a novel application of flow cytometry. Lasers Surg Med. 2003;32(1):3–9.
22. Choi IS, Chae YS, Zemek A, Protsenko DE, Wong B. Viability of human septal cartilage after 1.45 micron diode laser irradiation. Lasers Surg Med. 2008;40:562–9.
23. Sobol E, Vorobieva N, Baum O, Shekhter A, Guller A. Is it possible to perform laser reshaping without dramatic effect on chondrocytes. Lasers Surg Med. 2011;43(S23):911.
24. Mo JH. Viability and regeneration of chondrocytes after laser cartilage reshaping using 1,460 nm diode laser. Clin Exp Otorhinolaryngol. 2013;6(2):82–9.
25. Shnirel'man AI, Sobol EN, Bagratashvili VN. A new mechanism for stress relaxation in cartilaginous tissue upon laser heating. Laser Phys. 2004;14(3):404–8.
26. Bagratashvili VN, Sobol EN, Shekhter AB, editors. Laser engineering of cartilage. Moscow: Fizmatlit; 2006.
27. Ignatieva N, Zakharkina O, Leroy G, Sobol E, Vorobieva N, Mordon S. Molecular processes and structural alterations in laser reshaping of cartilage. Laser Phys Lett. 2007;4(10):749–53.
28. Sobol EN. Phase transformations and ablation in laser-treated solids. New York: Wiley; 1995.
29. Bagratashvili VN, Ovchinnikov YM, Omelchenko AI, Sviridov AP, Svistushkin VM, Sobol EN, Tsypina SI. Laser instrument for septochondrocorrection. Eurasian patent 009501; 2005.
30. Sobol E, Sviridov A, Svistushkin V, Vorobieva N. Feedback controlled laser system for safe and efficient reshaping of nasal cartilage. In: Proceedings of SPIE 7548, photonic therapeutics and diagnostics VI, 75482H; 2010. doi:10.1117/12.842347.
31. Youn J, Vargas G, Wong BJF, Milner TE. Depth-resolved phase retardation measurements for laser-assisted non-ablative cartilage reshaping. Phys Med Biol. 2005;50:1937–50.
32. Ovchinnikov Y, Sobol E, Svistushkin V, Shekhter A, Bagratashvili V, Sviridov A. Laser septochondrocorrection. Arch Facial Plast Surg. 2002;4(3):180–5.
33. Helidonis E, Sobol E, Ovchinnikov Y, Svistushkin V, Manevich I, Velegrakis G. Non-invasive correction of septonasal cartilage deformities. In: 2-nd meeting of European Academy of ORL-HNS and CE ORL_HNS Ortorinolaryngology & Head and Neck Surgery, Nice, France, 27–30 Apr 2013.
34. Bourolias C, Prokopakis E, Sobol E, et al. Septal cartilage reshaping with the use of an erbium doped glass fiber laser. Preliminary results. Rhinology. 2008;46(1):62–5.
35. Sobol E, Helidonis E, Ovchinnikov Y, et al. Nasal septal cartilage reshaping, using an Erbium doped glass fiber laser. ENT News. 2008;16(6):57–9.

36. Petropoulos I, Buys B, Mordon S, Leclère FM. Laser assisted septal cartilage reshaping (LASCR): a prospective study in 12 patients. Lasers Surg Med. 2010;42(8):693–8. doi:10.1002/lsm.20958.
37. Bourolias C, Hajiioannou J, Sobol E, Velegrakis G, Helidonis E. Epiglottis reshaping using CO2 laser: a minimally invasive technique and its potent applications. Head Face Med. 2008;4:15.
38. Baum OI, Soshnikova YM, Sobol EN, Korneychuk AY, Obrezkova MV, Svistushkin VM, Timofeeva OK, Lunin VV. Laser reshaping of costal cartilage or transplantation. Lasers Surg Med. 2011;43:511–5.
39. Velegrakis G, Volitakis M, Naumidi I, Bizakis J, Christodoulou P, Andhelidonis E. Thermochondroplasty of rabbit ear cartilage using the carbon dioxide laser. Lasers Med Sci. 1994;9:265–72.
40. Wang Z, Pankratov MM, Perrault DF, Shapshay SM. Laser-assisted reshaping of collapsed tracheal cartilage. A laboratory study. Ann Otol Rhinol Laryngol. 1996;105:176–81.
41. Mordon S, Wang T, Fleurisse L, Creusy C. Laser cartilage reshaping in an in vivo rabbit model using a 1.54 micron Er:glass laser. Lasers Surg Med. 2004;34(4):315–22.
42. Trelles MA, Mordon SR. Correction of ear malformations by laser-assisted cartilage reshaping (LACR). Lasers Surg Med. 2006;38(7):659–68.
43. Leclère FM, Trelles M, Mordon SR. Cartilage reshaping for protruding ears: a prospective long term follow-up of 32 procedures. Lasers Surg Med. 2011;43(9):875–80. doi:10.1002/lsm.21126.

Chapter 16

Low Level Laser (Light) Therapy (LLLT) in Otolaryngology

Chung-Ku Rhee

Low Level Laser (Light) Therapy

Recently, biotechnology has provided various new medical knowledge, tools, and techniques to generate treatments for diseases that were previously incurable or difficult to treat. Low level laser (light) therapy (LLLT) is one of these kinds of new medical technique that made it possible to treat many medical conditions that were difficult to treat previously.

LLLT, also known as photobiomodulation, has a wavelength-dependent capability to alter cellular behavior in the absence of significant heat. LLLT involves exposing lesions to low levels of red and near infrared laser or light in the range of 1–1000 mW and referred to low level because its light energy density is low compared to other forms of high energy laser that are used to cut, ablate, or thermally coagulate tissues. Traditionally, low power laser has been referred for LLLT, but recently, the light-emitting diode (LED) also has been used for LLLT in place of laser. LED produces lights that are similar to those of lasers, but its wavelength has broader output peaks and lacks the coherence that is a particular feature of laser light. LED has the advantage of being less expensive [1], safer to use, and easier to manufacture than laser.

Phototherapy (light therapy) was practiced in ancient Egypt, Greece, China, and India. The Egyptians utilized sunlight as well as color for healing [2]. Color has been investigated as medicine since 2000 BC [3]. LLLT was noticed to stimulate hair growth in 1967, wound healing in mice in 1971, and the wound healing effect was soon applied to human patients [4–7]. LLLT is being

Brian J.-F. Wong and Justus Ilgner (eds.), *Biomedical Optics in Otorhinolaryngology: Head and Neck Surgery*,
DOI 10.1007/978-1-4939-1758-7_16, © Springer Science+Business Media New York 2016

used to treat musculoskeletal injury, pain, inflammatory arthritis, tendinitis, neuropathic pain, orofacial pain, sports injuries, Buerger's disease, headache, nerve repair, sympathetic nervous system dysfunction, hemangiomas, immune modulation, bacterial infections, inflammation, and tinnitus [8]. LLLT has become a popular treatment modality and is finding a variety of uses in medical practice. In the past decade, LLLT has been approved by the United States Food and Drug Administration (FDA) in treating diseases such as carpal tunnel syndrome [9] and alopecia [10].

Mechanisms of LLLT

LLLT effects are due to photochemical effects unlike high powered laser. The photons of light must be absorbed by some molecular photoreceptors on chromophores for photochemistry to occur [11] as chlorophyll in plants responding to light and activating photosynthesis. Within the cells, there is strong evidence to suggest that LLLT acts on the mitochondria to increase adenosine triphosphate (ATP) production, modulation of reactive oxygen species (ROS), and induction of transcription factors. Several transcription factors are regulated by changes in cellular redox state. Among them, redox factor-1 (Ref-1) dependent activator protein-1 (AP-1) (a heterodimer of c-Fos and c-Jun), nuclear factor kappa B (NF-κ(kappa)B), p53 activating transcription factor/cAMP-response element-binding protein (ATF/CREB), hypoxia-inducible factor (HIF)-1, and HIF-like factor are those regulated [12]. These transcription factors then cause protein synthesis that triggers further effects downstream, such as increased cell proliferation and migration, modulation in the levels of cytokines, growth factors, and inflammatory mediators, and increased tissue oxygenation [13]. Figure 1 shows the proposed cellular and molecular mechanisms of LLLT [12].

Biphasic Dose Response

It is well established that if the light applied is not of sufficient irradiance or the irradiation time is too short then there is no response. If the irradiance is too high or irradiation time is too long then the response may be inhibited [14–16]. Somewhere in between is the optimal combination of irradiance and time for stimulation [12]. At present there has been no convincing report of biphasic dose responses occurring in patients, but several systematic reviews and meta analyses of randomized controlled trials in LLLT have found that some ineffective trials may be explained

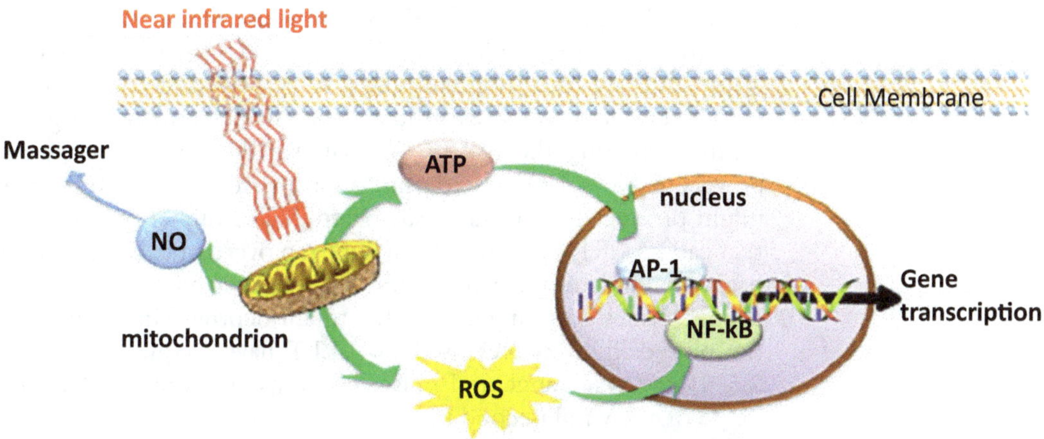

Fig. 1 Cellular mechanisms of LLLT. Schematic diagram showing the absorption of red or near infrared (NIR) light by specific cellular chromophores or photoacceptors localized in the mitochondrial. During this process in mitochondria respiration chain ATP production will increase and reactive oxygen species (ROS) are generated; nitric oxide is released or generated. These cytosolic responses may in turn induce transcriptional changes via activation of transcription factors (e.g., NF-κ(kappa) B and AP1) (from Ann Biomed Eng. 2012 40: 516–33, with permission from Springer)

by over-dosing, in that the guidelines set by World Association for Laser Therapy were exceeded. Moreover, it is unknown to what extent the parameters are needed for the onset of the biphasic dose response, and it will vary in a highly heterogeneous patient population as compared with a highly uniform population of experimental animals [16].

Pulsing in LLLT

Pulsed light offers numerous potential benefits. Because there are "quench periods" (pulse OFF times) following the pulse ON times, pulsed lasers can generate less tissue heating. In instances where it is desirable to deliver light to deeper tissues, increased powers are needed to provide adequate energy at the target tissue. This increased power can cause tissue heating at the surface layers and in this instance, pulsed light could be very useful. Whereas continuous wave (CW) causes an increase in temperature of the intervening and target tissues or organ, pulsed light has been shown to cause no measurable change in the temperature of the irradiated area for the same delivered energy density.

Aside from safety advantages, pulsed light might simply be more effective than CW. The "quench period" (pulse OFF times) reduces tissue heating, thereby allowing the use of potentially much higher peak power densities than those that could be safely used in CW. For example, when CW power densities at the skin of ≥ 2 W/cm^2 are used, doubling the CW power density would only marginally increase the treatment depth while potentially significantly increasing the risk of thermal damage; in contrast, peak powers of ≥ 5 W/cm^2 pulsed using appropriate ON and OFF times might produce little or no tissue heating. The higher peak powers that can be safely used by pulsing light can overcome tissue heating problems and improve the ability of the laser to penetrate into deeper tissues achieving greater treatment depths. The majority of the pulsed light sources used for LLLT have frequencies in the 2.5–10,000 Hz range and pulse durations are commonly in the range of a few millisecond [1].

Penetration Depth

The most important parameter that governs the depth of penetration of laser light into tissue is wavelength. Both the absorption and scattering coefficients of living tissues are higher at lower wavelength, so near-infrared light penetrates more deeply than red. It is often claimed that pulsed lasers penetrate more deeply into tissue than CW lasers with the same average power. There is no consensus on the effects of different frequencies and pulse parameters on the physiologic and therapeutic response of the various disease states that are often treated with laser therapy. This has allowed manufacturers to claim advantages of pulsing without hard evidence to back up their claims. CW light is the gold standard and has been used for most of LLLT applications. However, review of the literature indicates that overall pulsed light may be superior to CW light with everything else being equal. This seemed to be particularly true for wound healing and post-stroke management. On the other hand, pulsed laser as a solo treatment may be less beneficial than CW in patients requiring nerve regeneration. Reviews of literatures indicate that pulsing will continue to play an important role in LLLT especially for applications where deep tissue penetration is required [1].

Transcanal LLLT on Noise-Induced Hearing Loss, Ototoxic Hearing Loss, Tinnitus, and Vestibular Dysfunction

Transcanal Penetration Rate and Side Effects of Transcanal LLLT

The penetration rate of low level laser (LLL) into perilymphatic space of cochlea through an external ear canal, tympanic membrane, and cochlear wall has been measured using 830 nm laser diode, and side effects of LLL on ear canal, tympanic membrane,

Table 1
Transmeatal penetration rate of LLL (80 mW transcanal irradiation)

	Penetration through tympanic membrane	Penetration through cochlea wall
Cadaver	4 mW (5 %)	1.6 mW (2 %)
Guinea Pig	6.4 mW (8 %)	4 mW (4 %)

No penetration of laser through mastoid bone was demonstrated

and cochlea have been studied. Laser diode of 80 mW was irradiated through an external ear canal of guinea pigs once daily for 2 weeks. Histopathologic study was done, and hearing tests were measured using auditory brain response (ABR). Transcanal penetration rates in guinea pigs were 6.4 mW (8 %) at the middle ear behind the tympanic membrane and 4 mW (5 %) at the perilymphatic space of cochlea. Histopathology studies of ear canal skin and tympanic membrane showed all normal findings. ABR hearing tests revealed all normal hearing after transcanal LLLT for 2 weeks. Separate penetration study using human cadaver temporal bones showed that transcanal penetration rate of LLL was 4 mW (5 %) at the middle ear and 1.6 mW (2 %) at the perilymphatic space. No laser penetration was measurable through mastoid bone (Table 1).

This study indicates that transcanal LLLT with 80 mW of 830 nm LD does not induce any side effects to ear canal skin, drum, and cochlea [8].

LLLT on Noise-Induced Hearing Loss

One of the most common factors that cause hearing disorders is noise trauma. Noise is an increasing hazard and it is pervasive, which makes it difficult to take precautions and prevent noise-induced hearing loss (NIHL). Many researches have been carried out to find ways to restore hearing, but no definite treatment has been established yet. The effects of lasers on hearing recovery have been investigated, and several studies using animals reported that LLLT using 830 nm infrared laser diode may improve NIHL, ototoxic hearing loss, tinnitus, and vestibular dysfunction [17, 18].

NIHL was induced by exposing rats to 116 dB noise centered at 16 kHz for 6 h. The rats were treated with transcanal LLLT using 830 nm diode laser with 165 mW for 60 min/day (594 J/day) for

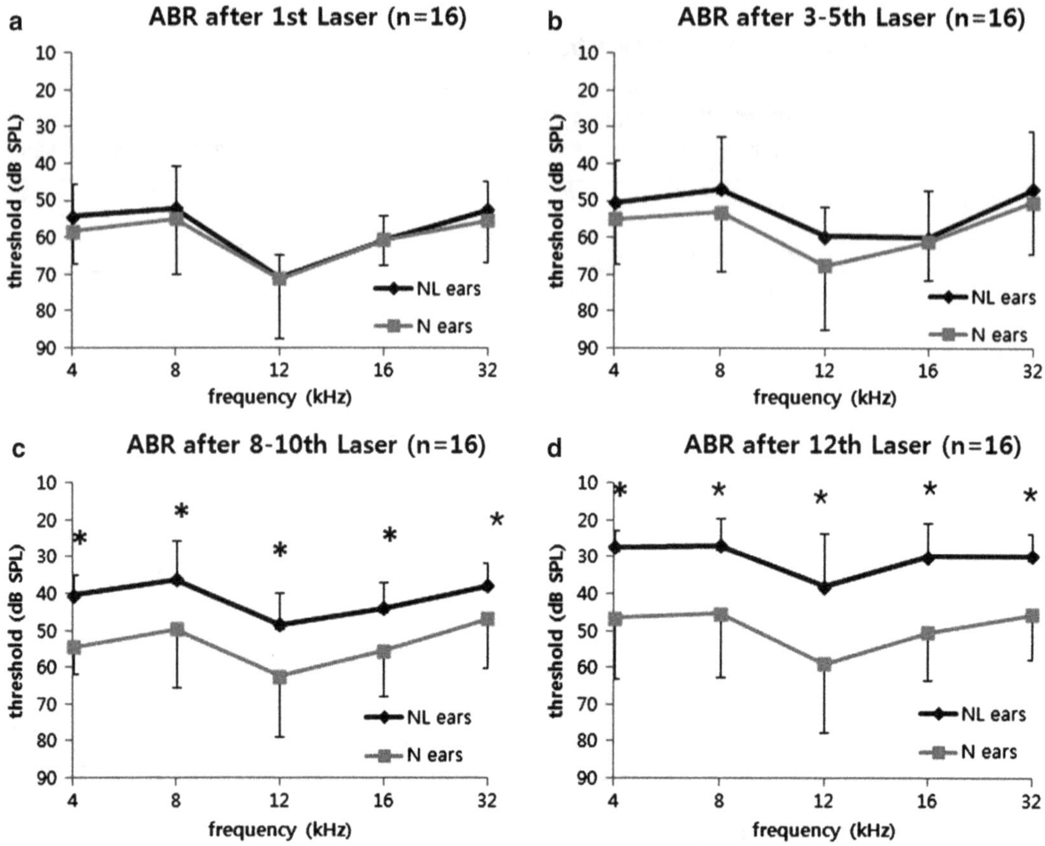

Fig. 2 Hearing threshold changes after repeated transcanal LLLT, 24 h after noise exposure (after the first LLLT), the ABR thresholds were increased markedly to 50–80 dB SPL for both N (noise only) and NL (noise and laser) ears. The hearing threshold between N and NL ears were almost the same at this time point. Signs of change were observed after 5 days of irradiation. After the 8th to 10th irradiation, a significant difference was found at all frequencies. After the 12th irradiation, the hearing threshold was significantly improved on the NL ears when compared to the N ears at all five frequencies ($p < 0.05$) (from J of Biomed Opt 17, 068002, 2012, with permission from SPIE)

12 days. Hearing has been evaluated by auditory brainstem response, and hair cells of cochlea were examined by SEM. The results are shown in Figs. 2 and 3 [17]. This study indicated that LLLT may have a positive effect on cochlear hair-cell recovery after acute acoustic trauma. The hearing threshold became lower (improved) after repeated laser irradiation, and the final hearing result was significantly better than that of the untreated ears. Considering that there is no definitive treatment for acute acoustic trauma in humans, LLLT evolves as a new treatment modality for noise-induced acute hearing loss once a human study is completed with positive result [17].

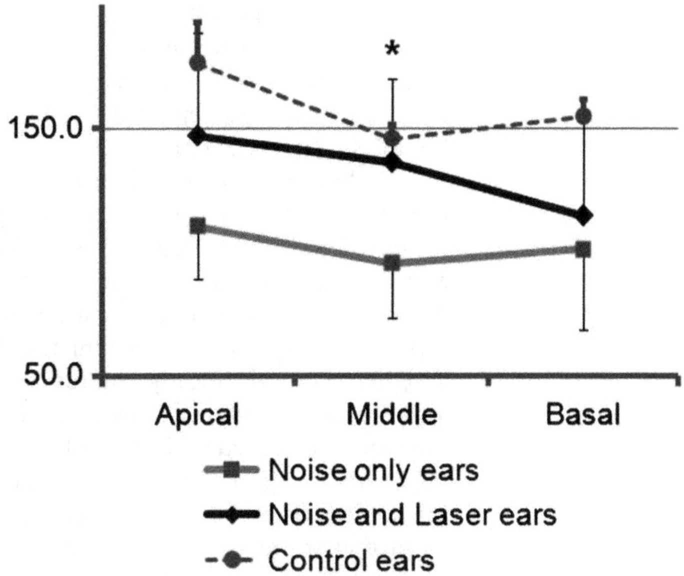

Fig. 3 Number of hair cells observed by scanning electron microscopy. The number of hair cells of the NL (noise and laser) ears was larger than that of the N (noise only) ears and this difference was statistically significant in the middle turn ($p < 0.05$). The number of hair cells of the C (control) ears was significantly larger than that of the N ears in the apical, middle, and the basal turn. The number of hair cells of the C ears was also significantly larger than that of the NL ears in the basal turn. But the number of hair cells of the C ear in the apical and middle turn was similar to that of the NL ears (from J of Biomed Opt 17, 068002, 2012, with permission from SPIE)

Before LLLT is applied to human ears, we need to consider two variations: the first one is the different penetration rate of humans; it is thought to be lower than that of rodents [8] (Rhee 2006 spie), therefore, more power needs to be delivered to the cochlea in humans, but without causing complications. The next consideration is local heating; this is presumed to be the only adverse effect [18]. Previous study showed that there is no damage with laser of power 200 mW, but there may be significant damages in human ears with irradiation of higher power than 200 mW [19].

LLLT on Tinnitus

Tinnitus is one of the most frequently encountered and the most enigmatic ear symptoms in otolaryngology clinic. Tinnitus has been known to develop from noise, aging, and many drugs such as salicylates, aminoglycoside, antibiotics, quinine, and cisplatin [20]. Even though many basic and clinical researches have been conducted to elucidate the mechanisms and to find ways to cure for decades, there is still no silver bullet for this bothersome ear problem. Since early 1990s, LLLT has been used to treat patients with tinnitus by several investigators. Significant reduction of tinnitus intensity was reported by different authors in a range of 15–80 % of patients [21–24].

A clinical study on tinnitus by transcanal LLLT applying 830 nm LD, 80.4 J/cm^2, three times per week for 4 weeks, demonstrated significant reductions of loudness and the degree of annoyance, while the duration of tinnitus was not significantly decreased in laser group. This study used VAS and tinnitus handicap inventory (THI) questionnaire for evaluation that is well accepted method to study tinnitus [8]. The results of clinical studies on tinnitus utilizing transcanal LLLT were mixed. Four previous studies reported positive result [23–26] and five studies showed negative result [21, 22, 27–29]. An optimal dosage of the LLLT for tinnitus or other various inner diseases needs to be established by further studies involving patients with tinnitus and other inner ear diseases.

Recently, phototherapy with transcanal LLLT on animal models has shown possible role of lasers in inner ear pathology [17, 30]. But, how laser irradiation is acting on inner ear hair cells and auditory nerves after various insults is yet to be elucidated, urging further mechanism study with animal model.

A study to quantify the effect of LLLT on the treatment of tinnitus in animal model has been carried out studying the effect of LLLT on salicylate-induced tinnitus in the rat model by means of Gap Prepulse Inhibition of Acoustic Startle (GPIAS). Tinnitus was elicited with salicylate intravenous injection daily. GPIAS was used to monitor tinnitus perception. Rats received transcanal LLLT, showed significantly higher GPIAS values throughout the experiment, indicating transcanal LLLT reduced tinnitus perception. The results of this study suggest that transcanal LLLT may provide a feasible therapeutic approach to control tinnitus. This is the first animal experiment to evaluate laser irradiation effects on tinnitus perception [31].

Effect of LLLT on Hearing and Cochlea Hair Cell Recovery After Ototoxic Hearing Loss

Gentamicin/furosemide-induced hearing loss animal models were established in rats using the modified method previously described [32]. The animals with gentamicin/furosemide-induced hearing loss were treated with transcanal LLLT using 830 nm diode laser at the fluence of 72 J (200 mW × 60 min) once a day for 10 days. Only 4.32 J (6 % of 72 J) is expected to reach into the cochlea. Hearing was measured with ABR, and quantitative scanning electron microscopic (SEM) observations were done by counting remaining hair cells. On SEM images, LLLT significantly increased the number of hair cells in middle and basal turn of the cochlea. Hearing was significantly improved by laser irradiation (from 57 to 44 dB). This study showed that LLLT improved gentamicin/furosemide-induced hearing loss and recovery of damaged cochlear hair cells. As for safety issues, transcanal LLLT in rats using the 830 nm laser irradiating 200 mW for 60 min has not induced any side effects [30].

Effects of Transcanal LLLT on Vestibular System After Gentamicin Ototoxicity

Vestibular disorders display high prevalence and can severely impact the daily life. Vertigo and dizziness rank among the most common reasons for consultation and referral to specialist care [33, 34]. However, pharmacological options that would efficiently relieve the vertigo symptoms without side effects are still lacking.

A bilateral vestibulopathy animal model using adult rats was developed by gentamicin (GM) intravenous injection once daily for 3 days. Bilateral vestibulopathy was confirmed by sinusoidal oscillation tests. Transcanal LLLT was irradiated to left ear canal for 7 days, starting 1 day post-GM injections for 3 days. The gain of LLLT left ear was decreased in 3 days post-LLLT but the decreased gain was improved significantly comparing to that of control right ear, and the improved gain of LLLT left ear was much closer to that of the pre-GM injection level. The average number of hair cells in the cupula of the laser treated left ear was significantly higher comparing to that of the control right ear and it was comparable to the cupula hair cells of the pre-GM injection level. This study demonstrated that LLLT restores vestibular dysfunction and damaged vestibular hair cells in rats post-gentamicin ototoxicity. Transcanal LLLT may have clinical implications in the treatment of various vestibular dysfunctions [35].

A study inducing unilateral vestibulopathy by GM injection into the middle ears of guinea pigs reported therapeutic effect of transcanal LLLT [8]. Unilateral left vestibulopathy was induced by injecting GM into left middle ears of both control and treated groups. Unilateral left vestibular dysfunction was confirmed by animal rotator in both groups. Transcanal LLLT was performed into the left ear canals of the treated-group, while the left ear of the control group was not treated. Unilateral vestibular dysfunction of the LLLT treated left ear was improved significantly, while the unilateral vestibular dysfunction in the left ear of the control group was not improved.

These two studies indicate that transcanal LLLT may be able to treat various vestibular dysfunctions of human patients.

Transnasal LLLT on Nasal Allergy

The number of patients with allergic rhinitis is still increasing, especially in the well-developed, industrialized countries. Although it is not associated with severe morbidity and mortality, allergic rhinitis has a major effect on the quality of life. Its increasing prevalence, its impact on the individual quality of life and social costs [36] and its role as a risk factor for asthma [37], underline the need for improved treatment options for this disorder.

Treatments for allergic rhinitis comprise allergen avoidance, pharmacotherapy, and immunotherapy. Although allergen avoidance may be the preferred treatment, total allergen avoidance may be an unrealistic approach, as it may require limited time spent outdoors. Thus, pharmacotherapy is preferable to allergen avoidance for symptom relief. Nonselective antihistamines can cause sedation and potentially cause other adverse effects such as dry mouth, dry eyes, urinary retention, constipation, and tachycardia. Nonselective antihistamines are associated with impaired sleep, learning, and work performance and with motor vehicle, boating, and aviation accidents [38]. Corticosteroids are recommended as first-line treatment for moderate/severe or persistent allergic rhinitis [39]. Adverse local effects may include increased intraocular pressure and nasal stinging, burning, bleeding, and dryness. Decongestants can be used only on healthy young patients for a limited period of time.

Since conventional therapy with antiallergic medications carries significant notable side effects and limitations, it would be worth to try LLLT to treat allergic rhinitis.

LLLT reduced delayed hypersensitivity reaction to ovalbumin in Balb/C mice in an animal study, and in a study with footpad histopathology, levels of TNF-α (alpha), INF-γ (gamma), and IL-10 analyses between control and hypersensitized animals. This study indicates that treatment with LLLT has an immunomodulatory effect on delayed hypersensitivity reaction to OVA [40].

The effects of intranasal LLLT on allergic rhinitis are not well established. The effects of intranasal LLLT on nasal allergy have been studied using rat allergy models [40] and patients with allergic rhinitis [42, 43].

The effect of LLLT in an experimental rat model of delayed hypersensitivity reaction in nasal cavity has been studied. Rats were sensitized with ovalbumin (OVA) and alum and challenged intranasally with OVA. The nasal rubbing symptom score was counted, spleen was emulsified, and cytokines IL-4, IL-5, IL-6, IL-10, IL-17, and IFN-γ in the splenocytes were assayed. Using 830 nm LD laser, 10 mW intranasal LLLT for 15 min daily for 10 days reduced allergic symptom and suppressed systemic cytokine production by splenocytes, while they were not decreased in no laser treated positive control group. This study demonstrated that intranasal LLLT with 10 mW LD laser into nasal cavity induced antiallergic effects by decreasing allergy symptoms and systemic cytokines production in an allergic rhinitis rat model. Intranasal LLLT with 50 mW was not effective to reduce allergy symptoms and cytokines. Biphasic dose response was applied here. Nasal LLLT may be considered as a potential therapeutic modality in treating allergic rhinitis [41].

In an open study, groups of patients with severe allergic rhinitis received intranasal LLLT with a 308 nm XeCl UVB excimer laser for 2 weeks. In the low-dose group, treatment was given twice weekly, starting with 0.25× the individual minimal erythema dose (MED), whereas patients in the medium-dose group were treated four times weekly, starting with 0.4× MED. In each group, the dosage was gradually increased. Evaluation was based on the symptom scores. The effect of the XeCl laser on the skin prick test reaction was also studied. In the low-dose group, there was no improvement in the nasal symptoms. In the medium-dose group, the XeCl UVB irradiation significantly inhibited the rhinorrhoea, the sneezing, the nasal obstruction, and the total nasal score ($p < 0.05$). The XeCl UVB excimer laser also inhibited the allergen-induced skin prick test in a dose-dependent manner. These results suggest that the XeCl UVB excimer laser might serve as a new therapeutic tool in the treatment of allergic rhinitis [42].

As these animal and human studies demonstrated, transnasal LLLT appears to be effective to improve status of allergic rhinitis without notable side effects, while most of the antiallergic medications may carry significant side effects.

LLLT on Oral Mucositis

Oral mucositis (OM) refers to erythematous and ulcerative lesions of the oral mucosa observed in patients with cancer being treated with chemotherapy and/or with radiation therapy to fields involving the oral cavity. OM can be very painful and can significantly affect nutritional intake, mouth care, increase risk for local and systemic infection, and quality of life [44, 45]. At the same time, OM is a major dose-limiting toxicity of chemotherapy and radiation therapy to the head and neck region. It was reported that 303 of 599 patients (51 %) receiving chemotherapy for solid tumors or lymphoma developed oral and/or GI mucositis [45]. OM developed in 22 % of 1236 cycles of chemotherapy and even higher percentage (approximately 75–80 %) of patients who receive high-dose chemotherapy prior to hematopoietic cell transplantation developed clinically significant OM [47]. Almost all patients treated with radiation therapy for head and neck cancer will develop some degree of OM. In the recent studies, severe OM occurred in 29–66 % of all patients receiving radiation therapy for head and neck cancer [48, 49].

Management of OM has been largely palliative to date. Management of OM is divided into the following sections: nutritional support, pain control, oral decontamination, palliation of dry mouth, management of oral bleeding, and therapeutic interventions for OM. Several agents have been tested to reduce the severity of, or prevent, mucositis. Conventional treatments of OM include cryotherapy, administration of growth factors, anti-inflammatory agents, and antioxidants [50]. LLLT has been tried by many clinicians and investigators for preventive and therapeutic purposes. Multiple studies have indicated that LLLT can reduce the severity of chemotherapy and radiation-induced OM [51–53]. Studies are difficult to compare due to varying laser types and parameters (such as wavelength and fluence). Nevertheless, success rate of 81 % when LLLT was given as a preventive treatment, and 83 % of therapeutic success rate have been reported [53].

Previous study revealed that no heterogeneity between trials with optimal doses for the red (630–670 nm) and the infrared (780–830 nm) subgroups. The optimal dose ranges for red and infrared wavelengths on OM are usually 1–8 J. The laser applications are usually performed daily, perpendicular to the lesions intraorally. LLLT needs to be performed at least every other day for the duration of chemoradiotherapy regimens or as long as OM ulcers are present. The trials which aimed at the prevention of OM started LLLT at 7 days before chemoradiotherapy regimens [50]. The newly available blue LED has potential for the management of OM, and research is warranted based on the known effects of this light therapy in wound healing [54].

Although the literatures suggest that lasers with wavelengths varying between 632 and 830 nm can have beneficial effects on preventing and treating OM, no specific protocols that investigated other parameters such as tissue fluency (energy density), ideal time of laser application, variations in cancer type, and cancer treatment regimens are available [55]. Extraoral application of LED, 4 J (total 12 J/treatment) to the extraoral bilateral cheeks and anterior throat tissues, was shown to have a significant reduction in pain but not for other mucositis scoring scales [56].

LLLT improved quality of life by reducing oral hygiene, difficulty of drinking, swallowing, speaking, and secondary infection [52, 57]. LLLT appears to be effective in improving OM, in controlling the intensity of mucositis, in relieving the OM related pain, and in improving the quality of life. All the studies investigated possible side effects, but none found side effects or adverse effects. LLLT was well tolerated among all patients with OM [51].

LLLT in the Management of Neck Pain

Chronic neck pain is a highly prevalent and costly condition affecting 10–24 % of the population [58–60] and for which pharmacological management has limited evidence of efficacy. LLLT is noninvasive treatment for neck pain, in which nonthermal laser irradiation is applied to sites of pain. The presenting neck pain can have several concurrent sources of pain from joints, muscles, and ligaments.

Transcutaneous application results in laser-energy scattering and spreading into a three-dimensional volume of tissue up to 5 cm for infrared laser [61]. Previous studies suggest that trigger points in the neck coincide with the location of acupuncture points in 70–80 % of patients [62, 63]. Since trigger points and acupuncture points are characterized by tenderness, the treatment effect of laser irradiation to tender points, trigger points, or acupuncture points is likely to be the same. Thus, when treating neck pain with LLLT, irradiation of known trigger points, acupuncture points, tender points, and symptomatic zygapophyseal joints is advisable [64]. A meta-analysis reported that at 820–830 nm, doses are most effective in the range of 0.8–9.0 J per point, with irradiation times of 15–180 s. At 904 nm, doses are slightly smaller (0.8–4.2 J per point) with slightly longer irradiation times (100–600 s) than at 820–830 nm [64]. The optimum mean dose per point for 820–830 nm was 5.9 J, with an irradiation time of 39.8 s, and for 904 nm, 2.2 J delivered with an irradiation time of 238 s. The same meta-analysis reported moderate statistical evidence for efficacy of LLLT in the treatment of acute and chronic neck pain in the short and medium term [64].

This positive relieving effect was maintained for 3 months after the treatment ended, while the effect of NSAIDs ends rapidly when drug is discontinued [65]. Another study of LLLT on acute neck pain with radiculopathy reported significant improvement for intensity of arm pain and neck extension. LLLT was applied to the skin projection at the anatomical site of the spinal segment involved with the following parameters: 905 nm at 5000 Hz, power density of 12 mW/cm^2, and dose of 2 J/cm^2, for 120 s, at whole dose of 12 J/cm^2 [66]. Side effects of tiredness, nausea, and stiffness have been reported post-LLLT [67]. LLLT does not generate any heat and safety issue relating mainly to potential eye damage, and safety glasses are required for the use of LLLT.

Mechanisms for LLLT-mediated pain relief are not fully understood. Anti-inflammatory effects of red and infrared laser irradiation have been shown by reduction in specific inflammatory markers (prostaglandin E, interleukin 1β (beta), TNF α in vivo and in vitro studies in animal and man [68]. Second possible mechanism is to reduce oxidative stress and skeletal muscle fatigue that has been reported in animal and human studies [69, 70]. Another mechanism for LLLT effects on myofascial pain and trigger points could be an inhibition of transmission at the neuromuscular junction [71]. Such effects could mediate the clinical finding that LLLT decreases tenderness in trigger points within 15 min of LLLT application [72]. LLLT studies on cervical pain compare favorable with other widely used therapies and especially with pharmacological interventions for which evidence is spare and side effects are common.

References

1. Hashmi JT, Huang YY, Osmani BZ, Shama SK, Naeser MA, Hamblin MR. Role of low-level laser therapy in neurorehabilitation. PM R. 2010;2 Suppl:S292–305.
2. Hansen HJ, Thoroe U. Low power laser biostimulation of chronic oro-facial pain: a double-blind placebo controlled cross-over study in 40 patients. Pain. 1990;43:169–79.
3. Basford JR. Low intensity laser therapy: still not an established clinical tool. Lasers Surg Med. 1995;16:331–42.
4. Mester E, Szende B, Tota JG. Effect of laser on hair growth of mice. Kiserl Orvostud. 1967; 19:628–31.
5. Mester E, Spiry T, Szende B, Tota JG. Effect of laser rays on wound healing. Am J Surg. 1971;122:532–5.
6. Mester E, Szende B, Spiry T, Scher A. Stimulation of wound healing by laser rays. Acta Chir Acad Sci Hung. 1972;13:315–24.
7. Mester E, Nagylucskay S, Doklen A, Tisza S. Laser stimulation of wound healing. Acta Chir Acad Sci Hung. 1976;17:49–55.
8. Rhee CK, Lim ES, Kim YS, Chung YW, Jung JY, Chung P. Effect of low-level laser (LLL) on cochlear and vestibular inner ear including tinnitus. Proc SPIE. 2006;6078:60781K-1-12.
9. Melkerson MN. K081166. Rockville: U.S. Food and Drug Administration; 2009.
10. Melkerson MN. K091496. Silver Spring: U.S. Food and Drug Administration; 2010.
11. Sutherland JC. Biological effects of polychromatic light. Photochem Photobiol. 2002;76: 164–70.
12. Chung H, Dai T, Sharma SK, Huang YY, Carrol JD, Hamblin MR. The nuts and bolts of low-level laser (light) therapy. Ann Biomed Eng. 2012;40:516–33.
13. Karu TI, Kolyakov SF. Exact action spectra for cellular responses relevant to phototherapy. Photomed Laser Surg. 2005;23:355–61.
14. Castano AP, Dai T, Yaroslavsky I, Cohen R, Apruzzese WA, Smotrich MH, Hamblin MR. Low-level laser therapy for zymosan-induced arthritis in rats: importance of illumination time. Lasers Surg Med. 2007;39: 543–50.
15. Lanzafame RJ, Stadler I, Kurtz AF, Connelly R, Peter Sr TA, Brondon P, Olson D. Reciprocity of exposure time and irradiance on energy density during photoradiation on wound healing in a murine pressure ulcer model. Lasers Surg Med. 2007;39:534–42.
16. Huang YY, Sharma SK, Carroll J, Hamblin M. Biphasic dose response in low level light therapy—an update. Dose Response. 2011; 9(4):602–18.
17. Rhee CK, Bahk CW, Kim SH, Ahn JC, Jung JY, Chung PS, Suh MW. Effect of low-level laser treatment on cochlea hair-cell recovery after acute acoustic trauma. J Biomed Opt. 2012;17:068002–6.
18. Rhee CK, He P, Jung JY, Ahn JC, Chung PS, Suh MW. Effect of low-level laser therapy on cochlear hair cell recovery after gentamicin-induced ototoxicity. Laser Med Sci. 2012;27: 987–92.
19. Suh MW, Jung JY, Ahn JC, Jung PS, Moon TH. External, middle and inner ear safety of trans-canal low level laser therapy. J Intern Adv Otol. 2013;9(3):105.
20. Jastreboff PJ. Phantom auditory perception (tinnitus): mechanisms of generation and perception. Neurosci Res. 1990;8:221–54.
21. Mirz F, Zachariae R, Andersen SE, Nielsen AG, Johansen LV, Bjerring P, Pedersen CB. The low-power laser in the treatment of tinnitus. Clin Otolaryngol Allied Sci. 1999;24: 346–54.
22. Partheniadis-Stumpf M, Maurer J, Mann W. Soft laser therapy in combination with tebonin i.v. in tinnitus. Laryngorhinootologie. 1993;72:28–31.

23. Plath P, Olivier J. Results of combined low-power laser therapy and extracts of Ginkgo biloba in cases of sensorineural hearing loss and tinnitus. Adv Otorhi-nolaryngol. 1995; 49:101–4.
24. Shiomi Y, Takahashi H, Honjo I, Kojima H, Naito Y, Fujiki N. Efficacy of trans-meatal low power laser irradiation on tinnitus: a preliminary report. Auris Nasus Larynx. 1997;24: 39–42.
25. Hahn A, Sejna I, Stolbova K, Cocek A. Combined laser-Egb 761 tinnitus therapy. Acta Otolaryngol Suppl. 2001;545:92–3.
26. Tauber S, Beyer W, Schorn K, Baumgartner R. Transmeatal cochlear laser treatment of cochlear dysfunction : a feasibility study for chronic tinnitus. Lasers Med Sci. 2003;18: 154–61.
27. von Wedel H, Calero L, Walger M, Hoenen S, Rutwalt D. Soft-laser/Ginkgo therapy in chronic tinnitus. A placebo-controlled study. Adv Otorhinolaryngol. 1995;49:105–8.
28. Rogowski M, Munich S, Gindzienska E, Lazarczyk B. Low-power laser in the treatment of tinnitus—a placebo-controlled study. Otolaryngol Pol. 1999;53:315–20.
29. Nakashima T, Ueda H, Misawa H, Suzuki T, Tominaga M, Ito A, Numata S, Kasai S, Asahi K, Vernon JA, Meikle MB. Transmeatal low-power laser irradiation for tinnitus. Otol Neurotol. 2002;23:296–300.
30. Rhee CK, He P, Jung JY, Ahn JC, Chung PS, Lee MY, Suh MW. Effect of low-level laser treatment on cochlea hair cell recovery after ototoxic hearing loss. J Biomed Opt. 2013; 18(12):128003.
31. Park YM, Na WS, Park IY, Suh MW, Rhee CK, Chung PS, Jung JY. Trans-canal laser irradiation reduces tinnitus perception of salicylate treated rat. Neurosci Lett. 2013;7(544): 131–5.
32. Liu HY, Chi FL, Gao WY. Taurine attenuates aminoglycoside ototoxicity by inhibiting inducible nitric oxide synthase expression in the cochlea. Neuroreport. 2008;19:117–20.
33. Nakashima K, Yokoyama Y, Shimoyama R, Saito H, Kuno N, Sano K. Prevalence of neurological disorders in a Japanese town. Neuroepidemiology. 1996;15:208–13.
34. Moulin T, Sablot D, Vidry E, Belahsen F, Berger E, Lemounaud P. Impact of emergency room neurologists on patient management and outcome. Eur Neurol. 2003;50:207–14.
35. Rhee CK, Hyun JH, Suh MH, Ahn JC, Jung JY. Effect of low level laser therapy (LLLT) on vestibular system after gentamicin ototoxicity. Proc SPIE. 2013;8565:85651S.
36. Law AW, Reed SD, Sundy JS, Schulman KA. Direct costs of allergic rhinitis in the United States: estimates from the 1996 Medical Expenditure Panel Survey. J Allergy Clin Immunol. 2003;111:296–300.
37. Togias A. Rhinitis and asthma: evidence for respiratory system integration. J Allergy Clin Immunol. 2003;111:1171–83.
38. Church MK, Maurer M, Simons FE, et al. Risk of first-generation H(1)-antihistamines: a GA(2)LEN position paper. Allergy. 2010; 65(4):459–66.
39. Wallace DV, Dykewicz MS, Bernstein DI, Blessing-Moore J, Cox L, Khan DA, Lang DM, Nicklas RA, Oppenheimer J, Portnoy JM, Randolph CC, Schuller D, Spector SL, Tilles SA, Joint Task Force on Practice; American Academy of Allergy; Asthma & Immunology; American College of Allergy; Asthma and Immunology; Joint Council of Allergy, Asthma and Immunology. The diagnosis and management of rhinitis: an updated practice parameter. J Allergy Clin Immunol. 2008;122(2 Suppl):S1–84.
40. Oliveira RG, Ferreira AP, Côrtes AJ, Aarestrup BJ, Andrade LC, Aarestrup FM. Low-level laser reduces the production of TNF-α, IFN-γ, and IL-10 induced by OVA. Lasers Med Sci. 2013;28(6):1519–25.
41. Rhee CK, Kim JH, Ahn JC, Mo JH. The effects of low level laser therapy on nasal allergy in SD rat allergy model on nasal allergy. Lasers Surg Med. 2012;44 Suppl 24:52.
42. Csoma Z, Ignacz F, Bor Z, Szabo G, Bodai L, Dobozy A, Kemeny L. Intranasal irradiation with the xenon chloride ultraviolet B laser improves allergic rhinitis. J Photochem Photobiol B. 2004;75:137–44.
43. Krespi YP, Kizhner V. Phototherapy for chronic rhinosinusitis. Lasers Surg Med. 2011; 43:187–91.
44. Lalla RV, Peterson DE. Oral mucositis. Dent Clin North Am. 2005;49(1):167–84.
45. Duncan GG, Epstein JB, Tu D, El Sayed S, Bezjak A, Ottaway J, Pater J, National Cancer Institute of Canada Clinical Trials Group. Quality of life, mucositis, and xerostomia from radiotherapy for head and neck cancers: a report from the NCIC CTG HN2 randomized trial of an antimicrobial lozenge to prevent mucositis. Head Neck. 2005;27(5): 421–8.
46. Elting LS, Cooksley C, Chambers M, Cantor SB, Manzullo E, Rubenstein EB. The burdens of cancer therapy. Clinical and economic outcomes of chemotherapy-induced mucositis. Cancer. 2003;98(7):1531–9.

47. Vera-Llonch M, Oster G, Ford CM, Lu J, Sonis S. Oral mucositis and outcomes of allogeneic hematopoietic stem-cell transplantation in patients with hematologic malignancies. Support Care Cancer. 2007;15(5):491–6.
48. Vera-Llonch M, Oster G, Hagiwara M, Sonis S. Oral mucositis in patients undergoing radiation treatment for head and neck carcinoma. Cancer. 2006;106(2):329–36.
49. Elting LS, Cooksley CD, Chambers MS, Garden AS. Risk, outcomes, and costs of radiation-induced oral mucositis among patients with head-and-neck malignancies. Int J Radiat Oncol Biol Phys. 2007;68(4): 1110–20.
50. Lalla RV, Sonis ST, Peterson DE. Management of oral mucositis in patients who have cancer. Dent Clin North Am. 2008;52(1):61–77.
51. Bjordal JM, Bensadoun RJ, Tuner J, Frigo L, Gjerde K, Lopes-Martins RAB. A systematic review with meta-analysis of the effect of low-level laser therapy (LLLT) in cancer therapy-induced oral mucositis. Support Care Cancer. 2011;19(8):1069–77.
52. Gautam AP, Fernandes DJ, Vidyasagar MS, Maiya AG, Nigudgi S. Effect of low-level laser therapy on patient reported measures of oral mucositis and quality of life in head and neck cancer patients receiving chemoradiotherapy—a randomized controlled trial. Support Care Cancer. 2012;21(5):1421–8.
53. Genot-Klastersky MT, Klastersky J, Awada F, Awada A, Crombez P, Martinez MD, Jaivenois MF, Delmelle M, Vogt G, Meuleman N, Paesmans M. The use of low-energy laser (LEL) for the prevention of chemotherapy- and/or radiotherapy-induced oral mucositis in cancer patients: results from two prospective studies. Support Care Cancer. 2008;16(12): 1381–7.
54. Adamskaya N, Dungel P, Mittermayr R. Light therapy by blue LED improves wound healing in an excision model in rats. Injury. 2011;42:917–21.
55. Migliorati C, Hewson I, Lalla RV, Antunes HS, Estilo CL, Hodgson B, Lopes NN, Schubert MM, Bowen J, Elad S. Systematic review of laser and other light therapy for the management of oral mucositis in cancer patients. Support Care Cancer. 2013;21(1): 333–41.
56. Hodgson BD, Margolis DM, Salzman DE, Eastwood D, Tarima S, Williams LD, Sande JE, Vaughan WP, Whelan HT. Amelioration of oral mucositis pain by NASA near-infrared light-emitting diodes in bone marrow transplant patients. Support Care Cancer. 2012;20(7): 1405–15.
57. Oton-Leite AF, Corrêa de Castro AC, Morais MO, Pinezi JC, Leles CR, Mendonça EF. Effect of intraoral low-level laser therapy on quality of life of patients with head and neck cancer undergoing radiotherapy. Head Neck. 2012;34(3):398–404.
58. Borghouts J, Koes B, Vondeling H, Bouter L. Cost-of-illness of neck pain in the Netherlands in 1996. Pain. 1999;80:629–36.
59. Webb R, Brammah T, Lunt M, Urwin M, Allison T, Symmons D. Prevalence and predictors of intense, chronic, and disabling neck and back pain in the UK general population. Spine. 2003;28:1195–202.
60. Fejer R, Kyvik KO, Hartvigsen J. The prevalence of neck pain in the world population: a systematic critical review of the literature. Eur Spine J. 2006;15:834–48.
61. Oshiro T. The laser apple: a new graphic representation of medical laser applications. Laser Ther. 1996;8:185–90.
62. Melzack R, Stillwell DM, Fox EJ. Trigger points and acupuncture points for pain: correlations and implications. Pain. 1977;3:3–23.
63. Dorsher PT. Can classical acupuncture points and trigger points be compared in the treatment of pain disorders? Birch's analysis revisited. J Altern Complement Med. 2008;14:353–9.
64. Chow RT, Johnson MI, Lopes-Martins RA, Bjordal JM. Efficacy of low-level laser therapy in the management of neck pain: a systematic review and meta-analysis of randomised placebo or active-treatment controlled trials. Lancet. 2009;374(9705):1897–908.
65. Chow RT, Heller GZ, Barnsley L. The effect of 300 mW, 830 nm laser on chronic neck pain: a double-blind, randomized, placebo-controlled study. Pain. 2006;124:201–10.
66. Konstantinovic LM, Cutovic MR, Milovanovic AN, Jovic SJ, Dragin AS, Letic MDj, Miler VM. Low-level laser therapy for acute neck pain with radiculopathy: a double-blind placebo-controlled randomized study. Pain Med. 2010;11(8):1169–78.
67. Gur A, Sarac AJ, Cevik R, Altindag O, Sarac S. Efficacy of 904 nm gallium arsenide low level laser therapy in the management of chronic myofascial pain in the neck: a double-blind and randomize-controlled trial. Lasers Surg Med. 2004;35(3):229–35.
68. Soriano F, Rios R. Gallium arsenide laser treatment of chronic low back pain: a prospective randomized and double blind study. Laser Ther. 1998;10:175–80.

69. Lopes-Martins RA, Marcos RL, Leonardo PS. Effect of low-level laser (Ga-Al-As 655nm) on skeletal muscle fatigue induced by electrical stimulation in rats. J Appl Physiol. 2006; 101:283–8.
70. Leal Junior EC, Lopes-Martins RA, Vanin AA. Effect of 830 nm low-level laser therapy in exercise-induced skeletal muscle fatigue in humans. Lasers Med Sci. 2009;24:425–31.
71. Nicolau RA, Martinez MS, Rigau J, Tomas J. Effect of low power 655nm diode laser irradiation on the neuromuscular junctions of the mouse diaphragm. Lasers Surg Med. 2004; 34:277–84.
72. Olavi A, Pekka R, Pertti K, Pekka P. Effects of the infrared laser therapy at treated and non-treated trigger points. Acupunct Electrother Res. 1989;14:9–14.

Chapter 17

Stimulation of Neurons with Infrared Radiation

Ken Zhao, Xiaodong Tan, Hunter Young, and Claus-Peter Richter

Introduction

The neurodevice market has been one of the fastest growing sectors in the medical device industry since Medtronic was granted FDA clearance and CMS reimbursement for treating Parkinson's disease in the late 1990s. The total worldwide market for neurostimulation devices (neuroprosthetics and neuromodulation) is estimated to be $3.1 billion in 2010 and is expected to grow substantially over the next several years, reaching approximately $10.2 billion by 2014 (Neuroinsights, Neurotechnology Report 2010). Devices that substitute for an impaired part of the nervous system make up the neuroprosthetic market, consisting of cochlear implants, retinal implants, and motor prostheses. There are over 100 million candidates worldwide that could benefit from these technologies. However, due to the infancy of this field and the limitations from existing stimulation technologies, the market is grossly underserved with less than 1 % market penetration. The goal for all neuroprostheses is to restore neural function to a condition having the fidelity of a healthy system. However, contemporary neuroprostheses, which use electric current to stimulate neurons, are not able to fully achieve this goal. As determined by the electrode configuration and the electric tissue properties, electric current spreads in tissue and consequently does not allow precise stimulation of focused neuronal populations. The result is an overlap of stimulation fields when neighboring electrode contacts are used [1]. Several strategies have been employed to increase the spatial selectivity of electrical stimulation (ES) over a conventional monopolar stimulation paradigm. Multipolar electrode

Brian J.-F. Wong and Justus Ilgner (eds.), *Biomedical Optics in Otorhinolaryngology: Head and Neck Surgery*, DOI 10.1007/978-1-4939-1758-7_17, © Springer Science+Business Media New York 2016

configurations have been employed to increase the spatial selectivity of stimulation [2–5] or to introduce virtual channels through current steering [6–9].

In cochlear implants, the use of either virtual channels or tripolar stimulation only showed marginal improvements in performance [7]. The limited improvement might be explained by the fact that multipolar stimulation and virtual channels did not result in an increase in the number of independent channels that can be used at the same time [7, 10, 11]. Cuff electrodes have been successfully used in several chronic animal and human studies to stimulate motor neurons and the optic nerve [12–14], but drawbacks of this method include nerve damage from contact with the cuff [15, 16]. Penetrating electrodes also allow for more spatially focused stimulation by inserting the stimulating source into the nerve tissue. However, by compromising the structure and integrity of the nerve, penetrating electrodes can cause inflammation and edema and, subsequently, impair neural conduction [17, 18]. An emerging technology in the field of neural excitation is the application of pulsed infrared (IR) light to precisely stimulate small populations of neurons. Laser light, of the appropriate parameter set, can reliably elicit neural action potentials in a non-contact manner [19]. This technology, due to the inherent ability to focus light on targets with spot sizes as small as hundreds of microns, presents a fundamental paradigm shift in the field of neural stimulation [19, 20]. Advantages of infrared neural stimulation (INS) include no stimulation artifact [21] and no tissue-electrode interface, with possible toxicity related to the electrode material and dependence of effective stimulation upon tissue impedance and coupling [22].

Pulsed Lasers for Neural Stimulation

The idea to stimulate neurons with a pulsed infrared laser was born at Vanderbilt University. The free-electron laser (FEL, $\lambda = 2100$–6100 nm) provided the ideal experimental tool to explore the possibility of stimulating nerves with light [19]. The selection of the initial radiation wavelengths was based on a Fourier transform infrared spectroscopy (FTIR) of rat sciatic nerve tissue. The free-electron laser was then tuned to deliver radiation at wavelengths corresponding to relative peaks and valleys based on FTIR measurements (Fig. 1a). Stimulation and ablation thresholds were determined. They varied significantly depending on the wavelength (Fig. 1b). Stimulation thresholds were typically below 1 J/cm^2 at wavelengths corresponding to high soft tissue absorption and were above 1 J/cm^2 at low soft tissue absorption. An increasing divergence was noted in stimulation, and ablation thresholds were noted as soft tissue absorption decreased (Fig. 1b). The greatest safety ratios were obtained at wavelengths ($\lambda = 2100$ and 4000 nm) corresponding to minima in the soft tissue absorption curve. Two reasons exist to select 2100 nm over 4000 nm. Firstly, the Ho:YAG laser ($\lambda = 2120$ nm) exists as a radiation source, and secondly, optical fibers to couple light at 2100 nm are readily available for the experiments. Moreover, small changes in wavelength result in significant changes in penetration depth. For example, the Aculight diode lasers cover wavelength ranges between 1844 and 1900 nm, which correspond to penetration depths between ~1000 and 100 nm, respectively.

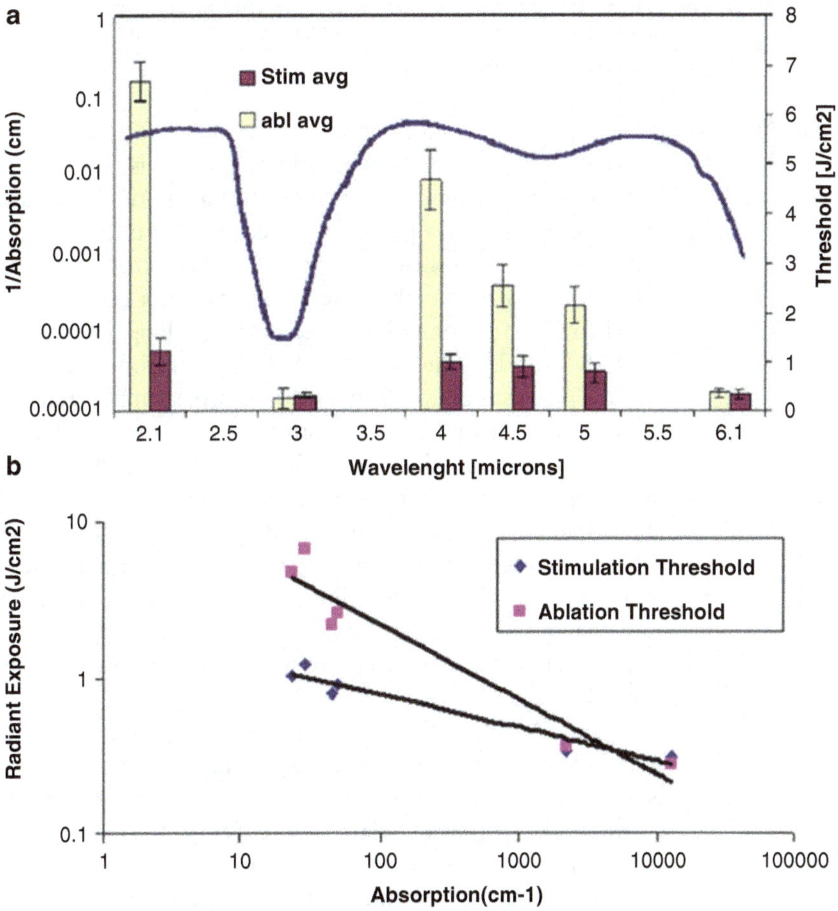

Fig. 1 (**a**) Wavelength dependence of stimulation. Free-electron laser (FEL) was employed to irradiate four different nerves for three trials each at six wavelengths: 2.1, 3.0, 4.0, 4.5, 5.0, and 6.1 μm (*columns*, right axis), each near a relative peak or valley of water absorption (*solid line*, left axis). (**b**) Log-log plot of ablation and stimulation radiant exposure thresholds as a function of the water absorption coefficient for each wavelength (from Wells et al. Application of infrared light for in vivo neural stimulation. J Biomed Opt. 2005;10(6):064003. With permission)

Mechanism of Infrared Neural Stimulation

Initial experiments have demonstrated that nerves can be stimulated with lasers. In spite of many efforts in clarifying the mechanism behind INS, the steps by which the absorption of the photons results in an action potential are not fully understood. Many advances have been made, yet it continues to be a topic of controversial debate. This is because laser-tissue interactions are complex, as they are determined by both laser parameters and tissue properties. Spot size, radiation wavelength, pulse duration, pulse repetition rate, and radiant energy characterize laser parameters, while absorption and scattering are important tissue properties. In general, three basic effects of photon tissue interaction are considered: photothermal, photochemical, and photomechanical effects.

Photothermal Effects

Current evidence supports photothermal effects as the mechanism behind INS; the absorbed radiant energy is converted to heat, which evokes a neural response. Initial work demonstrated that neural activation via pulsed infrared light is induced by a thermal transient [21]. To show that the key factor is the temperature transient, instead of the absolute temperature, a cold saline bath was used to vary the temperature of northern leopard frogs between 0 and 25 °C [21]. The frog sciatic nerve was stimulated in vivo using a Ho:YAG laser coupled to a 600 μm fiber submerged in the saline bath with fiber tip 0.4 mm from the nerve surface. The results did not show any statistically significant changes in the threshold radiant exposure with changes in resting nerve temperature. This indicates that there is no set threshold tissue temperature for initiation of action potentials. Similarly, recordings from single vestibular nerve fibers in the toadfish demonstrated a lack of afferent responses to changes in whole organ temperature and persistence of IR-evoked responses after the animal's temperature was lowered by 6–7 °C [23].

The degree of thermal change required to evoke neural responses with IR light varies depending on the type of neural tissue being stimulated. Thermal measurements from in vivo stimulation of the rat sciatic nerve demonstrated a minimum surface temperature increase of 6 °C for stimulation [21]. With regard to INS of the auditory nerve, the required thermal transient seems to be much lower than for peripheral nerves. Threshold radiant exposures for INS of the gerbil auditory nerve were 5 mJ/cm^2, corresponding to a calculated temperature rise of ~0.08 °C [24].

The importance of thermal transients was further highlighted by a study demonstrating that heating of the tissue reversibly alters the electrical capacitance of the plasma membrane by altering the ionic double layers around the membrane [25]. The authors demonstrated that the mechanism is highly ubiquitous by using IR light to evoke similarly shaped currents in oocytes, human embryonic kidney (HEK) cells, and an artificial 1:1 phosphatidylethanolamine and phosphatidylcholine bilayer. Larger radiant energies yielded greater capacitance changes. After IR stimulation, the increases in capacitance decayed on a timescale of 100–200 ms, consistent with the rate of thermal relaxation in water. These findings are supported by a recent study, with initial results showing that pulsed IR radiation rapidly alters the capacitance of the membrane through charge redistribution and evokes mitochondrial Ca^{2+} currents [26]. A recent computational model by Peterson et al. suggests that capacitive changes are unlikely to be the sole mechanism underlying INS, as the model's determined thresholds of activation were higher than capacitance changes observed in previous work [27]. Their parameter space consisted of beam diameter, pulse width, and dependence on illuminating nodes of Ranvier, yet their lowest membrane capacitive change required to elicit activation (15 %) was still twice the magnitude of those values reported by Shapiro et al. (2–8 %).

An alternative proposed photothermal mechanism involved in INS is the activation of heat-sensitive ion channels. These channels are the transient receptor potential (vanilloid) or TRPV channels [28]. The best-known example is TRPV1, which is activated by capsaicin, the compound in chili peppers, which produces a burning sensation [29]. TRPV1 is expressed in small diameter neurons within sensory ganglia and is also stimulated by acid ($pH \leq 5.9$), noxious heat (>43 °C), and other vanilloid compounds. TRPV channels have also been identified in the sciatic nerve, the dorsal root and trigeminal ganglia of rats [29], cochlear structures of the rat, guinea pig and mice [30–32], and vestibular neurons of mice and rats [33].

Activation of TRPV channels with IR light has been demonstrated to be highly dependent upon extracellular calcium influx in TRPV1 and TRPV4 channels. Rhee et al. isolated inferior ganglia neurons expressing TRPV1, a nonselective cation channel, from the rat vagus nerve [34]. Using radiation at $\lambda = 1850$ nm from a diode laser, which was delivered through 200 μm silica fiber, they successfully elicited transient rises in intracellular calcium concentration with brief 2 ms pulses. Significantly diminished responses were observed in the absence of extracellular calcium or upon application of capsazepine, a TRPV1 blocker, demonstrating the integral role of extracellular calcium and the TRPV1 channel. The role of TRPV1 was supported by another study which observed that the auditory nerve of most TRPV1 knockout mice could not be stimulated with infrared laser, while all control animals were successfully stimulated [32]. In isolated retinal ganglion cells from mice and in vestibular ganglion cells from rats, IR radiation at 1875 nm from a pulsed diode laser was delivered via a 105 μm fiber and successfully generated transient membrane potential variations in sensory neurons with 7–10 ms pulses [33]. These laser-evoked neuronal voltage variations (LEVVs) typically consisted of an initial humplike depolarization, on top of which a spike component occurred. Application of TTX, a blocker of voltage-gated sodium channels, abolished the spike component, while application of Ni/Cd solution, a blocker of voltage-gated calcium channels, diminished the initial humplike component and prevented the sodium-based spike. This suggests that the IR-evoked action potential is triggered by an initial calcium influx as represented by the humplike component. Unlike the experiments in the rat vagus by Rhee et al., capsazepine had no effect on LEVVs. However, application of RN 1734, a TRPV4 channel blocker, prevented induction of LEVVs in both the mice retinal and rat vestibular ganglion cells [33].

In contrast to the thermal transient driving the general electrostatic mechanism, it seems that absolute temperature is required for activation of TRPV channels. Bec and coworkers [35] performed a follow-up study to Albert et al. [33], in which they stimulated mice retinal and rat vestibular ganglion cells. Although the threshold radiant energy for stimulation varied depending on parameters such as pulse duration and wavelength, generation of action potentials consistently corresponded with a temperature rise to 55–60 °C. According to the authors, irradiation of the neurons did not result in tissue damage.

In contrast to the studies described above, Katz et al. [36] found evidence against activation of TRPV channels with IR light. In more than 85 % of the rat dorsal root and nodose ganglia, INS evoked depolarizations lasting for hundreds of milliseconds [36]. This is not consistent with stimulation of TRPV1 channels, because TRPV1 expression has been observed in only 32 % of cutaneous dorsal root ganglion neurons in rats [37] and less than 38 % of nodose neurons in mice [38]. Furthermore, the broad range of observed reversal potential values (−20 to −55 mV) does not correspond to those for nonselective cation channels such as the TRPV receptors (reversal potential should be approximately 0 mV). The range of reversal potentials suggests that IR produces depolarization through interactions with more than one ionic channel.

Photochemical Effects

A photochemical interaction occurs when a molecular chromophore absorbs a photon and converts it to chemical energy. The chromophore may be endogenous, such as amino acids, peptides, and pigments or may be exogenous molecules introduced into the tissue. This concept was demonstrated by Farber and Grinvald [39]. They synthesized a photosensitive dye that bound to the nerve membrane. Neurons stained with the compound could be reversibly depolarized by irradiation with a He-Ne laser ($\lambda = 632.8$ nm, $P = 11$ mW) [39]. Production of oxygen free radicals at the membrane was thought to drive depolarization and cause irreversible photochemical damage to neural tissue.

Neural activation through a photochemical reaction can also occur through a "caged" molecule that is released upon activation. These are molecules that were rendered inert by chemically modifying the structure of the bioactive molecule, typically the addition of nitrobenzyl groups. Irradiation transforms and/or cleaves the caged molecule to restore the biological activity. These activated molecules can be agonists or antagonists. In this manner, the photolysis of caged molecules is a method for utilization of light to switch biological processes on or off. Glutamate is commonly used as the caged bioactive molecule because of its ability to stimulate virtually every mammalian CNS neuron. Many investigators have taken advantage of photolabile neurotransmitter precursors in their research, especially for the study of cortical circuitry [40, 41]. It should be noted that investigators used lasers delivering low wavelength ($\lambda < 510$ nm) optical radiation to uncaged glutamate [42–44].

It is unlikely that pulsed, mid-infrared lasers, such as the FEL ($\lambda = 2100$–6100 nm), Ho:YAG ($\lambda = 2120$ nm), or Aculight diode lasers ($\lambda \approx 1860$ nm), can evoke neural responses via a photochemical reaction. The photon energies emitted by these lasers are significantly lower than the energies required to move an electron to the excited state, as is needed for a photochemical reaction. For example, the energy in individual photons from the Ho:YAG is ~0.58 eV, corresponding to ~56 kJ/mol bond energy. Typical bond energies are larger, in the range of 100–1000 kJ/mol.

Photomechanical Effects

Photomechanical reactions, such as laser-induced pressure waves from rapid heating and volumetric thermal expansion, were considered as a mechanism for stimulation. This view was investigated by measuring cell surface displacement attributable to heat-induced volumetric expansion using differential phase optical coherence tomography [21]. The surface displacement near stimulation threshold (0.4 J/cm^2) was measured to be 300 nm, and the precise relationship between the amplitude and duration of pressure transients secondary to temperature changes from pulsed laser irradiation was obtained. A piezoelectric probe was created to indent the surface of the cells, with which volumetric stress waves can be elicited without induction of laser temperature effects. A variety of mechanical pulses with amplitudes up to 9 μm, 30 times those measured for the optical nerve stimulation threshold, were delivered.

They found no evidence that pressure transients were able to initiate action potentials, concluding that the effect of volumetric stress is trivial.

With regard to INS of the cochlea, it has been demonstrated that the rapid heating of a small volume in front of the optical fiber results in optophonic events as expansion and stress relaxation occur. In a study by Teudt et al. [45], the Capella diode laser ($\lambda = 1850$ nm) generated an optophonic click up to a maximum of 62 dB SPL close to the 200 μm optical fiber's tip in air. This recorded pressure wave was most likely generated by the absorption of laser radiation in water vapor. Since the cochlea is filled by endo- and perilymph, measurements in a swimming pool were obtained to determine to what extent the laser-induced sound waves exist in water. Maximum radiant exposures of 0.35 J/cm^2, achieved with the laser at 100 μs pulse durations, generated a pressure of 31 mPa in water. This pressure corresponds to 89.8 dB (reference 1 μPa) and 63.8 dB SPL (reference 20 μPa). Note that the stimulation threshold for INS in the cochlea is about 0.01 J/cm^2, which is about 30 times smaller. Nevertheless, it is possible that this acoustic event is contributing to measured compound action potential (CAP) amplitudes during INS of the auditory nerve. Experiments that directly measure the intracochlear pressure during INS are necessary.

Whether optophonic events are of significant impact during infrared laser stimulation of the cochlea is a subject of much debate. It has been argued that the energy required for a primary photomechanical mechanism is much higher than that used for INS [21, 46]. Valid arguments also include that the parameter space of INS is outside of stress confinement. Stress confinement occurs when the optical energy accumulates in the tissue before a laser-induced stress wave can propagate out of the irradiated area. On the other hand, work by [47] convincingly indicates that optophonic stimulation of hair cells is the dominating mechanism for cochlear INS. They successfully elicited auditory CAPs in normal-hearing guinea pigs using an optical parametric oscillator delivering pulses of laser light, $\lambda = 420$–2150 nm [47]. However, CAP responses were drastically diminished in guinea pigs that underwent hair cell abolishment by acute deafening with intracochlear neomycin. Furthermore, a report from [48] also showed when INS was used to stimulate the cochlear nucleus, the evoked auditory brainstem responses were significantly reduced by cutting the auditory nerve, suggesting that it is merely an acoustic events stimulating the cochlea. In addition, results by Baumhoff et al. [49] suggest that INS in the cochlea is dominated by a direct stimulation of remaining hair cells. The discrepancies are not completely resolved at this point [49].

Target Tissues for INS

Auditory Nerve

Inspired by experiments by Wells and coworkers, acute in vivo experiments were conducted in gerbils to demonstrate that optically evoked CAPs could be obtained from the auditory nerve [46]. Stimulation was spatially selective, fast enough to encode acoustic information, and sustainable over extended periods of time.

Normal-hearing and deafened animals were stimulated with different laser models, the Ho:YAG laser ($\lambda = 2120$ nm) and several Aculight diode lasers ($\lambda = 1844$–1873, 1920–1940 nm). The lasers were coupled to optical fibers, 100–200 μm in diameter, and were inserted at the basal turn of the cochlea through the cochleostomy. Optically evoked CAPs were qualitatively similar to acoustically evoked CAPs. Note that responses from INS lack cochlear microphonics, the electrical potentials generated by hair cells in response to an acoustic stimulus (Fig. 2). In spite of drastically reduced acoustically evoked CAP amplitudes following deafening procedures, the optically evoked responses remained largely intact in acutely deafened animals and were reduced in chronically deaf animals. Histology revealed a lack of inner and outer hair cells and greatly reduced spiral ganglion cell density in chronically deafened cochleae [50]. The reduction in spiral ganglion cell density is presumed to be the driving factor behind the diminished optically evoked CAPs.

Selectivity Several approaches have been used to demonstrate that INS is spatially selective. The methods used are (1) immunohistochemical staining for c-FOS protein, (2) spatial tuning curves, which were constructed from neural responses in the ICC obtained with multichannel recordings, and (3) tone-on-light masking tuning curves. *c-fos* is a gene expressed in neuronal cells in response to membrane electrical signals, and its protein provides a cellular method to label activated neurons [51, 52]. To activate c-FOS expression, gerbil cochleae were stimulated optically using a Ho:YAG laser ($\lambda = 2120$ nm) coupled to a 100 μm optic fiber directed at the basal turn of the cochlea, electrically with electrodes inserted into the basal turn of the cochlea, or acoustically with tone pips. Poststimulation cochlear sections were prepared with immunohistochemical stains for c-FOS, and expression was demonstrated in spiral ganglion cells in response to optic, electric, and acoustic stimuli. Laser stimulation resulted in c-FOS expression primarily in tissue directly in the beam path (Fig. 3), whereas electrically stimulated cochleae expressed c-FOS in all turns of the cochlea throughout every tissue section examined (Fig. 4).

A study in guinea pigs demonstrated the spatial selectivity of INS by recording neural activity in the inferior colliculus while

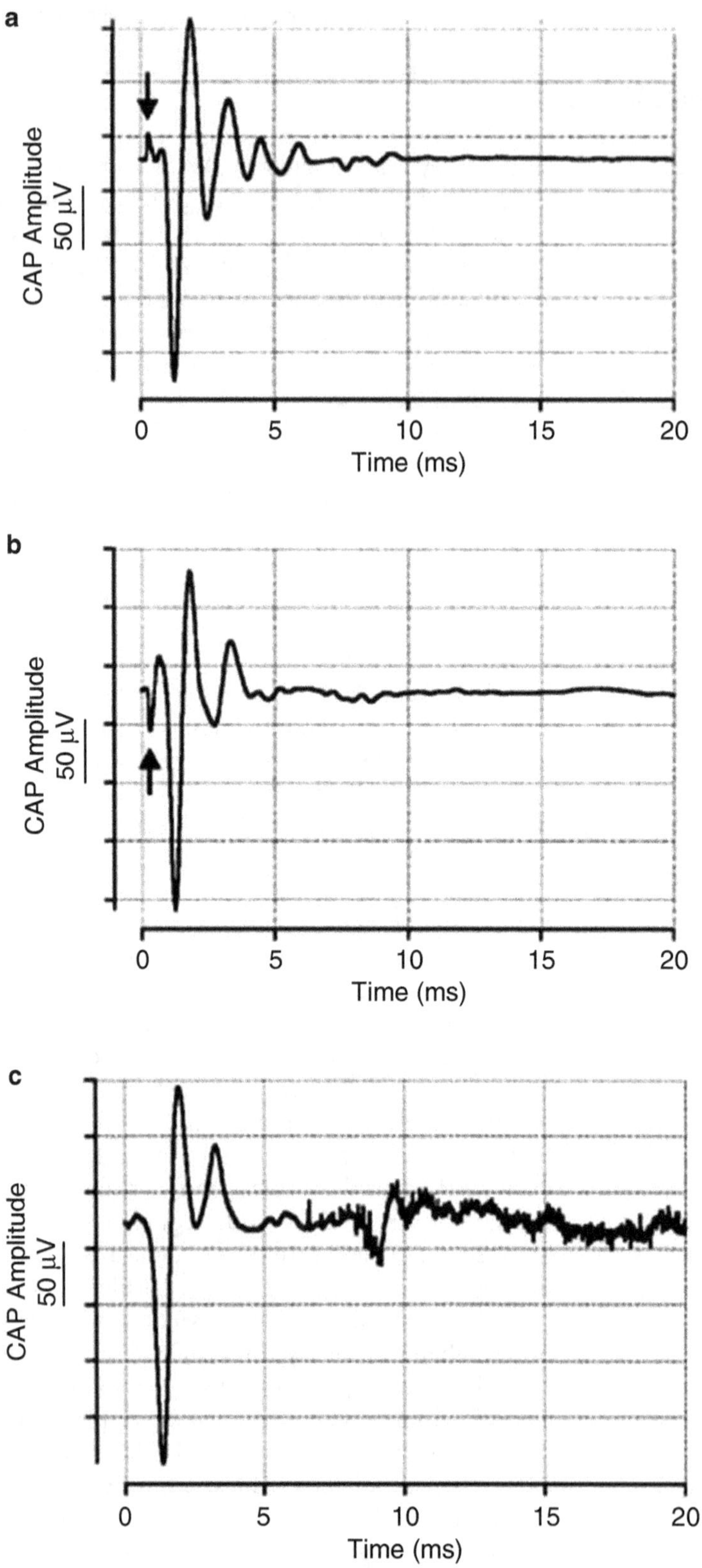

Fig. 2 Acoustically and optically evoked action potentials. (**a**, **b**) CAPs evoked from two acoustic click stimuli (81 dB SPL peak pressure), presented 180° out of phase, are shown. Note the presence of the cochlear microphonic as indicated by the *arrow*. This inverts when clicks are presented in opposite phase.

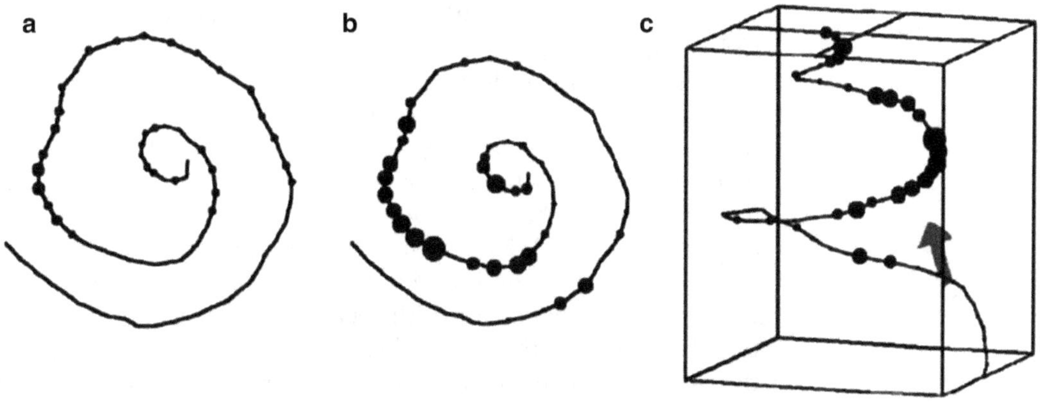

Fig. 3 c-FOS staining of representative optically stimulated cochleae indicates that the only cells stimulated were those directly in the optical path. (**a**, **b**) When the optical fiber is inserted through the round window and directed parallel to the modiolus, the optical path interacts with the upper base and upper middle turn. The amount of staining in the upper base was larger than in the upper middle. There was no staining evident at other turns in the cochlea. (**c**) Note the orientation of the optical fiber as shown by the *gray arrow*. *Filled circles* indicate where c-FOS staining was observed, with the size of the circle indicating the percent of stimulated cells (from Izzo et al. Selectivity of neural stimulation in the auditory system: a comparison of optic and electric stimuli. J Biomed Opt. 2007;12(2):021008. With permission)

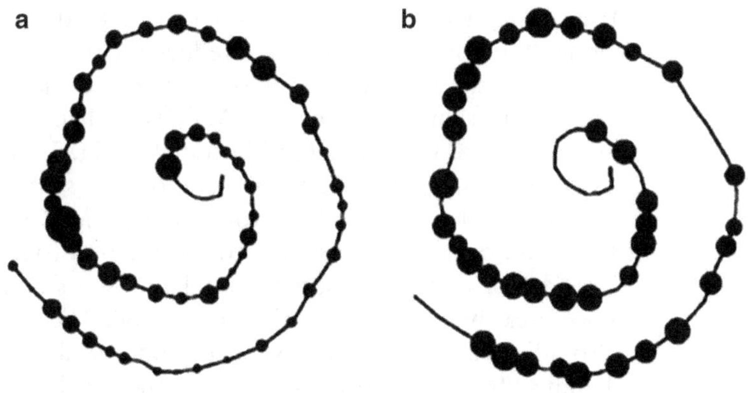

Fig. 4 c-FOS staining of representative electrically stimulated cochleae reveals staining throughout every tissue section across every turn. (**a**) In this electrically stimulated cochlea, a local maximum of stimulation is seen in the upper middle turn, with a significant amount of staining more basally from this maximum as well as in the apex. (**b**) A local maximum of c-FOS staining is seen in the base of the cochlea as well as one full turn higher. There seems to be spread of neural excitation from the middle of the cochlea toward both the apical and basal directions. *Filled circles* indicate where c-FOS staining was observed, with the size of the circle indicating the percent of stimulated cells (from Izzo et al. Selectivity of neural stimulation in the auditory system: a comparison of optic and electric stimuli. J Biomed Opt. 2007;12(2):021008. With permission)

Fig. 2 (continued) (**c**) A representative optical stimulation CAP with 0.06 J/cm^2 obtained from the same animal as (**a**, **b**). There is no cochlear microphonic present in the optical CAP. Noise seen from 6 to 20 ms in the optical CAP trace is electrical noise from the laser power supply (from Izzo et al. Laser stimulation of the auditory nerve. Laser Surg Med. 2006;38(8):745–53. With permission) stimulating the cochlea with pure tone stimuli and with laser pulses [53]. Responses were obtained from hearing and acutely deafened animals with intracochlear neomycin injection. Neural activity was recorded with a 16-channel penetrating electrode array from neurons in the central nucleus of the inferior colliculus (ICC) and was used to generate spatial tuning curves (STCs). The average width for pure tone-evoked STCs was 383 ± 131 μm and for optically evoked STCs was 357 ± 206 μm. The width of the response measured in the ICC for optical stimulation was similar to, and in some cases narrower than, the width measured for pure tone stimulation. Narrower widths indicate better spatial selectivity and suggest the possibility of an increased number of perceptual channels with cochlear implants based on optical stimulation. In our latest unpublished study in guinea pigs, the population of single units recorded in the ICC that responded to INS with a single tungsten electrode were limited to a range of ~600 μm along the isofrequency contours of the ICC. This distance corresponds to a frequency range of 0.6 octaves. The results confirmed spatial selectivity in response to INS.

In another approach, the response to INS in the cochlea was masked acoustically. Masking refers to the ability of a pure tone, presented simultaneously or shortly after a probe stimulus (here, a laser pulse), to reduce the response evoked by the probe stimulus alone. Pure tone masker levels to reduce the response to INS were plotted versus the stimulus frequency of the masker tone. The resultant masking tuning curves (MTC) can then be quantitatively analyzed based on parameters illustrated in Fig. 5, such as the best frequency, $Q_{10\ dB}$ ratio, tip-to-tail ratio, and slope of the high-frequency side. The resulting tone-on-light MTCs were qualitatively and quantitatively similar to the tone-on-tone MTCs [54]. This demonstrates that optical stimulation was stimulating a confined area similar to a fixed frequency tone. The best frequencies also adjusted appropriately when the optical fiber was moved; a 1 mm shift of the optical fiber toward the cochlear base yielded a best frequency shift from 5.3 to 10.8 kHz. This was expected, considering that high-frequency sounds are detected at the cochlear base, while lower frequency sounds are detected at the apex. This demonstrates that optical fiber orientation determines the location of stimulation and thus the frequency.

Laser parameter It is important to optimize the parameter space of INS for stimulation of the auditory nerve to reduce the energy and heat load delivered at the site of stimulation. Results show that the radiant exposure required to stimulate gerbil spiral ganglion cells increases as pulse duration increases [55]. For example, the stimulation threshold required to evoke a 50 μV CAP was 5.29 ± 0.6 mJ/cm^2 at 35 μs pulse duration and 58.38 mJ/cm^2 at 1 ms [55]. Interestingly, when the stimulation level data was calculated in

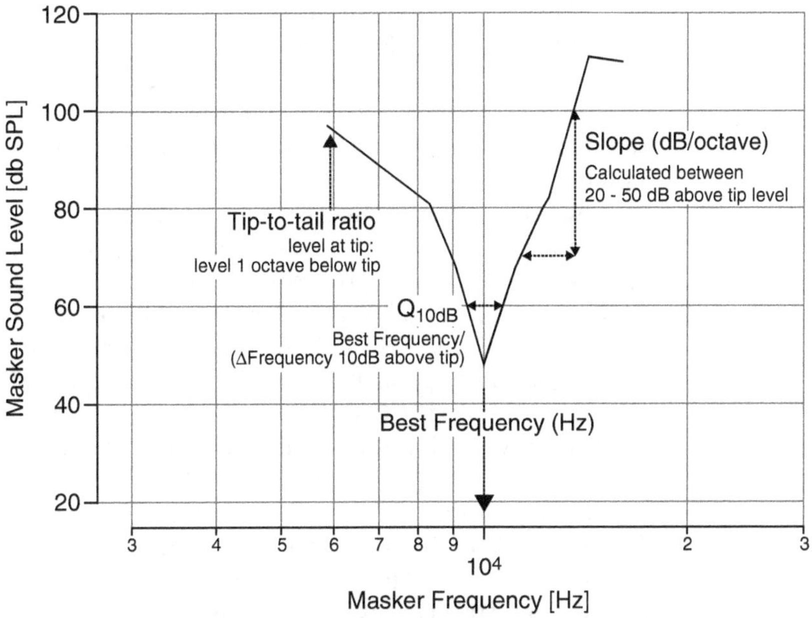

Fig. 5 Representative tone-on-tone masking tuning curve (MTC) with calculations for data analysis. This tone-on-tone MTC shows the best frequency (tip of the tuning curve) and the sharpness of tuning, $Q_{10\ dB}$, which was determined by the ratio of the BF to the MTC width at 10 dB sound level above BF level. The slope was measured as the rise/run between 20 and 50 dB above the BF level. When the high-frequency side of a curve did not extend 50 dB above BF level, we calculated the slope to the highest masker level. The tip-to-tail ratio is measured as the ratio between the masker level at the BF to the masker level one octave below the BF. When the low-frequency tail did not extend one full octave below the best frequency, the masker level at the lowest frequency of the tail was used (from Matic et al. Spatial extent of cochlear infrared neural stimulation determined by tone-on-light masking. J Biomed Opt. 2011;16(11):118002. With permission)

terms of peak optical power, it revealed a constant peak power across all pulse durations, except for at the shortest pulse duration of 35 μs, in which the peak power increased. This suggests that the time over which energy is deposited is more impactful than total energy deposition for auditory nerve INS, an observation fitting with the thermal transient mechanism. A follow-up study, utilizing pulse durations as low as 5 μs, found that the radiant exposure required to evoke a CAP of equal magnitude was the same for the 5, 10, and 30 μs pulses [24], suggesting that at lower pulse durations, total energy is the driving INS.

The effect of varying wavelength is largely a result of the optical penetration depth (OPD). OPD is defined as the distance over which the incident light is reduced in magnitude by $1/e$ and is a function of the absorption coefficient of the tissue. Since the cochlea is filled by endo- and perilymph, optical properties derived from the study of mid-infrared lasers and water can be applied [56]. From $\lambda = 1840$ to 1880 nm, where the OPD is inversely proportional to wavelength, evoked CAPs increased substantially over the initial 300 μm increase in OPD [55]. However, further increases in OPD yielded only slight increases in CAP amplitude. This corresponds well with the approximate length of the optical path through the spiral ganglion cell population in the upper basal turn of the gerbil cochlea (~250 μm). Further increases in OPD likely resulted in irradiation of nonneural tissue, explaining the saturation in response.

More recently, the effect of pulse shape on response to INS has been established. Initial work was done in gerbils using a diode laser ($\lambda = 1860$ nm) delivering square, triangle, ramp-up, and ramp-down pulse shapes of peak powers from 80 to 1500 mW. At the lower peak powers of 80 and 160 mW, square pulses evoked CAPs with significantly greater amplitude than the other shapes [57]. For instance, average CAP amplitude for the square pulse was 47 μV at 80 mW peak power, while the average results for the other shapes fell between 6 and 12 μV at 80 mW peak power. These results suggest that square pulses are the most efficient stimulus. Unpublished results from INS of the cat cochlea with the same various pulse shapes demonstrated that, at shorter pulse durations of less than 100–150 μs, square pulses required less peak power than other shapes to reach threshold CAP amplitudes. No major differences in peak powers were observed for the pulse shapes at larger pulse durations. These results are consistent with total energy deposition being the driving factor for INS at shorter pulse durations, because, due to geometric considerations, square pulses deliver at least double the radiant energy of the triangle, ramp-up, and ramp-down pulses at any given peak power and pulse duration. Interestingly, results from cat cochleae show that CAP amplitudes from triangle pulse shapes saturate at significantly lower CAP amplitudes as radiant energy is increased when compared to the other shapes (Fig. 6). Further investigation is required to explain this finding.

Safety Several studies were conducted using a cochlea model to demonstrate safety of INS. Tissue damage, caused by transient temperature increases and accumulation of thermal energy as a result of laser pulses, is the primary concern. The first safety studies were done by Izzo et al. using the gerbil cochlea [46, 55]. The cochleae were continuously stimulated with a Ho:YAG ($\lambda = 2120$ nm; $\tau_p = 250$ μs; $f = 2$ Hz, $Q = 0.06$ J/cm^2) or a diode laser ($\lambda = 1870$ nm, $\tau_p = 35$ μs; $f = 13$ Hz, $Q = 0.01$ J/cm^2) for 6 h. If neurons were damaged by the optical stimulation, a decrease in the CAP amplitude would be expected. The CAP amplitude remained stable during continual stimulation, indicating no damage was inflicted by IR stimulation.

A follow-up study characterizing damage thresholds was performed in the guinea pig animal model [58]. Optical stimulation was delivered by a diode laser ($\lambda = 1869$ nm) operated at 100 μs pulse duration, 250 Hz repetition rate, and delivering 0–127 μJ/pulse [58]. The cochleae were stimulated continuously for up to 5 h.

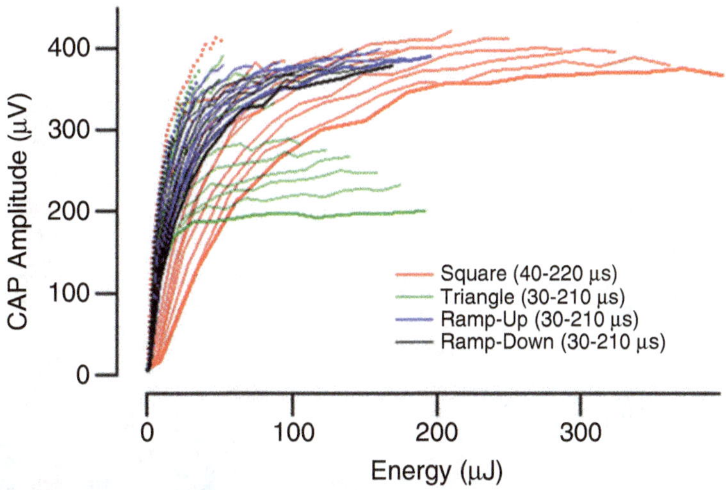

Fig. 6 Representative CAPs from a cat cochlea stimulated with various pulse shapes of varying pulse duration and radiant energy. Triangle pulses saturated at significantly lower CAP amplitude than the other shapes, with triangle pulses of greater pulse duration saturating at a relatively lower amplitude. *Red*, *green*, *blue*, and *black lines* represent data from square, triangle, ramp-up, and ramp-down waveforms, respectively. *Bolded* and *dotted lines* refer to data from the longest and shortest pulse durations of a pulse shape, respectively. In general, *lines* toward the *right* represent greater pulse durations. Range of pulse durations tested indicated in the figure legend

No cochlear damage, defined as decrease in CAP amplitude of greater than 25 % compared to baseline, was observed when the radiant energy was 25 μJ/pulse or lower. The likelihood for damage rose as radiant energy increased past 25 μJ/pulse, with almost 100 % likelihood at 80 μJ/pulse. It should be noted that the 250 Hz repetition rate used in this study is far greater than necessary for stimulation.

Recently, a long-term study of chronic cochlear INS was conducted in normal-hearing cats. The animals were chronically implanted with an optical fiber coupled to a battery-powered laser operated at parameters of 1850 nm wavelength, 100 μs pulse duration, 200 Hz repetition rate, and 12 μJ/pulse radiation energy [59]. Chronic stimulation was delivered for 4–8 h/day for up to 30 days. Optically evoked auditory brainstem responses (ABRs) were successfully attained postoperatively and 2 weeks into chronic stimulation, indicating that the brain received neural input from INS of spiral ganglion neurons. Shortly after activation of stimulation, the animals displayed an increase in head turning and ambulation toward the implanted side, suggesting ipsilateral perception of sound (Fig. 7). Electrophysiological recordings from gerbils, guinea pigs, and cats, as well as the behavior of the cats after activation of a chronically implanted device, provide evidence that stimulation of INS is possible and results in an auditory percept.

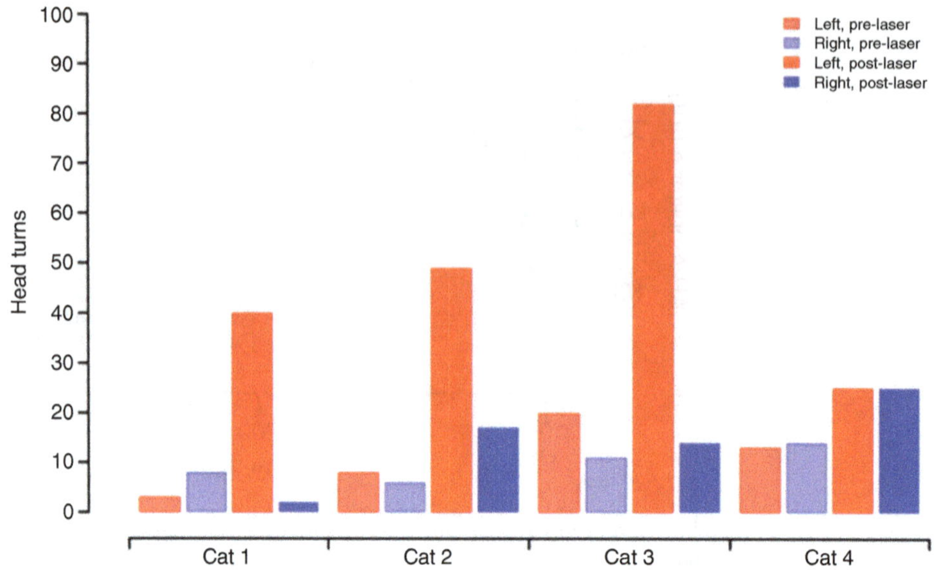

Fig. 7 Behavioral analysis of cats following after laser activation. In three animals, there is a drastic increase in head turns toward the left (implanted) side following the laser activation. The total time of head turns shows some variability between animals for the same ear and same time period. In one animal, cat 4, there was no evidence of a behavioral response, as measured by head turns. The counts for head turns are the same for the right and left side post laser activation. *Red bars* indicate head turns toward the left (implanted) side and *blue bars* indicate head turns toward the right. *Shaded bars* represent the 2 min prior to laser activation, and *solid bars* represent the 2 min after laser activation (from Matic et al. Behavioral and electrophysiological responses evoked by chronic infrared neural stimulation of the cochlea. PLoS One. 2013;8(3):e58189. With permission)

Vestibular Nerve

At present, it is not possible to directly stimulate the vestibular nerve. Responses from the vestibular nerve resulted from INS of vestibular hair cells. INS of the vestibular system has been investigated as a means to overcome the spread of electric current. Electrical stimuli and optical radiation at 1840 nm wavelength ($\tau_p = 10$ μs–1 ms) were delivered to the guinea pig VIIIth nerve, directed at the superior branch of the vestibular nerve, or the ampullae of the superior and lateral semicircular canals [60]. Both stimuli were effective at evoking CAPs from the VIIIth nerve. Optical power levels as low as 200 mW produced evoked potentials. The response amplitudes increased with increasing peak power but remained relatively constant as pulse duration was decreased from 1 ms to 200 μs. In contrast to electrical stimulation, optical stimulation of the ampullae did not evoke detectable eye movements. In a different set of experiments, Bradley stimulated Scarpa's ganglion in gerbils with diode lasers ($\lambda = 1844$–1877 nm; $\tau_p = 5$ μs–1 ms; $f = 2$–1000 Hz, $Q = 0$–127 μJ/pulse) while recording neural activity from single vestibular nerve fibers. INS did not result in detectable changes of single fiber activities.

The effects of INS have also been studied in single vestibular nerves [23, 61, 62]. In the toadfish, *Opsanus tau*, single-unit semicircular canal afferent responses were recorded from the lateral canal branch of the VIIIth nerve during irradiation of the lateral canal sensory epithelium with IR light ($\lambda = 1862$ nm). The recorded afferents exhibited excitatory, inhibitory, or mixed responses. Excitatory neurons increased their firing rate, and inhibitory neurons decreased their firing rate. The mixed response ($n = 7$) comprised of an onset inhibitory response followed by an excitatory phase with tonic stimulation. The time course for the excitatory phase of the mixed units was similar to that of the excitatory afferents. Sinusoidal mechanical indentation of the lateral semicircular canal limb (to simulate head turning) with a glass rod attached to a piezoelectric actuator and servo controller was delivered alone and then concurrently with IR light to determine how INS affects physiological stimuli. Sinusoidal mechanical stimulation by itself yielded a sinusoidal firing pattern. Once IR light was added, a phase advance was observed for both excitatory and inhibitory neurons. However, inhibitory afferents generally displayed greater phase advance. The excitatory versus inhibitory afferent responses may correlate with the dynamic adaptive properties of afferent responses observed during mechanical stimulation [63]. Highly phase-advanced afferent responses are absent in mammalian semicircular canals, but present in toadfish due to convergent inhibitory (GABA) and excitatory (glutamate) synaptic input from hair cells that ultimately shape the afferent discharge response [64, 65]. Data from those studies indicated that afferents receiving only glutamatergic inputs may increase their discharge rate with INS. This is consistent with depolarization of hair cells and increased tonic release of glutamate. On the other hand, afferents that synapse on combinations of glutamatergic and GABAergic hair cells were observed to reduce their discharge rate with INS.

The results obtained in the toadfish have been confirmed in the chinchilla [66]. Since these single-unit responses included a mix of large excitatory, inhibitory, and mixed responses from canal afferents, it is unclear whether infrared stimulation can evoke significant vestibulo-ocular reflex (VOR) eye movement responses. Experiments were conducted to test whether a robust VOR can be evoked with INS. Initial results of INS ($\lambda = 1870$ nm; $\tau_p = 200$–350 μs, $f = 200$–400 Hz) in the chinchilla demonstrated eye movements during IR stimulation in about 50 % of the animals [66].

Despite the fact that studies show responses to INS in vestibular nerve fibers, no study has yet demonstrated direct stimulation of the nerve, selectivity of the stimulation, or robust VORs.

Facial Nerve

Damage to the facial nerve is a serious complication of head and neck surgery. Surgeons in the United States commonly employ facial nerve monitoring in an effort to prevent inadvertent damage. Contemporary cranial nerve monitors inject current into tissue to stimulate the nerve. The resulting current spread and unselective stimulation of the nerve can lead to "false responses." For instance, a severed facial nerve may still be stimulated distally from the site of transection by current spread through surrounding tissue [67]. Furthermore, the physical contact required of a stimulation probe may also damage nerve function. Optical stimulation may offer a spatially precise, non-contact method of stimulation. A study by Teudt et al. demonstrated INS of the facial nerve. A Ho:YAG ($\lambda = 2120$ nm) laser was coupled to a 600 μm fiber, which delivered radiation to the dissected facial nerve trunk and branches of gerbils [20]. Stimulation with an electrode was done for comparison. Compound muscle action potentials (CmAPs) were successfully recorded at three facial muscles (m. orbicularis oculi, m. levator nasolabialis, and m. orbicularis oris) following radiant exposures of 0.71–1.77 J/cm^2 at the nerve trunk or branches, demonstrating successful INS. Spatial selectivity was demonstrated by stimulation of individual nerve bundles within the main trunk when the radial location of the stimulation site was varied (Fig. 8). This could not be reproduced with electrical stimulation of the nerve. INS of the facial nerve could be performed safely with a safety ratio of approximately 2.6 for stimulation with the Ho:YAG laser. Threshold radiant exposures for INS were approximately 0.71 and 0.88 J/cm^2 for the facial nerve trunk and branches, respectively. Histologic evidence of optic nerve damage, such as carbonization and disruption within nerve tissue, occurred above radiant exposures of 2.0 J/cm^2.

Cavernous Nerves

The close proximity of the cavernous nerves to the prostate puts them at significant risk of injury during dissection and resection of the prostate gland. Damage to the cavernous nerves can impair a man's ability to achieve spontaneous erections. Unfortunately, the microscopic nature of these nerves makes them difficult to locate and identify [68]. Conventional electrical stimulation underlies intraoperative nerve-mapping devices used to assist in the preservation of the cavernous nerve during prostatectomy. Results from these mapping devices have been shown to correlate poorly with precise anatomical location and poorly predict postsurgical outcomes [69, 70]. Optical nerve stimulation may present a potential intraoperative technique to aid nerve sparing in prostate surgery.

Successful optical stimulation of the cavernous nerve with a continuous-wave (cw) thulium fiber laser ($\lambda = 1870$ nm) was confirmed by intracavernosal pressure (ICP) measurements [68, 71]. ICP responses similar in shape and duration to conventional electrical stimulation were obtained at radiation wavelengths of 1860–1870 nm, 10 and 100 Hz pulse repetition rates, and pulse energies greater than 2.7 mJ/pulse [72]. Thermal imaging showed that ICP response time was closely correlated to the amount of time necessary to heat neural tissue to a threshold temperature of approximately 43 °C, with cw irradiation producing the most rapid temperature gains.

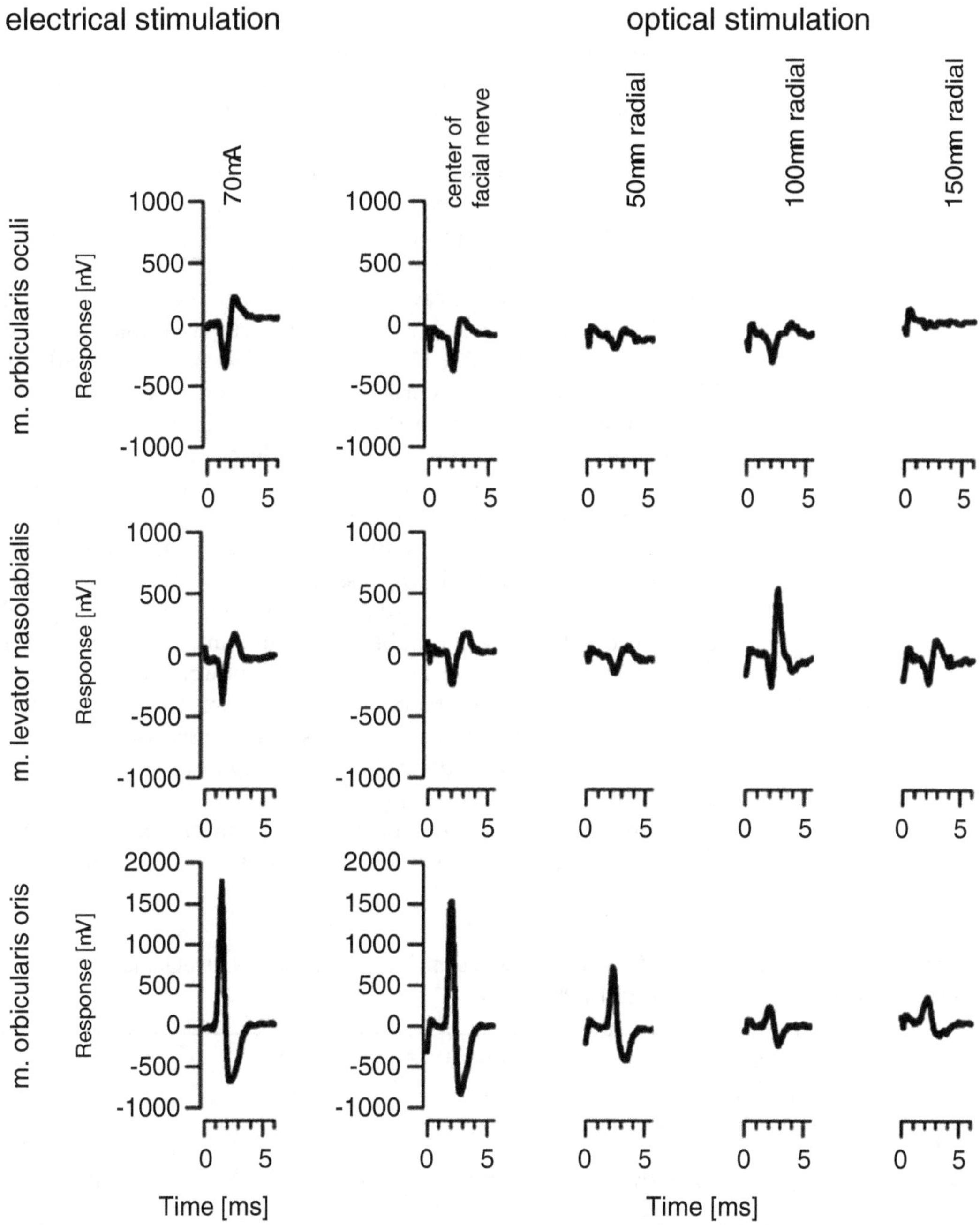

Fig. 8 Compound muscle action potentials (CmAPs) measured in three facial muscles. CmAP response evoked by an electrical stimulus (70 μA) on facial nerve trunk (*left column*). CmAP responses after optical radiation (0.88 J/cm^2) at the same stimulation site as for electrical stimulation (*four right columns*). Both CmAPs are an average of ten recordings. After the first recording (nerve center), the optical fiber was moved by 50 μm steps radially away from the nerve center, and additional measurements were performed. Note the isolated maximal response of the m. levator nasolabialis after moving the fiber 50 μm from the initial nerve center (from Teudt et al. Optical stimulation of the facial nerve: a new monitoring technique? Laryngoscope. 2007;117(9):1641–7. With permission)

The importance of the wavelength and the optical penetration depth of the ability for stimulation has been shown. Human cavernous nerves lie beneath the fascia, whereas rat cavernous nerves lie on the prostate surface. An optical radiation-based cavernous nerve stimulator must be able to deliver sufficient energy through a thin fascial layer. A diode laser, which was operated in cw mode, was used to stimulate the rat cavernous nerve with radiation at a wavelength of 1490 nm and power from 20 to 80 mW [73]. Testicular fascia layers of variable thickness (150–600 μm) were transplanted over the rat cavernous nerve. The required power for stimulation threshold increased as the fascia layer thickness was increased, from 40 mW at 150–160 μm to 53 mW at 360–380 μm. No ICP response was recorded at a thickness of 500–600 μm. This is not surprising given the thickness of the cavernous nerve (~200 μm) and the optical penetration depth (520 μm) in water for laser radiation at a wavelength of 1490 nm [74]. The results were compared to data from a previous study utilizing wavelengths of 1455 and 1550 nm, corresponding to optical penetration depths in water of 344 and 935 μm, respectively (Table 1) [75]. It has been observed that wavelengths corresponding to longer optical penetration depths are capable of stimulating through thicker fascial layers, but require greater input of power for stimulation. This suggests that penetration depths that are too deep are less efficient because energy deposition is not focused on the neural tissue, illustrating the importance of selecting an appropriate wavelength for optical stimulation.

Concerns regarding potential thermal damage led to a recent follow-up study, in which the efficacy of a prototype

Table 1
Comparison of surface and subsurface optical nerve stimulation threshold parameters for rat cavernous nerves as a function of laser wavelength

Laser wavelength (nm)	1455	1490	1550
Absorption coefficient in water (cm^{-1})	29.1	19.3	10.7
OPD in water (μm)	344	518	935
Power-to-surface stimulation (mW)	28.3 ± 5.2	38.8 ± 5.2	55.0 ± 4.1
Threshold IPC response time (s)	12.7 ± 1.0	12.6 ± 1.4	13.6 ± 1.6
Fascia thickness (μm)	100–110	360–380	420–450
Power-to-subsurface stimulation (mW)	45	53	80
Threshold IPC response time (s)	13.7 ± 0.7	10.4 ± 1.8	13.1 ± 0.5
Sample size (*N*)	9	8	8

ICP intracavernous pressure, *OPD* optical penetration depth

From Tozburun et al. Continuous-wave infrared subsurface optical stimulation of the rat prostate cavernous nerves using a 1490-nm diode laser. Urology. 2013;82(4):969–73. With permission temperature-controlled optical nerve stimulation (TC-ONS) system was tested. The TC-ONS system was composed of three main components: a single-mode fiber laser ($\lambda = 1455$ nm, continuous-wave irradiation) with a mechanical shutter, a laparoscopic laser probe, and a radiometer with a temperature feedback control system [76]. During stimulation, the mechanical shutter would rapidly open and close, maintaining the temperature within ±1 °C from a predetermined set point, in response to temperature feedback from the IR sensor. The TC-ONS system successfully maintained temperatures within ±1 °C of the set point (42–48 °C), even when laser powers were increased from 79 to 94 mW. The study demonstrated that the prototype TC-ONS was capable of maintaining a constant and precise nerve temperature suitable for safe INS.

Cortex

Successful application of INS in the brain could impact numerous clinical applications, including cortical mapping during craniotomies, tumor resection, and deep brain stimulation. Cayce et al. demonstrated that IR light could successfully stimulate cortical brain structures, however resulting in neuronal inhibition. A diode laser ($\lambda = 1875$ nm) was coupled to a 400 μm optical fiber and delivered radiation to the forepaw and barrel fields of the rat somatosensory cortex [77]. Intrinsic signal optical imaging was performed using a CCD camera to detect effects on neural activity. Recordings were done with tungsten microelectrodes. The optical intrinsic signals induced by INS were found to correspond to focal regions of activation, approximately 1.5–2 mm in diameter, demonstrating high spatial selectivity. The magnitude of evoked optical intrinsic signals was positively correlated with repetition rate and radiation energy. The optical responses induced in the somatosensory cortex were similar to those obtained with natural tactile stimulation, indicating successful neuronal stimulation. Electrophysiological measurements of neurons revealed that INS led to a reduction in firing rate, lasting for approximately 1.5–2.0 s that was followed by a return to baseline levels. This is the first example of INS causing inhibition, whereas INS resulted in neuronal excitation in studies involving peripheral and cranial nerves. This unusual effect could have been caused by excitation of inhibitory neurons in the superficial layers of the cortex. Normal neuronal tactile responses remained intact even after repeated presentation of INS for greater than 2 h, indicating that INS does not damage the cortex, which would impair neuronal activity. This study demonstrates that INS can be safely used to modulate neuronal activation in vivo.

A similar study demonstrated efficacy of INS in the primary visual cortex. A diode laser ($\lambda = 1875$ nm) was coupled to a 100, 200, or 400 μm fiber and delivered optical radiation to the primary visual cortex of macaque monkeys [78]. Just as in the above study, increasing radiant exposures resulted in greater magnitudes of the optical intrinsic signals. Unlike results from the rat somatosensory cortex, electrophysiological measurements revealed that INS evoked excitatory activity. Confinement of optical radiation to a single ocular dominance column (400 μm in width) using the 100 μm fiber resulted in stimulation effects contained within one ocular dominance cycle and no significant responses at distant locations, demonstrating the spatial selectivity of INS. Application of INS to the left eye ocular dominance column enhanced visually evoked responses to the left eye column and diminished responses to the right eye column. This indicates that INS of the visual cortex can modulate visual responses in an eye-specific manner. IR stimulation with the 100 and 200 μm fiber combined with visual stimulation resulted in an enhanced effect compared to visual stimuli alone; however, utilization of the 400 μm fiber led to a relatively suppressed response. This suggests that the 400 μm fiber's spot size is too large to target specific ocular dominance columns and resulted in activation of inhibitory surrounds. This study showed that INS can be used to either enhance or diminish visual cortical response, and this can be done in a targeted, domain-specific manner.

Infrared Stimulation of In Vitro and Nonneural Preparations

Lobsters

A diode laser ($\lambda = 1865$ nm) was coupled to a 600 μm fiber to deliver optical radiation to extracted nerves from the walking legs of lobsters, *Homarus americanus* [79]. Successful stimulation, per electrical and birefringent responses, of the nerve was achieved using optical stimulation at maximum power setting of the laser with 2 ms pulse width. The electrical and birefringent responses to optical stimulation were one order of magnitude smaller than responses to electrical stimulation, indicating that optical energy recruited far fewer axons than electrical stimulation. However, only 2–4 trials of optical stimulation were possible before thermal damage occurred. Shorter pulse widths delivering less radiant energy did not generate a detectable birefringence signal. Perhaps unmyelinated nerves, such as those found in the lobster leg, are more susceptible to thermal damage secondary to increased water content and higher wavelength absorption. Of note, energy output and spot size were not reported in this study.

Cardiomyocytes and Hearts

It has been demonstrated that pulsed laser light can stimulate cardiomyocytes, resulting in cell depolarization and visible contraction [80, 81]. A recent study showed that INS can be used to pace embryonic quail hearts in vivo [82]. A pulsed infrared diode laser ($\lambda = 1875$ nm) was coupled to a 400 μm diameter fiber that was positioned in close proximity to the quail embryo, illuminating an approximately 0.3 mm^2 area on the inflow region of the heart tube [82]. Optical stimuli of 1 ms pulse duration and 0.92 J/cm^2

radiant energy successfully locked the heart rate to the repetition rate of the laser (2–3 Hz). Standard transmission electron microscopy (TEM) was used to assess ultrastructural detail of cardiomyocytes at the inflow region of the heart tube where the laser was aimed. Comparisons were made between a control embryo that did not receive optical radiation, an embryo paced slightly above stimulation threshold (0.81 J/cm^2), and an embryo paced well above threshold (4.33 J/cm^2). Evidence of damage, such as vacuolated mitochondria, was only seen in the embryo paced well above threshold. No clear indication of cellular damage was observed in the embryo paced slightly above threshold or the control. This demonstrates that safe optical pacing of embryonic hearts is feasible. Optical pacing has great potential as a tool for study of developmental cardiology, as control of heart rate results in alteration of stresses and mechanically transduced signaling. Optical pacing could also have clinical applications if it is capable of pacing the adult heart.

Outer Hair Cells

While much of cochlear INS has focused on the auditory nerve, a recent study showed that prestin is responsive to fast temperature perturbations induced by IR laser. Prestin is a molecular motor abundantly expressed in cochlear outer hair cells that allows the hair cells to rapidly alter their length and stiffness, in this manner modulating amplifications of vibrations within the cochlea. Recently, patch-clamp recordings were conducted in HEK293 cells while using the Capella diode laser ($\lambda = 1850$ nm) to deliver rapid temperature jumps to cells within the recording chamber [83]. Some cells had prestin expression induced with tetracycline. Stimulation of control cells that did not express prestin revealed a linear temperature and capacitance change consistent with the double-layer electrostatic mechanism described by Shapiro et al. [25]. Stimulation of the prestin-expressing cells yielded a voltage-dependent nonlinear capacitance (NLC) that followed rapid changes in temperature. Stimulation after application of salicylate, an inhibitor of prestin, abolished the NLC but left intact linear capacitance changes. These results demonstrate that prestin's ability to respond to temperature changes is on par with double-layer susceptibility and may be used as a target for modulation of hearing using INS.

Costimulation with Electrical and Optical Stimuli

Thermal damage from heat deposition remains the primary concern for INS. Methods to reduce the necessary optical radiation would improve safety of INS. The threshold radiant exposure for infrared pulsed light can be lowered with concurrent application of a subthreshold electric stimulus. The initial study used a diode laser ($\lambda = 1875$ nm) and a bipolar hook electrode to deliver stimuli to the sciatic nerve of rats [84]. Results showed that delivery of subthreshold electric stimuli decreased the required optical energy in a manner best predicted by a logarithmic relationship (Fig. 9a).

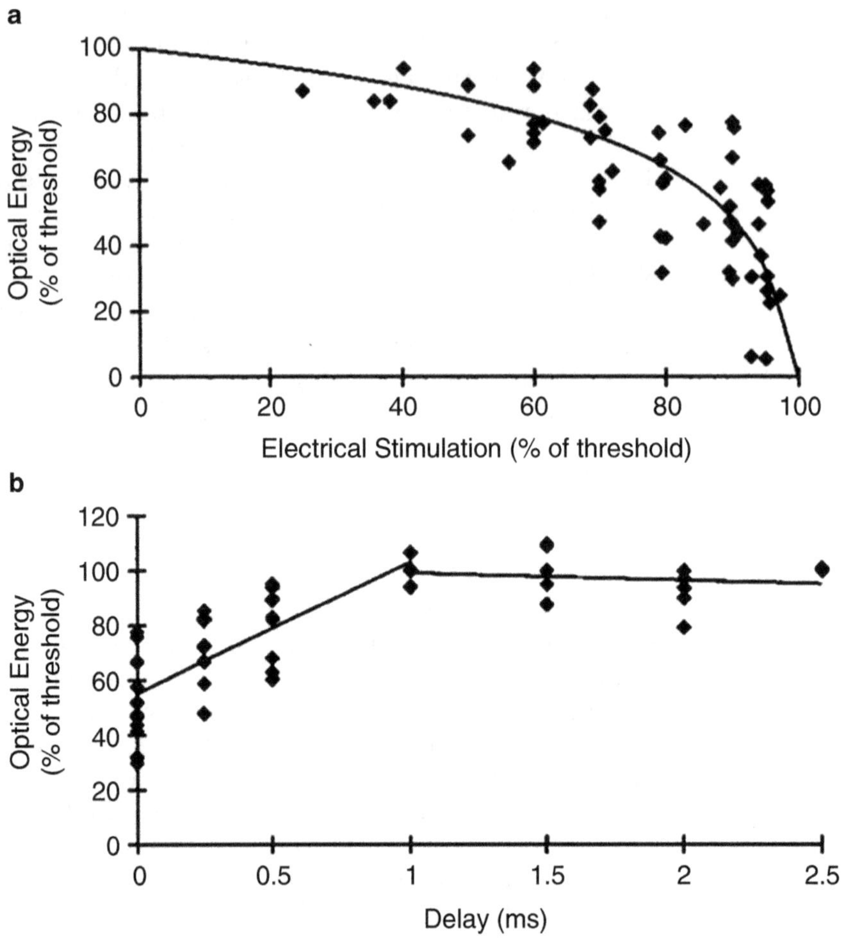

Fig. 9 Results of combining optical and electrical stimulation. (**a**) Optical energy (% of stimulation threshold) required to reach stimulation threshold as a function of subthreshold electrical stimulus. (**b**) Optical energy (% of stimulation threshold) required to reach stimulation threshold as a function of delay between electrical (90 % of stimulation threshold) and optical stimuli (from Duke et al. Combined optical and electrical stimulation of neural tissue in vivo. J Biomed Opt. 2009;14(6):060501. With permission)

This suggests that electrical stimulation and INS do not occur by the same mechanism. Otherwise a linear superposition would be expected, such as seen when two simultaneous electrical pulses are delivered [85]. According to the best fit logarithmic model based off the data ($R^2 = 0.56$), electric stimuli applied at 80 % or 90 % of threshold reduced the optical threshold by 1.54-fold and 2.03-fold, respectively. Such a reduction in optical threshold significantly increases the margin of safety for INS. With regard to the timing of stimuli, the greatest reduction in optical threshold was found during simultaneous administration of optical and electric stimuli (Fig. 9b). No benefit is observed when the optical stimuli were delayed for >1 ms, demonstrating the importance of timely stimuli delivery. Despite utilization of electric current, costimulation was shown to be spatially selective. Individual fascicles were successfully stimulated per recordings of CmAPs in isolated muscle groups.

A recent follow-up study by Duke et al. identified spatial and temporal factors contributing to variability in hybrid-electrical stimulation. Both the Ho:YAG ($\lambda = 2120$ nm) and a diode laser ($\lambda = 1875$ nm) were used as optical sources to stimulate rat sciatic and *Aplysia californica* buccal nerves [86]. A bipolar electrical stimulus was produced using glass pipettes. While translating the optical fiber back and forth across the nerve, a finite region of excitation (ROE) between the cathode and anode where costimulation was possible was found. This ROE tended to increase in size with increasing radiant exposure and was located adjacent to the cathode of the bipolar electrode (Fig. 10). Reversing the polarity of the bipolar electrode would result in the ROE shifting adjacent to the new cathode location. Thus, the relative location of the two stimuli affects the efficacy of stimulation. Repeated stimulation over 60 min revealed that thresholds for electrical and hybrid stimulation fluctuated with time and exhibited a negative correlation. For example, as the nerve became more sensitive to electrical stimulation, its response to optical stimuli decreased. This further indicates that electrical and optical neural stimulation have different underlying mechanisms, because the respective thresholds would be expected to correlate positively if the mechanism were similar.

The recent experiments by Duke et al. also revealed that increases in radiant energy could result in the inhibition of neuronal firing. At higher radiant exposures, the probability of action

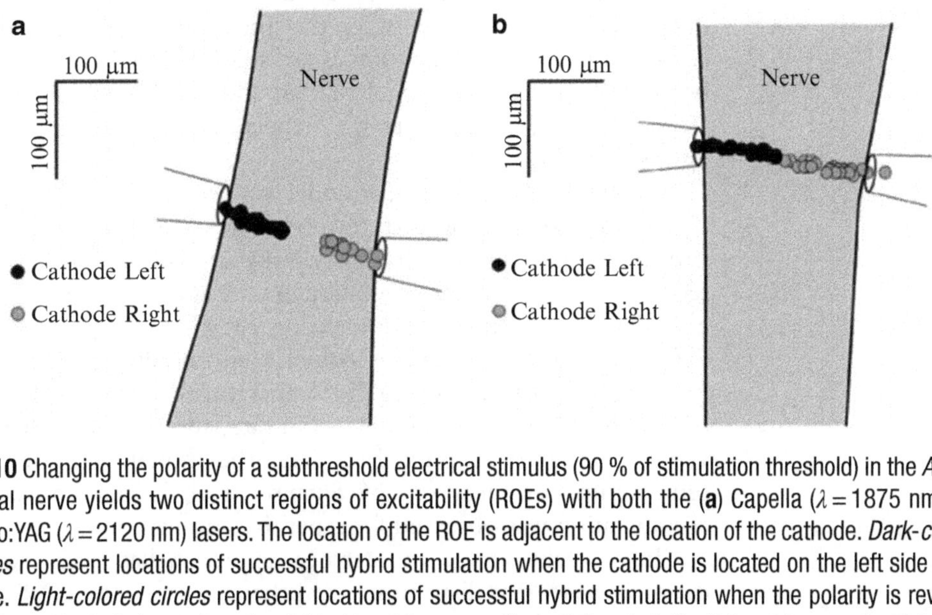

Fig. 10 Changing the polarity of a subthreshold electrical stimulus (90 % of stimulation threshold) in the *Aplysia* buccal nerve yields two distinct regions of excitability (ROEs) with both the (**a**) Capella ($\lambda = 1875$ nm) and (**b**) Ho:YAG ($\lambda = 2120$ nm) lasers. The location of the ROE is adjacent to the location of the cathode. *Dark-colored circles* represent locations of successful hybrid stimulation when the cathode is located on the left side of the nerve. *Light-colored circles* represent locations of successful hybrid stimulation when the polarity is reversed and the cathode is located on the right side of the nerve (from Duke et al. Spatial and temporal variability in response to hybrid electro-optical stimulation. J Neural Eng. 2012;9(3):036003. With permission)

potential generation decreased, instead of asymptotically approaching 100 % as expected. This inhibitory effect was only observed in *Aplysia* but not the rat. It is currently unclear why this inhibition occurred.

Modeling of INS

INS has been tested in many neural systems and laser parameters differ largely for stimulation among the different systems. An approach to explain the differences could come from modeling of INS. A Monte Carlo modeling approach was used to simulate light transport and absorption in tissue during INS [87]. The results of the modeling suggest that the optimal optical fiber (numerical aperture = 0.22) for INS has a diameter of 200 μm. The model also predicts a temperature rise at the spiral ganglion of 0.1 °C. This temperature rise is similar to what has been previously estimated from INS in the gerbil cochlea [24]. Thompson et al. also used their model to study the temporal effects of heating during INS [88]. Their model predicts two regimes of action: (1) for pulse durations up to 100 μs, a pulse energy-limited regime, and (2) for pulses longer than 100 μs, a temperature gradient-limited regime. The model was also used to determine the influence of the distance of the stimulation sources and the stimulus repetition rates on the local heating. With the assumption that the stimulus is delivered at 250 Hz, INS in the cochlea will lead to a local temperature increase of about 2.3 °C. The calculation was done for one stimulation site. When multiple stimulation sites are used, the temperature increase depends on the spacing between the stimulation sources. With the assumption that the light sources are separated by 750 μm, it has been predicted by the model that an additional 20 % increase in temperature will occur over the temperature increase of a single light source [89].

In a different approach, a model was created using multiphysics software from COMSOL to model the change in temperature and the temperature distribution during irradiation with an infrared laser at $\lambda = 1550$ nm radiation wavelength [90]. The model considers conduction and convection for heat transport. Results show that the distribution is complex and nonlinear. The maximum rise in temperature and the temperature distribution depends on the fiber size, the pulse repetition rate, and the radiant energy. When compared to published data, the model predicted low temperatures as measured by Shapiro et al. [25]. Temperature accumulation was observed for repetitive stimulation.

In a recent paper, an analytical approach has been used to determine the heat distribution and thermal criteria for INS [89]. A solution for the heat diffusion equation was combined with optical fluences. The developed framework could then be applied to existing experimental data to determine the necessary thermal parameters to evoke stimulation. A key conclusion that has been drawn from the model is that the rate in temperature change, and not the absolute temperature, is essential for INS [91].

Considerations for INS-Based Neural Prosthesis

INS can confine the stimulated volume of tissue and may be another means of increasing spatial selectivity of neural stimulation. Another advantage of INS is the lack of an electrochemical junction. The fluid interface between the active electrode and the tissue, which is not needed for INS, is a common location for device failure [92]. However, before implementing a prosthesis using INS, several design considerations must be made. While an optical fiber-based prosthesis may be suitable for a low-density prosthesis application (stimulation of 1–5 distinct sites), prostheses that encode more dense information, such as cochlear implants and visual prostheses, would be difficult to implement with 50–100 or more individually addressed optical fibers. Possible design solutions for these applications include a scanning optical source that sequentially addresses multiple stimulating sites or a high-density array of small solid-state optical sources that can simultaneously stimulate multiple neural populations. In addition to the type of source used, the placement of the optical source has implications for the prosthesis design. An external source would allow for higher power, larger battery capacity, and easier modifications to the stimulating source. However, by transmitting the optical energy transcutaneously, a significant portion of the optical power would be lost. Percutaneous links, while possible, are much less desirable due to the risk of infection. A fully implantable INS prosthesis is desirable, because it eliminates the transcutaneous link, except for battery charging. Hardware upgrades are difficult with a fully implantable device. Furthermore, implanted optical sources need to be more efficient than externally mounted sources to reduce the heat generated by powering the device. It remains to be seen if a solid-state device can be constructed with the size and power requirements to be fully implantable and stimulate neurons.

Conclusions and Future Directions

The experiments to characterize INS have demonstrated that optical radiation can be used to stimulate neurons. For the facial nerve, the sciatic nerve, and the nervus pudendus, direct stimulation upon irradiation with infrared light is obvious. For the cochlea, it has to be characterized whether the stimulation comes from a mechanical event to the hair cells or a direct interaction with auditory nerve and the radiation. For the vestibular system, it appears a direct interaction between the radiation and the hair cells is responsible. For the cortex, it remains unclear whether the radiation results in a modulation or whether action potentials can be evoked. With the recent development of a compact pulsed IR laser to evoke neural responses, it has been validated that stimulation with optical radiation is spatially selective. Stimulation with optical radiation has advantages over stimulation with electric current. The differences between stimulation modalities could be selectively exploited for the next generation of neural interfaces and as a neurophysiology research tool. INS, as a tool, could advance our understanding of many research-based neuroscience questions and lead to significant findings that would otherwise not be possible with conventional stimulation paradigms. In addition, the possibility of using INS for a neural prosthesis has its appeal. Many steps are required between technological conception and maturity of an INS-based prosthesis. The steps include biological safety and compatibility, as well as the engineering of a practicable device. With the objective to design and build INS prostheses, it is also extremely important to understand the underlying mechanism of stimulation. It will allow optimization of the laser parameter space and will aid the long-term safety of INS. Further work to understand the effect of beam quality (e.g., focused beam vs. collimated beam) on stimulation will aid in the design of efficient research and clinical stimulators.

Most of the work, to date, has been executed in vivo, and as such it would be useful to determine any differences with INS in vitro. Many neural systems and neuron types have yet to be stimulated with IR radiation, and it is unknown if INS will work on all neurons or only a subset. While there are many questions yet to be answered, INS provides a unique application of biomedical optics that may foster significant advances in neuroscience.

Acknowledgments

This project has been funded with federal funds from the National Institute on Deafness and Other Communication Disorders, R01 DC011855.

References

1. Grill WM, Norman SE, Bellamkonda RV. Implanted neural interfaces: biochallenges and engineered solutions. Annu Rev Biomed Eng. 2009;11:1–24.
2. Bierer JA, Middlebrooks JC. Auditory cortical images of cochlear-implant stimuli: dependence on electrode configuration. J Neurophysiol. 2002;87:478–92.
3. Snyder RL, Bierer JA, Middlebrooks JC. Topographic spread of inferior colliculus activation in response to acoustic and intracochlear electric stimulation. JARO. 2004;5:305–22.
4. Mens LH, Berenstein CK. Speech perception with mono- and quadrupolar electrode configurations: a crossover study. Otol Neurotol. 2005;26(5):957–64.

5. Srinivasan AG, Landsberger DM, Shannon RV. Current focusing sharpens local peaks of excitation in cochlear implant stimulation. Hear Res. 2010;270(1–2):89–100.
6. Koch DB, Downing M, Osberger MJ, Litvak L. Using current steering to increase spectral resolution in CII and HiRes 90K users. Ear Hear. 2007;28(2 Suppl):38S–41.
7. Berenstein CK, Mens LH, Mulder JJ, Vanpoucke FJ. Current steering and current focusing in cochlear implants: comparison of monopolar, tripolar, and virtual channel electrode configurations. Ear Hear. 2008;29(2): 250–60.
8. Choi CT, Hsu CH. Conditions for generating virtual channels in cochlear prosthesis systems. Ann Biomed Eng. 2009;37(3):614–24.
9. Landsberger DM, Srinivasan AG. Virtual channel discrimination is improved by current focusing in cochlear implant recipients. Hear Res. 2009;254(1–2):34–41.
10. McDermott HJ, McKay CM. Pitch ranking with nonsimultaneous dual-electrode electrical stimulation of the cochlea. J Acoust Soc Am. 1994;96(1):155–62.
11. Donaldson GS, Dawson PK, Borden LZ. Within-subjects comparison of the HiRes and Fidelity120 speech processing strategies: speech perception and its relation to place-pitch sensitivity. Ear Hear. 2011;32(2): 238–50.
12. Veraart C, Grill WM, Mortimer JT. Selective control of muscle activation with a multipolar nerve cuff electrode. IEEE Trans Biomed Eng. 1993;40:640–53.
13. Polasek KH, Hoyen HA, Keith MW, Kirsch RF, Tyler DJ. Stimulation stability and selectivity of chronically implanted multicontact nerve cuff electrodes in the human upper extremity. IEEE Trans Neural Syst Rehabil Eng. 2009;17(5):428–37.
14. Veraart C, Raftopoulos C, Mortimer JT, et al. Visual sensations produced by optic nerve stimulation using an implanted self-sizing spiral cuff electrode. Brain Res. 1998;813:181–6.
15. Larsen JO, Thomsen M, Haugland M, Sinkjaer T. Degeneration and regeneration in rabbit peripheral nerve with long-term nerve cuff electrode implant: a stereological study of myelinated and unmyelinated axons. Acta Neuropathol. 1998;96:365–78.
16. Grill WM, Mortimer JT. Neural and connective tissue response to long-term implantation of multiple contact nerve cuff electrodes. J Biomed Mater Res. 2000;50:215–26.
17. Bowman BR, Erickson RC. Acute and chronic implantation of coiled wire intraneural electrodes during cyclical electrical stimulation. Ann Biomed Eng. 1985;13:75–93.
18. Lefurge T, Goodall E, Horch K, Stensaas L, Schoenberg A. Chronically implanted intrafascicular recording electrodes. Ann Biomed Eng. 1991;19:197–207.
19. Wells J, Kao C, Jansen ED, Konrad P, Mahadevan-Jansen A. Application of infrared light for in vivo neural stimulation. J Biomed Opt. 2005;10(6):064003.
20. Teudt IU, Nevel AE, Izzo AD, Walsh Jr JT, Richter CP. Optical stimulation of the facial nerve: a new monitoring technique? Laryngoscope. 2007;117(9):1641–7.
21. Wells J, Kao C, Konrad P, et al. Biophysical mechanisms of transient optical stimulation of peripheral nerve. Biophys J. 2007;93(7): 2567–80.
22. Geddes LA, Roeder R. Criteria for the selection of materials for implanted electrodes. Ann Biomed Eng. 2003;31(7):879–90.
23. Rajguru SM, Richter CP, Matic AI, et al. Infrared photostimulation of the crista ampullaris. J Physiol. 2011;589(Pt 6):1283–94.
24. Izzo AD, Walsh Jr JT, Ralph H, et al. Laser stimulation of auditory neurons: effect of shorter pulse duration and penetration depth. Biophys J. 2008;94(8):3159–66.
25. Shapiro MG, Homma K, Villarreal S, Richter CP, Bezanilla F. Infrared light excites cells by changing their electrical capacitance. Nat Commun. 2012;3:736.
26. Liu Q, Jorgensen E, Holman H, Frerck M, Rabbitt RD. Miniature post synaptic currents are entrained by infrared pulses. Abstr Assoc Res Otolaryngol. 2013;36:464.
27. Peterson EJ, Tyler DJ. Activation using infrared light in a mammalian axon model. Conf Proc IEEE Eng Med Biol Soc. 2012; 2012:1896–9.
28. Harteneck C, Plant TD, Schultz G. From worm to man: three subfamilies of TRP channels. Trends Neurosci. 2000;23(4):159–66.
29. Caterina MJ, Schumacher MA, Tominaga M, Rosen TA, Levine JD, Julius D. The capsaicin receptor: a heat-activated ion channel in the pain pathway. Nature. 1997;389(6653):816–24.
30. Balaban CD, Zhou J, Li HS. Type 1 vanilloid receptor expression by mammalian inner ear ganglion cells. Hear Res. 2003;175(1–2): 165–70.
31. Zheng J, Dai C, Steyger PS, et al. Vanilloid receptors in hearing: altered cochlear sensitivity by vanilloids and expression of TRPV1 in the organ of corti. J Neurophysiol. 2003;90(1): 444–55.

32. Suh E, Matic AI, Otting M, Walsh JT, Richter CP. Optical stimulation in mice lacking the TRPV1 channel. Proc Soc Photo Opt Instrum Eng. 2009;7180:1–5.
33. Albert ES, Bec JM, Desmadryl G, et al. TRPV4 channels mediate the infrared laser-evoked response in sensory neurons. J Neurophysiol. 2012;107(12):3227–34.
34. Rhee AY, Li G, Wells J, Kao YPY. Photostimulation of sensory neurons of the rat vagus nerve. Proc SPIE. 2008;6854: 68540E68541.
35. Bec JM, Albert ES, Marc I, et al. Characteristics of laser stimulation by near infrared pulses of retinal and vestibular primary neurons. Lasers Surg Med. 2012;44(9):736–45.
36. Katz EJ, Ilev IK, Krauthamer V, Kim do H, Weinreich D. Excitation of primary afferent neurons by near-infrared light in vitro. Neuroreport. 2010;21(9):662–6.
37. Hwang SJ, Oh JM, Valtschanoff JG. Expression of the vanilloid receptor TRPV1 in rat dorsal root ganglion neurons supports different roles of the receptor in visceral and cutaneous afferents. Brain Res. 2005;1047(2):261–6.
38. Zhang L, Jones S, Brody K, Costa M, Brookes SJ. Thermosensitive transient receptor potential channels in vagal afferent neurons of the mouse. Am J Physiol Gastrointest Liver Physiol. 2004;286(6):G983–91.
39. Farber IC, Grinvald A. Identification of presynaptic neurons by laser photostimulation. Science. 1983;222(4627):1025–7.
40. Callaway EM, Yuste R. Stimulating neurons with light. Curr Opin Neurobiol. 2002;12(5):587–92.
41. Eder M, Zieglgansberger W, Dodt HU. Shining light on neurons—elucidation of neuronal functions by photostimulation. Rev Neurosci. 2004;15(3):167–83.
42. Callaway EM, Katz LC. Photostimulation using caged glutamate reveals functional circuitry in living brain slices. Proc Natl Acad Sci U S A. 1993;90(16):7661–5.
43. Staiger JF, Kotter R, Zilles K, Luhmann HJ. Laminar characteristics of functional connectivity in rat barrel cortex revealed by stimulation with caged-glutamate. Neurosci Res. 2000;37(1):49–58.
44. Katz LC, Dalva MB. Scanning laser photostimulation: a new approach for analyzing brain circuits. J Neurosci Methods. 1994;54(2):205–18.
45. Teudt IU, Maier H, Richter CP, Kral A. Acoustic events and "optophonic" cochlear responses induced by pulsed near-infrared laser. IEEE Trans Biomed Eng. 2011;58(6):1648–55.
46. Izzo AD, Richter C-P, Jansen ED, Walsh JT. Laser stimulation of the auditory nerve. Laser Surg Med. 2006;38(8):745–53.
47. Schultz, M., Baumhoff, P., Maier, H., Teudt, I.U., Kruger, A., Lenarz, T., Kral, A. Nanosecond laser pulse stimulation of the inner ear-a wavelength study. Biomed Opt Express 2012;3:3332–45
48. Verma RU, Guex AA, Hancock KE, Durakovic N, McKay CM, Slama MC, Brown MC, Lee DJ. Auditory responses to electric and infrared neural stimulation of the rat cochlear nucleus. Hearing research 2014;310C:69–75.
49. Baumhoff P, Schultz M, Kallweit N, et al. Midbrain activity evoked by pulsed laser light. In: 2013 Conference on implantable auditory prostheses; 2013. p. 135.
50. Richter C-P, Bayon R, Izzo AD, Otting M, Suh E, Goyal S, Hotaling J, Walsh Jr., JT. Optical stimulation of auditory neurons: effects of acute and chronic deafening. Hear Res 2008;242:42–51.
51. Sagar SM, Sharp FR, Curran T. Expression of c-fos protein in brain: metabolic mapping at the cellular level. Science. 1988;240(4857):1328–31.
52. Izzo AD, Suh E, Pathria J, Walsh JT, Whitlon DS, Richter CP. Selectivity of neural stimulation in the auditory system: a comparison of optic and electric stimuli. J Biomed Opt. 2007;12(2):021008.
53. Richter CP, Rajguru SM, Matic AI, et al. Spread of cochlear excitation during stimulation with pulsed infrared radiation: inferior colliculus measurements. J Neural Eng. 2011; 8(5):056006.
54. Matic AI, Walsh Jr JT, Richter CP. Spatial extent of cochlear infrared neural stimulation determined by tone-on-light masking. J Biomed Opt. 2011;16(11):118002.
55. Izzo AD, Walsh JT, Jansen ED, et al. Optical parameter variability in laser nerve stimulation: a study of pulse duration, repetition rate, and wavelength. IEEE Trans Biomed Eng. 2007;54(6 Pt 1):1108–14.
56. Walsh Jr JT, Cummings JP. Effect of the dynamic optical properties of water on midinfrared laser ablation. Lasers Surg Med. 1994;15(3):295–305.
57. Banakis RM, Matic AI, Rajguru SM, Richter CP. Optical stimulation of the auditory nerve: effects of pulse shape. Proc SPIE. 2011;7883(788358):1–8.
58. Goyal V, Rajguru S, Matic AI, Stock SR, Richter CP. Acute damage threshold for infrared neural stimulation of the cochlea:

functional and histological evaluation. Anat Rec (Hoboken). 2012;295(11):1987–99.

59. Matic AI, Robinson AM, Young HK, et al. Behavioral and electrophysiological responses evoked by chronic infrared neural stimulation of the cochlea. PLoS One. 2013;8(3):e58189.

60. Harris DM, Bierer SM, Wells JD, Phillips JO. Optical nerve stimulation for a vestibular prosthesis. Proc SPIE. 2009;7180:71800R.

61. Rajguru SM, Rabbitt RR, Matic AI, Highstein SM, Richter CP. Selective activation of vestibular hair cells by infrared light. In: Biophysical Society 54th annual meeting. San Fransisco, CA: Biophysical Society; 2010.

62. Rajguru SM, Rabbitt RR, Matic AI, Highstein SM, Richter CP. Inhibitory and excitatory vestibular afferent responses induced by infrared light stimulation of hair cells. In: 33rd Midwinter meeting. Anaheim, CA: Association for Research in Otolaryngology; 2010.

63. Rabbitt RD, Boyle R, Highstein SM. Mechanical indentation of the vestibular labyrinth and its relationship to head rotation in the toadfish, Opsanus tau. J Neurophysiol. 1995;73(6):2237–60.

64. Holstein GR, Martinelli GP, Boyle R, Rabbitt RD, Highstein SM. Ultrastructural observations of efferent terminals in the crista Ampullaris of the toadfish, opsanus tau. Exp Brain Res. 2004;155(3):265–73.

65. Holstein GR, Rabbitt RD, Martinelli GP, Friedrich Jr VL, Boyle RD, Highstein SM. Convergence of excitatory and inhibitory hair cell transmitters shapes vestibular afferent responses. Proc Natl Acad Sci U S A. 2004; 101(44):15766–71.

66. Boutros PJ, Ahn J, Fridman GY, Dai C, Lasker D, DC DS. Vestibulo-ocular reflex eye movement responses to infra-red laser stimulation of the mammalian labyrinth. Abstr Assoc Res Otolaryngol 2013;36:255.

67. Hanekom JJ, Shannon RV. Gap detection as a measure of electrode interaction in cochlear implants. J Acoust Soc Am. 1998;104(4): 2372–84.

68. Fried NM, Lagoda GA, Scott NJ, Su LM, Burnett AL. Laser stimulation of the cavernous nerves in the rat prostate, in vivo: optimization of wavelength, pulse energy, and pulse repetition rate. Conf Proc IEEE Eng Med Biol Soc. 2008;2008:2777–80.

69. Kim HL, Stoffel DS, Mhoon DA, Brendler CB. A positive caver map response poorly predicts recovery of potency after radical prostatectomy. Urology. 2000;56(4):561–4.

70. Holzbeierlein J, Peterson M, Smith JJ. Variability of results of cavernous nerve stimulation during radical prostatectomy. J Urol. 2001;165(1):108–10.

71. Fried NM, Lagoda GA, Scott NJ, Su LM, Burnett AL. Noncontact stimulation of the cavernous nerves in the rat prostate using a tunable-wavelength thulium fiber laser. J Endourol. 2008;22(3):409–13.

72. Tozburun S, Cilip CM, Lagoda GA, Burnett AL, Fried NM. Continuous-wave infrared optical nerve stimulation for potential diagnostic applications. J Biomed Opt. 2010;15(5): 055012.

73. Tozburun S, Stahl CD, Hutchens TC, Lagoda GA, Burnett AL, Fried NM. Continuous-wave infrared subsurface optical stimulation of the rat prostate cavernous nerves using a 1490-nm diode laser. Urology. 2013;82(4):969–73.

74. Hale GM, Querry MR. Optical constants of water in the 200 nm to 200 μm region. Appl Opt. 1973;12:555–63.

75. Tozburun S, Lagoda GA, Burnett AL, Fried NM. Subsurface near-infrared laser stimulation of the periprostatic cavernous nerves. J Biophotonics. 2012;5(10):793–800.

76. Tozburun S, Hutchens TC, McClain MA, Lagoda GA, Burnett AL, Fried NM. Temperature-controlled optical stimulation of the rat prostate cavernous nerves. J Biomed Opt. 2013;18(6):067001.

77. Cayce JM, Friedman RM, Jansen ED, Mahavaden-Jansen A, Roe AW. Pulsed infrared light alters neural activity in rat somatosensory cortex in vivo. Neuroimage. 2011;57(1):155–66.

78. Cayce JM, Friedman RM, Chen G, Jansen ED, Mahadevan-Jansen A, Roe AW. Infrared neural stimulation of primary visual cortex in non-human primates. Neuroimage. 2013;84C:181–90.

79. Wininger FA, Schei JL, Rector DM. Complete optical neurophysiology: toward optical stimulation and recording of neural tissue. Appl Opt. 2009;48(10):218–24.

80. Smith NI, Kumamoto Y, Iwanaga S, Ando J, Fujita K, Kawata S. A femtosecond laser pacemaker for heart muscle cells. Opt Express. 2008;16(12):8604–16.

81. Dittami GM, Rajguru SM, Lasher RA, Hitchcock RW, Rabbitt RD. Intracellular calcium transients evoked by pulsed infrared radiation in neonatal cardiomyocytes. J Physiol. 2011;589(Pt 6):1295–306.

82. Jenkins MW, Duke AR, Gu S, et al. Optical pacing of the embryonic heart. Nat Photonics. 2010;4:623–6.

83. Okunade O, Santos-Sacchi J. IR laser-induced perturbations of the voltage-dependent solute carrier protein SLC26a5. Biophys J. 2013;105(8):1822–8.

84. Duke AR, Cayce JM, Malphrus JD, Konrad P, Mahadevan-Jansen A, Jansen ED. Combined

optical and electrical stimulation of neural tissue in vivo. J Biomed Opt. 2009;14(6):060501.

85. Bostock H, Rothwell JC. Latent addition in motor and sensory fibres of human peripheral nerve. J Physiol. 1997;498(Pt 1):277–94.

86. Duke AR, Lu H, Jenkins MW, Chiel HJ, Jansen ED. Spatial and temporal variability in response to hybrid electro-optical stimulation. J Neural Eng. 2012;9(3):036003.

87. Thompson AC, Wade SA, Brown WG, Stoddart PR. Modeling of light absorption in tissue during infrared neural stimulation. J Biomed Opt. 2012;17(7):075002.

88. Thompson AC, Wade SA, Cadusch PJ, Brown WG, Stoddart PR. Modeling of the temporal effects of heating during infrared neural stimulation. J Biomed Opt. 2013; 18(3):035004.

89. Thompson A, Wade S, Pawsey N, Stoddart P. Infrared neural stimulation: influence of stimulation site spacing and repetition rates on heating. IEEE Trans Biomed Eng. 2013; 60(12):3534–41.

90. Liljemalm R, Nyberg T, von Holst H. Heating during infrared neural stimulation. Lasers Surg Med. 2013;45(7):469–81.

91. Norton BJ, Bowler MA, Wells JD, Keller MD. Analytical approaches for determining heat distributions and thermal criteria for infrared neural stimulation. J Biomed Opt. 2013;18(9):98001.

92. Brummer SB, Robblee LS, Hambrecht FT. Criteria for selecting electrodes for electrical stimulation: theoretical and practical considerations. Ann N Y Acad Sci. 1983;405: 159–69.

Part III

Photodynamic Therapy

Dick Sterenborg

Introduction

Reference to the use of photosensitizing plants for treatment of skin diseases are found in the earliest documents of the several ancient cultures, such as the book Veda from ancient India and the Ebers Papyrus from ancient Egypt. Primitive forms of Photodynamic Therapy have probably been around since the dawn of mankind. More systematic research on the backgrounds of PDT and its application dates from more recent times. From the early beginning of the twentieth century, there have been occasional scientific reports on PDT experiments and even some early clinical work. From the 1940s, however, the scientific interest in PDT really takes off. A quick survey in Pubmed reveals that the number of peer-reviewed papers has since then exponentially increased over the years until roughly 1000 per year in 2010. A similar survey in the patent database Espacenet shows that a wave of patents on PDT sets off starting in the late 1970s. Again an exponential increase with time, but now a steeper one, growing to roughly 200 patents per year in 2010. The number of registered clinical trials on PDT follows a similar pattern, but, logically, sets in a few years later, roughly around 1980 and reached roughly 100 per year in 2010. This dramatic growth has been fuelled by the advancement of technology and especially in optics. It started with the appearance of lasers and fiberoptics in the late 1970s and is still an accelerating field. The path to routine clinical practice, however, is treacherous, and only a very small fraction of all these efforts eventually lead to a registered photosensitizer, which is an indication of a clinical application that has become routine. In 1993, the first clinically approved photosensitizer appeared on the market, but in 2010 this number still lingered around ten.

This shows that to come to successful clinical application of photodynamic therapy, we need more than the advancement of science alone. We need to bridge not just the gap between science and clinical practice, but, due to the very multidisciplinary nature of Photodynamic Therapy, also make the different scientific, technological, and medical specialties (pharmacology, biology, physics and medicine) work together successfully and over an extended period of time. The numbers quoted above illustrate that this is not easy and only rarely successful.

Nevertheless, in the field of Head and Neck Cancer, we have been very active to beat these odds. What lies before you is a book on the current state of Photodynamic Therapy for Head and Neck Malignancies. It shows that a relatively small but highly motivated and dedicated multidisciplinary international community can do. For people new to the field, from any of the disciplines or with a general interest, this is an excellent introduction to the basic concepts, the possibilities and the broadness of the applications. For members of the medical field experienced in treatment of Head and Neck malignancies, this book gives an excellent overview of what is currently possible with Photodynamic Therapy. I hope this book will stimulate critical discussions on Photodynamic Therapy and will help giving it the position in everyday medicine that it deserves.

Chapter 18

Physics of Photodynamic Therapy

Steen J. Madsen

Introduction

Photodynamic therapy (PDT) uses light-activated drugs (photosensitizers) for the treatment of neoplastic and non-neoplastic diseases. Administration of the photosensitizer constitutes the first step in the PDT process. Then, following a waiting period (minutes to days) to allow for selective accumulation in the target tissue, the sensitizer is activated via light (usually from a laser) of a wavelength matching a prominent absorption resonance in the red or near-infrared part of the visible spectrum. Absorption of this light by the photosensitizer results in photochemical processes which ultimately produce the cytotoxic species (e.g., singlet molecular oxygen) responsible for the biological damage.

The beginning of photodynamic therapy (PDT) is generally attributed to Raab in 1900 [1] who noted that the combination of dyes and light of certain wavelengths was toxic to microorganisms; however, it wasn't until the 1970s that this therapeutic approach was introduced into the clinic [2, 3]. At that time PDT dosimetry was in a primitive state and it was recognized that, in order for PDT to gain clinical acceptance, a more rigorous dosimetric approach requiring a better understanding of PDT physics was required. A number of pioneering studies laying the foundation for PDT dosimetry were initiated in the 1980s. These studies focused primarily on gaining a better understanding of PDT dosimetry along with developing noninvasive (or minimally invasive) techniques for determining the three essential dosimetry components: light, photosensitizer, and oxygen. An excellent summary of the state of PDT physics in the 1980s, along with a recent update, can be found in [4] and [5], respectively.

Brian J.-F. Wong and Justus Ilgner (eds.), *Biomedical Optics in Otorhinolaryngology: Head and Neck Surgery*,
DOI 10.1007/978-1-4939-1758-7_18, © Springer Science+Business Media New York 2016

The purpose of this review is to provide an overview of the physics of PDT as it relates to dosimetry. Of the three dosimetry parameters, light interactions/propagation cannot be understood without a rudimentary knowledge of optical physics and transport theory and, as such, these topics are discussed in significant detail and they provide a good starting point for the review. Knowledge of the optical properties of biological tissues is important for predicting light distributions and their in vivo measurement is considered in section "Optical Property Measurements In Vivo." This is followed by an in-depth examination of various dosimetric approaches that can be used to predict biological response during PDT. The review concludes with an examination of dose-rate effects and associated strategies for improving PDT response.

Fundamental Light Interactions in Tissue

Knowledge of light distributions in biological tissue is critical for accurate PDT dosimetry. There are four fundamental types of interactions between light and tissue: refraction, reflection, absorption, and scattering. Reflection and refraction occur when light propagates between two different media and they are described by Fresnel's Law and Snell's law, respectively. The loss of light intensity between the interfaces is determined by the difference in refractive indices between the two media. From a practical point of view, light loss can be minimized by perpendicular light application [6].

Scattering is the most dominant interaction in tissues accounting for approximately 90–99 % of the total light attenuation [7]. This is in stark contrast to X-ray interactions in tissue where attenuation due to scattering and absorption is approximately equivalent. The dominance of light scattering in tissues makes optical imaging significantly more difficult than X-ray imaging. Light scattering can be either elastic (incident and scattered photons have the same energy) or inelastic (incident and scattered photons have different energy). In PDT applications, inelastic scattering (e.g., Brillouin and Raman) is negligible and can be ignored. The dominant elastic interactions in tissues are Rayleigh and Mie scattering: the type of interaction is determined by the ratio of the scattering particle size to the wavelength of light and the shape of the particle. Mie scattering dominates in situations where the wavelength and particle size are approximately equal, while Rayleigh scattering dominates for wavelengths much larger than the particle size. In practice, neither type of elastic scattering completely describes the situation in biological tissues and, as such, a number of closely related scattering formulations have been developed [8].

Compared to scattering, light absorption in tissues is relatively straightforward and can be described by the Beer–Lambert law [9]:

$$I = I_0 e^{-\varepsilon CL} \tag{1}$$

where I and I_0 are the transmitted and incident light intensities, respectively, ε is the molar extinction coefficient, C is the concentration of the solution, and L is the sample thickness. The Beer–Lambert Law is valid only under the following assumptions [10]: (1) the absorbing compounds are independent, (2) the concentration of the absorber is constant along the light path (generally not true in case of a complex material such as tissue), (3) atomic effects such as multiphoton absorption, optical saturation, or stimulated emission can be ignored (this is the case for the relatively low light intensities used in PDT), and (4) the incident light consists of parallel rays that traverse the sample without scattering (not the case for biological tissues). Since some of these assumptions are invalid in scattering media, the Beer–Lambert law has limited utility in biological media and, therefore, more sophisticated models of light transport are required to accurately determine the optical properties.

Light absorption in tissue is due primarily to a few highly absorbing molecules (chromophores) including water, oxyhemoglobin, deoxyhemoglobin, melanin, and cytochromes. The absorption spectra of these molecules are illustrated in Fig. 1 which shows that there is an "optical window" between 600 and 1400 nm where the absorbance of each chromophore is relatively low. This optical window provides the rationale for using red to near-infrared absorbing photosensitizers since these wavelengths have the deepest penetration in tissues.

Light Transport in Biological Tissues

Tissues are considered optically turbid since they scatter and absorb light and, as such, light propagation can be modeled using the radiation transport equation (RTE), also known as the Boltzmann transport equation [11]. Solution of the RTE requires knowledge of the fundamental optical properties (absorption, scattering, and scattering anisotropy). Once the tissue optical properties have been determined, the RTE can be used to calculate the light distribution (fluence rate) at any point for a given source geometry. Analytical solutions to the RTE exist in only a few limiting cases, thus necessitating the use of approximate methods.

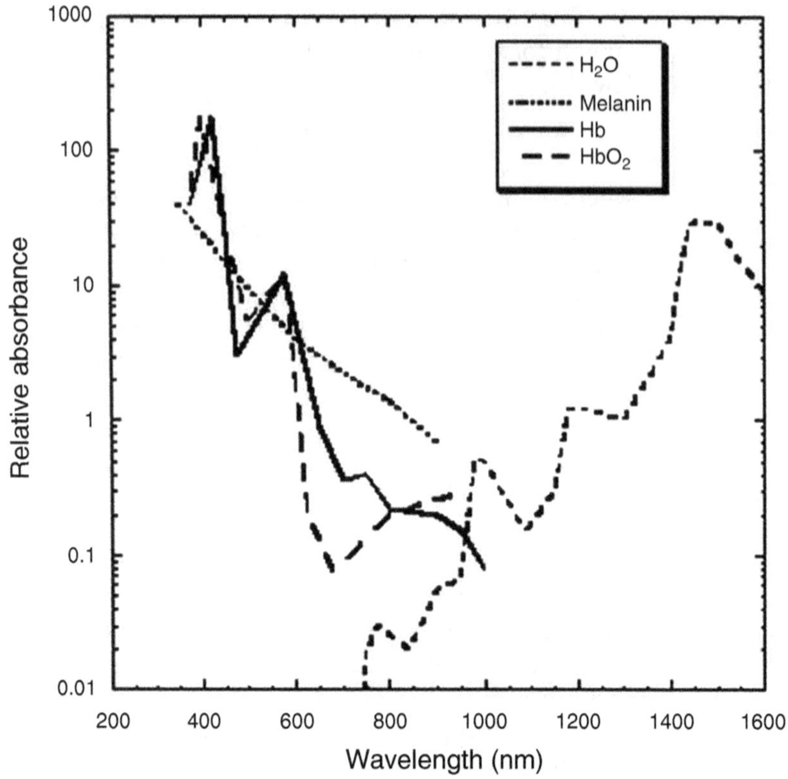

Fig. 1 Absorption spectra of common tissue chromophores. An optical window corresponding to reduced scattering and absorption is evident from 600 to 1400 nm. *Hb* hemoglobin, *HbO2* oxyhemoglobin

Radiation Transport Equation

The time-dependent RTE describing light transport in a turbid medium can be expressed as [5]:

$$\frac{1}{v}\frac{\partial}{\partial t}L(\mathbf{r},\Omega,t)+\Omega\cdot\nabla L(\mathbf{r},\Omega,t)+[\mu_a(\mathbf{r})+\mu_s(\mathbf{r})]L(\mathbf{r},\Omega,t) = \mu_s\int_{4\pi}p(\Omega,\Omega')L(\mathbf{r},\Omega',t)\mathrm{d}\Omega'+S(\mathbf{r},\Omega,t) \quad (2)$$

where $L(\mathbf{r}, \boldsymbol{\Omega})$ is the energy radiance which is the radiant power transported at location $\mathbf{r}$ in a given direction $\boldsymbol{\Omega}$ per unit solid angle per unit area perpendicular to that direction [W m^{-2} sr^{-1}]. The energy radiance is considered the fundamental quantity of interest in the RTE. The energy fluence rate, $E_0(\mathbf{r})$ [W m^{-2}], can be determined simply by integrating the radiance over 4π solid angle. This is an important parameter in a number of applications including PDT. The absorption coefficient is denoted by μ_a, while the scattering coefficient is given by μ_s. $S(\mathbf{r}, \boldsymbol{\Omega}, t)$ is a source term, v is the speed of light in tissue, and $p(\boldsymbol{\Omega}, \boldsymbol{\Omega}')$ is the phase function which gives the probability that a photon moving in the direction of unit vector $\mathbf{\Omega}$ is scattered in the direction $\mathbf{\Omega}'$. The phase function can be expanded as a series in Legendre polynomials, Pn [12]:

$$p(\Omega,\Omega') = \frac{1}{4\pi}\sum_{\infty}^{n=0}(2n+1)b_n P_n(\Omega,\Omega') \tag{3}$$

The first term accounts for normalization ($b_0 = 1$) and the second term yields $b_1 = g$, the mean cosine of the scattering angle. Accurate values for higher order terms in the expansion of the phase function are very difficult to obtain for biological tissues. The value of g varies from −1 to 1: $g = 0$ corresponds to isotroptic scattering, while values of 1 and −1 correspond to total forward and backward scattering, respectively. Light scattering in most tissues is highly forwardly directed ($g \approx 0.7$–0.9), thus requiring several scattering events to randomize the direction of light propagation. The most commonly used phase function to describe light scattering in tissues is the Henyey–Greenstein phase function which is defined by $bn = gn$ in Eq. (1) [13]. This phase function was originally developed to describe light scattering in stellar atmospheres and can be applied to biological tissue in a very straightforward manner since it only depends on one parameter (g).

Solution to the Transport Equation

Exact Solutions

Solution of the RTE assumes that the wave properties of light are ignored and therefore light photons propagating in biological tissues are considered as neutral particles, much like neutrons in a nuclear reactor. Analytical solutions to the RTE can be found in only a few limiting cases. Chandrasekhar [14] solved the case of a homogeneous, semi-infinite, isotropically scattering medium irradiated with a collimated beam of infinite extent, while Rybicki [15] solved the RTE in a similar medium irradiated with a narrow collimated beam. Due to the geometrical constraints and the simple assumptions regarding medium composition, these techniques are not relevant for clinical PDT.

Numerical Techniques: Monte Carlo Simulations

The most commonly used numerical technique for solving the RTE is Monte Carlo (MC) modeling. Although the Monte Carlo approach was introduced in the late 1940s to investigate neutron transport in various materials [16], it wasn't until the early 1980s that it was applied to tissue optics [17]. The MC technique is capable of solving the RTE to a high degree of accuracy and, as such, it has become the gold standard for modeling light propagation in tissue [18]. For example, MC simulations are commonly used to verify the accuracy of analytical models such as diffusion theory [19].

The algorithms used in MC simulations are relatively straightforward and codes for simulating light propagation in tissues are readily available (e.g., [20]). MC simulations track the history of individual photons in the medium, and parameters such as the distance between interactions and the scattering angle are sampled from appropriate probability distributions which depend on the optical properties of the medium [17]. The fluence can be determined from the number of photon interactions recorded in each volume element. In addition to obtaining light distributions from known optical properties (the forward problem), MC modeling can also be used to estimate optical properties by fitting simulated light distributions to experimental data (the inverse problem).

The primary advantage of the MC approach is that it can be used to simulate light propagation under realistic conditions (e.g., variety of light sources, multiple tissue types, and complex geometries); however, this flexibility comes with a price: simulations can be computationally intensive as they typically require millions of photon histories to obtain the desired accuracy—the higher the degree of accuracy required, the longer the simulation time. A number of techniques have been introduced to increase the speed of MC simulations including scaling and perturbation methods, hybrid approaches, variance reduction techniques, and parallel computation methods [21]. Parallel computation methods are particularly intriguing since they have the potential to significantly reduce computation times. In essence, this approach involves running an MC simulation simultaneously on many computers with the goal of using the dead time of networked computers to increase the speed of MC simulations. A variation of this approach is to use a multiple processor MC code that can be run on one computer with multiple processors, i.e., parallelization [22]. Other techniques for increasing computation speed include (1) the implementation of MC codes in graphic processing unit (GPU) environments [23], (2) using field-programmable gate arrays [24], and (3) using Internet-based parallel computation (cloud computing) [25]. Some of these approaches have been shown to reduce computation times by a factor of 1000 compared to conventional CPU-based approaches [21].

MC modeling of light propagation in biological tissues has been used to simulate a number of common optical measurements including fluorescence and diffuse transmittance and reflectance. MC modeling is ideally suited for PDT applications since it can be used in realistic treatment situations involving multiple sources, complex geometries, and heterogeneous tissues. For example, MC simulations have been used to characterize PDT dosimetry in a variety of oncologic applications including prostate [26] and skin cancers [27–29]. In this context, MC modeling is particularly useful since it has the ability to simulate both the temporal and spatial distributions of the fundamental dosimetric PDT parameters (light distribution and photosensitizer and oxygen concentrations).

The Diffusion Approximation

Under the assumption that the radiance is only weakly direction dependent (i.e., linearly anisotropic), the integro-differential equation [Eq. (1)] can be expressed as a partial differential equation that can be solved using standard techniques. Specifically, the radiance is expanded in terms of spherical harmonics, $\Upsilon_{n,m}$, with only the first two terms considered. In terms of the fluence rate, $E_0(\mathbf{r})$, the diffusion equation can be expressed [5]:

$$\frac{1}{v}\frac{\partial}{\partial t}E_0(\mathbf{r},t)-\nabla\cdot[3(1-g(\mathbf{r}))\mu_s(\mathbf{r})]^{-1}\nabla E_0(\mathbf{r},t)+\mu_a(\mathbf{r})E_0(\mathbf{r},t)=S(\mathbf{r},t) \tag{4}$$

In the diffusion approximation, the source-free equations are invariant for changes in μ_s and g that leave $\mu_s(1-g)$ constant [30]. Therefore, the precise value of g might not be required in regions where the diffusion approximation holds, i.e., far from boundaries and sources and in highly scattering media ($\mu_s\,(1-g)\gg\mu_a$). This represents a significant simplification since g is very difficult to measure. Thus, for determination of light distribution in tissues, it is sufficient to know μ_a and $\mu_s(1-g)$ accurately and g only approximately [31]. $\mu_s(1-g)$ is typically denoted by μ_s', the so-called reduced (or transport) scattering coefficient. Accurate values of g may only be important close to boundaries and sources, i.e., under conditions where the diffusion approximation is invalid. In such instances, alternative approximation methods are required, e.g., higher-order analytic solutions using spherical harmonics for the angular parameters in Eq. (1) and expansion of the phase function in Legendre polynomials [Eq. (3)] [32]. Analytic solutions to the diffusion equation exist only for very simple conditions (optically homogeneous tissue) and geometries (infinite, semi-infinite, and slab) [33].

Other Approximation Methods

Kubelka and Munk developed a simple two-flux model to describe the propagation of a uniform diffuse irradiance in a one-dimensional slab with no reflection at the boundaries [34, 35]. It is assumed that the slab is illuminated by a Lambertian source and that the radiance remains isotropic with depth. The model has been used primarily for determining the optical properties of tissues in simple layered models; however, the underlying assumptions of isotropic scattering, matched boundaries, and diffuse irradiance are unrealistic for many light-tissue applications.

The inverse adding doubling (IAD) technique is a numerical solution to the one-dimensional RTE that is applicable to homogeneous turbid slabs with any optical thickness, albedo, or phase function [36–38]. The method is a reversal of the usual procedure of calculating reflection and transmission from optical properties, hence the term "inverse." The IAD approach is ideally suited to measurements involving biological tissues placed between glass slides, and it has been used to determine the optical properties of a wide variety of tissues. Since this technique applies only to uniformly illuminated homogenous slabs, it is difficult to envision its use for in vivo determination of optical properties.

Optical Property Measurements In Vivo

A number of methods have been employed to measure the optical properties of biological tissues. These include direct methods requiring tissue samples sufficiently thin such that single scattering dominates. This requires measurements on excised tissues. Unfortunately, the results are fraught with uncertainty due to preparation and handling artifacts such as blood loss and freezing/thawing. These types of measurements are ill suited to the clinic since they are time intensive and cannot be used for real-time optical property monitoring during PDT. For these reasons, the focus has been on in vivo measurements using either invasive or noninvasive approaches. Invasive methods involve the insertion of fiber optic sources and detectors directly into the tissue of interest for measurements of the light distribution. A model of light propagation in a homogeneous medium is then employed to estimate the interaction coefficients from a set of measurements (e.g., the fluence rate at a number of distances from the internal source). Such measurements are commonly employed in PDT. In noninvasive approaches, the sources and detectors are placed in contact with the external boundary. Although this is less intrusive, the accuracy of the optical properties is often difficult to estimate since the light travels through different tissue types.

Spectroscopic techniques for in vivo determination of tissue optical properties can be divided into three categories: steady-state (or continuous wave), time-resolved, and frequency domains. In the vast majority of cases, the diffusion approximation is used to extract the optical properties (μ_a and μ_s').

Steady-State Spectroscopy

Reflectance Measurements

In diffuse reflectance measurements, light is collected by a detector fiber at a known distance from a source fiber (Fig. 2a). Both fibers are placed in contact with the surface of the medium and the measured reflectance is fitted to a model of light propagation (i.e., the diffusion approximation) in order to extract the optical properties of the medium. Nonlinear least squares fitting routines (e.g., Levenberg–Marquardt algorithm) are commonly used to fit the measured data to the model [39]. Analytic expressions based on the diffusion approximation have been derived by a number of groups applicable in simple geometries such as semi-infinite homogeneous media [19, 40, 41]. Using the diffusion theory solution of Kienle and Patterson [41], the diffuse reflectance as a function of fiber separation (ρ) is given by

$$R(\rho) = C_1\psi(\rho) + C_2 j_z(\rho) \tag{5}$$

where $\psi(\rho)$ is the fluence rate at the surface and $jz(\rho)$ is the reflected flux exiting the surface from the tissue. C_1 and C_2 are constants which depend on the relative refractive index mismatch at the tissue/detector interface and the numerical aperture of the detection fibers.

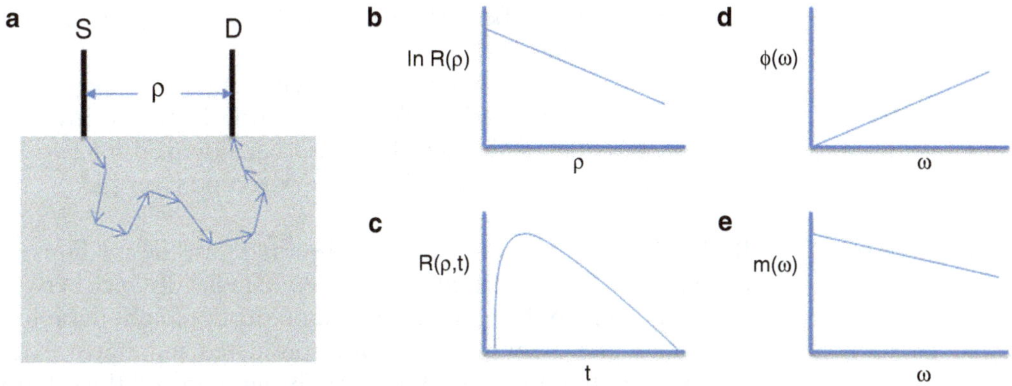

Fig. 2 Noninvasive spectroscopic approaches for determining optical properties. (**a**) Photons are introduced into a homogeneous semi-infinite tissue-like medium via an optical fiber (S) and detected by an optical fiber (D). In the steady-state approach (**b**), diffusely reflected photons are collected as a function of source-detector fiber separation (ρ). In time-resolved spectroscopy (**c**), diffusely reflected photons are detected as a function of time. In the frequency domain, the phase shift (ϕ) (**d**) and demodulation amplitude (m) (**e**) are determined as a function of modulation frequency (ω). In all cases, the tissue optical properties (μ_a and μ_s') can be determined by fitting the diffusion approximation to the experimental data illustrated in (**b**)–(**e**)

If the index of refraction of tissue is 1.4, the numerical aperture of the detection fiber is 0.22, and if the index of refraction of the detector fiber is 1.46, then C_1 is 1.46 and C_2 is 0.0389 [42]. In Eq. (5), $\psi(\rho)$ and $jz(\rho)$ are given by

$$\psi(\rho) = \frac{1}{4\pi D}\left(\frac{\exp(-\mu_{\text{eff}} r_1(\rho))}{r_1(\rho)} - \frac{\exp(-\mu_{\text{eff}} r_2(\rho))}{r_2(\rho)}\right) \tag{6}$$

and

$$j_z(\rho) = \frac{1}{4\pi\mu_t'}\left[\left(\mu_{\text{eff}} + \frac{1}{r_1(\rho)}\right)\frac{\exp(-\mu_{\text{eff}} r_1(\rho))}{r_1^2(\rho)} + \left(\frac{1}{\mu_t'} + 2z_b\right)\left(\mu_{\text{eff}} + \frac{1}{r_2(\rho)}\right)\frac{\exp(-\mu_{\text{eff}} r_2(\rho)}{r_2^2(\rho)}\right] \tag{7}$$

where D is the diffusion coefficient ($= [3(\mu_a + \mu_s')]^{-1}$), μ_{eff} is the effective attenuation coefficient ($= [3\mu_a(\mu_a + \mu_s')]^{1/2}$), and μ_t' is the total interaction coefficient ($= \mu_a + \mu_s'$). The parameter z_b is the extrapolated boundary position, i.e., the location of an imaginary boundary a distance of $2AD$ above the surface of the medium, where A is a dimensionless constant determined by the relative refractive index mismatch at the boundary [40]. The parameter $r_1(\rho)$ is the distance from a detection point on the surface of the medium to an imaginary point source located one transport mean free path ($= 1/\mu_t'$) directly below the source fiber, while $r_2(\rho)$ is the distance from the detection point on the surface to a negative image source located at a distance of $1/\mu_t' + 2z_b$ directly above the source fiber. The rationale for using these parameters is discussed in detail in [40]. The use of reflectance measurements and steady-state diffusion theory has been shown to yield values of μ_a and μ_s' to an accuracy of around 10 %.

Equation (18.5) applies to a semi-infinite homogeneous medium. Solutions to the diffusion equation in the steady-state, time, and frequency domains have also been derived for two-layered turbid media with an infinitely thick second layer [43].

Interstitial Measurements

Both source and detector fibers are inserted into the medium and the fluence rate is measured as a function of radial distance between the fibers. Due to the limited penetration depth of light in biological tissues, the medium is typically considered infinite in extent and, as such, boundary conditions can be ignored and the solution to the diffusion equation is thus relatively trivial. In this case, the fluence rate ϕ at a distance r around an isotropic point source delivering a radiant power P into the infinite turbid medium is given by [44]:

$$\phi(r) = \frac{P}{4\pi Dr}\exp(-\mu_{\text{eff}} r) \tag{8}$$

The equation can be modified to account for tissue heterogeneity and extended sources [45].

Time-Resolved Spectroscopy

In time-resolved (or time-of-flight) spectroscopy, the temporal spreading of a short light pulse ($\leq 10^{-12}$ s) is measured in reflectance or transmittance mode as it travels through a scattering medium such as tissue (Fig. 2c). The temporal spreading of the light pulse is related to the optical properties of the medium which may be extracted via application of a model of light propagation. For example, the time-dependent diffusion equation has been solved for semi-infinite and finite homogeneous tissue slabs [46] as well as spherical and cylindrical geometries [47]. A particularly useful quantity is the time-resolved diffuse reflectance from a homogeneous semi-infinite tissue slab:

$$R(\rho,t) = (4\pi Dc)^{-3/2} z_0 t^{-5/2} \exp(-\mu_a ct)\exp(-\frac{\rho^2 + z_0^2}{4Dct}) \tag{9}$$

where ρ is the source–detector fiber separation, c is the speed of light in tissue (=0.214 mm ps^{-1} assuming that $n = 1.4$), and z_0 is the depth at which the incident photons are initially scattered ($= 1/\mu_s'$). Time-resolved spectroscopy has been investigated in a wide variety of geometries [43, 46, 48] and the accuracy of the derived optical properties (μ_a and μ_s') is similar to that obtained with steady-state techniques ($\approx$10 %). The high cost of instrumentation required for time-resolved spectroscopy is a significant limitation.

Frequency Domain Spectroscopy

In frequency domain spectroscopy the intensity of light incident on biological tissue is modulated at a high frequency (10^8–10^9 Hz) and the diffusely reflected or transmitted signal is measured with a phase-sensitive detector (Figs. 2d,e). It has been shown that intensity-modulated light propagates through multiple scattering media as diffuse photon density waves with a coherent front [49–51]. Since density wave dispersion is a function of the optical properties of the material interrogated, the absorption and transport scattering coefficients can be determined simply by fitting the measured frequency and distance-dependent behavior to analytical expressions derived from diffusion theory [40, 51, 52]. For example, Fourier transformation of Eq. (18.9) yields analytic expressions for the modulation and phase as functions of the optical properties of the tissue.

Compared to time-resolved techniques, frequency domain spectroscopy offers several advantages including (1) cheaper instrumentation, especially for frequencies below 200 MHz [53, 54], (2) the possibility of determining the optical properties (μ_a and μ_s') from modulation and phase measurements at a single frequency, and (3) the potential of monitoring dynamic phenomena (e.g., hemoglobin oxygenation) since both modulation and phase can be measured over short time periods. For these reasons, frequency domain spectroscopy has become the preferred method for diffuse optical spectroscopy applications.

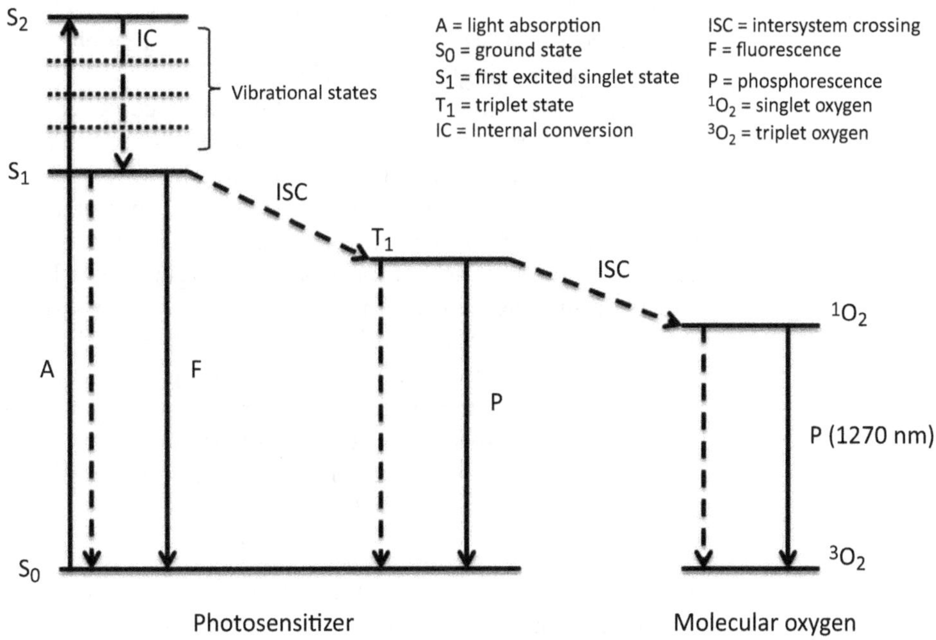

Fig. 3 Abbreviated Jablonski diagram showing the most relevant energy levels and transitions for singlet oxygen-mediated PDT. *Solid* and *dashed arrows* denote radiative and non-radiative transitions, respectively. De-excitation of singlet molecular oxygen to ground-state triplet molecular oxygen is accompanied by 1270 nm phosphorescence which can be used as a direct dose metric during PDT

PDT Dosimetry

Introduction

In comparison to ionizing radiation, PDT dosimetry is not well developed. This can be attributed to the complexity of the PDT process which is illustrated in Fig. 3. A photosensitizer in its ground state is characterized by paired electrons with a total spin $(S)=0$ and a corresponding spin multiplicity of 1. This ground-state configuration is termed a singlet state (S_0). Upon absorption of photons of appropriate energy, the photosensitizer is raised to an electronically excited singlet state Sn $(n=1, 2, 3...)$ which contains additional vibrational modes. The photosensitizer may return to its ground state resulting in prompt fluorescence emission; however, efficient photosensitizers typically undergo an intersystem crossing (ISC) through rearrangement of electronic spin resulting in a triplet excited state (T_1). This triplet state has a relatively long lifetime in biological tissues (typically tens of microseconds) and, in well-oxygenated conditions, de-excites via energy transfer to ground-state molecular oxygen in a triplet state $(^3O_2)$. If sufficient energy is provided in this transfer, singlet excited oxygen $^1O_2$ is produced. For example, typical sensitizers yield approximately one molecule of singlet oxygen for every two photons absorbed [55]. There is strong evidence showing that singlet oxygen is the primary cytotoxic species in PDT [56, 57]; however, reactions yielding other reactive species have also been demonstrated [58]. PDT-induced tissue necrosis requires the production of approximately 10^{18}–10^{19} molecules $cm^{-3}$of singlet oxygen [59].

Clinical PDT dosimetry has traditionally been accomplished based on the amount of photosensitizer administered followed by measurement of the incident light exposure. This is a very simplistic and inadequate approach due to intra- and inter-patient variability in sensitizer concentrations. Second, the light distribution is dependent on the optical properties of the target tissue. Third, the yield of singlet oxygen depends on the oxygenation state of the tissue. Finally, the photosensitizer concentration, light distribution, and tissue oxygenation may change during treatment and one parameter may interact with the other. These factors must be accounted for in a successful PDT dosimetry scheme.

Assuming that singlet oxygen is responsible for the biological response, Wilson et al. [60] have proposed three dosimetry approaches:

1. Explicit dosimetry which typically involves separate measurements of light, photosensitizer, and oxygen during PDT. These measurements are then incorporated into a dose model. Although this is a cumbersome approach fraught with uncertainties, it has nevertheless been used by a number of groups [61–63].

2. Implicit dosimetry in which a combination of treatment parameters are incorporated into a single dose metric, e.g., photosensitizer photobleaching which can be determined by monitoring photosensitizer fluorescence during PDT. Fluorescence spectroscopic measurements of photoproducts associated with photobleaching have also been proposed as an implicit dosimetry technique [64–66].
3. Direct dosimetry in which the cytotoxic species, single oxygen, is measured.

Strategies for measuring the individual components (light photosensitizer and oxygen) required for explicit dosimetry will be summarized in sections "Light Dosimetry," "Photosensitizer Dosimetry," and "Oxygen Dosimetry," while implicit dosimetry techniques and direct singlet oxygen measurements will be discussed in sections "Implicit Dosimetry" and "Direct Dosimetry," respectively.

Light Dosimetry

Determination of light fluence was discussed in section "Light Transport in Biological Tissues." It was shown that the fluence (and fluence rate) can be determined from knowledge of the tissue optical properties and the irradiation geometry. Another approach involves the direct measurement of the fluence rate which is typically accomplished at discrete points within the tissue. Rather than generating a complete fluence rate profile, which would require many invasive measurements, the goal is usually to verify the results of calculations and/or to determine the fluence rate at clinically critical locations where calculations may be suspect (e.g., near boundaries). Measurements are typically accomplished using small diameter (≈200 μm-dia.) optical fibers with isotropic scattering tips. Using commercially available fiber probes with highly uniform angular response (±5 %), fluence rate measurements can be made with an accuracy of around 5–10 % [5].

Photosensitizer Dosimetry

A number of approaches have been used to measure photosensitizer concentration in tissues. The most promising techniques involve optical methods based on absorption, fluorescence, or Raman scattering which can yield the concentration at discrete points or the mean concentration over a tissue volume.

Since most photosensitizers fluoresce, the fluorescence emission from a tissue can be used to infer the concentration of the photosensitizer. The relationship between emission and concentration is not straightforward since the emission may be affected by the local environment of the photosensitizer including pH. Another complication is that both the excitation and emission light typically propagate through thick tissue layers and, therefore, the detected fluorescence will depend on the tissue optical properties. This effect can be minimized by delivering the excitation light and collecting the fluorescence via an optical fiber inserted directly into the tissue [67]. Although this approach is capable of yielding photosensitizer concentrations to an accuracy of about 10 %, it is limited by the small tissue volumes sampled. Larger sample volumes have been accomplished using surface probes consisting of fiber bundles [68].

In the case of non-fluorescing or low quantum yield photosensitizers, absorption spectroscopy is commonly used. The objective is to determine the photosensitizer concentration from its specific contribution to the total absorption coefficient. This is typically accomplished by determining the absorption coefficient over a range of wavelengths so that the sensitizer peaks can be differentiated from the tissue background absorption. A system for performing quantitative absorption spectroscopy to estimate photosensitizer concentration in vivo has been described by Farrell et al. [69].

A number of other approaches have been developed for quantifying sensitizer concentration. The most promising of these is Raman scattering which has been used for ex vivo measurements [70], although fiber optic-based Raman systems developed for in vivo diagnostics could be used for this purpose.

Oxygen Dosimetry

In situ measurements of tissue oxygenation require thin probes. Commercially available metal-based microelectrodes for measuring pO_2 in tissues have tip diameters of a few μm [71]. Although these microelectrodes are capable of measuring pO_2 with excellent spatial and temporal resolution, they are rather fragile and can easily be broken during clinical measurements. Similar to fluence rate measurements discussed in section "Light Dosimetry," pO_2 measurements are made at discrete points in the tissue and therefore placement of electrodes requires careful consideration of the tissue to be monitored. A combination fiber optic probe for measuring pO_2, pCO_2, and pH was approved for clinical use in 2000 [71]. Advantages of these luminescence-based sensors include their non-chemical and reversible mechanism of sensing in which both the probe and the analyte are not consumed, high sensitivity and selectivity, rapid response times (ms), and the possibility of contactless measurements through a (semi) transparent material [72]. Additionally, due to their larger tip diameters (ca. 500 μm), optical probes are also more robust. Some studies have found that the larger fiber optic probes consistently measure a higher fraction of hypoxic pO_2 values in both tumors and normal tissues compared to microelectrodes [73]. This may be due to damage to the microcirculation by the larger optic probes.

Although direct microelectrode/fiber optic measurements of tissue oxygenation have not been attempted during clinical PDT, spectroscopic techniques, such as those described in section "Optical Property Measurements In Vivo," have been investigated. For example,

Zhu et al. [63] used a continuous wave spectroscopy approach (section "Interstitial Measurements") to measure both oxy- and deoxyhemoglobin concentrations in human prostate during PDT. Knowledge of these parameters allows evaluation of tissue oxygenation.

Implicit Dosimetry

In most instances, implicit dosimetry is accomplished via detection of photobleaching or photoproducts. In this context, photobleaching refers to the photochemical destruction of the sensitizer rendering it incapable of further fluorescence. For some photosensitizers, photobleaching is mediated by $^1O_2$ and, therefore, it should be possible to infer its concentration based on the initial and final sensitizer concentrations. For example, Dysart and Patterson [74] have developed an expression for the total amount (i.e., dose) of singlet oxygen generated during a PDT treatment starting at $t=0$ and ending at $t=T$:

$$\text{Dose} = \frac{1}{\tau}\int_T^0 [^1\text{O}_2]dt = \frac{1}{\tau\ k_{\text{os}}}\log_e \frac{[S_0]_{t=0} + \gamma}{[S_0]_{t=T} + \gamma} \qquad (18.10)$$

where τ_Δ is the singlet oxygen lifetime in the tissue, k_{os} is the sensitizer bleaching rate constant, and γ is the effective minimum sensitizer concentration. Therefore, only a few parameters are required to determine the absolute dose, namely, the initial and final sensitizer concentrations, $[S_0]t_{=0}$ and $[S_0]t_{=}T$, and τ_Δ, k_{os}, and γ.

This model has been verified in simple in vitro systems using the sensitizer mTHPC. The model is accurate only under well-oxygenated conditions ($pO_2 > 5$ μM) [75] and it cannot be applied to commonly used photosensitizers such as Photofrin and ALA-PpIX since they can be photobleached by non-$^1O_2$ pathways under hypoxic conditions [74, 76, 77]. The results of these studies suggest that there are likely two different photobleaching mechanisms for sensitizers such as Photofrin: one mediated by singlet oxygen and the other by the sensitizer triplet state. The relative importance of each depends on the ambient oxygen concentration. Furthermore, it has been postulated that the fluorescent photoproduct of Photofrin is due exclusively to singlet oxygen-mediated bleaching and, as such, determination of the concentration of the photoproduct would be more reliable than measuring Photofrin photobleaching [76]. Similarly, the photoproducts of PpIX [77] and BPD [64] have been found to be more reliable predictors of PDT response in vitro and in vivo.

In summary, implicit dosimetry is still in its infancy: the majority of studies have been performed in relatively simple systems consisting of cell suspensions and multicell spheroids. Additional in vivo studies will be required in order to determine the clinical potential of this approach.

Direct Dosimetry

Direct dosimetry involves measurement of the 1270 nm phosphorescence resulting from the de-excitation of singlet oxygen to its ground state. Although measurement of this signal is trivial in vitro, its detection in complex media such as biological tissue is challenging due to its short lifetime (30–200 ns) and weak emission. As a result, singlet oxygen luminescence detection requires sensitive and rapid time response detection systems. Early systems employing liquid nitrogen-cooled germanium detectors and lock-in detection techniques were capable of measuring singlet oxygen luminescence in cell suspensions, but lacked the sensitivity for reliable measurements in vivo [78–80]. With the introduction of sensitive near-infrared photomultiplier tubes in the late 1990s, in vivo singlet oxygen detection became possible and two groups reported positive results in animals [57, 81]. In subsequent studies, Niedre et al. [82] showed that the total singlet oxygen signal detected during PDT of tumor cell suspensions correlated well with cell survival over a wide range of treatment conditions. These results have been confirmed in animals which also show a good correlation between cumulative singlet oxygen signals and biological response [83]. There are no reports of measurements during PDT in humans even though this is highly feasible for easily accessible lesions such as skin cancers.

Even with state-of-the-art instrumentation, singlet oxygen luminescence detection is difficult. This is due to a combination of factors including the weakness of the luminescence and the low quantum efficiency (~1 %) of the detectors [75]. As a result, the luminescence is difficult to measure since the overall signal also contains stronger sources of luminescence, including photosensitizer and cell tissue fluorescence [84]. Due to the low signal, fiber optic probes cannot be used to collect the singlet oxygen luminescence and acceptable signal-to-noise ratios can only be obtained by integrating the signal over a significant volume of irradiated tissue [5]. In addition, the instrumentation is very complex and significantly more expensive compared to that required for continuous wave fluorescence measurements in the visible spectrum.

Dose-Rate Effects

The biological response to PDT depends not only on light fluence but also on the rate at which light is delivered. Dose-rate effects may be due to biological and/or physical mechanisms. As fluence rates are reduced (corresponding to longer treatment times), cell repair and responses to oxidative stress become important [85–87]. Additionally, physical mechanisms involving photosensitizer ground-state depletion during pulsed irradiation and fluence-rate-dependent photochemical oxygen depletion are also important factors influencing biological response to PDT.

PDT with short-pulse lasers has been shown to be less effective compared to continuous wave irradiation for equivalent average fluence rates [88]. This is attributed to the finite number of sensitizer molecules in the tissue volume. If a significant fraction of these is excited during the initial part of the laser pulse, photons in the remainder of the pulse will be wasted due to the reduced likelihood of absorption and subsequent singlet oxygen production.

Oxygen depletion, the second physical mechanism for dose-rate effects, typically occurs on a timescale of seconds and depends on the average fluence rate. Simply stated, oxygen depletion occurs when PDT-induced photochemical oxygen consumption exceeds the ability of the microvasculature to deliver oxygen to the irradiated tissue. Tromberg et al. [89] were the first to show that oxygen concentration was reversibly reduced during PDT irradiation. Subsequently, biophysical models have shown that oxygen depletion is likely under typical PDT treatment conditions [90, 91]. These modeling studies have been verified by a number of other groups [92–95]. There is now substantial evidence that PDT is less effective at high fluence rates [66, 90, 92, 96, 97].

Delivery of light and/or photosensitizer at very low dose rates is a potential strategy for overcoming the ineffectiveness of PDT at high fluence rates. This has been termed metronomic PDT (mPDT) [98] and must be distinguished from treatments in which the light dose rate is only slightly reduced (by a factor of 2 or 3) in order to avoid oxygen depletion. Metronomic PDT using ALA in a rat brain tumor model has been shown capable of producing tumor cell (glioma) killing through apoptosis without inducing any measurable damage to normal brain. Furthermore, no necrotic cell death was found in the tumor. This is a particularly interesting observation since necrotic cell death triggers inflammatory responses which may result in additional secondary damage to normal brain. With regard to intracranial treatments, another rationale for mPDT is that single high dose-rate PDT treatments are unlikely to result in the delivery of a tumoricidal dose beyond about 2 cm with current photosensitizers. This is due to an inability to deliver a sufficiently high light dose at depth in a clinically acceptable treatment time, especially when PDT is given intraoperatively to the surface of the resection bed. However, delivering the light over a much longer period (hours, days, or weeks) relaxes this constraint. Such a protracted delivery scheme requires specialized indwelling applicators such as those used for intracranial brachytherapy (Fig. 4a, b) [99].

The low dose-rate PDT regime has been explored extensively in vitro using human glioma spheroids [100]. Specifically, enhanced efficacy of ALA-PDT at $\leq$10 mW cm^{-2} was demonstrated and repetitive low fluence rate treatments resulted in much higher tumor cell kill than single treatments (Fig. 4c). Collectively, the photobiological findings from the mPDT and low dose-rate studies provide a compelling rationale for investigating low and very low dose rate PDT, especially for the treatment of high-grade glioma.

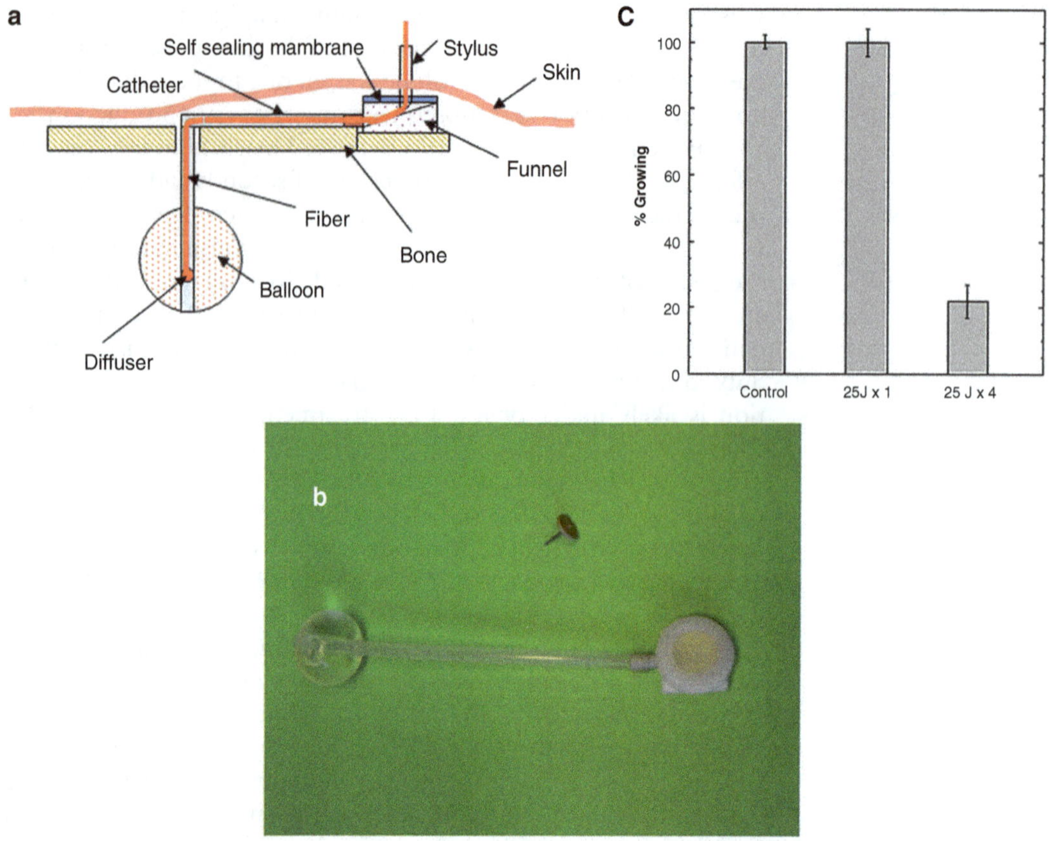

Fig. 4 Low dose-rate PDT. (**a**) Schematic and (**b**) photograph of indwelling balloon applicator for prolonged light delivery to the surgical resection cavity. The optical fiber is connected to a laser and the applicator is left in place following wound closure, (**c**) in vitro ALA-PDT responses in glioma spheroids showing suppression of spheroid growth following single low dose-rate (2.5 mW cm^{-2}) treatment or repetitive treatments (at weeks 0, 1, 2, and 3). Each data point represents % growth 12 weeks after the first treatment

Summary

PDT dosimetry is complex as it depends on a number of difficult-to-measure parameters. A further confounding factor is the dynamic interplay between these parameters. There are a number of established dosimetric techniques of varying degrees of complexity. The method chosen is typically dictated by the application and the level of physics support.

Widespread clinical acceptance of PDT will require strategies for accurate determination of the PDT dose. In contrast to radiation therapy, the dose is not measured directly in PDT—it is inferred from a number of indirect measurements including sensitizer photobleaching, oxygen perfusion, and light fluence rate. Direct dosimetry approaches involving measurement of the 1270 nm singlet oxygen luminescence appear promising. Unfortunately, with current state-of-the-art singlet oxygen luminescence detection systems, the weak 1270 nm emission can only be measured at tissue surfaces. This limitation may be overcome with the development of fiber-coupled nanostructure detectors facilitating interstitial detection of singlet oxygen [101].

Rigorous PDT dosimetry approaches have been implemented recently in a number of clinical trials involving prostate cancer [61, 102] and basal cell carcinoma [62]. Such approaches, based on the principles discussed herein, may help establish PDT as a viable treatment option to radiation therapies such as the brachytherapy techniques used in the treatment of prostate cancer.

References

1. Raab O. Über die Wirkung fluoreszierender Stoffe and Infusorien. Z Biol. 1900;39: 524–46.
2. Dougherty TJ, Kaufman JE, Goldfarb A, Weisshaupt KR, Boyle D, Mittleman A. Photoradiation therapy for the treatment of malignant tumors. Cancer Res. 1978;38: 2628–35.
3. Dougherty TJ, Lawrence G, Kaufman JH. Photoradiation in the treatment of recurrent breast carcinoma. J Natl Cancer Inst. 1979;62:231–7.
4. Wilson BC, Patterson MS. The physics of photodynamic therapy. Phys Med Biol. 1986;31:327–60.
5. Wilson BC, Patterson MS. The physics, biophysics and technology of photodynamic therapy. Phys Med Biol. 2008;53:R61–109.
6. Hecht E. Optics. Reading, MA: Addison-Wesley; 1987.
7. Cheong W, Prahl SA, Welch AJ. A review of the optical properties of biological tissues. IEEE J Quant Electron. 1990;26:2166–85.
8. van de Hulst HC. Light scattering by small particles. New York: Dover; 1981.
9. Beer A, Lambert J. Einleitung in die höhere Optik. 1854.
10. Huppert TJ. History of diffuse optical spectroscopy of human tissue. In: Madsen SJ, editor. Optical methods and instrumentation in brain imaging and therapy. New York: Springer; 2013. p. 23–56.
11. Ishimaru A. Wave propagation and scattering in random media. New York: Academic; 1979. Ch 7 and 9.
12. Star WM. Diffusion theory of light transport. In: Welch AJ, van Gemert MJC, editors. Optical thermal response of laser-irradiated tissue. New York: Plenum; 1995. p. 131–206.
13. Henyey LG, Greenstein JL. Diffuse radiation in the galaxy. Astrophys J. 1941;93:70–83.
14. Chandrasekhar S. Radiative transfer. London: Oxford University Press; 1950.
15. Rybicki G. The searchlight problem with isotropic scattering. J Quant Spectros Radiat Transf. 1971;11:827–49.
16. Metropolis N, Ulam S. The Monte Carlo method. J Am Stat Assoc. 1949;44:335–41.
17. Wilson BC, Adam G. A Monte Carlo model for the absorption and flux distributions of light in tissue. Med Phys. 1983;10:824–30.
18. Flock ST, Patterson MS, Wilson BC, Wyman DR. Monte-Carlo modeling of light-propagation in highly scattering tissues. I. Model predictions and comparison with diffusion theory. IEEE Trans Biomed Eng. 1989;36:1162–8.
19. Farrell TJ, Patterson MS, Wilson BC. A diffusion theory model of spatially resolved, steady-state diffuse reflectance for the noninvasive determination of tissue optical properties *in vivo*. Med Phys. 1992;19:879–88.
20. Wang LH, Jacques SL, Zheng LQ. MCML—Monte Carlo modeling of light transport in multilayered tissues. Comput Methods Programs Biomed. 1995;47:131–46.
21. Zhu C, Liu Q. Review of Monte Carlo modeling of light transport in tissues. J Biomed Opt. 2013;18:050902.
22. Colasanti A, Guida G, Kisslinger A, Liuzzi R, Quarto M, Riccio P, Roberti G, Villani F. Multiple processor version of a Monte Carlo code for photon transport in turbid media. Comput Phys Commun. 2000;132:84–93.

23. Alerstam E, Svensson T, Andersson-Engels S. Parallel computing with graphic processing units for high-speed Monte Carlo simulation of photon migration. J Biomed Opt. 2008;13:060504.
24. Lo WCY, Redmond K, Lilge L, Luu J, Chow P, Rose J. Hardware acceleration of a Monte Carlo simulation for photodynamic therapy treatment planning. J Biomed Opt. 2009;14:014019.
25. Pratx G, Xing L. Monte Carlo simulation of photon migration in a cloud computing environment with MapReduce. J Biomed Opt. 2011;16:125003.
26. Barajas O, Ballangrud AM, Miller GG, Moore RB, Tulip J. Monte Carlo modeling of angular radiance in tissue phantoms and human prostate: PDT light dosimetry. Phys Med Biol. 1997;42:1675–87.
27. Liu B, Farrell TJ, Patterson MS. A dynamic model for ALA-PDT of skin: simulation of temporal and spatial distributions of ground-state oxygen, photosensitizer and singlet oxygen. Phys Med Biol. 2010;55:5913–32.
28. Valentine RM, Brown CTA, Moseley H, Ibbotson SH, Wood K. Monte Carlo modeling of *in vivo* protoporphyrin IX fluorescence and singlet oxygen production during photodynamic therapy for patients presenting with superficial basal cell carcinomas. J Biomed Opt. 2011;16:048002.
29. Valentine RM, Wood K, Brown CTA, Ibbotson SH, Moseley H. Monte Carlo simulations for optimal light delivery in photodynamic therapy of non-melanoma skin cancer. Phys Med Biol. 2012;57:6327–45.
30. Wyman DR, Patterson MS, Wilson BC. Similarity relations for the interaction parameters in radiation transport. Appl Opt. 1989;28:5243–9.
31. Star WM. Light dosimetry *in vivo*. Phys Med Biol. 1997;42:763–87.
32. Hull EL, Foster TH. Steady-state reflectance spectroscopy in the P_3 approximation. J Opt Soc Am A. 2001;18:584–99.
33. Patterson MS, Wilson BC, Wyman DR. The propagation of optical radiation in tissue. 1. Models of radiation transport and their application. Lasers Med Sci. 1991;6:155–68.
34. Kubelka P, Munk F. Ein beitrag zur optic der farbanstriche. Z Tech Phys. 1931;12:593–601.
35. Kubelka P. New contributions to the optics of intensely light scattering materials. J Opt Soc Am. 1948;38:448–57.
36. Prahl SA, van Gemert MJC, Welch AJ. Determining the optical properties of turbid media using the adding-doubling method. Appl Opt. 1993;32:559–68.
37. Pickering JW, Prahl SA, van Wieringen N, Beek JF, Sterenborg HJ, van Gemert MJC. Double-integrating-sphere system for measuring the optical properties of tissue. Appl Opt. 1993;32:339–410.
38. Pickering JW, Bosman S, Posthumus P, Blokland P, Beek JF, van Gemert MJC. Changes in the optical properties (at 632.8 nm) of slowly heated myocardium. Appl Opt. 1993;32:367–71.
39. Press WH, Teukolsky SA, Vetterling WT, Flannery BP. Numerical recipes in C: the art of scientific computing. New York: Cambridge University Press; 1992. p. 213–4.
40. Haskell RC, Svaasand LO, Tsay T-T, Feng T-C, McAdams MS, Tromberg BJ. Boundary conditions for the diffusion equation in radiative transfer. J Opt Soc Am A. 1994; 11:2727–41.
41. Kienle A, Patterson MS. Improved solutions of the steady-state and time-resolved diffusion equations or reflectance from a semi-infinite turbid medium. J Opt Soc Am A. 1997;14:246–54.
42. Hull EL, Nichols MG, Foster TH. Quantitative near-infrared spectroscopy of tissue-simulating phantoms containing erythrocytes. Phys Med Biol. 1998;43:3381–404.
43. Kienle A, Patterson MS, Dognitz N, Bays R, Wagnieres G, van den Bergh H. Noninvasive determination of the optical properties of two-layered turbid media. Appl Opt. 1998; 37:779–91.
44. Driver I, Lowdell CP, Ash DV. In vivo measurements of the optical interaction coefficients of human tumours at 630 nm. Phys Med Biol. 1991;36:805–13.
45. Li J, Zhu TC. Determination of *in vivo* light fluence distribution in a heterogeneous prostate during photodynamic therapy. Phys Med Biol. 2008;53:2103–14.
46. Patterson MS, Chance B, Wilson BC. Time resolved reflectance and transmittance for the non-invasive measurement of tissue optical properties. Appl Opt. 1989;28:2331–6.
47. Moulton JD. Diffusion theory modelling of picosecond laser pulse propagation in turbid media. M. Eng. Thesis, McMaster University, Hamilton, ON, Canada; 1990.
48. Madsen SJ, Wilson BC, Patterson MS, Park YD, Jacques SL, Hefetz Y. Experimental tests of a simple diffusion model for the estimation of scattering and absorption coefficients of turbid media from time resolved diffuse

reflectance measurements. Appl Opt. 1992;31:3509–17.

49. Fishkin J, Gratton E, vandeVen MJ, Mantulin WW. Diffusion of intensity modulated near-infrared light in turbid media. Proc SPIE. 1991;1431:122–35.
50. O'Leary MA, Boas DA, Chance B, Yodh AG. Refraction of diffuse photon density waves. Phys Rev Lett. 1992;69:2658–61.
51. Tromberg BJ, Svaasand LO, Tsay T-T, Haskell RC. Properties of photon density waves in multiple-scattering media. Appl Opt. 1993;32:607–16.
52. Patterson MS, Moulton JD, Wilson BC, Berndt KW, Lakowicz JR. Frequency-domain reflectance for the determination of the scattering and absorption properties of tissue. Appl Opt. 1991;30:4474–6.
53. Madsen SJ, Anderson ER, Haskell RC, Tromberg BJ. Portable, high-bandwidth frequency-domain photon migration instrument for tissue spectroscopy. Opt Lett. 1994;19:1934–6.
54. Pham TH, Coquoz O, Fishkin JB, Anderson E, Tromberg BJ. Broad bandwidth frequency domain instrument for quantitative tissue optical spectroscopy. Rev Sci Inst. 2000; 71:2500–13.
55. Redmond RW, Gamlin JN. A compilation of singlet oxygen yields from biologically relevant molecules. Photochem Photobiol. 1999;70:391–475.
56. Weishaupt KR, Gomer CJ, Dougherty TJ. Identification of singlet oxygen as cytotoxic agent in photoinactivation of a murine tumor. Cancer Res. 1976;36:2326–9.
57. Niedre M, Patterson MS, Wilson BC. Direct near-infrared luminescence detection of singlet oxygen generated by photodynamic therapy in cells *in vitro* and tissues *in vivo*. Photochem Photobiol. 2002;75:382–91.
58. Foote CS. Definition of type-I and type-II photosensitized oxidation. Photochem Photobiol. 1991;54:659.
59. Farrell TJ, Wilson BC, Patterson MS, Olivo MC. Comparison of the *in vivo* photodynamic threshold dose for Photofrin, mono- and tetrasulfonated aluminum phthalocyanine using a rat liver model. Photochem Photobiol. 1998;68:394–9.
60. Wilson BC, Patterson MS, Lilge L. Implicit and explicit dosimetry in photodynamic therapy: a new paradigm. Lasers Med Sci. 1997; 12:182–99.
61. Weersink RA, Bogaards A, Gertner M, Davidson SR, Zhang K, Netchev G, Trachtenberg J, Wilson BC. Techniques for delivery and monitoring of TOOKAD (WST09)-mediated photodynamic therapy of the prostate: clinical experience and practicalities. J Photochem Photobiol B. 2005; 79:211–22.
62. Thompson MS, Johansson A, Johansson T, Andersson-Engels S, Svanberg S, Bendsoe N, Svanberg K. Clinical system for interstitial photodynamic therapy with combined on-line dosimetry measurements. Appl Opt. 2005;44:4023–31.
63. Zhu TC, Finlay JC, Hahn SM. Determination of the distribution of light, optical properties, drug concentration, and tissue oxygenation *in vivo* in human prostate during motexafin lutetium-mediated photodynamic therapy. J Photochem Photobiol B. 2005;79:231–41.
64. Zeng H, Korbelik M, McLean DI, MacAulay C, Lui H. Monitoring photoproduct formation and photobleaching by fluorescence spectroscopy has the potential to improve PDT dosimetry with a verteporfin-like photosensitizer. Photochem Photobiol. 2002;75:398–405.
65. Georgakoudi I, Nichols MG, Foster TH. The mechanism of Photofrin photobleaching and its consequences for photodynamic dosimetry. Photochem Photobiol. 1997;65:135–44.
66. Robinson DJ, de Bruijn HS, van der Veen N, Stringer MR, Brown SB, Star WM. Fluorescence photobleaching of ALA-induced protoporphyrin IX during photodynamic therapy of normal hairless mouse skin: the effect of light dose and irradiance and the resulting biological effect. Photochem Photobiol. 1998;67:140–9.
67. Diamond KR, Patterson MS, Farrell TJ. Quantification of fluorophore concentration in tissue-simulating media by fluorescence measurements with a single optical fiber. Appl Opt. 2003;42:2436–42.
68. Pogue BW, Burke G. Fiber-optic bundle design for quantitative fluorescence measurement from tissue. Appl Opt. 1998;37:7429–36.
69. Farrell TJ, Patterson MS, Hayward JE, Wilson BC, Beck ER. A CCD and neural network based instrument for the non-invasive determination of tissue optical properties *in vivo*. Proc SPIE. 1994;2135:117–28.
70. Synytsya A, Kral V, Matejka P, Pouckova P, Volka K, Sessler JL. Biodistribution assessment of a lutetium (III) texaphyrin analogue in tumor-bearing mice using NIR Fourier-transform Raman spectroscopy. Photochem Photobiol. 2004;79:453–60.

71. Buerk DG. Measuring tissue PO_2 with microelectrodes. Methods Enzymol. 2004;381: 665–90.
72. Papkovsky DB. Methods in optical oxygen sensing: protocols and critical analyses. Methods Enzymol. 2004;381:715–35.
73. Braun RD, Lanzen JL, Snyder SA, Dewhirst MW. Comparison of tumor and normal tissue oxygen tension measurements using OxyLite or microelectrodes in rodents. Am J Physiol Heart Circ Physiol. 2001;280:H2533–44.
74. Dysart JS, Patterson MS. Characterization of Photofrin photobleaching for singlet oxygen dose estimation during photodynamic therapy of MLL cells *in vitro*. Phys Med Biol. 2005;50:2597–616.
75. Jarvi MT, Patterson MS, Wilson BC. Insights into photodynamic therapy dosimetry: simultaneous singlet oxygen luminescence and photosensitizer photobleaching measurements. Biophys J. 2012;102:661–71.
76. Finlay JC, Mitra S, Patterson MS, Foster TH. Photobleaching kinetics of Photofrin *in vivo* and in multicell tumor spheroids indicate two simultaneous bleaching mechanisms. Phys Med Biol. 2004;49:4837–60.
77. Dysart JS, Patterson MS. Photobleaching kinetics, photoproduct formation, and dose estimation during ALA induced PpIX PDT of MLL cells under well oxygenated and hypoxic conditions. Photochem Photobiol Sci. 2006;5:73–81.
78. Rodgers MAJ. On the problem involved in detecting the luminescence from singlet oxygen in biological specimens. J Photochem Photobiol B Biol. 1988;1:371–3.
79. Patterson MS, Madsen SJ, Wilson BC. Experimental tests of the feasibility of singlet oxygen luminescence monitoring *in vivo* during photodynamic therapy. J Photochem Photobiol. 1990;5:69–84.
80. Gorman AA, Rodgers MAJ. Current perspectives of singlet oxygen detection in biological environments. J Photochem Photobiol B Biol. 1992;14:159–76.
81. Hirano T, Kohno E, Nishiwaki M. Detection of near infrared emission from singlet oxygen in PDT with an experimental tumor bearing mouse. J Jpn Soc Laser Surg Med. 2002;22:99–108.
82. Niedre MJ, Secord AJ, Patterson MS, Wilson BC. *In vitro* tests of the validity of singlet oxygen luminescence measurements as a dose metric in photodynamic therapy. Cancer Res. 2003;63:7986–94.
83. Niedre MJ, Yu CS, Patterson MS, Wilson BC. Singlet oxygen luminescence as an *in vivo* photodynamic therapy dose metric: validation in normal mouse skin with topical aminolevulinic acid. Br J Cancer. 2005;92:298–304.
84. Jimenez-Banzo A, Ragas X, et al. Time-resolved methods in biophysics. 7. Photon counting vs. analog time-resolved singlet oxygen phosphorescence detection. Photochem Photobiol Sci. 2008;7:1003–10.
85. Luna MC, Wong S, Gomer CJ. Photodynamic therapy mediated induction of early response genes. Cancer Res. 1994;54:1374–80.
86. Oleinick NL, Evans HH. The photobiology of photodynamic therapy: cellular targets and mechanisms. Radiat Res. 1998;150:S146–56.
87. Veenhuizen RB, Stewart FA. The importance of fluence rate in photodynamic therapy—is there a parallel with ionizing radiation dose-rate effects. Radiother Oncol. 1995;37:131–5.
88. Sterenborg HJCM, vanGemert MJC. Photodynamic therapy with pulsed light sources: a theoretical analysis. Phys Med Biol. 1996;41:835–49.
89. Tromberg BJ, Orenstein A, Kimel S, Barker SJ, Hyatt J, Nelson JS, Berns MW. *In vivo* tumor oxygen-tension measurements for the evaluation of the efficiency of photodynamic therapy. Photochem Photobiol. 1990;52: 375–85.
90. Foster TH, Murant RS, Bryant RG, Knox RS, Gibson SL, Hilf R. Oxygen consumption and diffusion effects in photodynamic therapy. Radiat Res. 1991;126:296–303.
91. Foster TH, Gao L. Dosimetry in photodynamic therapy—oxygen and the critical importance of capillary density. Radiat Res. 1992;130:379–83.
92. Busch TM. Local physiological changes during photodynamic therapy. Lasers Surg Med. 2006;38:494–9.
93. Chen Q, Chen H, Hetzel FW. Tumor oxygenation changes post-photodynamic therapy. Photochem Photobiol. 1996;63: 128–31.
94. Chen Q, Huang Z, Chen H, Shapiro H, Beckers J, Hetzel FW. Improvement of tumor response by manipulation of tumor oxygenation during photodynamic therapy. Photochem Photobiol. 2002;76:197–203.
95. Henderson BW, et al. Photofrin photodynamic therapy can significantly deplete or preserve oxygenation in human basal cell carcinomas during treatment depending on fluence rate. Cancer Res. 2000;60:525–9.
96. Coutier S, Bezdetnaya LN, Foster TH, Parache RM, Guillemin F. Effect of irradiation fluence rate on the efficacy of photodynamic therapy and tumor oxygenation in meta-

tetra(hydroxyphenyl)chlorine (mTHPC)-sensitized HT29 xenografts in nude mice. Radiat Res. 2002;158:339–45.

97. Henderson BW, Gollnick SO, Snyder JW, Busch TM, Kousis PC, Cheney RT, Morgan J. Choice of oxygen-conserving treatment regimen determines the inflammatory response and outcome of photodynamic therapy in tumors. Cancer Res. 2004;64: 2120–6.

98. Bisland SK, Lilge L, Lin A, Rusnov R, Wilson BC. Metronomic photodynamic therapy as a new paradigm for photodynamic therapy: rationale and pre-clinical evaluation of technical feasibility for treating malignant brain tumors. Photochem Photobiol. 2004;80: 2–30.

99. Madsen SJ, Sun C-H, Tromberg BJ, Hirschberg H. Development of a novel indwelling balloon applicator for optimizing light delivery in photodynamic therapy. Lasers Surg Med. 2001;29:406–12.

100. Madsen SJ, Sun C-H, Tromberg BJ, Hirschberg H. Repetitive 5-aminolevulinic acid-mediated photodynamic therapy on human glioma spheroids. J Neurooncol. 2003;62:243–50.

101. Gemmell NR, McCarthy A, Liu B, Tanner MG, Dorenbos SD, Zwiller V, Patterson MS, Buller GS, Wilson BC, Hadfield RH. Singlet oxygen luminescence detection with a fiber-coupled superconducting nanowire single-photon detector. Opt Express. 2013;21: 5005–13.

102. Du KL, Mick R, Busch TM, Zhu TC, Finlay JC, Yu G, Yodh AG, Malkowicz SB, Smith D, Whittington R, Stripp D, Hahn SM. Preliminary results of interstitial motexafin lutetium-mediated PDT for prostate cancer. Lasers Surg Med. 2006;38:427–34.

Chapter 19

Light Sources, Drugs, and Dosimetry

Jarod C. Finlay and Arash Darafsheh

Introduction

This chapter will address the technical and physical aspects of the light sources, delivery devices, and photosensitizers used in ENT photodynamic therapy (PDT). Effective delivery of treatment light to the target tissue requires appropriate matching of the light source to the tissue, the sensitizer, and the delivery device. The delivery device, typically an optical fiber with a directional or diffusing termination, must be chosen to match the target area and the surrounding geometry.

In order for photodynamic action to occur, the photosensitizer accumulated in the target tissue must be activated by light possessing enough optical power and appropriate wavelength. The emission wavelength of the light source should match the absorption wavelength of the photosensitizer. Most photosensitizers, particularly those derived from porphyrins and chlorins, have multiple absorption peaks: a Soret Band around 400 nm and several Q-bands in 500–700 nm range. The absorption in the Soret band is often an order of magnitude greater than that in the Q-bands; however, selecting a peak in the longer wavelengths is favorable due to the longer penetration depth of light in tissue, so that a larger volume of target tissue can be treated.

Tissue optics also plays a critical role in the distribution of treatment light in tissue. Optical penetration depth (OPD) in a medium is defined as the distance over which the intensity of light decreases to $1/e$ (~37 %) of its initial intensity. OPD in tissue is limited due to scattering and absorption of light and is wavelength dependent, as shown in Fig. 1. For example, the

Brian J.-F. Wong and Justus Ilgner (eds.), *Biomedical Optics in Otorhinolaryngology: Head and Neck Surgery*,
DOI 10.1007/978-1-4939-1758-7_19, © Springer Science+Business Media New York 2016

OPD in the 600–800 nm spectral range is more than twice that in 500–600 nm range [1]. Scattering is the dominant mechanism of light attenuation in tissue, except in highly pigmented tissues and short wavelengths, where absorption is the dominant attenuation process. It should be noted that biological effects are not limited to a distance corresponding to 1 OPD; they can still be observed at ~3 OPD [2].

As mentioned in the previous chapter, there is an "optical window" in tissue between 600 and 1400 nm, where the absorption of light is minimal. However, as the wavelength of light increases, the photon energy decreases and consequently for wavelengths longer than approximately 850 nm the efficiency of the photodynamic process decreases [3–5]. The fundamental limit for longer wavelengths is imposed by the energy required to excite an oxygen molecule from its triplet to singlet excited state. Therefore, the "therapeutic window" for PDT is between 600 and 800 nm.

An "ideal" photosensitizer is assessed based on various biological/physiological, chemical/biochemical/photochemical, physical/photophysical, and economic considerations [8, 9]. Low dark toxicity, high target selectivity, non-mutagenicity, pain-free therapy, appropriate administration method (oral, systemic, or topical), short cutaneous photosensitivity period, high chemical stability, water solubility for easy transport in the body, availability of chemical compounds and ease of synthesis, high quantum yield of singlet oxygen, long enough activation wavelength to assure deep optical

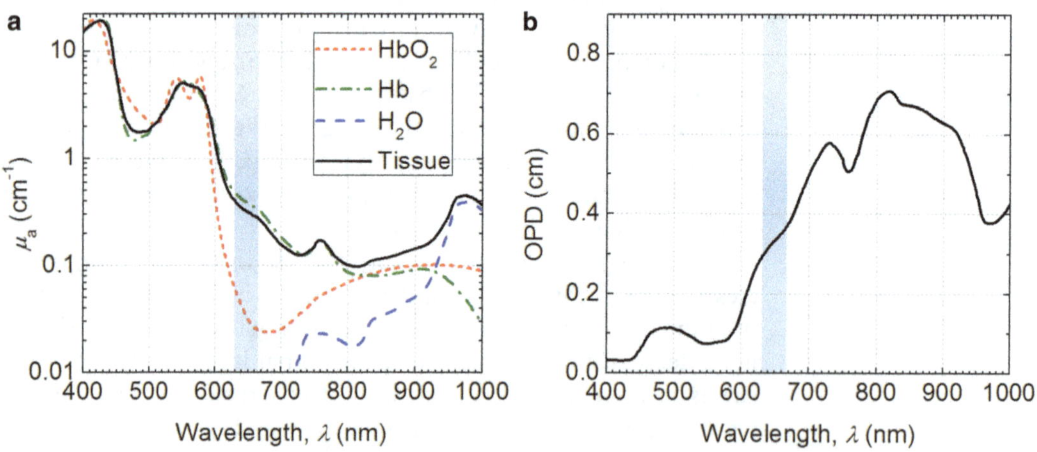

Fig. 1 (**a**) Absorption coefficients, μ_a, of oxy- and deoxyhemoglobin, water, and of tissue composed of 80 % water with 80 % hemoglobin oxygen saturation and (**b**) optical penetration depth of the same tissue. The typical range treatment wavelengths of sensitizers used in ENT PDT are indicated on both figures. Hemoglobin and water absorption data are taken from Finlay et al. [6] and Kou et al. [7], respectively

penetration in tissue, and appropriate fluorescent yield for drug monitoring are some of these considerations. In practice, there is a trade-off among these considerations in development of a photosensitizer for PDT.

PDT photosensitizers have been classified into three categories: (1) first-generation photosensitizers which are porphyrin-based, such as hematoporphyrin derivative (H_pD) developed in the 1970s and early 1980s, (2) second-generation photosensitizers which are modified porphyrin compounds with long absorption wavelength, and (3) third-generation photosensitizers which are modified photosensitizers for selective tumor uptake. Based on their chemical structures, PDT photosensitizers belong to three families: porphyrins, chlorins, or dyes [8].

Photofrin® (porfimer sodium) [10–16], Levulan® (5-ALA, 5-aminolevulinic acid) [17–20], Foscan® (*m*-THPC, *m*-tetrahydroxyphenylchlorin) [21–30], and Photochlor® (HPPH, 2-[1-hexyloxyethyl]-2-devinyl pyropheophorbide-a) [14, 31] at excitation wavelengths of 630, 635, 652, and 665 nm, respectively, have been used in various PDT studies, including head and neck cases. Among them, Photofrin® and Foscan® have been used extensively for head and neck cases [29, 32–41]. It should be noted that ALA is not a sensitizer itself; however, it induces the formation of the sensitizer protoporphyrin IX (PpIX) in vivo through the heme biosynthetic pathway.

Lasers, light-emitting diodes (LEDs), and lamps are three main conventional categories of light sources used for PDT applications. Tumor location, photosensitizer, and optical dose are determining factors for the choice of the light source for PDT [42]. Head and neck cases present a particular challenge, as the geometry is often minimally accessible to external optical fibers.

Light Sources

Lasers

Lasers (an acronym for light amplification by stimulated emission of radiation) are the most commonly used light source for both superficial and interstitial PDT applications. Lasers generate monochromatic light with high power, narrow bandwidth, and precisely controlled wavelength corresponding to a specific photosensitizer. Unlike LED or lamp sources, lasers produce collimated light with small (submillimeter) spot sizes. Lasers can therefore be coupled efficiently with optical fibers for endoscopic or interstitial use. For superficial PDT, the output of the laser is expanded by a set of lenses, known as beam expander, to cover a larger tumor area with uniform irradiance.

A laser fundamentally consists of three components: a gain medium, a resonant cavity, and an energy source, as schematically illustrated in Fig. 2. The resonant cavity is essentially a pair of mirrors facing each other with the gain medium between them. The energy source, or pump, provides energy which excites the molecules of the gain medium to an excited state. Under normal conditions, these molecules would spontaneously emit fluorescence, which would be incoherent and poorly collimated. In a laser, however, the fluorescence light emitted by the gain medium is reflected within the cavity such that it passes through the gain medium multiple times, generating stimulated emission of photons from the gain medium on each pass. Because the stimulated emission is in phase with the light field that stimulated it, this amplification process produces coherent, monochromatic light. One of the mirrors in the cavity is partially transmitting, so a fraction of the light amplified in the cavity is extracted on each reflection, producing a useful beam. Different types of lasers such as dye, metal vapor, and diode lasers have been used for PDT, as detailed below [42, 43]. Currently, diode lasers are the most commonly used laser source in PDT applications. Both pulsed and CW lasers have been used in PDT and the advantage of one over the other is still under investigation.

Dye Lasers

In dye lasers [44], organic dye molecules, such as rhodamine or kiton red, with emission wavelengths in the 600–650 nm range, matching the absorption wavelength of a specific photosensitizer, are used as the lasing medium. The dye is typically a liquid

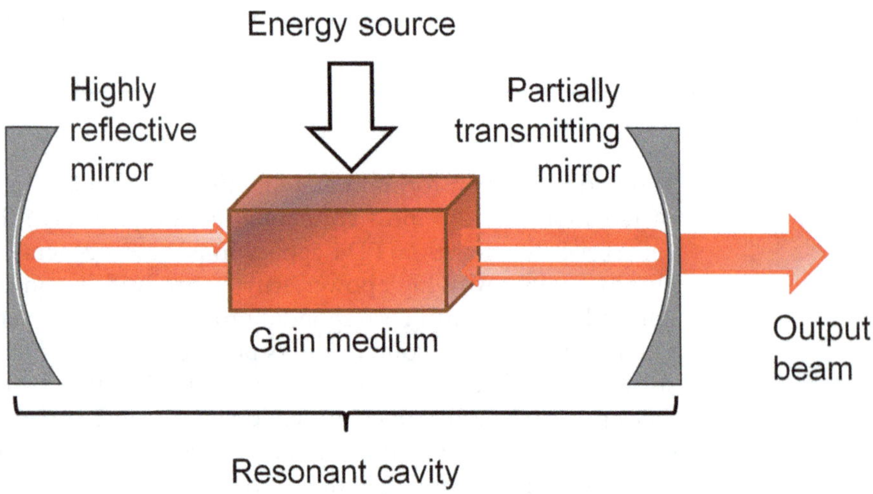

Fig. 2 Schematic illustration of fundamental components of a laser, including gain medium, energy source, and resonant cavity

that is circulated continuously to prevent overheating. Only a small fraction of the dye is in the resonant cavity at any one time. A pump laser, such as an argon, Nd:YAG, copper vapor, or KTP laser, serves as the energy source. In general, practical dye lasers require pump powers of tens of watts. Pump lasers capable of sufficient output power often require high current, high voltage power supplies and water-cooled heat exchangers, limiting their portability, although surgical laser systems have been adapted to pump dye lasers. The absorption wavelength of the laser dye must match the emission wavelength of the pump laser. One particular advantage of dye lasers is that the gain medium generally emits over a wide range of wavelengths. The wavelength at which light amplification is achieved is determined by the geometry of resonant cavity and by tunable filters placed in the beam to narrow the wavelength range over which lasing can occur. Therefore, the dye laser's emission wavelength can be tuned to cover a range of wavelengths corresponding to different photosensitizers. This makes dye lasers versatile and ideally suited to laboratory work; however, due to their large size, difficult portability, high cost, and high maintenance requirements [45], dye lasers have been replaced by diode lasers in most clinical PDT applications.

Diode Lasers

Diode lasers are electrically pumped semiconductor lasers. The energy source in this case is electrical current, which directly excites the semiconductor gain medium. The semiconductor gain medium and the resonant cavity can be manufactured in one compact, solid-state unit. Low-power semiconductor lasers are used in many consumer applications, from laser pointers to optical disk readers. Higher power diode lasers are the main light source currently used in PDT applications. Their advantages, in addition to general advantages of laser sources, are their lighter weight, compactness, portability, stability, and low economic cost. Diode lasers generating up to 8 W of optical power can generally be powered by standard electrical supplies and use air-cooled thermoelectric coolers to maintain temperature. High-power output is often accomplished by combining or "stacking" laser diodes. The result is output with a larger spot size and greater beam divergence than that produced by a dye laser. Coupling into optical fibers can still be efficient, but larger fiber cores may be required in some cases. The disadvantage of diode lasers compared to dye lasers is that a separate diode laser is required for each sensitizer. Modular dye lasers have been proposed [46] to deal with this limitation; however, none are currently approved for clinical use.

LEDs

LEDs are semiconductor light sources. The mechanism of light generation in an LED is similar to that in a diode laser; however, an LED lacks the resonant cavity necessary for stimulated emission and instead emits light spontaneously. LEDs can produce light of a specific wavelength with wider bandwidth (~5 % of the central wavelength) compared to the output spectra of diode lasers, which leads to lower efficiency absorption by the photosensitizer. Their output power is generally lower than that of diode lasers. The main advantage of LEDs over diode lasers is their lower cost. LEDs can be manufactured in different sizes and can be arranged in different configurations. LEDs are suitable for irradiation of superficial tumors [19, 47, 48]. However, arrays of LEDs [49] can be designed for endoscopic or interstitial use [50, 51]. Due to low electrical to optical conversion efficiency of LEDs, thermal effect is a drawback, especially for interstitial applications.

Lamps

Lamps were the earliest artificial light sources used in PDT studies [52, 53]. Incandescent, fluorescent, halogen, xenon arc, metal halide, and sodium lamps have been used in PDT. Although lamps, in principle, can be coupled to light guides, they suffer from huge coupling losses, so they are generally used to directly irradiate the tumor in case of superficial tumors, such as skin or oral cavity. Due to the broadband output spectrum of the lamps, heavy spectral filtering is needed to effectively select the photoactivating wavelength spectral band matching the absorption band of the photosensitizer and to remove the unnecessary infrared and ultraviolet radiations. Simplicity, economic considerations, and a wide illumination field are main advantages of lamps as light sources [54]. However, the use of broadband sources, such as lamps, complicates dosimetry. Because the absorption of light by tissue varies with wavelength, tissue irradiated by a broad beam lamp will effectively see a different spectrum at depth than at the surface. For most sensitizers, this has the effect of adding excitation from shorter wavelengths with shallower penetration in tissue, reducing the overall depth of treatment. In some cases, where very superficial treatment is desired, this is an advantage, but this is not often the case for ENT lesions.

A side effect of ability of lamps to excite photosensitizers is that the lamps used to visualize the tissue during intraoperative PDT procedures can cause unwanted photodynamic effects. The intensity and duration of illumination should therefore be minimized, and surgical lights, which are typically very intense and contain a significant spectral component in the sensitizers' Soret band, should be filtered whenever possible.

Delivery Devices

Successful PDT depends on the ability of localized light delivery throughout the entire treatment region. The tumor, therefore, should be optically accessible either directly, endoscopically, or interstitially through specially designed light delivery probes. Based on the mode of light delivery to the target tissue, PDT optical delivery devices are categorized into three groups: noncontact, contact, and interstitial probes.

Optical fibers are the main component of flexible light delivery systems. Optical fibers are, fundamentally, composed of two concentric dielectric cylinders: core and cladding. Usually, there is a protective buffer layer (plastic) around the cladding and a protective jacket around the fiber. As schematically shown in Fig. 3, the core is surrounded by the cladding and has slightly higher refractive index than the cladding ($n_c > n_{cl}$); therefore, a ray of light incident within the "acceptance cone" of the fiber on the entrance surface of the core (red ray in Fig. 3b) will impinge on the core-cladding boundary at an angle greater than the critical angle, $\theta_c = \mathrm{Sin}^{-1}(n_{cl}/n_c)$, and is "trapped" inside the core, totally internally reflected at the core-cladding boundary and guided through the core. Rays incident on the entrance face of the fiber

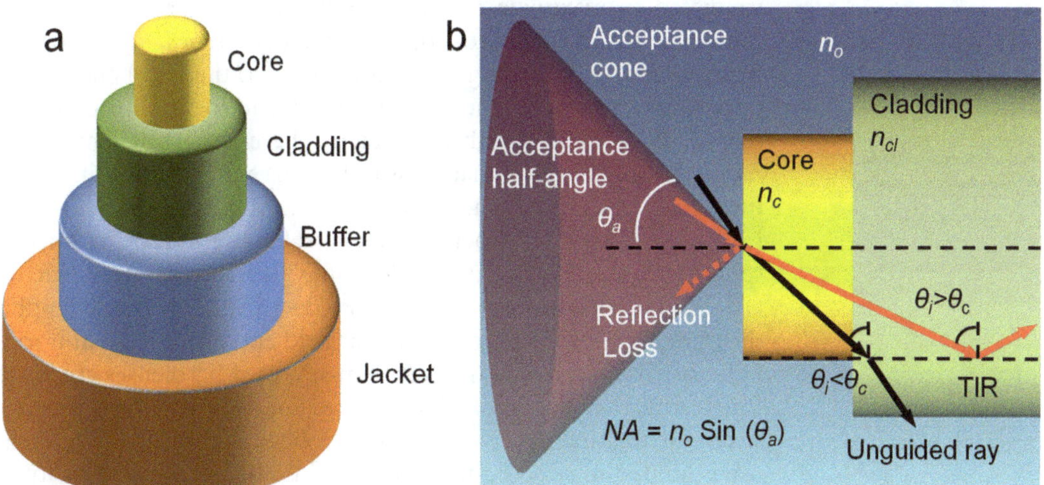

Fig. 3 (**a**) Structure of an optical fiber and (**b**) illustration of the acceptance cone of the fiber. A ray of light incident within the acceptance cone on the entrance face of the fiber will strike the core-cladding interface with an angle (θ_i) greater than the critical angle (θ_c) and is guided through the fiber by total internal reflection (TIR). Panel (**b**) is reproduced from Darafsheh [55] with permission

with angles greater than the acceptance angle will impinge on the core-cladding boundary at angles smaller than θ_c, will be only partially reflected at each encounter with the core-cladding boundary and will quickly leak out of the fiber. The acceptance angle defines a cone of angles (acceptance cone) within which all rays are guided in the fiber. For optical power delivery, multimode fibers, which can be considered "light pipes," are used.

Transmission loss in optical fibers is extremely small for short-haul applications. Coupling loss and reflection losses at both ends of the fiber are minimized by antireflection coating of the fiber ends. As a result, for practical applications, the fiber can be made long enough to accommodate any treatment configuration (including having the laser in a separate room from the patient), with negligible loss of power in transmission. Special couplers are designed to optimize the coupling between laser and fiber by matching their numerical apertures (NA). The NA is a quantitative parameter of optical fibers and is related to the critical angle in the fiber that defines a cone of angles within which all rays are guided in the fiber by total internal reflection, as shown in Fig. 3b. Mathematically, $\mathrm{NA} = n_o \sin\theta_a = \sqrt{n_c^2 - n_{cl}^2}$, where n_o is the refractive index of the medium in which the fiber's tip is inserted ($n_o = 1$ for air) and θ_a is the half-angle of the fiber's acceptance cone, as illustrated in Fig. 3b. Practically, the NA is defined as the sine of the angle at which the output optical power falls to 5 % of the peak value.

In PDT applications, since the treatment area should be uniformly irradiated to maximize the damage to the malignant tissues and minimize the damage to adjacent healthy tissues, a micro (or macro)-lens or a diffusing cap is connected to the distal end of the optical fiber to modify the output optical field to a uniform illumination. Back focal length of a microsphere-lens (ball lens) with radius $R >> \lambda$ (λ is illumination wavelength) and refractive index n, measured from its "shadow-side" pole, is given by $R(2-n)/[2(n-1)]$; therefore, depending on its refractive index, the microsphere focuses light on its "shadow-side" surface ($n \approx 2$), inside of ($n > 2$), and outside of the lens ($n < 2$) [55]; the focused light diverges while propagating to the far field and produces a uniform light distribution over a desired circular area. Microlenses are ideal for treatment of flat, accessible surfaces and have been used extensively for treatment of skin lesions. In head and neck PDT, their use is limited to superficial disease, for instance in the oral cavity.

On the other hand, diffusing tips uniformly distribute the transmitted light along their length. Fibers with diffusing tips are made by introducing surface roughness or scattering particles in the cladding-core boundary along the desired length of the tip. The resulting applicator emits light approximately isotropically and uniformly along its length. Probes with diffusing tips can be applied interstitially into the tissue via transparent catheters. Interstitial PDT can take advantage of the mature technology already developed for interstitial brachytherapy. In brachytherapy, radioactive seeds incorporated into plastic strands or ribbons are inserted into plastic catheters implanted in the tissue and deliver a dose of ionizing radiation. Because the radioactive seeds in most common use are of similar diameter to a diffusing optical fiber, these same catheters can accommodate optical fibers with little or no modification. Furthermore, two- and three-dimensional imaging techniques developed to localize radioactive seeds within tissue can be applied to optical fibers with only minor modification. Some manufacturers supply optical fibers with radio-opaque markers at their ends specifically to facilitate X-ray imaging for this purpose. Although commercially available diffusors are generally designed to provide uniform emission over their length, it is possible to make custom diffusors, with light emission profiles designed to match specific treatment plans [56].

For hollow organs, such as larynx [20] or esophagus [57], diffuser balloons [58] are used to provide uniform illumination over the interior tissue surface. These devices consist of a linear diffuser inserted into a cylindrical balloon. The balloon serves two purposes: it ensures that the diffuser is centered in the organ so that all sides receive equal irradiance, and also provides a uniform, smooth surface by dilating the tissue. This is particularly important in tissues such as the esophagus which might otherwise fold and contract around the applicator, partially shielding some areas of tissue, while overexposing others.

Specific treatment geometries may require specialized delivery devices. For instance, for the treatment of nasopharyngeal disease, Nyst et al. [59] have developed a delivery device consisting of dual catheters for the insertion of diffusing fibers and isotropic detectors and black silicone shielding designed to protect the soft palate.

Detectors and Dosimetry

Dosimetry by definition refers to the measurement of dose delivered to the target tissue. In the case of PDT, "dose" in its simplest form is taken to be the light energy delivered per unit mass of tissue (in J/kg). This definition of dose is consistent with that used in ionizing radiation therapy (i.e., Gy). However, sometimes the term dose or optical dose is used to indicate delivered radiant energy fluence, i.e., optical energy delivered to unit surface of the target tissue (in J/cm^2), that makes the term "optical dose" context dependent. Nevertheless, throughout this section, we will use "PDT dose" to mean energy delivered per unit mass of tissue. More sophisticated measures of photodynamic dose will be discussed in detail later in the chapter. Any definition of dosimetry, however, must include accurate quantification of the intensity of light delivered to the tissue, as described in the previous chapter. This includes accurate calibration of the light source and delivery devices, as well as any measurements made during treatment.

Light Source Calibration

Proper calibration of the light source used for PDT is essential to accurate light delivery. Clinical dye and diode lasers are generally digitally controlled, allowing the output power to be set using a digital display. Internal monitoring electronics ensure constant output; however, they generally are not capable of monitoring transmission losses in the fiber or changes in fiber output. Therefore, care should be taken to ensure that the power delivered to the treatment device is accurate. Guidelines for calibration of PDT light sources have recently been published by the American Association of Physicists in Medicine (AAPM) [60]. The following discussion generally follows these guidelines.

Most light sources require some warm-up time to stabilize before they should be calibrated. Dye lasers may exhibit instability in power until they reach thermal equilibrium. Incandescent lamps exhibit highly temperature-dependent power consumption. These sources should be allowed to warm up before setting the source power.

Diode lasers have the additional complication that their output wavelength is temperature dependent. Diode lasers are typically actively cooled and maintain their wavelength via precise thermal regulation. However, at high power, the temperature, and therefore the wavelength, may drift. Therefore, it is recommended that diode lasers be warmed up and both the power and wavelength allowed to stabilize before power or wavelength calibration measurements are made.

The power transmitted to the tissue will depend on the delivery device being used. If possible, the delivery device and the laser should be calibrated together, and the power should be measured at the output of the delivery device. If the delivery device produces collimated output, as with flat-cut fibers and microlenses, the output can be measured with a calibrated optical power meter. In general, thermopile detectors are appropriate for measuring clinically relevant laser power. The geometry for measuring the power of a fiber with flat-cut and microlens tip is shown in Fig. 4a, b. The power meter should be sufficiently large and positioned close enough to the fiber termination that the light field under-fills the detector and the entire beam is collected. The irradiance at any point in the light field can then be calculated by dividing the measured optical power by the area of the projected beam. This calculation assumes that the beam is spatially uniform, which should be verified by independent measurement.

When a diffusing applicator is used, an optical power meter will generally only measure a fraction of the light output from the device. In this case, an integrating sphere should be used to

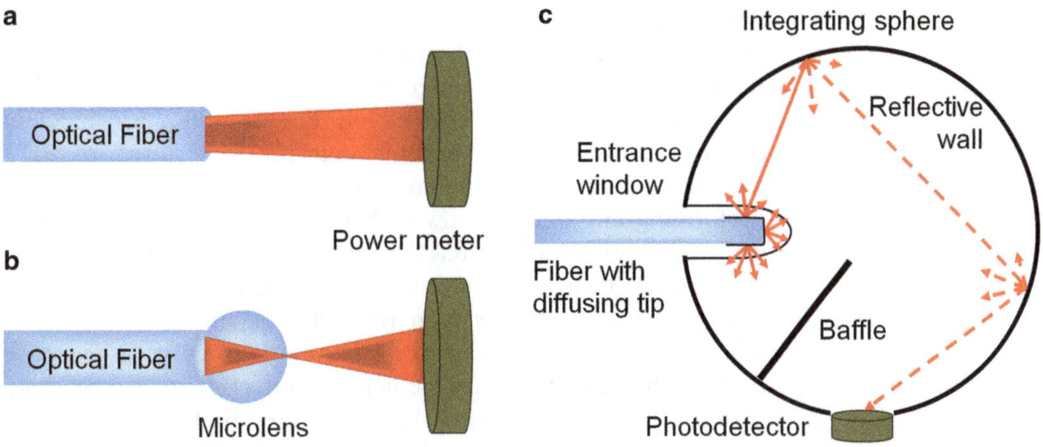

Fig. 4 Schematic of output power measurement for a fiber with (**a**) flat-cut, (**b**) microlens, and (**c**) diffusing tip

calibrate the device. The integrating sphere, illustrated in Fig. 4c, is a hollow sphere of sufficient size to contain the entire source, internally coated with a highly diffuse reflective material, so any light originating within the sphere will be scattered multiple times and have an approximately uniform probability of intersecting the detector, regardless of its position or direction of origin. To properly calibrate an integrating sphere, it is essential that the source be separated from the detector by a baffle whose geometry ensures that only multiply scattered light reaches the detector. The combination of sphere and detector can be calibrated by measuring a source of known power and establishing the relationship between the total power injected into the sphere and the reading measured by the detector. In general, this relationship will be independent of source geometry.

In Vivo Light Dosimetry

While it is essential to calibrate the output of the light sources and delivery devices, this calibration ignores the largest source of variability in PDT treatment, namely the patient. Because tissues can vary widely in absorption and scattering coefficients, geometry, and accessibility, the dose delivered to two different patients by the same light source and delivery device may be significantly different. Fortunately, it is possible to measure the optical energy fluence delivered to the tissue, either on the surface or at depth. The most suitable device for these in vivo measurements is the fiber optic-based isotropic detector. This detector consists of an optical fiber terminating in a spherical tip with a very high scattering coefficient, as shown in Fig. 5. Its operation is essentially the reverse of that of a diffusing optical fiber delivery device. Instead of diffusing light from the fiber into the surrounding tissue, the isotropic detector collects light isotropically and conducts some fraction of it via multiple scattering into the core of the fiber. Because their detection is isotropic, these detectors measure fluence rate, including both incident irradiance and light scattered from tissue. Because photosensitizer molecules on average absorb light isotropically, the photodynamic effect is dependent on fluence rate, not incident irradiance, making the isotropic detector well suited to PDT dosimetry. It has been shown that significant errors can result from performing in vivo dosimetry with a flat (irradiance) detector that does not capture backscattered light [61].

Because isotropic detectors rely partially on multiple reflection at the interface between the detector and the medium in which they are embedded to collect light, their sensitivity depends on the refractive index mismatch at that interface [62]. The likelihood of a photon scattering, being reflected back into the sphere and making its way into the fiber, as shown by green path in Fig. 5, is greater when the index mismatch is greatest. The difference in sensitivity between air and water, for example, can be as much as 80 %, making index-appropriate calibration essential.

Isotropic detectors can be made small enough to insert interstitially via catheters and robust enough to be placed directly on the tissue surface or sutured into the walls of cavities. They have become the gold standard for in vivo light dosimetry and should be used whenever possible. In addition, measurements made at multiple locations can be used to determine the detailed light distribution in tissue and, when coupled with an appropriate light source, to determine tissue optical properties [63].

Beyond Light Dosimetry

Light dosimetry is essential, but neglects the effects of variable sensitizer concentration and tissue oxygenation. Several strategies have been proposed to address this deficiency, as described in the previous chapter. They can generally be categorized as explicit,

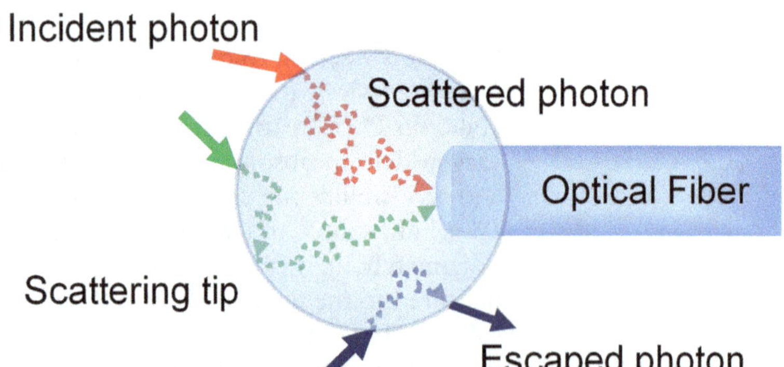

Fig. 5 Schematic of an isotropic detector. Incident photons from all directions are scattered inside the sphere. Some photons reach the fiber through diffusion and some escape the sphere. The index of refraction mismatch at the boundary influences the probability of scattering back into the sphere and therefore the sensitivity of the detector

implicit, or direct dosimetry [64]. Explicit dosimetric techniques rely on characterization of the sensitizer concentration, tissue oxygenation, and light dose independently, and a model of photodynamic effect capable of combining them into a prediction of tissue response. While each component required for explicit dosimetry can be measured using well-established techniques, measuring all of them simultaneously in a clinical setting is challenging. Several approaches to near-real-time explicit dosimetry have been developed. If the sensitizer is fluorescent, a beamsplitter can be used to separate the signal collected by an isotropic detector into treatment light (for light dosimetry) and fluorescence emission (for sensitizer distribution measurement) [65]. It has been shown that optical properties, light dose, and tissue oxygenation can be measured using one or more isotropic detectors coupled to spectrometers, with a separate fiber-based detector for sensitizer fluorescence [66]. Similar measurements have been obtained with flat-cut fibers coupled to a system with internal fiber switches that allow each fiber to provide treatment light, white light, or fluorescence excitation or to act as a detector [67].

Regardless of the methods for determining sensitizer concentration, oxygenation, and light dose, a theoretical model is required to combine them into a predictor of response. If singlet oxygen is the primary cytotoxic agent responsible for tissue response, then the net photochemical consumption of oxygen (or, equivalently, the concentration of singlet oxygen reactions) is a reasonable predictor of outcome. In simple cell models, this metric can be spatially quantified, and predicts cell killing on the scale of single cells. Extension to clinical use, however, presents a challenge: The scale of variability of photochemical reactions is much smaller than the typical treated volume, and only volume-averaged measurements of sensitizer, oxygenation, and light dose are generally available. This has led to the development of approximate macroscopic models of singlet oxygen deposition [68, 69]. The photophysical parameters required for these models (see section "Photosensitizers") may differ from their corresponding microscopic values, but the model has the potential to overcome some of the limitations of drug–light product dosimetry.

Implicit dosimetry, in contrast, uses a measurable surrogate for tissue damage. The originally proposed metric was the photobleaching of the sensitizer itself [64]. If the sensitizer is bleached primarily by the singlet oxygen it generates, the extent of photobleaching will be predictive of the local tissue response. This effect has been confirmed in tumor spheroid models [70, 71], and animal models [72, 73], and used as a metric to reduce pain in clinical treatment of skin cancer [74]. The caveat remains that it is valid only when the bleaching and tissue damage are mediated by the same mechanism. Sensitizers may exhibit photobleaching that is not predictive of dose for a variety of reasons [75–77]. Therefore, care must be taken to verify the accuracy of implicit dosimetry prior to clinical implementation. As in the case of explicit dosimetry described above, it is possible to quantify photobleaching based on measurements of sensitizer fluorescence excited by the treatment light [20].

Photosensitizers

The final parameter over which the clinician has direct control is the choice of sensitizer. At a fundamental level, the sensitizer's role in photodynamic therapy depends on a small number of key photophysical parameters. In the following discussion, we will use the notation of the Foster laboratory [70, 71]. The fundamental parameters and the relationships between them are summarized in Fig. 6.

A molecule at room temperature normally resides in the ground state. The ground state in almost all molecules is a singlet state but molecular oxygen is an exception. There exist two unpaired electrons in the outermost orbital of ground-state molecular oxygen that makes it a spectroscopic triplet state since

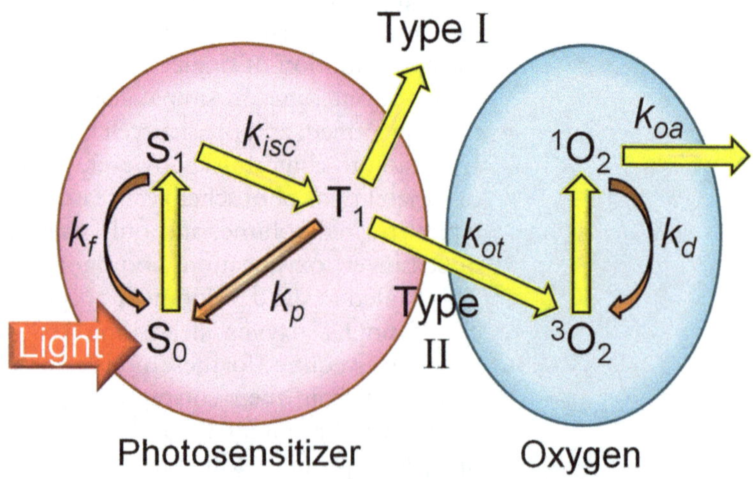

Fig. 6 Graphical illustration of fundamental photophysical parameters during photodynamic action. Photosensitizer in its ground state (S_0) is excited to its singlet state (S_1) by absorption of light. Through intersystem crossing (ISC) process the sensitizer decays to its triplet excited state (T_1). In Type I photochemical reaction pathway, interaction of excited sensitizer and surrounding molecules leads to production of free radicals. In Type II pathway, energy is transferred through the decay of T_1 state sensitizer to ground-state molecular oxygen ($^3O_2$) that creates reactive singlet oxygen ($^1O_2$). k_f, k_{isc}, k_p, k_{ot}, k_d, and k_{oa} are, respectively, rate constants for fluorescence, intersystem crossing, spontaneous relaxation of T_1 state, collision with ground-state oxygen, spontaneous relaxation of $^1O_2$, and reaction of $^1O_2$ with cellular targets

the combined spin of electrons can acquire any of three quantum states. In contrast, molecular singlet oxygen constrained to have only one spin quantum state because it has two paired electrons in a single orbital. Singlet and triplet states refer to the multiplicity of the molecule. Transition from the triplet to the lowest lying singlet state in molecular oxygen requires ~0.98 eV energy [78]. It should be noted that although visible light has enough energy ($3.1 > E > 1.65$ eV for $400 < \lambda < 750$ nm) to derive this transition, direct transition by optical means is forbidden due to molecular quantum selection rules. According to quantum selection rules, triplet–singlet interactions are spin forbidden, while triplet–triplet interactions are spin allowed. Therefore, it is necessary to use a photosensitizer that is elevated to a triplet state by absorption of optical energy and transfers the energy to molecular oxygen through collision. This interaction is spin allowed because both excited-state photosensitizer and ground-state molecular oxygen are triplet states.

The PDT process begins with absorption of light by the photosensitizer that initiates reactions generating cytotoxic species, such as singlet oxygen, free radicals, and peroxides. The sensitizer, initially in its singlet ground state (S_0), absorbs a photon and is elevated to its first excited state (S_1), which is also a singlet state. The absorption spectrum of the sensitizer is determined by the energy gaps between the ground state and the excited states of the sensitizer. It is possible to excite higher-energy states (S_2, S_3, etc.), but in most sensitizers, these higher-energy states quickly decay to the S_1 or an excited triplet state (T_1), so they result in the same photochemistry as excitation to S_1. The rate of excitation to S_1 state depends on the fluence rate of light, the extinction coefficient of the sensitizer at the wavelength of the treatment light (ε), and the concentration of ground-state sensitizer. The light fluence rate is the only parameter that is under direct control at the time of treatment.

Once in the S_1 state, the sensitizer can either spontaneously decay back to the S_0 state, often with the emission of a fluorescence photon, or transition to an excited triplet state (T_1) with a change in the spin of one electron, a process known as intersystem crossing (ISC). These two processes are simultaneous and competitive. A sensitizer with a very high fluorescence quantum yield necessarily has a low intersystem crossing yield, and vice versa. If the sensitizer has a sufficiently high intersystem crossing yield, it will accumulate a population in the T_1 state. Reactions of T_1 state with surrounding medium are more favorable due to its longer lifetime (~μs) compared with that of the S_1 state (~ns) and have been classified in two pathways. In the Type I reaction pathway, free radicals are produced due to hydrogen-atom abstraction or electron transfer between the excited sensitizer and surrounding molecules; the produced free radicals can react with oxygen molecules to form reactive oxygen species (ROS). In the Type II reaction pathway, singlet oxygen ($^1O_2$) is generated due to energy transfer between the triplet-state sensitizer and ground-state molecular triplet oxygen ($^3O_2$). As mentioned earlier, triplet–triplet interactions are spin allowed according to quantum selection rules. It should be noted that both Type I and II reactions can occur simultaneously; type of photosensitizer and the concentrations of substrate and oxygen determine the ratio between these pathways [79]. Nevertheless, the Type II pathway is the dominant mechanism of PDT and is discussed in more detail in the following. Photosensitizer molecules in the T_1 state can decay spontaneously to the S_0 state with the emission of a phosphorescent photon. Alternatively, the decay of sensitizer molecules in T_1 state to their ground state can be accompanied by transfer of energy, via collision, to ground-state triplet molecular oxygen present in the tissue to form singlet oxygen. These processes are competitive. In the absence of oxygen, the decay is dominated by phosphorescence, and the lifetime of T_1 state is long. When oxygen is present, it rapidly interacts with molecules in the T_1 state, so the T_1 state lifetime is short and the phosphorescence yield is low. This makes it possible to use a sensitizer with detectable phosphorescence emission as an oxygen sensor [80], or, conversely, a phosphorescence-based oxygen sensor as a sensitizer [81]. The goal of clinical PDT is to produce singlet oxygen, so it is advantageous to have a low rate constant for spontaneous relaxation of T_1 state (k_p) and hence a long T_1 lifetime.

Singlet oxygen is relatively stable in the absence of reaction targets, with a 45 min lifetime in the gas phase [82] and a 2–200 μs lifetime in liquids [83]. Although singlet oxygen molecules can, in principle, decay to their ground states, in a target-rich environment they will generally react before they have enough time to spontaneously decay. It is the reaction with targets that cause the cellular damage responsible for the PDT effect. The short lifetime of singlet oxygen (~ns) in biological environments constrains singlet oxygen-mediated damage to the immediate vicinity within tens to hundreds of nanometers of its generation [84, 85]. Therefore, the cellular location of the sensitizer will determine the site of singlet oxygen damage.

In general, the generation of singlet oxygen returns the sensitizer molecule to its ground state, so no sensitizer is consumed in the process. However, there are several potential reactions that can degrade the sensitizer, collectively known as photobleaching. They can involve reaction of singlet oxygen generated by a sensitizer with the sensitizer molecule itself, directly or via intermediate reactions, or reactions of excited-state sensitizer molecules with cellular targets. These different reactions can have very different consequences for PDT dosimetry [70], particularly in the case of implicit dosimetry [64].

Comparison of Photophysical Parameters and Dosimetric Consequences

Over the last half-century, there have been many attempts to develop better sensitizers. In general, the differences between sensitizers can be understood in terms of their basic photophysical parameters and their localization within cells and tissues, all of which can be modified via changes in their chemical structure or delivery vehicle. These differences can explain the clinically observed differences in biological effectiveness of different sensitizers.

The first parameter that can be adjusted in the development of photosensitizers is the absorption spectrum. The ideal sensitizer would have a high extinction coefficient in regions of the spectrum where tissue is not highly absorbing. This has led to the development of photosensitizers with absorption peaks at longer wavelengths. As shown in Fig. 1, the optimal wavelength is in the near-infrared region around 750 nm. Light penetration is limited by hemoglobin and melanin absorption at shorter wavelengths and by water absorption at longer wavelengths.

Triplet formation quantum yield, defined by the number of photosensitizer molecules excited to T_1 state per absorbed photon, can also vary among photosensitizers. The ideal photosensitizer would have a large triplet quantum yield; however, a triplet yield very close to 1 precludes fluorescence, which may be a disadvantage, as fluorescence is useful for both implicit and explicit dosimetry. The product of the sensitizer's extinction coefficient, its local concentration in tissue, and its quantum yield give the rate of triplet production per unit fluence rate of light. While this argues for sensitizers with high extinction coefficients and triplet yields, low extinction coefficient can be compensated by an increase in sensitizer concentration, as long as the sensitizer's dark toxicity is not a limiting factor. Therefore, a sensitizer with a moderate extinction coefficient but a very low dark toxicity might be preferable to a highly absorbing but toxic sensitizer.

The limited diffusion distance of singlet oxygen means that the subcellular location of photodynamic damage is determined primarily by the sensitizer's subcellular localization. Sensitizers localize in different subcellular locations depending on their structure and route of administration. Many porphyrin-based sensitizers accumulate in mitochondrial membranes. This makes them particularly likely to cause mitochondrial damage and loss of mitochondrial membrane potential, which in turn triggers apoptotic cell death. Of particular interest is the prodrug ALA. ALA itself is not a sensitizer, but it enters the heme biosynthesis pathway downstream of its usual regulatory feedback steps. ALA is synthesized into a series of porphyrins culminating in PpIX, which is an effective photosensitizer. The final step in the biosynthetic pathway, incorporation of iron into the PpIX ring to form heme, is limited by the available supply of ferrochelatase and is overwhelmed by an excess of ALA, leading to a temporary accumulation of PpIX. Because these synthesis steps take place in and around the mitochondrial membrane, PpIX accumulates preferentially in the mitochondria.

Other sensitizers have been shown to accumulate in various other organelles, including lysosomes, Golgi apparatus, and endoplasmic reticulum [79]. The site of localization may vary among cell types. The localization can also be dynamic. For instance, some sensitizers can change their localization in response to the singlet oxygen that they themselves generate upon exposure to light [86]. A similar effect has been exploited for photochemical internalization [87], in which a sensitizer is used to enhance the delivery of another agent.

On a macroscopic level, the distribution of sensitizers among different organs depends on a number of factors. When sensitizers are administered intravenously, the time interval between the administration of the sensitizer and the start of irradiation (the drug–light interval) is critical. At early times after injection, many sensitizers are confined to the vasculature. Irradiation at short times can be used to target vasculature specifically. This approach has been used for treatment of prostate cancer [88] and macular degeneration [89]. At later times, the sensitizer is more likely to be distributed in tissue. Therefore, tuning the timing of irradiation can enhance or suppress the vascular effect in PDT [90]. Vascular response to PDT can be remarkably complicated [91, 92] and it is not always clear what the ideal drug–light interval is.

In addition to the drug–light interval, the duration of cutaneous photosensitivity is an important consideration. First-generation sensitizers can cause unwanted skin sensitivity for as long as 2 months. While the consequences of skin photosensitivity can be managed, they cause inconvenience for patients. As a result, many newer sensitizers have been designed to have faster clearance from the skin. Perhaps the most successful of these is ALA/PpIX. The excess PpIX is rapidly consumed as the heme biosynthetic pathway comes back into equilibrium. The skin sensitivity resulting from PpIX sensitization therefore can be as short as a few days.

Finally, we mention typical doses of drug and light energies used in PDT. As mentioned earlier, Foscan® and Photofrin® are two photosensitizers that have been most extensively used in PDT of head and neck cancers. The typical drug dose of Foscan® for head and neck PDT is 0.15 mg/kg body weight administered intravenously; the drug–light interval is 90–110 h and then the target tissue is illuminated at wavelength of $\lambda = 652$ nm to deliver optical energy fluence of 20 J/cm^2 at fluence rate of 100 mW/cm^2. The exposure time (in seconds) is given by the ratio of energy fluence (in J/cm^2) and fluence rate (in W/cm^2). Note that not only the light fluence but also the fluence rate affects the PDT response [93]. Therefore, for each specific tumor, the total energy fluence and fluence rate are predetermined values based on clinical trials. Systemic elimination of Foscan® and Photofrin® takes approximately 3 and 6 weeks, respectively. In the case of Photofrin®, depending on tumor type, various combinations of drug dose and light fluence have been used clinically: drug dose in the range of 1.5–5 mg/kg administered intravenously, drug–light intervals of 24–48 h, and the light fluence in the range of 50–150 J/cm^2 at fluence rate of 100–150 mW/cm^2 at $\lambda = 630$ nm [33]. ALA-mediated PDT for head and neck cases has been reported in fewer studies than Foscan® and Photofrin®. In ALA-mediated PDT for head and neck mucosal dysplasia, a drug dose of 60 mg/kg administered systemically, drug–light intervals between 3 and 5 h, and optical energy fluence of 100 J/cm^2 at fluence rates of 100–150 mW/cm^2 at illumination wavelength of $\lambda = 635$ nm have been reported with posttreatment skin photosensitivity of less than 24 h [39].

New Technologies

New Light Sources and Drug Delivery Methods

There are various avenues of research in progress in the design of localized and flexible light sources, delivery methods, and devices for PDT. Within the paradigm of cancer nanotechnology [94, 95] ongoing effort has been aimed at targeted delivery of drugs. This direction relies on the ability to identify and grow nanoparticles with high tumor uptake selectivity. Certain nanoparticles can potentially be used to carry photosensitizer molecules and be actively taken up by tumor cells [96], attach to tumor cells and deliver singlet oxygen while maintaining the embedded photosensitizer [97], or act as a light source [98–100] (quantum dots).

Another research direction is connected with the combination of PDT and radiotherapy [101–105]. Scintillating nanoparticles attached to photosensitizers and molecular targeting agents were proposed as in vivo light sources for simultaneous PDT and radiotherapy [106, 107]. Scintillation or persistent luminescence of such nanoparticles, when exposed to ionizing radiation, such as X-rays, activates the photosensitizer and initiates the PDT. In this way, deep tumors can be treated due to the penetration of X-rays and cellular targeting of PDT [108]. This direction can be further developed by exploiting Čerenkov radiation for simultaneous PDT and radiotherapy. Čerenkov radiation occurs when charged particles travel faster than the phase velocity of light in a given dielectric medium [109–112]. It has been demonstrated that Čerenkov radiation induced by external beam irradiation can lead to molecular fluorescence [113]. In principle, such a fluorescence emission can be used to excite a photosensitizer. However, due to the very low intensity of the Čerenkov radiation, the PDT would be probably done under ultralow [114] fluence rate which requires the photosensitizer to be highly selectively taken up by the tumor. In any application involving simultaneous PDT and radiotherapy, it is important to be aware of the significant differences in the total energy deposited by the standard treatments in each modality. The typical total energy delivered in a stand-alone PDT treatment is 4–5 orders of magnitude higher than that in a typical course of ionizing radiation therapy. Hence, any strategy that relies on ionizing radiation to power PDT, even with 100 % conversion efficiency, must depend on very low dose rate PDT and synergy with radiation damage.

Another research avenue in developing new localized light sources is connected with in vivo chemiluminescence (bioluminescence) [115, 116]. For example, it was proposed [115] that sufficient photoactivation light to release singlet oxygen is generated as a consequence of the intracellular proximity of D-luciferin and a photosensitizer, when they are taken up by luciferase-transfected cells. While this mechanism is potentially feasible, it further complicates the dosimetry by adding another factor (the luciferase transfection vector) that must be included in the calculation of dose. In addition, because this method relies on transfection of cells with luciferase genes, it is useful for animal research, but unlikely to be applied in patients.

In terms of development in light delivery devices, they are under continuous development to match different tumor site geometries. For instance, a flexible light source has been designed using a light patch [117] based on high-intensity chemiluminescence for topical activation of ALA. Upon activation, the light patch emits blue light (431–515 nm), and due to its short wavelength, it has a shallow penetration in tissue that makes is suitable for superficial treatments, such as actinic keratosis [118].

Another flexible light delivery system is designed based on a textile diffusor composed of plastic optical fibers [119–121]. Due to its flexibility, it can cover the tumor site while irradiating it. To reduce the complexity of the design, a "light blanket" has been designed by coiling a single diffusing optical fiber in a rectangular region inside flexible plastic layers (PVC) to achieve a uniform irradiation field [122, 123]. The proximal end of the fiber is coupled with the desired laser source and the portion of its length which is swirled inside the plastic blanket is side-emitting.

Recently, "point source" delivery of photosensitizer and singlet oxygen by using a microoptic device has been suggested to improve the localization of the PDT. In this method, 669 nm light from a diode laser and oxygen gas are transmitted through a hollow core optical fiber; light–drug interactions in the microprobe lead to the formation of singlet oxygen molecules that emerge from the mesoporous fluorinated silica tip toward the target tissue [124]. Clinical application of this method involves several challenges; for example, due to extremely short diffusion length of singlet oxygen, the probe must be held in almost contact with the target tissue, which might not be feasible for all tumors and also requires a very precise monitoring and mechanical system. Since the treatment area is determined by the size of the tip, either a large size tip or a scanning tip is required.

Two-photon PDT [125] is an approach to extend PDT to near-infrared region of the spectrum based on simultaneous absorption of two photons whose total energy is sufficient for photosensitizer excitation. Two-photon excitation has been extensively used in microscopy [126] because of its ability to localize excitation to a small volume. Similarly, two-photon excitation for PDT can localize the region of generation of singlet oxygen to a very small volume. This allows PDT-driven microsurgery of superficial lesions [125]. It should be noted that two-photon excitation does not necessarily address the problem of optical penetration depth; because the rate of sensitizer excitation depends on the square of the light intensity, the optical penetration depth is effectively halved for two-photon PDT. Research in this direction is toward producing new photosensitizers, some of which is based on advances in nanotechnology.

In addition to the aforementioned research directions related to PDT light sources and delivery methods, various research avenues related to improving photosensitizers are aimed at synthesizing drugs with higher tumor selectivity; rapid accumulation in target tissue to reduce drug–light interval; and rapid clearance from the patient to minimize posttreatment cutaneous photosensitivity period.

References

1. Detty M, Gibson S, Wagner S. Current clinical and preclinical photosensitizers for use in photodynamic therapy. J Med Chem. 2004; 47:3897–915.
2. Dougherty TJ, Marcus SL. Photodynamic therapy. Eur J Cancer. 1992;28A:1734–42.
3. Sharman W, Allen C, van Lier JE. Photodynamic therapeutics: basic principles and clinical applications. Drug Discov Today. 1999;4:507–17.
4. Oleinick NL, Kessel D, Principles of photodynamic therapy-induced killing of tumor cells. In: Biel MA (ed) Photodynamic Therapy of Diseases of the Head and Neck, Plural Publishing Inc., Abingdon, 2008. p. 19–31.
5. Zhu TC, Finlay JC. The role of photodynamic therapy (PDT) physics. Med Phys. 2008;35:3127–36.
6. Finlay JC, Foster TH. Effect of pigment packaging on diffuse reflectance spectroscopy of samples containing red blood cells. Opt Lett. 2004;29:965–7.
7. Kou L, Labrie D, Chylek P. Refractive indices of water and ice in the 0.65- to 2.5-μm spectral range. Appl Optics. 1993;32:3531–40.
8. Allison RR, Downie GH, Cuenca R, Hu X-H, Childs CJ, Sibata CH. Photosensitizers in clinical PDT. Photodiagnosis Photodyn Ther. 2004;1:27–42.
9. Wilson BC, Patterson MS. The physics, biophysics and technology of photodynamic therapy. Phys Med Biol. 2008;53:R61–109.
10. Dougherty TJ, Gomer CJ, Henderson BW, et al. Photodynamic therapy. J Natl Cancer Inst. 1998;90:889–905.
11. Hopper C. Photodynamic therapy: a clinical reality in the treatment of cancer. Lancet Oncol. 2000;1:212–9.
12. Tanaka H, Hashimoto K, Yamada I, et al. Interstitial photodynamic therapy with rotating and reciprocating optical fibers. Cancer. 2001;91:1791–6.
13. Rigual NRN, Thankappan K, Cooper M, et al. Photodynamic therapy for head and

neck dysplasia and cancer. Arch Otolaryngol Head Neck Surg. 2009;135:784–8.

14. Schweitzer VG, Somers ML. PHOTOFRIN-mediated photodynamic therapy for treatment of early stage (Tis-T2N0M0) SqCCa of oral cavity and oropharynx. Lasers Surg Med. 2010;42:1–8.
15. Quon H, Finlay JC, Cengel K, Zhu TC, O'Malley B, Weinstein G. Transoral robotic photodynamic therapy for the oropharynx. Photodiagnosis Photodyn Ther. 2011;8: 64–7.
16. Ikeda H, Tobita T, Ohba S, Uehara M, Asahina I. Treatment outcome of Photofrin-based photodynamic therapy for T1 and T2 oral squamous cell carcinoma and dysplasia. Photodiagnosis Photodyn Ther. 2013;10: 229–35.
17. Fan KFM, Hopper C, Speight PM, Buonaccorsi G, MacRobert AJ, Bown SG. Photodynamic therapy using 5-aminolevulinic acid for premalignant and malignant lesions of the oral cavity. Cancer. 1996;78: 1374–83.
18. Sieroń A, Adamek M, Kawczyk-Krupka A, Mazur S, Ilewicz L. Photodynamic therapy (PDT) using topically applied delta-aminolevulinic acid (ALA) for the treatment of oral leukoplakia. J Oral Pathol Med. 2003;32: 330–6.
19. Chen H-M, Chen C-T, Yang H, et al. Successful treatment of oral verrucous hyperplasia with topical 5-aminolevulinic acid-mediated photodynamic therapy. Oral Oncol. 2004;40:630–7.
20. Grossman C, Zhu T, Finlay J, et al. Targeted laryngeal photodynamic therapy with a balloon diffusing light source. Photodiagnosis Photodyn Ther. 2010;7:158–61.
21. Dilkes MG, DeJode ML, Rowntree-Taylor A, McGilligan JA, Kenyon GS, McKelvie P. m-THPC photodynamic therapy for head and neck cancer. Lasers Surg Med. 1996;11: 23–9.
22. Fan KF, Hopper C, Speight PM, Buonaccorsi GA, Bown SG. Photodynamic therapy using mTHPC for malignant disease in the oral cavity. Int J Cancer. 1997;73(1):25–32.
23. Copper MP, Triesscheijn M, Tan IB, Ruevekamp MC, Stewart FA. Photodynamic therapy in the treatment of multiple primary tumours in the head and neck, located to the oral cavity and oropharynx. Clin Otolaryngol. 2007;32:185–9.
24. Jerjes W, Upile T, Hamdoon Z, et al. Photodynamic therapy: the minimally invasive surgical intervention for advanced and/or recurrent tongue base carcinoma. Lasers Surg Med. 2011;43:283–92.
25. Nyst HJ, Wildeman MA, Indrasari SR, et al. Temoporfin mediated photodynamic therapy in patients with local persistent and recurrent nasopharyngeal carcinoma after curative radiotherapy: a feasibility study. Photodiagnosis Photodyn Ther. 2012;9: 274–81.
26. Karakullukcu B, Nyst HJ, van Veen RLP, et al. mTHPC mediated interstitial photodynamic therapy of recurrent nonmetastatic base of tongue cancers: development of a new method. Head Neck. 2012;34:1597–606.
27. Karakullukcu B, van Veen RLP, Aans JB, et al. MR and CT based treatment planning for mTHPC mediated interstitial photodynamic therapy of head and neck cancer: description of the method. Lasers Surg Med. 2013;45:517–23.
28. Story W, Sultan AA, Bottini G, Vaz F, Lee G, Hopper C. Strategies of airway management for head and neck photo-dynamic therapy. Lasers Surg Med. 2013;45:370–6.
29. de Visscher SAHJ, Melchers LJ, Dijkstra PU, et al. mTHPC-mediated photodynamic therapy of early stage oral squamous cell carcinoma: a comparison to surgical treatment. Ann Surg Oncol. 2013;20:3076–82.
30. de Visscher SAHJ, Dijkstra PU, Tan IB, Roodenburg JLN, Witjes MJH. mTHPC mediated photodynamic therapy (PDT) of squamous cell carcinoma in the head and neck: a systematic review. Oral Oncol. 2013; 49:192–210.
31. Rigual NR, Shafirstein G, Frustino J, et al. Adjuvant intraoperative photodynamic therapy in head and neck cancer. JAMA Otolaryngol Head Neck Surg. 2013;139: 706–11.
32. Schweitzer VG. Photodynamic therapy for treatment of head and neck cancer. Otolaryngol Head Neck Surg. 1990;102: 225–32.
33. Biel MA. Photodynamic therapy in head and neck cancer. Curr Oncol Rep. 2002;4(1): 87–96.
34. Dolmans DEGJ, Fukumura D, Jain RK. Photodynamic therapy for cancer. Nat Rev Cancer. 2003;3:380–7.
35. Brown SB, Brown EA, Walker I. The present and future role of photodynamic therapy in cancer treatment. Lancet Oncol. 2004;5: 497–508.
36. Huang Z. A review of progress in clinical photodynamic therapy. Technol Cancer Res Treat. 2005;4:283–93.

37. Biel MA (ed), Photodynamic Therapy of Diseases of the Head and Neck, Plural Publishing Inc., Abingdon, 2008.
38. Biel MA, Photodynamic therapy of head and neck cancers. In: Gomer CJ (Ed) Photodynamic Therapy, Vol. 635 of the series Methods in Molecular Biology, Springer, New York, 2010. p. 281–93.
39. Quon H, Grossman CE, Finlay JC, et al. Photodynamic therapy in the management of pre-malignant head and neck mucosal dysplasia and microinvasive carcinoma. Photodiagnosis Photodyn Ther. 2011;8: 75–85.
40. Jerjes W, Hamdoon Z, Hopper C. Photodynamic therapy in the management of potentially malignant and malignant oral disorders. Head Neck Oncol. 2012;4:1–7.
41. Green B, Cobb ARM, Hopper C. Photodynamic therapy in the management of lesions of the head and neck. Br J Oral Maxillofac Surg. 2013;51:283–7.
42. Brancaleon L, Moseley H. Laser and non-laser light sources for photodynamic therapy. Lasers Med Sci. 2002;17:173–86.
43. Mang TS. Lasers and light sources for PDT: past, present and future. Photodiagnosis Photodyn Ther. 2004;1:43–8.
44. Schäfer FP. Dye lasers. Berlin: Springer; 1990.
45. Wilson BC. Photodynamic therapy: light delivery and dosage for second-generation photosensitizers. Ciba Found Symp. 1989; 146:60–73.
46. Wilson B, Patterson M. The physics, biophysics and technology of photodynamic therapy. Phys Med Biol. 2008;53:61–109.
47. Yu C-H, Lin H-P, Chen H-M, Yang H, Wang Y-P, Chiang C-P. Comparison of clinical outcomes of oral erythroleukoplakia treated with photodynamic therapy using either light-emitting diode or laser light. Lasers Surg Med. 2009;41:628–33.
48. Tsai J-C, Chiang C-P, Chen H-M, et al. Photodynamic therapy of oral dysplasia with topical 5-aminolevulinic acid and light-emitting diode array. Lasers Surg Med. 2004; 34:18–24.
49. Schmidt MH, Bajic DM, Reichert KW, Martin TS, Meyer GA, Whelan HT. Light-emitting diodes as a light source for intraoperative photodynamic therapy. Neurosurgery. 1996;38:552–6.
50. Chen J, Keltner L, Christophersen J, et al. New technology for deep light distribution in tissue for phototherapy. Cancer J. 2002; 8:154–63.
51. Lustig RA, Vogl TJ, Fromm D, et al. A multicenter phase I safety study of intratumoral photoactivation of talaporfin sodium in patients with refractory solid tumors. Cancer. 2003;98:1767–71.
52. Diamond I, McDonagh AF, Wilson CB, Granelli SG, Nielsen S, Jaenicke R. Photodynamic therapy of malignant tumors. Lancet. 1972;2:1175–7.
53. Wilson BC, Patterson MS. The physics of photodynamic therapy. Phys Med Biol. 1986; 31:327–60.
54. Morton CA, McKenna KE, Rhodes LE. Guidelines for topical photodynamic therapy: update. Br J Dermatol. 2008;159:1245–66.
55. Darafsheh A. Optical super-resolution and periodical focusing effects by dielectric microspheres. PhD dissertation, University of North Carolina at Charlotte; 2013.
56. Rendon A, Weersink R, Lilge L. Towards conformal light delivery using tailored cylindrical diffusers: attainable light dose distributions. Phys Med Biol. 2006;51:5967–75.
57. Panjehpour M, Overholt BF, Photodynamic therapy for Barrett's esophagus. In: Mönkemüller K, Wilcox CM, Muñoz-Navas M (eds) Interventional and Therapeutic Gastrointestinal Endoscopy. Front Gastrointest Res. vol 27, Karger, Basel, 2010, p. 128–39.
58. Dwyer PJ, White WM, Fabian RL, Anderson RR. Optical integrating balloon device for photodynamic therapy. Lasers Surg Med. 2000;26:58–66.
59. Nyst HJ, van Veen RLP, Tan IB, et al. Performance of a dedicated light delivery and dosimetry device for photodynamic therapy of nasopharyngeal carcinoma: phantom and volunteer experiments. Lasers Surg Med. 2007;39:647–53.
60. Zhu TC, Bonnerup C, Colussi VC, et al. Absolute calibration of optical power for PDT: report of AAPM TG140. Med Phys. 2013;40:081501.
61. Vulcan TG, Zhu TC, Rodriguez C, et al. Comparison between isotropic and nonisotropic dosimetry systems during intraperitoneal photodynamic therapy. Lasers Surg Med. 2000;26:292–301.
62. Marijnissen JPA, Star WM. Calibration of isotropic light dosimetry probes based on scattering bulbs in clear media. Phys Med Biol. 1996;41:1191–208.
63. Dimofte A, Finlay JC, Zhu TC. A method determination of the absorption and scattering properties interstitially in turbid media. Phys Med Biol. 2005;50:2291–311.

64. Wilson B, Patterson M, Lilge L. Implicit and explicit dosimetry in photodynamic therapy: a new paradigm. Lasers Med Sci. 1997;12: 182–99.
65. Sharikova AV, Finlay JC, Liang X, Zhu TC, PDT dose dosimetry for pleural photodynamic therapy, Proc. SPIE, Vol. 8568, 856817, 2013.
66. Finlay JC, Zhu TC, Dimofte A, et al. Interstitial fluorescence spectroscopy in the human prostate during motexafin lutetium-mediated photodynamic therapy. Photochem Photobiol. 2006;82:1270–80.
67. Soto-Thompson M, Johansson A, Johansson T, et al. Clinical system for interstitial photodynamic therapy with combined on-line dosimetry measurements. Appl Optics. 2005; 44:4023–31.
68. Wang KK-H, Finlay JC, Busch TM, Hahn S, Zhu TC. Explicit dosimetry for photodynamic therapy: macroscopic singlet oxygen modeling. J Biophotonics. 2010;3:304–18.
69. Hu XH, Feng Y, Lu JQ, et al. Modeling of a type II photofrin-mediated photodynamic therapy process in a heterogeneous tissue phantom. Photochem Photobiol. 2005;81(6): 1460–8.
70. Georgakoudi I, Foster TH. Singlet oxygen-versus nonsinglet oxygen-mediated mechanisms of sensitizer photobleaching and their effects on photodynamic dosimetry. Photochem Photobiol. 1998;67:612–25.
71. Georgakoudi I, Nichols MG, Foster TH. The mechanism of photofrin photobleaching and its consequences for photodynamic dosimetry. Photochem Photobiol. 1997;65:135–44.
72. Robinson DJ, de Bruijn HS, de Wolf WJ, Sterenborg HJ, Star WM. Topical 5-aminolevulinic acid-photodynamic therapy of hairless mouse skin using two-fold illumination schemes: PpIX fluorescence kinetics, photobleaching and biological effect. Photochem Photobiol. 2000;72(6):794–802.
73. Robinson DJ, de Bruijn HS, van der Veen N, Stringer MR, Brown SB, Star WM. Fluorescence photobleaching of ALA-induced protoporphyrin IX during photodynamic therapy of normal hairless mouse skin: the effect of light dose and irradiance and the resulting biological effect. Photochem Photobiol. 1998;67(1):140–9.
74. Cottrell WJ, Paquette AD, Keymel KR, Foster TH, Oseroff AR. Irradiance-dependent photobleaching and pain in δ-aminolevulinic acid-photodynamic therapy of superficial basal cell carcinomas. Clin Cancer Res. 2008;14(14):4475–83.
75. Finlay JC, Mitra S, Patterson MS, Foster TH. Photobleaching kinetics of Photofrin in vivo and in multicell tumour spheroids indicate two simultaneous bleaching mechanisms. Phys Med Biol. 2004;49:4837–60.
76. Baran TM, Foster TH. Fluence rate-dependent photobleaching of intratumorally administered Pc 4 does not predict tumor growth delay. Photochem Photobiol. 2012;88: 1273–9.
77. Finlay JC, Mitra S, Foster TH. In vivo mTHPC photobleaching in normal rat skin exhibits unique irradiance-dependent features. Photochem Photobiol. 2002;75:282–8.
78. Derosa MC, Crutchley RJ. Photosensitized singlet oxygen and its applications. Coord Chem Rev. 2002;233–234:351–71.
79. Castano AP, Demidova TN, Hamblin MR. Mechanisms in photodynamic therapy: part one—photosensitizers, photochemistry and cellular localization. Photodiagnosis Photodyn Ther. 2004;1:279–93.
80. Sterenborg H, de Wolf J, Koning M, Kruijt B, van den Heuvel A, Robinson D. Phosphorescence-fluorescence ratio imaging for monitoring the oxygen status during photodynamic therapy. Opt Express. 2004;12: 1873–8.
81. Mitra S, Foster TH. Photochemical oxygen consumption sensitized by a porphyrin phosphorescent probe in two model systems. Biophys J. 2000;78:2597–605.
82. Arnold SJ, Kubo M, Ogryzlo EA. Relaxation and reactivity of singlet oxygen. Adv Chem Ser. 1968;77(77):133–42.
83. Merkel PB, Kearns DR. Remarkable solvent effects on the lifetime of $^1\Delta g$ oxygen. J Am Chem Soc. 1972;94:1029–30.
84. Moan J, BERG K. The photodegradation of porphyrins in cells can be used to estimate the lifetime of singlet oxygen. Photochem Photobiol. 1991;53:549–53.
85. Skovsen E, Snyder JW, Lambert JDC, Ogilby PR. Lifetime and diffusion of singlet oxygen in a cell. J Phys Chem B. 2005;109:8570–3.
86. Georgakoudi I, Foster TH. Effects of the subcellular redistribution of two nile blue derivatives on photodynamic oxygen consumption. Photochem Photobiol. 1998;68(1):115–22.
87. Berg K, Selbo PK, Prasmickaite L, et al. Photochemical internalization: a novel technology for delivery of macromolecules into cytosol. Cancer Res. 1999;59(6):1180–3.
88. Weersink RA, Bogaards A, Gertner M, et al. Techniques for delivery and monitoring of TOOKAD (WST09)-mediated photodynamic therapy of the prostate: clinical

experience and practicalities. J Photochem Photobiol B. 2005;79:211–22.

89. Schmidt-Erfurth U, Hasan T. Mechanisms of action of photodynamic therapy with verteporfin for the treatment of age-related macular degeneration. Surv Ophthalmol. 2000;45(3):195–214.

90. Chen B, Pogue BW, Hoopes PJ, Hasan T. Combining vascular and cellular targeting regimens enhances the efficacy of photodynamic therapy. Int J Radiat Oncol Biol Phys. 2005;61(4):1216–26.

91. Yu G, Durduran T, Zhou C, et al. Real-time in situ monitoring of human prostate photodynamic therapy with diffuse light. Photochem Photobiol. 2006;82:1279–84.

92. Mesquita RC, Han SW, Miller J, et al. Tumor blood flow differs between mouse strains: consequences for vasoresponse to photodynamic therapy. PLoS One. 2012;7:e37322.

93. Henderson BW, Busch TM, Snyder JW. Fluence rate as a modulator of PDT mechanisms. Lasers Surg Med. 2006;38:489–93.

94. Ferrari M. Cancer nanotechnology: opportunities and challenges. Nat Rev Cancer. 2005;5:161–71.

95. Ryu JH, Koo H, Sun I-C, et al. Tumor-targeting multi-functional nanoparticles for theragnosis : new paradigm for cancer therapy. Adv Drug Deliv Rev. 2012;64:1447–58.

96. Roy I, Ohulchanskyy TY, Pudavar HE, et al. Ceramic-based nanoparticles entrapping water-insoluble photosensitizing anticancer drugs: a novel drug-carrier system for photodynamic therapy. J Am Chem Soc. 2003;125:7860–5.

97. Yan F, Kopelman R. The embedding of meta-tetra(hydroxyphenyl)-chlorin into silica nanoparticle platforms for photodynamic therapy and their singlet oxygen production and pH-dependent optical properties. Photochem Photobiol. 2003;78:587–91.

98. Bakalova R, Ohba H, Zhelev Z, Ishikawa M, Baba Y. Quantum dots as photosensitizers? Nat Biotechnol. 2004;22:1360–1.

99. Weng J, Ren J. Luminescent quantum dots: a very attractive and promising tool in biomedicine. Curr Med Chem. 2006;13:897–909.

100. Samia ACS, Dayal S, Burda C. Quantum dot-based energy transfer: perspectives and potential for applications in photodynamic therapy. Photochem Photobiol. 2006;82:617–25.

101. Schnitzhofer GM, Krammer B. Photodynamic treatment and radiotherapy: combined effect on the colony-forming ability of V79 Chinese hamster fibroblasts. Cancer Lett. 1996;108:93–9.

102. Luksiene Z, Kalvelyte A, Supino R. On the combination of photodynamic therapy with ionizing radiation. J Photochem Photobiol B. 1999;52:35–42.

103. Allman R, Cowburn P, Mason M. Effect of photodynamic therapy in combination with ionizing radiation on human squamous cell carcinoma cell lines of the head and neck. Br J Cancer. 2000;83:655–61.

104. Madsen SJ, Sun C-H, Tromberg BJ, Yeh AT, Sanchez R, Hirschberg H. Effects of combined photodynamic therapy and ionizing radiation on human glioma spheroids. Photochem Photobiol. 2002;76:411–6.

105. Pogue BW, O'Hara JA, Demidenko E, et al. Photodynamic therapy with verteporfin in the radiation-induced fibrosarcoma-1 tumor causes enhanced radiation sensitivity. Cancer Res. 2003;63:1025–33.

106. Chen W, Zhang J. Using nanoparticles to enable simultaneous radiation and photodynamic therapies for cancer treatment. J Nanosci Nanotechnol. 2006;6:1159–66.

107. Liu Y, Chen W, Wang S, Joly AG. Investigation of water-soluble x-ray luminescence nanoparticles for photodynamic activation. Appl Phys Lett. 2008;92:043901.

108. Morgan NY, Kramer-Marek G, Smith PD, Camphausen K, Capala J. Nanoscintillator conjugates as photodynamic therapy-based radiosensitizers : calculation of required physical parameters. Radiat Res. 2009;171: 236–44.

109. Čerenkov PA. Visible emission of clean liquids by action of γ radiation. Comptes Rendus (Dokl) Acad Sci URSS. 1934;2:451–4.

110. Čerenkov P. Visible radiation produced by electrons moving in a medium with velocities exceeding that of light. Phys Rev. 1937; 52(4):378–9.

111. Frank I, Tamm I. Coherent visible radiation of fast electrons passing through matter. Comptes Rendus (Dokl) Acad Sci URSS. 1937;14:109–14.

112. Jelley JV. Čerenkov radiation and its applications. New York: Pergamon; 1958.

113. Axelsson J, Davis SC, Gladstone DJ, Pogue BW. Cerenkov emission induced by external beam radiation stimulates molecular fluorescence. Med Phys. 2011;38:4127.

114. Mathews MS, Angell-Petersen E, Sanchez R, et al. The effects of ultra low fluence rate single and repetitive photodynamic therapy on glioma spheroids. Lasers Surg Med. 2009;41: 578–84.

115. Theodossiou T, Hothersall JS, Woods EA, Okkenhaug K, Jacobson J, Macrobert AJ.

Firefly luciferin-activated rose bengal: in vitro photodynamic therapy by intracellular chemiluminescence in Transgenic NIH 3T3 Cells. Cancer Lett. 2003;63:1818–21.

116. Bown SG. Photodynamic therapy for photochemists. Philos Trans R Soc A. 2013; 371(1995):Article No. UNSP20120371.

117. Zelickson B, Counters J, Coles C, Selim M. Light patch: preliminary report of a novel form of blue light delivery for the treatment of actinic keratosis. Dermatol Surg. 2005;31: 375–8.

118. Smits T, Moor ACE. New aspects in photodynamic therapy of actinic keratoses. J Photochem Photobiol B. 2009;96:159–69.

119. Selm B, Rothmaier M, Camenzind M, Khan T, Walt H. Novel flexible light diffuser and irradiation properties for photodynamic therapy. J Biomed Opt. 2007;12:034024.

120. Rothmaier M, Selm B, Spichtig S, Haensse D, Wolf M. Photonic textiles for pulse oximetry. Opt Express. 2008;16:12973–86.

121. Cochrane C, Mordon SR, Lesage JC, Koncar V. New design of textile light diffusers for photodynamic therapy. Mater Sci Eng C Mater Biol Appl. 2013;33:1170–5.

122. Hu Y, Wang K, Zhu TC. A light blanket for intraoperative photodynamic therapy. Proc SPIE. 2009;7380:73801W.

123. Liang X, Kundu P, Finlay J, Goodwin M, Zhu TC, Maximizing fluence rate and field uniformity of light blanket for intraoperative PDT, Proc. SPIE, Vol. 8210, 82100X, 2012.

124. Ghogare AA, Rizvi I, Hasan T, Greer A. "Pointsource" delivery of a photosensitizer drug and singlet oxygen: eradication of glioma cells in vitro. Photochem Photobiol. 2014;90(5):1119–25.

125. Bhawalkar JD, Kumar ND, Zhao CF, Prasad PN. Two-photon photodynamic therapy. J Clin Laser Med Surg. 1997;15(5):201–4.

126. Denk W, Strickler JH, Webb WW. Two-photon laser scanning fluorescence microscopy. Science. 1990;248(4951):73–6.

Chapter 20

Guidelines on Clinical Management

Waseem Jerjes and Colin Hopper

Multidiscipline Involvement and Informed Consent

The management of head and neck malignancies is coordinated through a multidisciplinary team approach. The suggested treatments are discussed and a decision is made regarding the most appropriate treatment to the patient. Many factors tend to influence the decision-making process and it is not unusual for this process to be dominated by surgeons if the patient was primarily referred for surgery, or by oncologists if the patient was referred for chemoradiation. This process is not straightforward and the decision-making is facilitated by further information about the histopathological and radiological status of the disease. Although Allied Health Care Professionals are less needed in the decision-making process, their preintervention assessments are vital and help toward better care. Treatment of malignancies depends on many factors including tumour size, nodal disease and surgical margins; the involvement of more than one modality is not uncommon especially in advanced, recurrent or palliative disease [1–24].

In general, clinicians are less informed when it comes to photodynamic therapy (PDT) compared to the conventional modalities and as such tend to recommend that the patient undergo traditional treatments (i.e. surgery, radiotherapy and/or chemotherapy). Very few surgeons and oncologists are trained in PDT which led to this technology being offered to a small group of patients (in comparison) giving the impression that PDT is less effective than these modalities. On the other hand, there has been very little clinical evidence comparing PDT effect to these

Brian J.-F. Wong and Justus Ilgner (eds.), *Biomedical Optics in Otorhinolaryngology: Head and Neck Surgery*, DOI 10.1007/978-1-4939-1758-7_20, © Springer Science+Business Media New York 2016

modalities; many problems have been identified including political, logistical, funding and difficulties in study designs and comparative technique [1–24].

In an ethical environment, the patient is informed of the discussions that took place in the multidisciplinary team meeting and is offered more than one intervention (if applicable) with all the pros and cons being highlighted, including information about quality of life and survival. The patient should be allowed some time to think this through and no immediate decision should be sought. The clinician should be neutral in presenting the treatment options and only recommend an option if directly asked by the patient. The clinician should not advance a clinical trial option ahead of other options unless there is a guaranteed higher benefit for the patient. The patient should be fully informed about what is required from him/her if took part in a clinical trial when it comes to extra samples, extra visits and all other investigations [1–24].

The consent needs to be signed by the patient and should be fully informed. The patient can change his/her decision at any time and their wishes should be respected and accommodated. The patient can choose to withdraw from a trial at any time without affecting the suitability of other treatment options, if any. End-stage disease patients should be told about the prognosis to allow a fully informed decision-making and their wishes about whether they would want resuscitation or not [1–24].

General UCL/UCLH Guidelines for Management of Superficial Disease

Surface illumination photodynamic therapy is offered under local or general anaesthesia, using 5-ALA (for thin mild-moderate dysplasia) and mTHPC (for thicker mild–moderate dysplasia, severe dysplasia and carcinoma in situ). A 60 mg/kg 5-ALA cream is applied topically 3–4 h prior to tissue illumination, while mTHPC is administered at a dose of (0.05–0.15 mg/kg) intravenously into the midcubital vein 96 h prior to treatment. This would allow the photosensitising chemotherapeutic agent to accumulate in the diseased area which would increase therapeutic effect. Patients are advised to avoid direct sunlight exposure for 2 weeks if the drug was administered intravenously to avoid systemic photosensitisation, while topically applied drugs required shielding of the treated area from sunlight rather than the whole body [1–24].

On the day of treatment, shielding of the macroscopically healthy surrounding tissue is employed when indicated to prevent collateral tissue damage (which can occur during photodynamic therapy). A safety margin of 2–3 mm around the suspicious lesion is included and illuminated as part of the treatment to eliminate any microscopic disease. For 5-ALA-PDT, a single-channel 628 nm diode laser is used for illumination. The laser light delivery fibre, with a core diameter of 400 μm, is held directly above the suspect area and light is delivered. Light is then delivered from the fibres to the target tissue at 100 or 200 J/cm^2 per site. For mTHPC-PDT, A single-channel 652 nm diode laser is used for illumination. The laser light delivery fibre, with a core diameter of 400 μm, is held directly above the suspect area (distance of 5 cm with 3 cm spot diameter). Light is then delivered from the fibres to the target tissue at 20 J/cm^2 per site [1–24].

Treatment is repeated to cover larger lesions and sometime needles are used to allow the optical fibres to deliver light to the base of the superficial disease (Figs. 1, 2 and 3). Special grids can be made, and with preoperative imaging, further rounds of treatment may be given, if indicated, where additional pathology necrosis and removal are deemed appropriate; the recommended minimum interval is 4 weeks between treatments [1–24].

General UCL/UCLH Guidelines for Management of Deep Pathology

The photosensitising agent used for deep-seated pathologies is mTHPC (Foscan™) which is licensed for the palliative treatment of advanced head and neck squamous cell carcinoma patients, who failed prior therapies and unsuitable for radiotherapy, surgery or systemic chemotherapy. The agent is administered in specialist surgical oncology centres under the supervision of surgeons experienced in photodynamic therapy. mTHPC is usually administered at a dose of 0.15 mg/kg intravenously into the midcubital vein 96 h prior to treatment. This would allow the agent to accumulate in the pathological area which would increase its effect. Patients are usually kept in a side room (with a dim light) to avoid systemic photosensitisation [1–24].

Contraindications of the drug include porphyria or other diseases exacerbated by light, hypersensitivity to temoporfin, known allergies to porphyrins, tumours known to be eroding into a major blood vessel in or adjacent to the illumination site, a planned surgical procedure within the next 30 days, coexisting ophthalmic disease likely to require slit-lamp examination within the next 30 days and existing therapy with a photosensitising agent. While its side effects include injection site reactions (i.e. injection site pain and burning sensation), tumour/local tissue reaction (i.e. pain, haemorrhage, facial pain and/or edema, scar formation and trismus, intraoral ulceration and/or necrosis, skin ulceration and/or

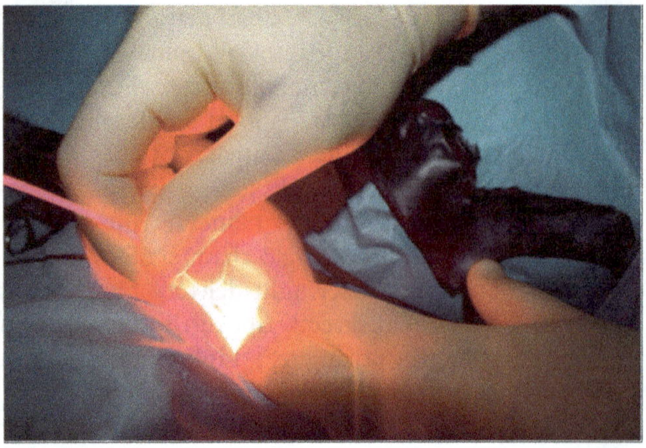

Fig. 1 Clinical image showing surface illumination photodynamic therapy of the oral cavity. Thick black thermal wax can be seen; this is usually used for shielding macroscopically healthy tissue in the oral cavity. The figure is adapted from authors' own article: Jerjes W, Upile T, Hamdoon Z, Alexander Mosse C, Morcos M, Hopper C. Photodynamic therapy outcome for T1/T2 N0 oral squamous cell carcinoma. Lasers Surg Med. 2011;43(6):463–9

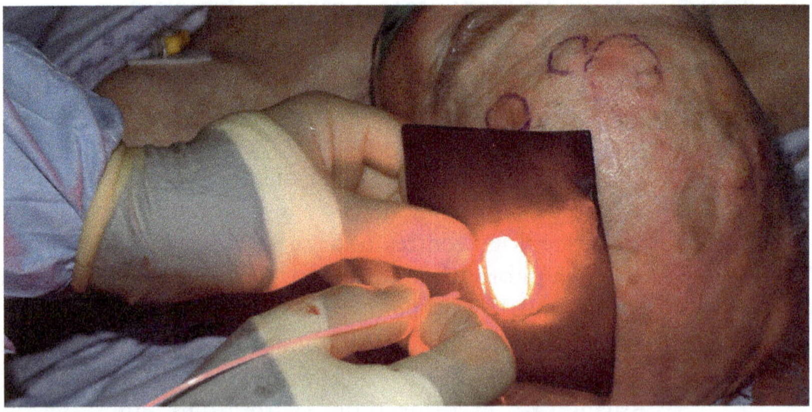

Fig. 2 Surface illumination PDT of multiple basal cell carcinomas and actinic keratosis

necrosis, dysphagia and localised infection), phototoxic events [i.e. skin burn (1st–3rd degree), hyperpigmentation and other photosensitive events] and other general events (i.e. anaemia, nausea, vomiting, constipation and giddiness) [1–24].

Advanced tumours and vascular anomalies can be treated, salvage or palliative with the aim to reduce the tumour bulk to alleviate symptoms and control bleeding, improve function and control pain. Healing usually occurs with minimal scarring and the procedure can be repeated with little cumulative toxicity. There is

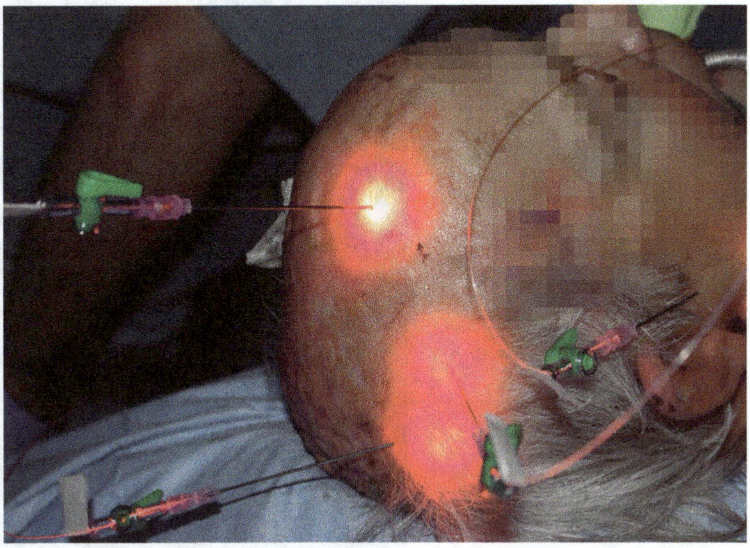

Fig. 3 Interstitial PDT of multiple skin squamous cell carcinomas

sparing of tissue architecture, providing a matrix for regeneration of normal tissue [1–24].

Intraoperative imaging-guided needle insertion into the tumour mass has enabled more accurate identification of tumour centre and periphery. Here a three-dimensional application therapy is enabled. This is usually aided by a specialist in head and neck interventional radiology. To date guiding modalities included two-dimensional-ultrasound (2D-US), magnetic resonance imaging (MRI), computed tomography (CT), nasoendoscopy, laryngoscopy and bronchoscopy. The model of US-guided photodynamic therapy is described here [1–24].

Intraoperatively, an ultrasound (EMP 1100 with high-resolution) probe is used to examine the pathological tissue (centre and periphery). The main aim here is to determine tumour volume, depth, invasion of vascular structures, hollow organs or hard tissue (Figs. 4, 5 and 6). This is usually followed by insertion of 18 Gauge 70 mm long spinal needles under US guidance into the pathological tissue. Great care is taken to ensure that the needles are inserted parallel to each other with 1 cm distance in between. If the treatment is close to a major blood vessel, a safety distance of 1 cm between the needle and the vessel is implemented to avoid any possible risk to promoting rupture in case the vessel wall contained tumour (Fig. 7) [1–24].

A four-channel 652 nm diode laser is used for illumination. Bare polished tip laser light delivery fibres with a core diameter of 400 μm are introduced through the spinal needles into the tumour.

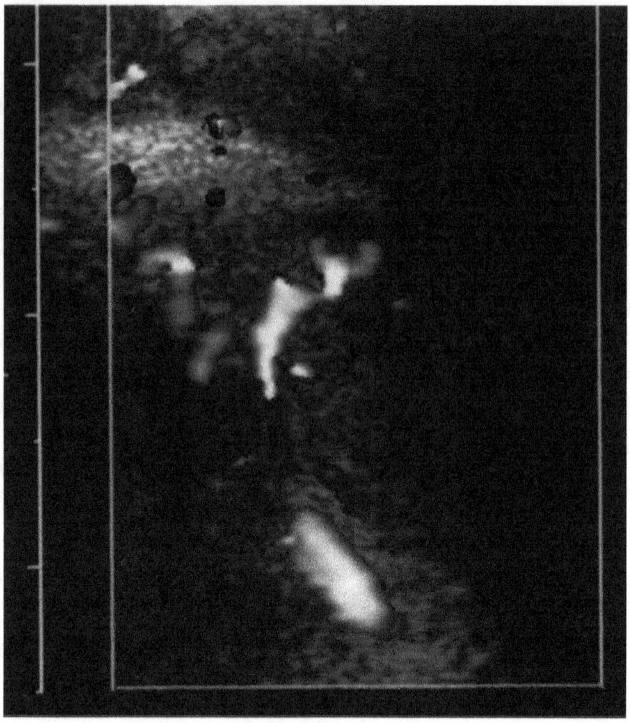

Fig. 4 Ultrasound image showing vascular malformation (haemangioma) of face and neck. The figure is adapted from authors' own article: Jerjes W, Upile T, Vincent A, Abbas S, Shah P, Mosse CA, McCarthy E, El-Maaytah M, Topping W, Morley S, Hopper C. Management of deep-seated malformations with photodynamic therapy: a new guiding imaging modality. Lasers Med Sci. 2009;24(5):769–75

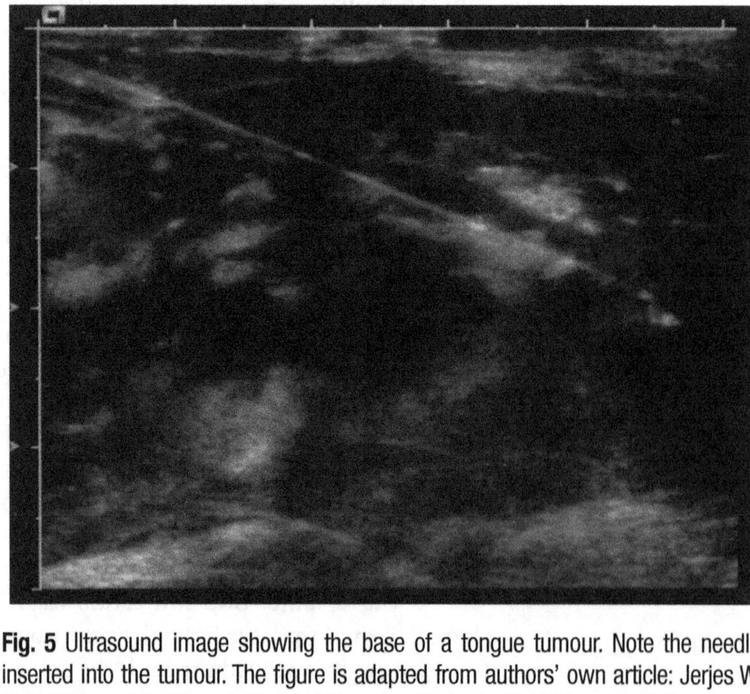

Fig. 5 Ultrasound image showing the base of a tongue tumour. Note the needle inserted into the tumour. The figure is adapted from authors' own article: Jerjes W, Upile T, Vincent A, Abbas S, Shah P, Mosse CA, McCarthy E, El-Maaytah M, Topping W, Morley S, Hopper C. Management of deep-seated malformations with photodynamic therapy: a new guiding imaging modality. Lasers Med Sci. 2009;24(5):769–75

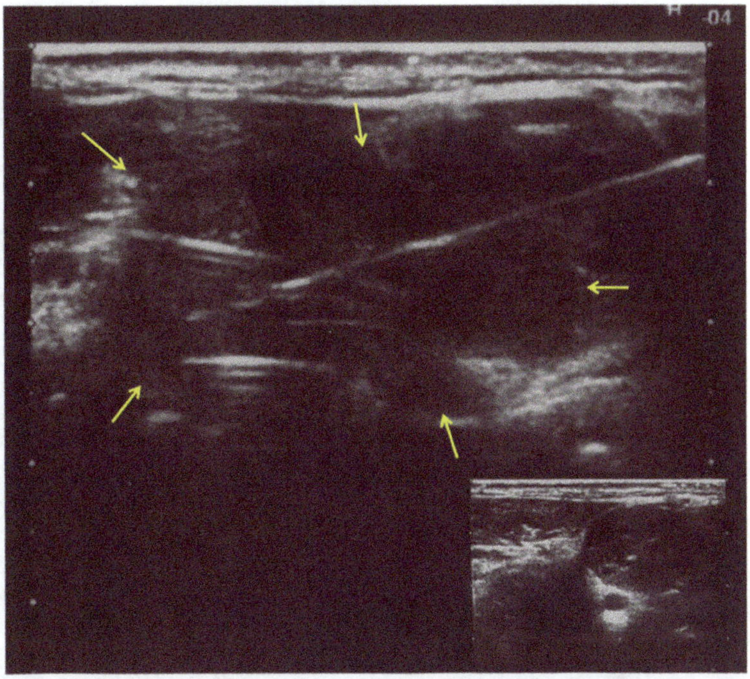

Fig. 6 Ultrasound image showing needle insertion in bilateral tongue base carcinoma followed by insertion of polished tip optical fibres. The patient also had necrotic cervical lymph node (*inset*) treated at the same time. The figure is adapted from authors' own article: Jerjes W, Upile T, Hamdoon Z, Abbas S, Akram S, Mosse CA, Morley S, Hopper C. Photodynamic therapy: The minimally invasive surgical intervention for advanced and/or recurrent tongue base carcinoma. Lasers Surg Med. 2011;43(4):283–92

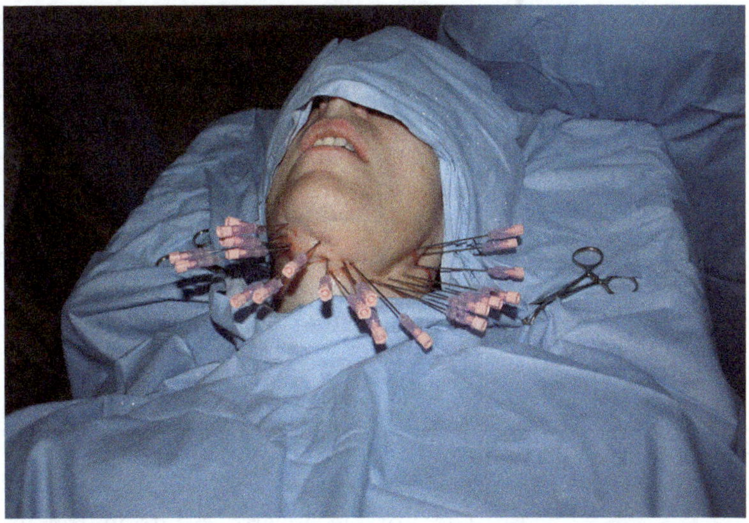

Fig. 7 Needle insertion under US guidance in a patient with bilateral tongue base and floor of mouth carcinoma with multiple reactive cervical lymph nodes. The figure is adapted from authors' own article: Jerjes W, Upile T, Akram S, Hopper C. The surgical palliation of advanced head and neck cancer using photodynamic therapy. Clin Oncol (R Coll Radiol). 2010;22(9):785–91

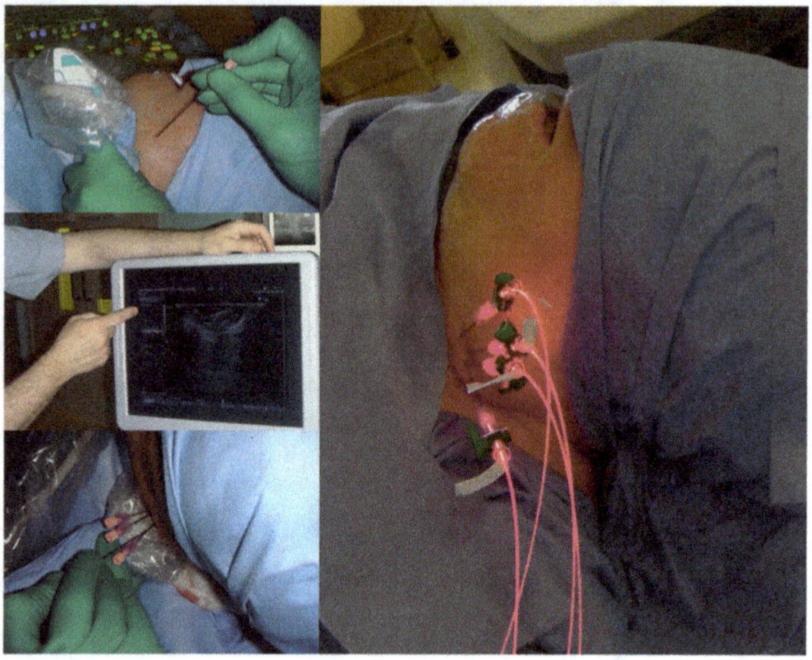

Fig. 8 Ultrasound-guided interstitial photodynamic therapy of peri-carotid disease. Note parallel array needle insertion, optical fibres feeding into the delivery needles and tissue illumination. The figure is adapted from authors' own article: Jerjes W, Upile T, Hamdoon Z, Nhembe F, Bhandari R, Mackay S, Shah P, Mosse CA, Brookes JA, Morley S, Hopper C. Ultrasound-guided photodynamic therapy for deep seated pathologies: prospective study. Lasers Surg Med. 2009;41(9):612–21

The fibres are allowed to protrude by 2–3 mm from the needle tip into tissue to ensure maximal tissue illumination. The incident light dose is 20 J/cm^2, delivered at an irradiance of 100 mW/cm^2 to the target tissue, implying an illumination time of approximately 200 s. Each bare tip fibre delivers an output power of ≈0.5 W. The delivery method of light to initiate the photochemical reaction depends on the tumour size and location (Figs. 8 and 9). Diffuser fibres are used when treating vascular tumours along with the bare polished tip fibres. The structure of the vascular tumours allows maximal tissue illumination when using those types of fibres (Fig. 10) [1–24].

Pain and Swelling Control

The notable adverse events in the immediate post-treatment phase include pain and swelling. Pain is experienced at some stage following PDT by all of the patients. Pain usually peaks at 48–72 h postoperatively. Special PDT pain protocols are followed. NSAIDs and opiates are usually supplied if not contraindicated when managing superficial disease. The standard regime, when managing a deep-seated disease in head and neck cancer patients,

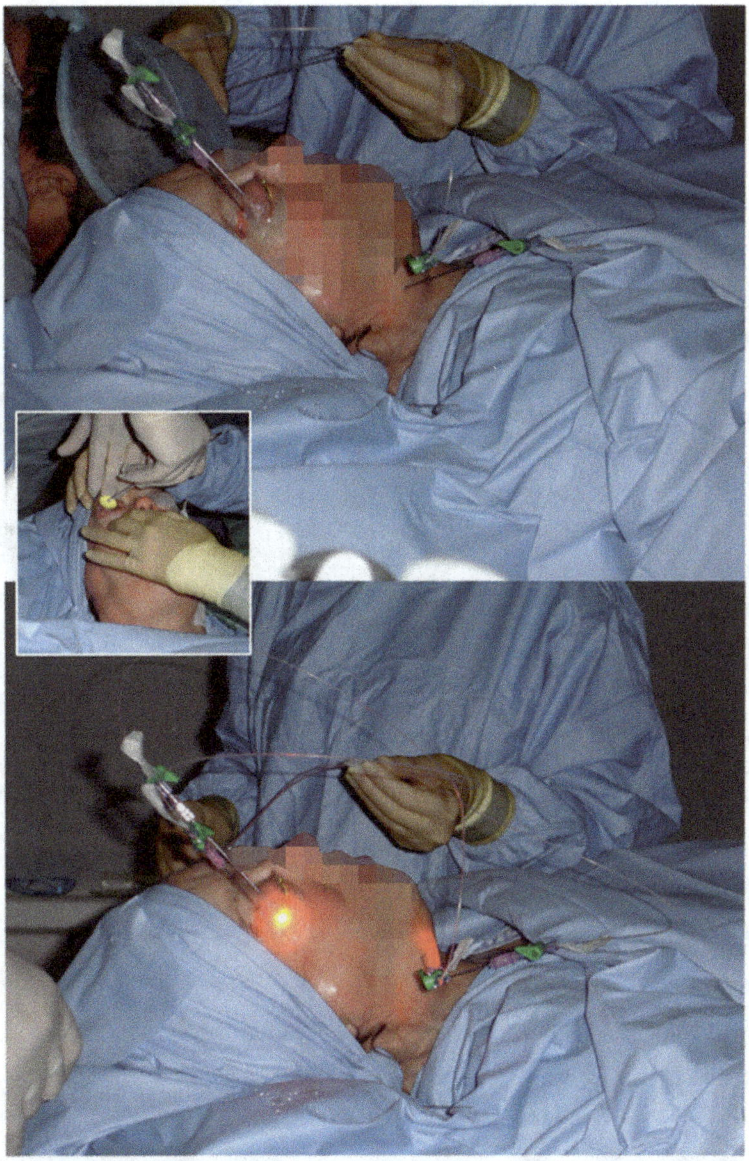

Fig. 9 *Top*: Needle insertion under US-guidance to the supraorbital region and submandibular lymph node. *Middle*: eye shield inserted prior to treatment. *Bottom*: tissue interstitial illumination with 652 nm diode laser. The figure is adapted from authors' own article: Hamdoon Z, Jerjes W, Upile T, Osher J, Hopper C. Lacrimal gland mantle lymphoma treated with photodynamic therapy: overview and report of a case. Photodiagnosis Photodyn Ther. 2010;7(2):129–33

involves a fentanyl transdermal patch 72 h 12 mcg/h with morphine sulphate (immediate release) as needed for breakthrough pain. Dose-escalating the patient's own pain medication or prescribing patient-controlled analgesics is implemented when indicated. Usually different specialist centres have different PDT pain-control protocols depending on experience and the areas treated [1–24].

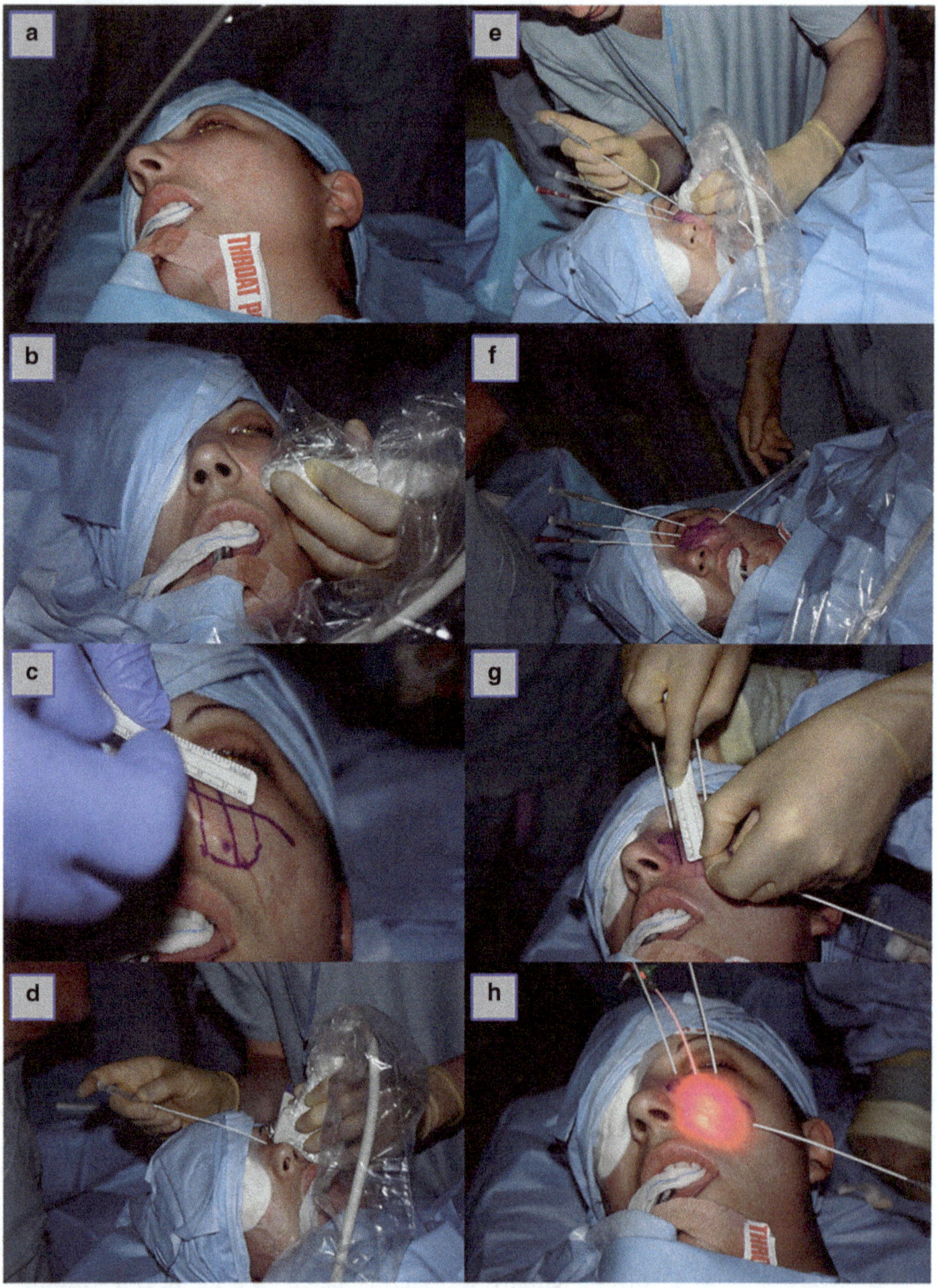

Fig. 10 US-guided interstitial photodynamic therapy of haemangioma of the left infraorbital region. (**a**) Patient draped, prepped and eye shield applied; (**b**) Intraoperative ultrasound scanning of the centre and periphery of the lesions; (**c**) marking the path for needle insertion; (**d**) first needle insertion under US-guidance; (**e**) further needles inserted; (**f**) complete needle insertion to ensure coverage of the whole lesion width and depth;

Airway control is a priority, when managing disease in the oropharyngeal–laryngeal region, as compromise can occur as part of the local inflammatory reaction. If a potential compromise is expected, an elective tracheostomy prior to interstitial PDT is implemented; this is commonly practised when managing advanced tumours. In this case, a tracheostomy tube is inserted intraoperatively and kept for 3–5 days postoperatively; intravenous steroids (i.e. dexamethasone) are also administered for 3 days to reduce local inflammatory responses and reduce swelling. The use of nasopharyngeal tubes has been found to be helpful in patients treated for oral pathologies using PDT [1–24].

Tissue Changes

To date, there is no exact scientific documentation about the stages that tissues go through following the initiation of the photodynamic process. Based on treating large cohorts of patients we have identified three stages:

1. Acute inflammatory/immunological tissue reactions. Usually pathologies undergo these changes within the first few hours and last for 2–3 days. This is usually associated with transient increase in inflammatory markers and significant pain and swelling, which may be due to histamine release. Superficial disease shows redness and peeling of oral tissues or skin with occasional blister formation, while peri-pathological inflammation on the MRI or CT has been identified when managing deep-seated pathologies.
2. Cellular death and tissue necrosis. Usually starts few hours post-illumination and may continue up to 5–6 weeks. Superficial disease shows tissue necrosis and slough formation which disintegrates after few weeks and this is usually associated with unpleasant odour. Deeper pathologies, on the other hand, display marked tissue necrosis on MRI or CT which a PDT-experienced radiologist to interpret these findings.
3. Healing and tissue regeneration (Fig. 11). Usually started from 2 to 3 weeks and lasted up to 6 weeks.

A common finding, adjacent macroscopically normal appearing tissue can become photosensitised and undergo necrosis or

Fig. 10 (continued) (**g**) measuring needle length inside the tissue to ensure that the tip is not too close to the skin surface which can lead to necrosis, this was followed by optical diffuser fibre insertion; and (**h**) light delivered to the diseased tissue. The figure is adapted from authors' own article: Jerjes W, Upile T, Alexander Mosse C, Hamdoon Z, Morcos M, Morley S, Hopper C. Prospective evaluation of 110 patients following ultrasound-guided photodynamic therapy for deep seated pathologies. Photodiagnosis Photodyn Ther. 2011;8(4):297–306

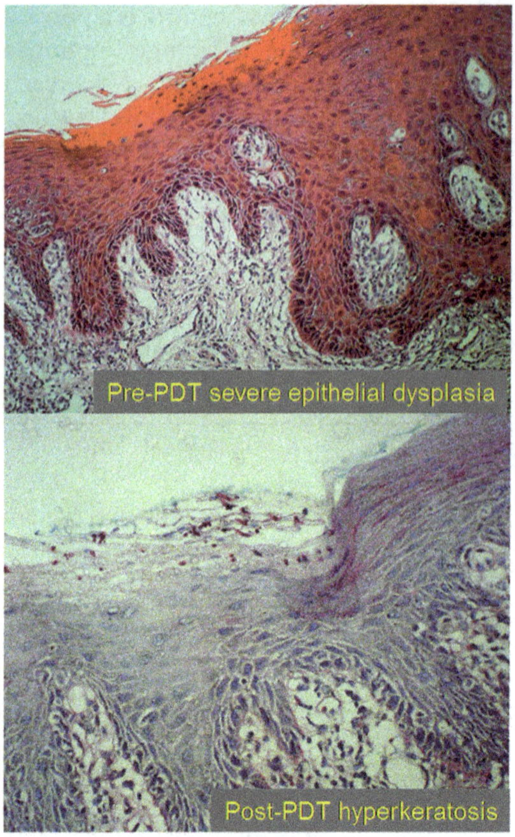

Fig. 11 Histopathology images of severe oral dysplasia subjected to PDT. Hyperkeratosis replaced most of the dysplastic tissue. The figure is adapted from authors' own article: Jerjes W, Upile T, Hamdoon Z, Mosse CA, Akram S, Hopper C. Photodynamic therapy outcome for oral dysplasia. Lasers Surg Med. 2011;43(3):192–9

apoptosis causing unfavourable outcome (i.e. ulceration of the mucosa and necrosis of the skin). The optimal way of reducing these effects is by ensuring that the light doesn't illuminate any adjacent areas either by using special probes or by shielding the adjacent tissues (i.e. skin or mucosa) [1–24].

Residual Systemic Photosensitisation

The major side effect of PDT is residual systemic photosensitisation, which lasts for several days or weeks depending on the administered photosensitiser. This is caused by minor concentrations of the photosensitiser in the skin and may lead to oedema, sunburn or even superficial skin necrosis when normal skin is exposed to bright light (Figs. 12, 13 and 14). So far 5-aminolevulinic acid (5-ALA) is the only photosensitiser that can be applied

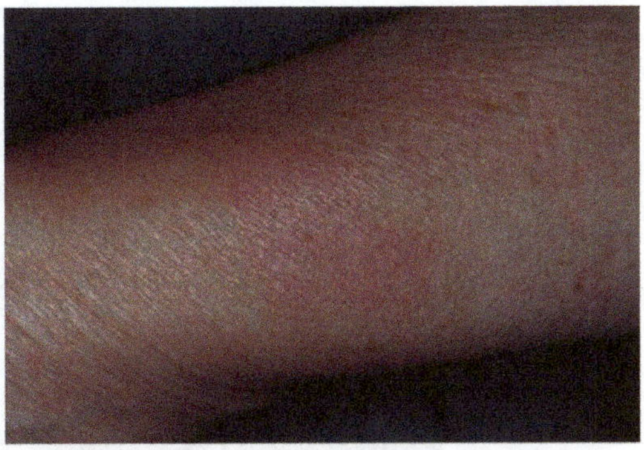

Fig. 12 Photosensitivity reactions—mild. The figure is adapted from authors' own article: Jerjes W, Upile T, Betz CS, El Maaytah M, Abbas S, Wright A, Hopper C. The application of photodynamic therapy in the head and neck. Dent Update. 2007;34(8):478–80, 483–4, 486

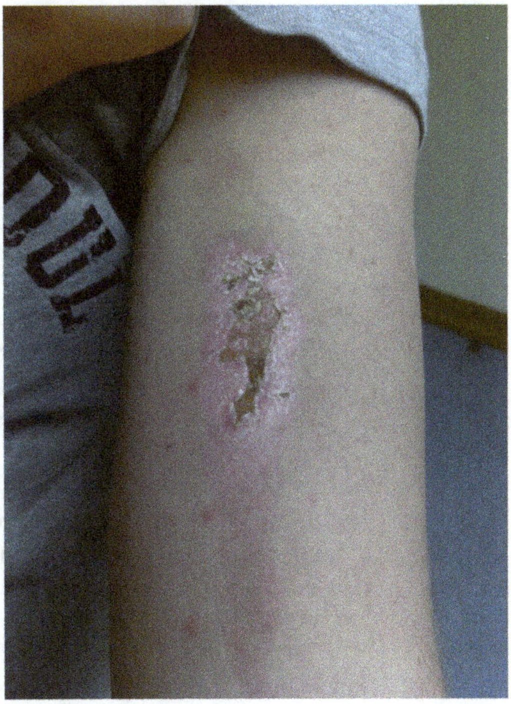

Fig. 13 Healing of third-degree skin burn following inadvertent sun exposure. This is the arm where the photosensitiser is administered. Patients are given pre- and post-treatment instructions (including written) regarding light exposure and complication avoidance and reporting. The figure is adapted from authors' own article: Jerjes W, Upile T, Hamdoon Z, Nhembe F, Bhandari R, Mackay S, Shah P, Mosse CA, Brookes JA, Morley S, Hopper C. Ultrasound-guided photodynamic therapy for deep seated pathologies: prospective study. Lasers Surg Med. 2009;41(9):612–21

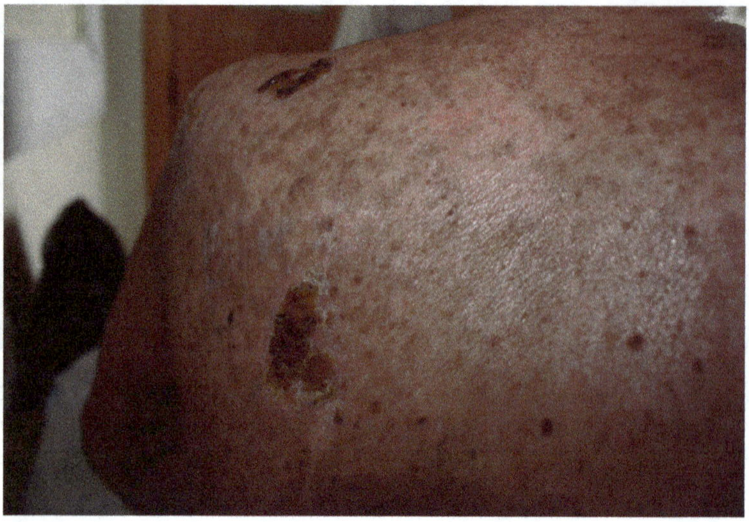

Fig. 14 Healing of third-degree skin burn following inadvertent sun exposure

topically; all others have to be given intravenously. The advantage of topically applied ALA is the complete lack of systemic photosensitivity and the fact that ALA-treated patients do not have to avoid exposure to light following treatment. The major disadvantage of a topically applied photosensitiser is the small treatment depth of only 1–2 mm that can be obtained. Therefore, only very superficial lesions of less than 1 mm can be treated successfully [1–24].

Gradual light re-exposure at an incremental rate of 100 lux/day is implemented. Every patient is instructed on the need to avoid direct sun exposure for up to 2 weeks after injection and is given light exposure guidelines. Patients, sometimes, fail to achieve a gradual re-exposure to sunlight and as a result they develop skin burn, 1st or 2nd degree, when they are exposed for the first time to direct sun light after 3–4 weeks of treatment. Also, the skin over the injection site (especially the arm area) is more sensitive to light and skin burn has been reported to occur up to 10 weeks after the photosensitisation in this area [1–24].

Assessment of Outcome

The patients' symptom-related disease included visual, breathing, swallowing and speech problems, as well as disfigurement and impeded limb function are documented. As there is no current verified assessment of quality of life in patients undergoing photodynamic therapy, the patients are asked only to report the nature of the complaint and not the severity. Patients are followed up and

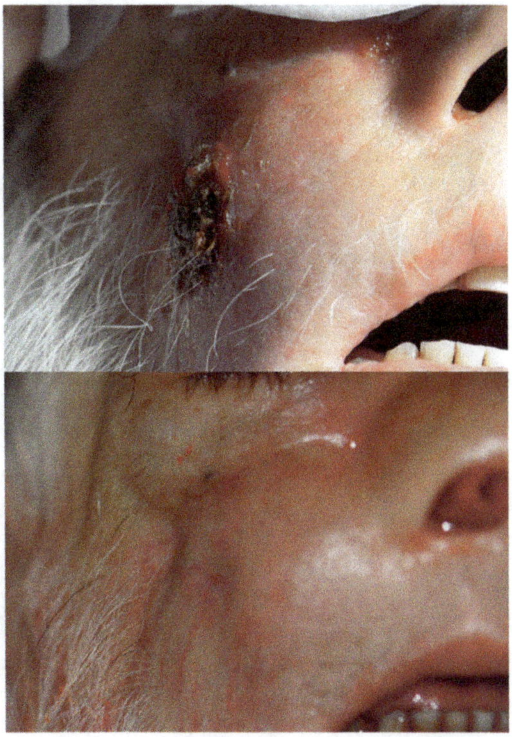

Fig. 15 Treatment of skin cancer with PDT. *Top*: fungating tumour mass of the right cheek which was subjected to subcutaneous interstitial photodynamic therapy. No surface illumination techniques were employed trying to avoid skin ulceration. *Bottom*: tumour mass necrosis and skin regeneration with minimal tethering and scaring and no ulceration. The figure is adapted from authors' own article: Hamdoon Z, Jerjes W, Upile T, Akram S, Hopper C. Metastatic renal cell carcinoma to the orofacial region: A novel method to alleviate symptoms and control disease progression. Photodiagnosis Photodyn Ther. 2010;7(4):246–50

asked to report on the outcome of their therapy if there is any improvement, no change or worsening of symptoms. Clinical assessment outcome is performed by a team of surgeons/physicians trained in photodynamic therapy at approximately 4–6 weeks postoperatively [1–24].

Lesion response evaluation is carried out according to RECIST: **complete response** (CR): disappearance of all target lesions for at least 4 weeks; **partial response** (PR): at least a 30 % decrease in the sum of the longest diameter (LD) of target lesions confirmed at 4 weeks; **stable disease** (SD): neither sufficient shrinkage to qualify for PR nor sufficient increase to qualify for progressive disease taking as references the smallest sum LD; and **progressive disease** (PD): at least a 20 % increase in the sum of LD of target lesions taking as references the smallest sum LD recorded since the treatment started or the appearance of one or more new lesions (Figs. 15 and 16) [1–24].

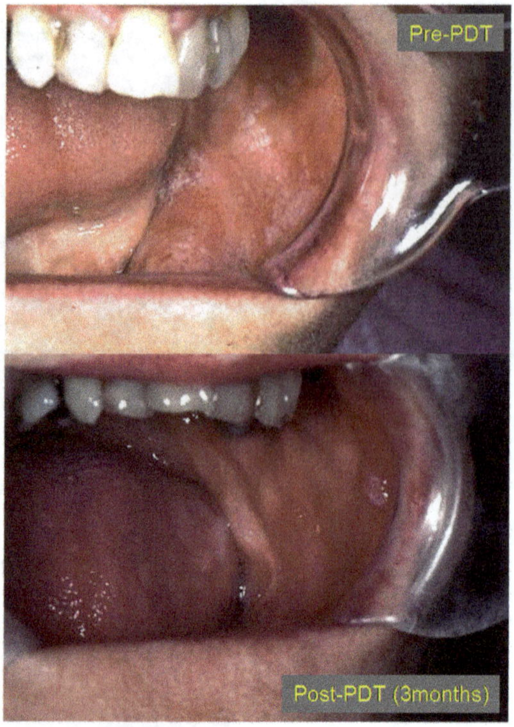

Fig. 16 Clinical images showing response of moderate oral dysplasia to photodynamic therapy. The figure is adapted from authors' own article: Jerjes W, Upile T, Hamdoon Z, Mosse CA, Akram S, Hopper C. Photodynamic therapy outcome for oral dysplasia. Lasers Surg Med. 2011;43(3):192–9

MRI or CT imaging is performed 5–6 weeks post-PDT. Comparisons are, then, made to assess radiological outcome. Radiological assessment parameters include no response (no change in pathology size), minimal response (reduce size by <25 %), moderate response (reduce size by <50 %) and significant response (reduce size by 50–75 %). Identification of peri-pathology or peri-lesional inflammation, assessing response to PDT, should also be reported (Figs. 17, 18 and 19) [1–24].

Our Experience

In order to encourage evidence-based practice in medicine and surgery, and to ensure that the treatment and processes are sound, we developed upon the work of our previous preliminary prospective studies, collecting data from a larger population treated. We evaluated the outcome following ultrasound-guided iPDT (US-iPDT) of deep-seated pathologies. Patients' reports on quality of life with clinical and radiological evaluation were the main parameters used to assess the outcome. Further factors influencing

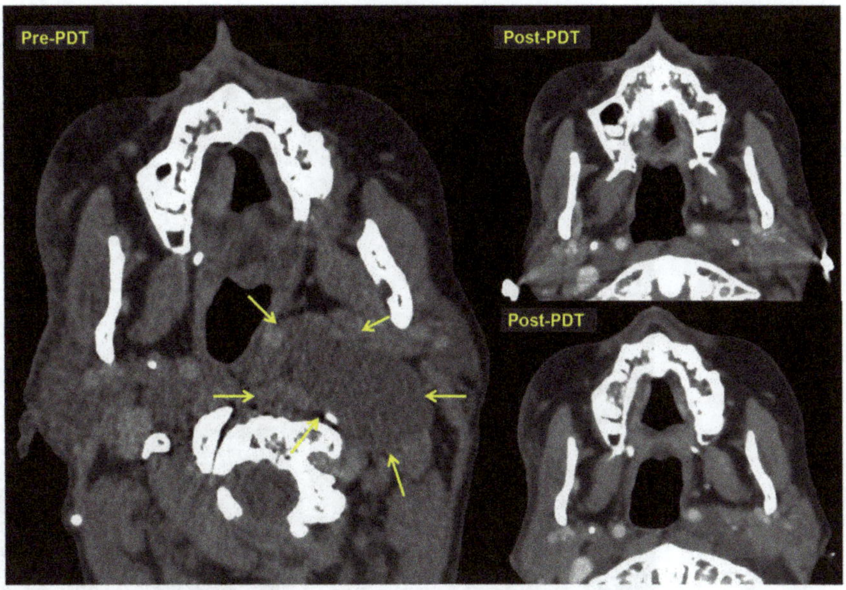

Fig. 17 Axial MRI scanning of neurofibroma of the neck. *Left*: pre-PDT showing extensive lesion compressing the airway. *Right* (*top* and *bottom*) post-PDT scans slightly upper and lower to the pre-PDT scan level showing significant shrinkage with increase in airway patency. The figure is adapted from authors' own article: Hamdoon Z, Jerjes W, Al-Delayme R, Hopper C. Solitary giant neurofibroma of the neck subjected to photodynamic therapy: case study. Head Neck Oncol. 2012;4(1):30

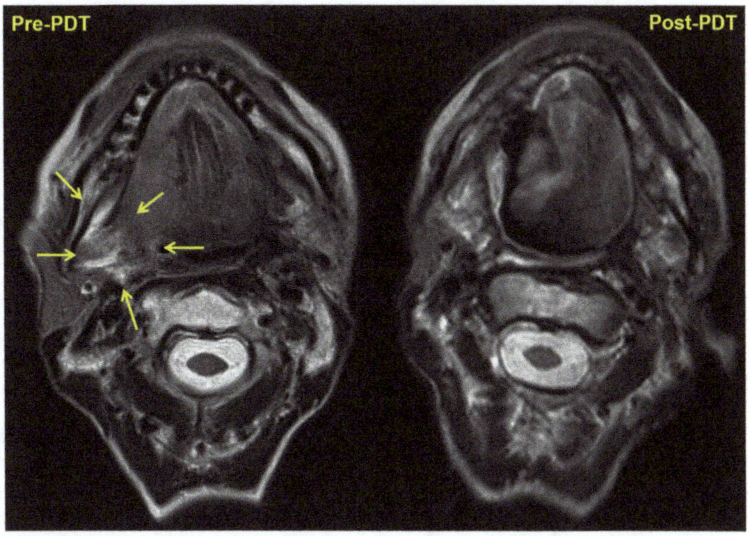

Fig. 18 Axial MRI scanning of SCC of the posterio-lateral tongue. *Left*: pre-PDT; *right*: post-PDT showing extensive necrosis of the tumour area. The figure is adapted from authors' own article: Jerjes W, Upile T, Akram S, Hopper C. The surgical palliation of advanced head and neck cancer using photodynamic therapy. Clin Oncol (R Coll Radiol). 2010;22(9):785–91

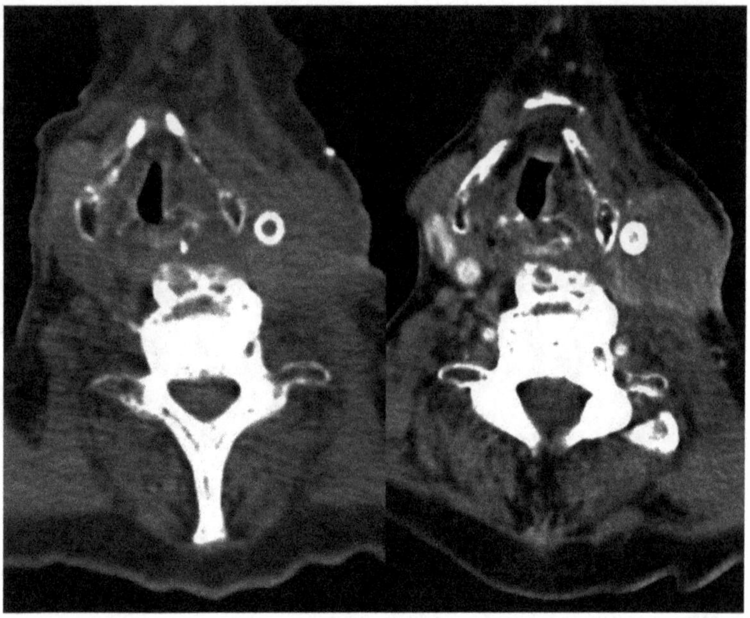

Fig. 19 PDT in the management of peri-carotid disease. *Left*: axial CT with contrast post stent insertion. Peri-carotid and left vocal cord disease can be seen with midline shift. *Right*: 4 weeks post-US-guided interstitial PDT, necrotic tissue formation can be seen with peri-tumour inflammation and improvement of airway patency. Granulation tissue formation can be seen in the stent area. The images are the best exact match that could be achieved. The figure is adapted from authors' own article: Hamdoon Z, Jerjes W, Upile T, Hoonjan P, Hopper C. Endoluminal carotid stenting prior to photodynamic therapy to pericarotid malignant disease: technical advance. Photodiagnosis Photodyn Ther. 2010;7(2):126–8

outcome, follow-up and the future of this modality are being discussed. One hundred and ten patients were referred to the UCLH Head and Neck Centre, London for treatment of a range of deep-seated pathologies related to the head and neck region, upper and lower limbs (from 2007 to 2009). The mean age was 53 years with three-quarters of the cohort being Caucasians. The most common primary sites were the oral and oropharyngeal regions, mid face and upper limbs. Fifty-two patients were diagnosed with carcinomas, 11 with sarcomas and 42 with vascular anomalies. Disease staging was carried out and showed that nearly all the malignant tumours were stage IV or of a high-grade nature; while all the vascular anomalies were regional rather than local. Tumour volume was assessed using preoperative imaging (CT or MRI). Thirty-nine patients were not suitable for conventional management (not including palliative), while 45 patients declined further treatment (Table 1) [6].

The patients' symptom-related disease included visual, breathing, swallowing and speech problems, as well as disfigurement and impeded limb function. Five patients reported visual problems due

Table 1
Demographic details of 110 patients with deep-seated pathologies treated with PDT

	No. (%)	Diagnosis	No. (%)
Gender			
Male	63 (57.3)	Squamous cell carcinoma	39 (35.5)
Female	47 (42.7)	Adenoid cystic carcinoma	4 (3.6)
		Adenocarcinoma	4 (3.6)
Age (years)		Acinic cell carcinoma	2 (1.8)
Mean	53.1	Mucoepidermoid carcinoma	2 (1.8)
Minimum–maximum	0.5–93	Metastatic carcinoma	1 (0.9)
St. deviation	24.1		
		Chondrosarcoma	1 (0.9)
Primary site		Osteosarcoma	2 (1.8)
Oral cavity	17 (15.5)	Rhabdomyosarcoma	2 (1.8)
Oropharynx	26 (23.6)	Fibromyxoid sarcoma	1 (0.9)
Larynx	2 (1.8)	Angiosarcoma	5 (4.6)
Lower respiratory tract	2 (1.8)		
		Arteriovenous malformation	9 (8.2)
Mid face	32 (29.1)	Haemangioma	14 (12.8)
Lower face	9 (8.2)	Lymphangioma	13 (11.9)
Neck	6 (5.5)	Neurofibroma	3 (2.7)
		Mixed hamartoma	3 (2.7)
Upper limb	12 (10.9)		
Lower limb	3 (2.7)	Kimura disease	1 (0.9)
Glans penis	1 (0.9)	Pleomorphic adenoma	2 (1.8)
		Malignant melanoma	1 (0.9)
		Mantle cell lymphoma	1 (0.9)

Modified from: Jerjes W, Upile T, Alexander Mosse C, Hamdoon Z, Morcos M, Morley S, Hopper C. Prospective evaluation of 110 patients following ultrasound-guided photodynamic therapy for deep seated pathologies. Photodiagnosis Photodyn Ther. 2011;8(4):297–306

to globe compression by external swelling caused by the pathology, or tumour invading the optic nerve or retinal vessels. Problems associated with pathological growth in the oropharyngeal/laryngeal region caused breathing problems in 32 patients, swallowing problems in 37 patients and speech problems in 29 patients. Disfigurement was reported by 52 patients (mostly with vascular anomalies) and impeded limb function was found in 9 patients (Table 2) [6].

Four out of the five patients who had visual problems reported improvement after treatment ($p<0.001$). Also 27/32 patients reported improvement of breathing ($p<0.001$), with one patient reporting worsening of symptoms. Improvement of swallowing was reported by 30/37 patients ($p<0.001$), with three patients reporting progressive dysphagia, indicating poor response. Speech improvement was evident in 22/29 patients ($p<0.001$) and 43/52 reported reduction in the disfigurement caused by their pathology

Table 2
Patient's response to PDT: clinical and radiological assessments

Patient's report	No. (%)	Clinical assessment	No. (%)
Visual problems	**5**	No response	3 (2.7)
Improved ($p<0.001$)	4 (80.0)	Minimal response	15 (13.6)
No change	1 (20.0)	Moderate response	39 (35.5)
Worse	0 (0.0)	Good response	48 (43.6)
		Free of disease	5 (4.6)
Breathing problems	**32**		
Improved ($p<0.001$)	27 (84.4)	**Radiological assessment**	
No change	4 (12.5)	No response—stable	6 (5.5)
Worse	1 (3.1)	No response—progressing	4 (3.6)
		Minimal response	23 (20.9)
Swallowing problems	**37**	Moderate response	45 (40.9)
Improved ($p<0.001$)	30 (81.1)	Significant response	32 (29.1)
No change	4 (10.8)		
Worse	3 (8.1)	**PEG**	12 (10.9)
		Nasopharyngeal	19 (17.3)
Speaking problems	**29**	**Tracheostomy**	18 (16.4)
Improved ($p<0.001$)	22 (75.9)	**NG feed**	25 (22.7)
No change	5 (17.2)		
Worse	2 (6.9)	**Complications**	
		Emergency airway	6 (5.5)
Disfigurement	**52**	Fistula	7 (6.4)
Improved ($p<0.001$)	43 (82.7)	Infection	11 (10.0)
No change	6 (11.5)	Skin necrosis	4 (3.6)
Worse	3 (5.8)	Skin burn	13 (11.8)
		Peripheral edema	2 (1.8)
Limb function	**9**	Motor nerve injury	4 (3.6)
Improved ($p<0.001$)	7 (77.8)	Severe haemorrhage/transfusion	2 (1.8)
No change	1 (11.1)	Stroke	2 (1.8)
Worse	1 (11.1)		

Modified from: Jerjes W, Upile T, Alexander Mosse C, Hamdoon Z, Morcos M, Morley S, Hopper C. Prospective evaluation of 110 patients following ultrasound-guided photodynamic therapy for deep seated pathologies. Photodiagnosis Photodyn Ther. 2011;8(4):297–306

($p < 0.001$). Seven out of nine patients reported improved of impeded limb function ($p < 0.001$) [6].

Clinical assessment showed that 48/110 patients had "good response" to the treatment and 39/110 had "moderate response" with five patients being "disease free." Radiological assessment comparing imaging 6-week post-PDT to the baseline showed stable pathology with no change in size in 6/110 patients, minimal response (<25 % reduction) in 23/110 patients, moderate response (<50 % reduction) in 45/110 patients and significant response (50–75 % reduction) in 32 patients. Unfortunately, four patients showed no response with pathology progression (noted in two squamous cell carcinoma, one angiosarcoma and one malignant melanoma patients). Peri-pathology inflammation was reported in all 110 patients indicating a successful photochemical reaction in all patients [6].

The clinical responses have almost in all cases were associated with reported improvement of symptoms of patients treated with PDT ; however, radiological response reported varying degree of disease shrinkage with this outcome. We have noticed that our guidance of successful treatment is the clinical assessment rather than the radiological one. Patients who suffered from pathologies in the oropharyngeal/laryngeal regions had undergone prophylactic nasopharyngeal tube insertion ($n = 19$) or elective tracheostomy ($n = 18$) to maintain airway. Unfortunately, postoperative complications resulted in emergency tracheostomy tube insertion in six further patients. No drug interactions have been observed [6].

Patients with superficial and deep-seated pathologies undergoing photodynamic therapy are likely to benefit from the intervention, especially in case of advanced and/or recurrent disease. Our studies have provided further evidence that PDT is a useful modality in the management of these pathologies that are otherwise resistant to conventional treatments and with minimal side effects [1–24].

References

1. Hamdoon Z, Jerjes W, Al-Delayme R, Hopper C. Solitary giant neurofibroma of the neck subjected to photodynamic therapy: case study. Head Neck Oncol. 2012;4(1):30.
2. Abbas S, Jerjes W, Upile T, Vaz F, Hopper C. The palliative role of PDT in recurrent advanced nasopharyngeal carcinoma: case series. Photodiagnosis Photodyn Ther. 2012;9(2):142–7.
3. Jerjes W, Hamdoon Z, Hopper C. Photodynamic therapy in the management of potentially malignant and malignant oral disorders. Head Neck Oncol. 2012; 4(1):16.
4. Abbas S, Jerjes W, Upile T, Vincent A, Hopper C. Treatment of Kimura disease with photodynamic therapy: a case study. Photodiagnosis Photodyn Ther. 2012;9(1):83–6.
5. Jerjes W, Upile T, Radhi H, Hopper C. Photodynamic therapy and end-stage tongue base cancer: short communication. Head Neck Oncol. 2011;3(1):49.
6. Jerjes W, Upile T, Alexander Mosse C, Hamdoon Z, Morcos M, Morley S, Hopper C. Prospective evaluation of 110 patients following ultrasound-guided photodynamic therapy for deep seated pathologies. Photodiagnosis Photodyn Ther. 2011;8(4):297–306.

7. Jerjes W, Upile T, Hamdoon Z, Alexander Mosse C, Morcos M, Hopper C. Photodynamic therapy outcome for T1/T2 N0 oral squamous cell carcinoma. Lasers Surg Med. 2011;43(6):463–9.
8. Jerjes W, Upile T, Hamdoon Z, Mosse CA, Akram S, Morley S, Hopper C. Interstitial PDT for vascular anomalies. Lasers Surg Med. 2011;43(5):357–65.
9. Jerjes W, Upile T, Hamdoon Z, Abbas S, Akram S, Mosse CA, Morley S, Hopper C. Photodynamic therapy: the minimally invasive surgical intervention for advanced and/or recurrent tongue base carcinoma. Lasers Surg Med. 2011;43(4):283–92.
10. Jerjes W, Upile T, Hamdoon Z, Mosse CA, Akram S, Hopper C. Photodynamic therapy outcome for oral dysplasia. Lasers Surg Med. 2011;43(3):192–9.
11. Osher J, Jerjes W, Upile T, Hamdoon Z, Morley S, Hopper C. Adenoid cystic carcinoma of the tongue base treated with ultrasound-guided interstitial photodynamic therapy: a case study. Photodiagnosis Photodyn Ther. 2011;8(1):68–71.
12. Nhembe F, Jerjes W, Upile T, Hamdoon Z, Vaz F, Hopper C. Subglottic carcinoma treated with surgery and adjuvant photodynamic therapy. Photodiagnosis Photodyn Ther. 2010; 7(4):284–7.
13. Hamdoon Z, Jerjes W, Upile T, Akram S, Hopper C. Metastatic renal cell carcinoma to the orofacial region: a novel method to alleviate symptoms and control disease progression. Photodiagnosis Photodyn Ther. 2010;7(4): 246–50.
14. Jerjes W, Upile T, Akram S, Hopper C. The surgical palliation of advanced head and neck cancer using photodynamic therapy. Clin Oncol (R Coll Radiol). 2010;22(9):785–91.
15. Shah P, Jerjes W, Upile T, Hopper C. The effective management of a leg hemangioma using ultrasound-guided interstitial photodynamic therapy. Photodiagnosis Photodyn Ther. 2010;7(3):201–3.
16. Hamdoon Z, Jerjes W, Upile T, Akram S, Hopper C. Cystic hygroma treated with ultrasound guided interstitial photodynamic therapy: case study. Photodiagnosis Photodyn Ther. 2010;7(3):179–82.
17. Hamdoon Z, Jerjes W, Upile T, Osher J, Hopper C. Lacrimal gland mantle lymphoma treated with photodynamic therapy: overview and report of a case. Photodiagnosis Photodyn Ther. 2010;7(2):129–33.
18. Hamdoon Z, Jerjes W, Upile T, Hoonjan P, Hopper C. Endoluminal carotid stenting prior to photodynamic therapy to pericarotid malignant disease: technical advance. Photodiagnosis Photodyn Ther. 2010;7(2):126–8.
19. Nhembe F, Jerjes W, Upile T, Hamdoon Z, Hopper C. Chondrosarcoma of the hyoid treated with interstitial photodynamic therapy: case study. Photodiagnosis Photodyn Ther. 2009;6(3-4):235–7.
20. Jerjes W, Upile T, Hamdoon Z, Nhembe F, Bhandari R, Mackay S, Shah P, Mosse CA, Brookes JA, Morley S, Hopper C. Ultrasound-guided photodynamic therapy for deep seated pathologies: prospective study. Lasers Surg Med. 2009;41(9):612–21.
21. Jerjes W, Upile T, Vincent A, Abbas S, Shah P, Mosse CA, McCarthy E, El-Maaytah M, Topping W, Morley S, Hopper C. Management of deep-seated malformations with photodynamic therapy: a new guiding imaging modality. Lasers Med Sci. 2009;24(5):769–75.
22. Jerjes W, Upile T, Abbas S, Hopper C. Photodynamic therapy role in the premalignancy/malignancy of the head and neck. Oncol News. 2008;2(5):8–10.
23. Jerjes W, Upile T, Abbas S, Vincent A, Hopper C. The developing role of photodynamic therapy in multidisciplinary oncological care. Oncol News. 2008;3(3):12–5.
24. Jerjes W, Upile T, Betz CS, El Maaytah M, Abbas S, Wright A, Hopper C. The application of photodynamic therapy in the head and neck. Dent Update. 2007;34(8):478–80, 483–4, 486.

Chapter 21

Oral Cavity: Early Lesions

Max J.H. Witjes, Sebastiaan A.H.J. de Visscher, and Jan L.N. Roodenburg

Introduction

From the early development of photosensitizers, the treatment of oral premalignancies and cancers has been a major field of research in photodynamic therapy. The first clinically available photosensitizer, hematoporphyrin derivative (HpD) was first tested in 1982 in several head and neck malignancies, including the oral cavity, shortly after availability for clinical studies in 1978 [1, 2]. Although PDT has been applied in a wide variety of head and neck cancers, this chapter will focus on the results of first, second, and third generation sensitizers in the treatment of early (superficial) oral and accessible oropharyngeal carcinoma and potentially malignant disorders of the oral mucosa.

The Clinical Problem in Oral and Oropharyngeal Squamous Cell Carcinoma and Potentially Malignant Disorders of the Oral Mucosa

In most cases, the development of oral and oropharyngeal tumors is preceded by a so-called potentially malignant disorder of the mucosa. The clinical appearance of such lesions of the mucosa is usually described as a white patch (homogenous leukoplakia), red patch (erythroplakia), or a mixed white/red appearance (inhomogenous leukoplakia or erythroleukoplakia). Leukoplakia is considered as a premalignant lesion of which the nomenclature

Brian J.-F. Wong and Justus Ilgner (eds.), *Biomedical Optics in Otorhinolaryngology: Head and Neck Surgery*, DOI 10.1007/978-1-4939-1758-7_21, © Springer Science+Business Media New York 2016

has been altered to potentially malignant disorders (PMDs) [3]. PMD comprises "all clinical presentations that carry a risk of cancer" [3]. Entities such as submucosal fibrosis have a distinct presentation that may not be described as any form of leukoplakia but can also be regarded as a potentially malignant disorder. Other lesions such as oral lichen planus or lichen like lesions have a less clear premalignant character and are therefore not considered as PMD but may transform into a carcinoma in rare cases. Several authors have tried to assess the rate of malignant transformation of PMD. Since transformation from PMD into an invasive carcinoma may take several years, it is very difficult to establish the percentage of these disorders that will ultimately become a cancer. Observational studies of transformation of oral leukoplakia have yielded a wide variety of percentages of 2–30 % [4–7]. However, it is generally agreed that certain lesions such as erythroplakia have a very high risk of malignant transformation and that certain lesions such as homogenous leukoplakia carry a low risk. Histopathological or molecular analysis has not yet provided clear markers that can predict malignant transformation. Histopathology is considered as the gold standard in the diagnosis of PMD which mainly focuses on the presence of dysplasia in the examined mucosa. Dysplasia is usually described in three stages from slight, moderate, to severe. The nomenclature of severe dysplasia and carcinoma in situ (CIS) is often used alternatively for describing a state of the mucosal tissue as being at the brink of conversion into a carcinoma. Although such classifications are elementary for studying these lesions, there is no consensus on when and how these lesions should be treated [8]. Clinicians should treat in case of severe dysplasia. However, there is no consensus that a wait and see policy in case of early stage dysplasia or nondysplastic PMD is acceptable or not and if treatment should always be considered [8, 9].

Clinically, these mucosal disorders can be challenging to treat. Removal of risk factors such as smoking or alcohol abuse is essential, but often not achieved [10]. Some lesions recur or are of considerable size, which creates considerable morbidity after treatment with surgery (Fig. 1a, b). Determining the margin of such lesions can be difficult. Radiotherapy is usually not considered as therapy when malignant transformation has not occurred. Other strategies such as CO_2 laser evaporation have been quite successful in small-sized PMD [11]. Chemoprevention with several compounds such as retinoids or vitamins A/E has not been successful and is currently not considered as treatment. Treatment of recurrent lesions or of widespread PMD remains a problem for clinicians. Alterations to the oral mucosa are often widespread and therefore treatment of a large field of mucosa around PMDs might be a necessity [12]. Photodynamic therapy has been identified as a modality that can effectively treat PMD [13].

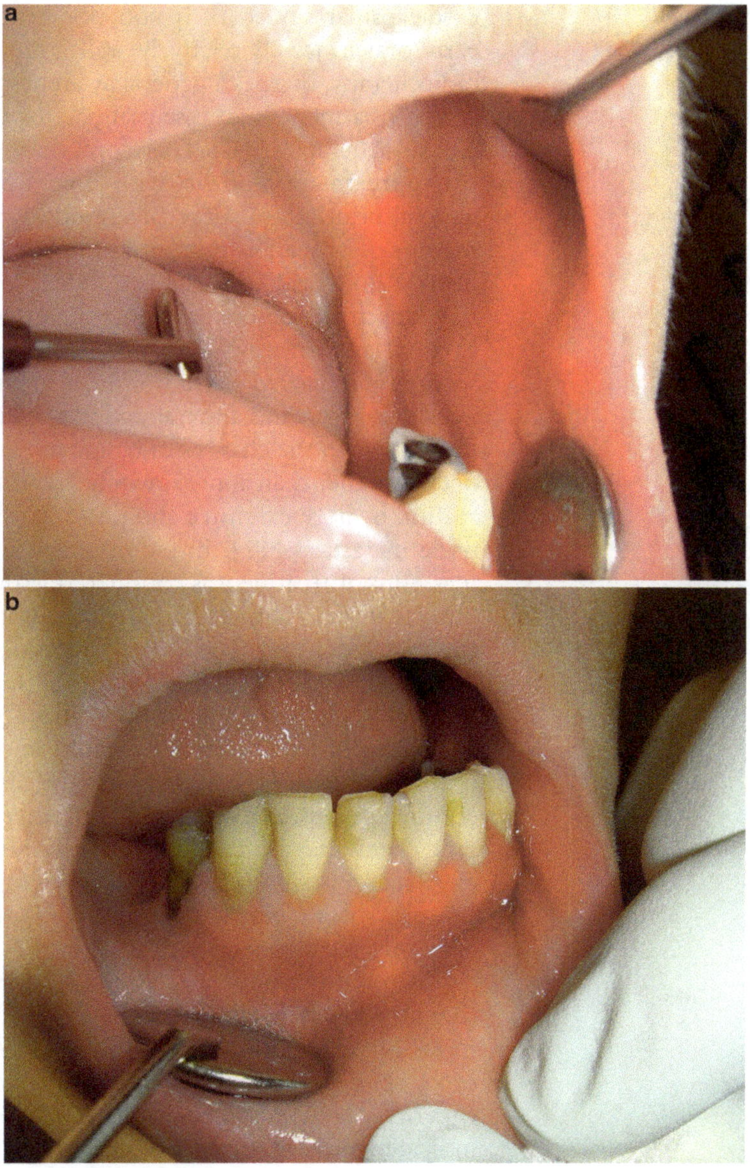

Fig. 1 Example of a widespread potentially malignant disorder of the oral mucosa in a patient with various degrees of dysplasia in the cheek (**a**) and gingiva of the lower mandible (**b**)

Oral and Accessible Oropharyngeal Squamous Cell Carcinoma

The current standard treatment of early oral squamous cell carcinoma is surgical removal, radiotherapy, or a combination of both. Overall survival in oral carcinoma is influenced by factors such as tumor size (T stage), the presence of lymph node metastasis (N stage), depth of infiltration, margin status after surgery, and extracapsular spread of lymph node metastasis [14, 15]. While early oral cancer is relatively well controlled by surgery and/or radiotherapy, there is a general awareness that reducing morbidity of the treatment is an essential part of the improvement of outcome of therapies [16]. Therefore, there is a rationale for an alternative treatment modality with fewer long-term side effects. The general principle of surgery is removal of the tumor with a clear margin of at least 5 mm in all directions which is measured on histopathological H&E stained slides [17]. In practice this means that due to tissue contraction after excision, the surgeon has to excise a larger margin sometimes close to 1 cm. When a neck dissection is indicated there is a differentiation between an elective neck dissection and a therapeutic neck dissection. The first is performed when the chances of lymphatic spread of the tumor to the neck is higher than approximately 20 %. The therapeutic neck dissection is more extensive and performed in case of proven lymph node metastasis [17]. In radiotherapy, a similar approach to primary tumor treatment is considered with regards to the total volume that needs to be radiated. Radiotherapists determine the tumor border on CT or MRI and add to that an extra margin, with exclusions of certain structures such as the eye, brain, or spine [18]. It is generally agreed that the strategy in oral cancer should be aimed at effective tumor removal with one modality in one attempt, to balance between the efficacy and morbidities. A combined approach of surgery and radiotherapy (or concommittant chemoradiation) should be used in high-risk cases, such as close margins after surgery, multiple lymph node metastasis, extra capsular spread, etc. The use of a combination of modalities leads to higher morbidity after treatment.

When the tumor burden is low, that is in superficial lesions, there is a low risk of metastasis to the lymph nodes. Usually squamous cell carcinomas of less than 4 mm invasive are regarded as such [19]. Therefore in most guidelines surgical removal of superficial (<4 mm invasion) oral squamous cell carcinoma is indicated without an elective neck dissection. Four millimeters of invasion still requires that an excision of at least 9 mm in depth is performed for obtaining surgical-free margins. After surgical removal of early superficial cancer long-term morbidity can be summarized as lack of mobility of the tongue, loss of sensation, or neuropathic pain of the tong or lower lip due to nerve damage. The consequences for patients can involve problems with propagation of food from the anterior of the mouth to the oropharynx, chronic pain syndromes in case of nerve damage, or oral incontinence due to the lack of sensation of the lower lip . Morbidities of radiotherapy of early squamous cell carcinoma of the oral cavity often include dry mouth due to loss of salivary secretion, altered or loss of taste due to nerve damage and of less incidence cases of long-term fibrosis with swallowing problems or (osteo) radionecrosis [20].

Photodynamic Therapy of Potentially Malignant Disorders of the Oral Mucosa

For treatment with PDT of potentially malignant disorders and squamous cell carcinoma several photosensitizers have been studied in preclinical studies. Four sensitizers have been studied used in clinical studies involving patient treatment, which will be the focus of this paragraph. The mechanisms of PDT and particular aspects of photosensitizers will not be discussed here. In PDT of PMD and early superficial squamous cell carcinoma, the illumination technique is that of superficial , which will be described further in this chapter. Studies of interstitial PDT will not be described in this chapter.

Several studies investigated the efficacy of photodynamic therapy as a treatment modality for PMD. The suggested benefit of PDT of PMD lies in the possibility of treating large areas of affected mucosa with minimal morbidity compared to an intervention such as surgery. The most investigated photosensitizer for PMD has been 5-Aminolevulinic acid (5-ALA) which can be administered intravenously, orally, or can be applied topically [21]. It is water soluble and therefore easy to dissolve for use. 5-ALA is the only drug in PDT that is not a photosensitizer but requires metabolization in the mitochondrion to the photosensitive compound protoporphyrin IX. In premalignant disorders of the skin, topical 5-ALA PDT is now routinely used with good results [22]. For treatment of PMD of the oral mucosa with 5-ALA as photosensitizer, 13 studies can be identified in the literature [23–36]. Because several groups published multiple papers, it is difficult to identify if the outcome of 5-ALA PDT of the same patients have repeatedly been described. The rationale is very clear for using a local treatment such as 5-ALA with little morbidity for patients suffering from potentially malignant disorders since a small proportion of PMD will develop into cancer but it cannot be predicted which lesions will. Most studies describe small patient numbers ($n = 10–15$) or some of less than 50 patients with relatively short follow-up time. Two studies have a large number of patients treated with 5-ALA ($n = 80$) [29, 37] or sufficiently long follow-up time (>60 months [13]. Treatment protocols differed substantially on major parameters which makes comparison between the studies difficult. In the 13 studies found, the concentration of 5-ALA differs from 10 to 20 %. The application time varies from 1 to 4 h. Some authors have used experimental gel-like application technique [37] and most of them used emulsions or cream. Illumination technique was fiber based using laser or LED light of 635 nm or close to that wavelength (628–630 nm). The early papers describe a one time illumination protocol, while more recently a different approach using a multiple of 5-ALA weekly treatment strategy which showed some interesting results with complete response rates over 90 % [35]. Authors have used different or no fractionated illumination schemes within one treatment. Next to that some authors use fluorescence spectroscopy to verify the presence of protoporphyrin IX, the PDT-active metabolite of 5-ALA. When comparing 5-ALA treatments, the outcome shows a significantly better response for multiple weekly treatments using fractionated illumination per treatment [37]. Multiple weekly treatments after 5-ALA application compensate for the limited penetration depth of ALA PDT which is found to be of a maximum around 1 mm [26]. It is largely depending on the penetration of 5-ALA into the mucosal layer which is influenced by factors such as the presence and)thickness of hyperkeratosis [32]. Impressive removal of very thick and extensive verrucous leukoplakia was achieved by multiple treatments with 5-ALA showing the possibility of this approach [34] (Fig. 2a–h). Authors describe that on average 3–4 treatments suffice to obtain a complete response with a maximum number of 8 weekly treatments. One nonrandomized study compared cryosurgery with single nonfractionated 5-ALA treatments showing comparable results of around 75 % complete response rates [24]. Side effects reported are mild with 5-ALA PDT. Sometimes there is pain during PDT treatment which can be solved by using local anesthetics. When studied, all authors report that postillumination pain is effectively controlled by NSAIDs. Generally, it can be concluded that topical 5-ALA PDT seems to provide clinicians with an interesting treatment strategy with little morbidity. Multiple fractionated treatments repeated once or twice in a weekly schedule after 2 h of 20 % topical application of 5-ALA seem to yield the best results. However, further detailed studies should clarify which treatment protocol is best and randomized comparative studies should be undertaken to compare the efficacy and morbidity of 5-ALA PDT treatments with modalities such as CO_2 laser evaporation or cryosurgery.

Hematoporphyrin derivatives (HpD, Photofrin) and meta-tetra(hydroxyphenyl)chlorine (mTHPC, temoporfin, Foscan) have been used to treat potentially malignant disorders of the oral mucosa as well [13, 38]. Fewer studies are available of these sensitizers and often the treated PMDs consist of high-grade dysplasia or carcinoma in situ. Often these studies include the treatment of high-grade dysplasia cases and small T1 carcinoma cases, due to the high risk nature of severe dysplasia. Since the introduction of HpD a number of studies included the treatment of high-grade dysplasia or CIS. The results were summarized in a review [39]

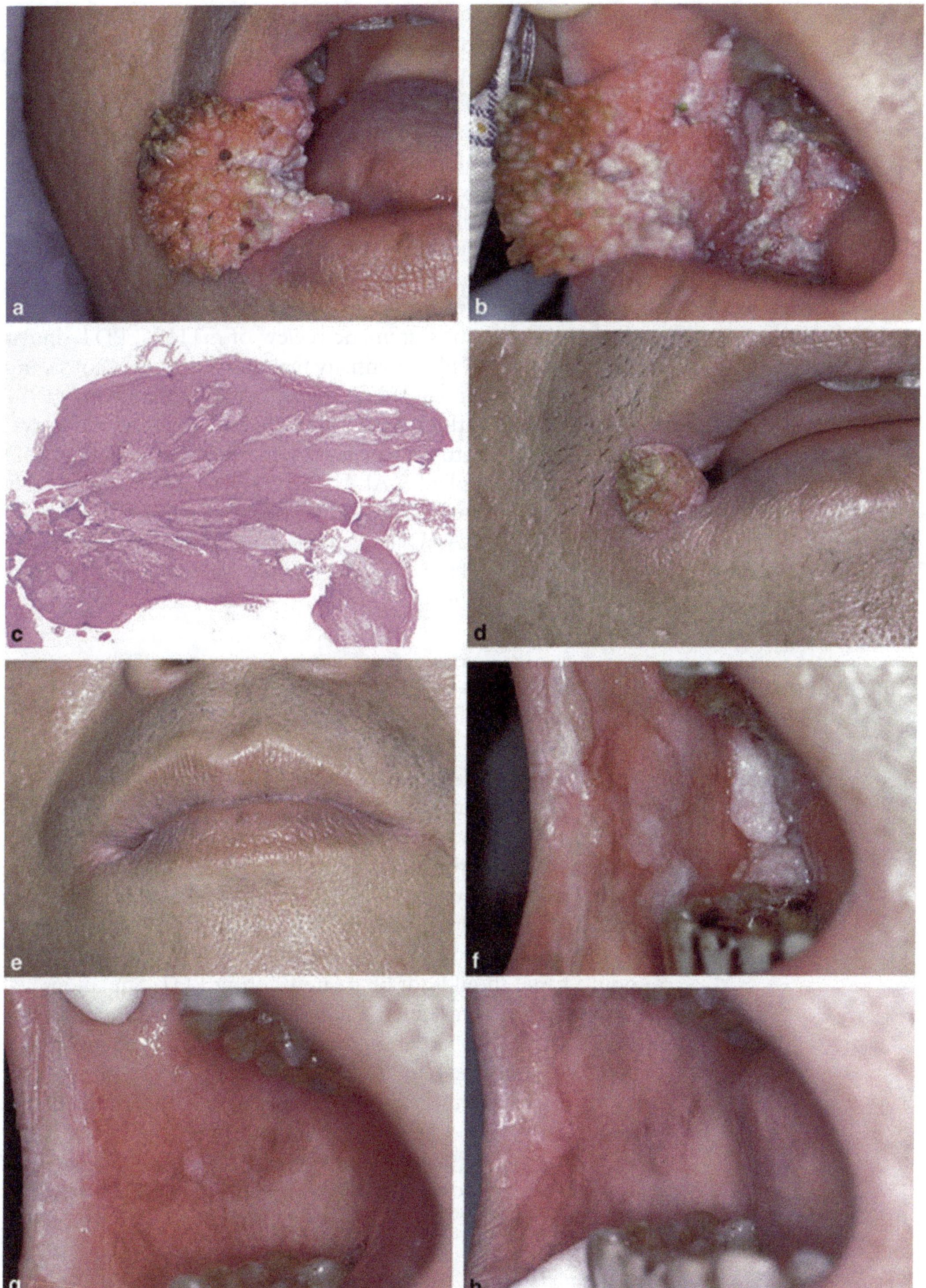

Fig. 2 5-ALA) treatment of widespread verrucous carcinoma of the buccal cheek, extending outside of the oral cavity (**a**, **b**) which was histologically proven (**c**). After 22 weekly treatments using topical 5-ALA the lesion gradually reduced in size (**e-h**) until a complete response was achieved (treatment performed by Dr Chen Department of Dentistry, National Taiwan University Hospital, Taipei, Taiwan). Reproduced with permission from the publisher from Chen et al. J Oral Pathol Med (2005) 34:253–6

showing a good response rate (>90 %) for CIS. Conversely, in a more recent study investigating the efficacy of photofrin-PDT in PMD and small oral tumors it was found that oral PMDs recurred more ($n = 3$ out of 9) than small oral carcinomas ($n = 10$ out of 11) [38]. It was hypothesized that this was due to insufficient photofrin uptake in small intraepithelial disorders or maybe by a light delivery problem due to the highly keratinized mucosa. A similar counterintuitive finding was published more recently with a different second generation photosensitizer 3-(10-hexyloxyethyl) pyropheophorbide-a (HPPH) [40]. It was found that PMDs showed a response of 46 %, while 82 % of the T1 carcinomas responded. In a recent systematic review of mTHPC PDT similar results were found [41]. Potentially malignant disorders consisting of carcinoma in situ, recurred significantly more than small oral T1 carcinoma treated with mTHPC PDT. Therefore it seems that systemically applied photosensitizers are less effective in treating PMD than the topically applied 5-ALA. The discrepancy can be possibly explained by the route of delivery and by the possibility of repeated treatment with 5-ALA, while systemic photosensitizers are usually administered once. However, the precise cause for this disparity has not been elucidated.

Photodynamic Therapy of Early Squamous Cell Carcinoma of the Oral Cavity

The objective of PDT of superficial oral or accessible oropharyngeal squamous cell carcinoma should be to induce necrosis of the tumor and a surrounding margin of at least 5 mm, including the tissue constituting the deep margin. Photodynamic therapy should not differ from the principles of tumor treatment applied in surgery or radiotherapy. In the past much of PDT research was devoted to find photosensitizers that are selectively taken up by tumor tissue. This, however, should not imply that a margin of surrounding tissue should not be treated during PDT. Squamous cell carcinomas of the oral mucosa are often developing in an area of mucosa with nonapparent potentially malignant changes [12]. Although it is not possible to clinically establish the presence or location of such areas it has been shown that the width of the resection margin is a predictor for recurrence of tumor [42]. Patients have higher survival rates when tumors are excised with 5 mm margin or more. The sensitizers that have been used for studying the efficacy of PDT in the treatment of early oral squamous cell carcinoma are photofrin and mTHPC. Recently a new sensitizer, HPPH was tested in a large phase 1 study showing promising results in the treatment of oral squamous cell carcinoma [40]. Photofrin is typically injected at a dose of 2 mg/kg body weight and illumination is performed 48 h later using 630 nm of incident light. The total light dose varies between authors but is mainly reported to be around 100 J/cm^2 (75–150 J/cm^2). In a retrospective analysis of 15 years of patient treatment the efficacy of removal of early squamous cell carcinoma (3 mm or less thick) with photofrin PDT was summarized [43]. The general finding was that superficial tumors respond well to photofrin PDT with 6 recurrences out of 112 patients (94 %) after an average of 80 months follow up. Because this was a retrospective analysis of results from a single institution, a prospective trial was designed to confirm the efficacy of photofrin PDT in oral squamous cell carcinoma [38]. In that study, 10 out of 11 patients with oral squamous cell carcinoma showed a complete response after photofrin PDT. Two retrospective studies using photofrin PDT in superficial (<5 mm thick) oral squamous cell carcinoma described a complete response in 24/25 patients (95 %) [44] and 80 % in 30 patients [45]. Other earlier reports of photofrin PDT describe small numbers of patients and were not prospective in design. Large phase 2 or 3 trial or randomized trials comparing surgery with HpD-PDT are not available. Photofrin is not registered for primary treatment of head and neck cancer but has been registered for early- and late-stage endobronchial tumors and minimally invasive esophageal adenocarcinomas and high-grade dysplasia associated with Barrett esophagus. Photofrin-based PDT seems to fulfill the criteria for minimally invasive yet effective treatment of oral squamous cell carcinoma. The pain is mild and after treatment very little problems occur with feeding. From the available literature it becomes apparent that comparing the morbidity of PDT vs. surgery may well be in favor of photofrin PDT since swallowing problems or loss of sensation in treated areas are not reported. However, data on long-term morbidity, such as tongue mobility, swallowing etc. are missing.

mTHPC is a second generation photosensitizer that is considered to be the most potent clinically available sensitizer at present. From the first clinical studies it became apparent that it has a high potential for inducing tumor necrosis up to 10 mm deep [46, 47]. Several large studies have been performed for primary treatment or palliative treatment of oral squamous cell carcinoma [48–50]. It is typically used at a dose of 0.15 mg/kg and illumination is performed 96 h later using 652 nm incident light at a dose rate of 100 mW/cm^2 and a total dose of 20 J/cm^2. mTHPC PDT has been used for skin cancer and nasopharyngeal cancer at shorter drug light intervals of 24 h, whereby the drug dose could be reduced to 0.05 mg/kg and the total light dose reduced to 10 J/cm^2 [51, 52]. Several prospective studies were published on the efficacy of mTHPC PDT of oral squamous cell carcinoma. In a recent systematic review, the efficacy of treatment of oral squamous cell carcinoma with mTHPC PDT has been analyzed [41]. After applying predetermined criteria, six prospective mTHPC PDT studies were selected, and patient data ($n = 301$) were obtained from the original files and these could be reliably pooled for analysis [49, 53–57]. It was found that T1 oral squamous cell carcinomas respond well to mTHPC with a sustained complete response rate of 86 %, while T2 tumors had a significantly lower cure rate of 63 %. One study described significant differences in response rates for different subsites in the oral cavity [57]. Oral tongue was reported with a significant better response rate and alveolar process with a significant lower response rate compared to the other oral subsites. This was attributed to the geometry of the oral subsites at which sometimes it is difficult to evenly distribute the incident light [58]. Two studies compared cohorts of early oral squamous cell carcinoma treated with surgery or mTHPC PDT [59, 60]. Although these studies have minimal partially overlapping patient data on mTHPC-treated patients the reference surgical databases were not. Both studies found no differences in complete response rates between surgery and mTHPC PDT. Although these studies were not randomized trials it presented convincing evidence that both modalities are equally effective in treating early oral squamous cell carcinoma. The main issue for future studies therefore should be on which advantage PDT possibly has over surgery or radiotherapy. The difference in morbidities of surgery and PDT has not been studied yet in detail. Clinicians involved in PDT of oral squamous cell carcinoma are usually trained as head and neck surgeons and report that the long-term morbidity of mTHPC PDT is considered lower than that of surgery, especially in preserving mobility of the muscular structures and sensation in the treated areas (Fig. 3a–d). In a recent study, mTHPC PDT was applied repeatedly until complete response was obtained [57]. In recurrent T1/T2 tumor cases, mTHPC PDT was applied up to three times with 6 months interval with little loss of function. It was decided not to change to surgical excision due to the anticipated morbidity of surgery. Even after three times of PDT the tissue healed well showing no cumulative toxicity in that study. For clinicians the anticipated lower morbidity of PDT than of surgery is the main incentive for offering patients suffering from early oral squamous cell carcinoma a treatment with PDT even though randomised clinical trials are lacking. It can be stated, however, that mTHPC PDT can be added as a primary treatment modality for early oral squamous cell carcinoma.

Selecting Cases for Primary Treatment of Oral Squamous Cell Carcinoma with mTHPC PDT

Case selection for mTHPC PDT of oral squamous cell carcinoma should be based on tumor factors as well as patient factors. Tumor factors should include the thickness of the lesion as well as the location of the lesion. Thickness of squamous cell carcinoma should

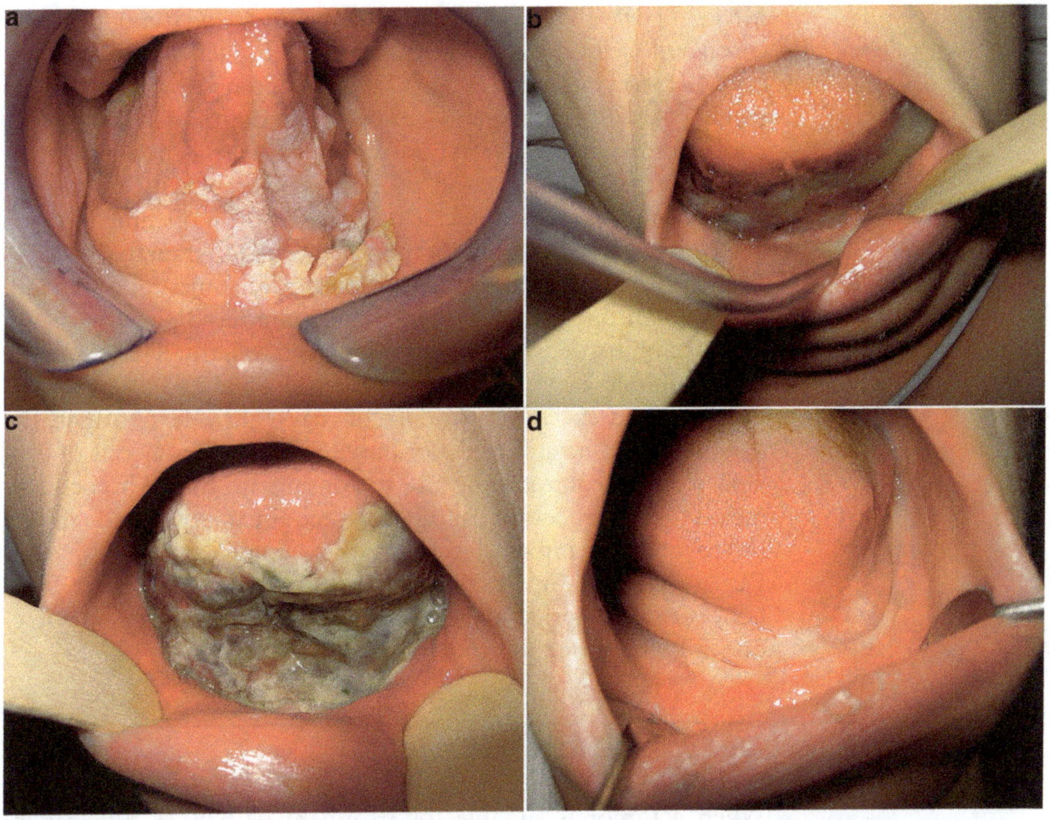

Fig. 3 Patient with a large squamous cell carcinoma of the floor of mouth (**a**) which was treated with mTHPC mediated PDT (0.15 mg/kg, 20 J/cm^2). The treatment response 2 h after illumination (**b**). Although the tongue and floor of mouth showed impressive swelling the patient retained oral intake and did not require tracheotomy. Treatment response 1 week after PDT (**c**). The swelling has been reduced and necrosis demarcated. Clinical view of floor of mouth 3 months after PDT showing normal oral mucosa (**d**). Tongue mobility was normal and a dental prosthesis could be worn. Sensory nerves of the treated area remained intact

not exceed beyond 5 mm in case of mTHPC. The limit to 5 mm stems from the measurement that red light around 652 nm can penetrate tissue and yield a PDT effect around 1 cm depth [47]. Light delivery to tissue is a science by itself addressed to in a different chapter. Histopathological analysis has shown that a higher risk of micrometastasis in the lymph nodes of the neck exist when a tumor has an infiltration depth of more than 4 mm. Therefore, most clinicians adopted the strategy to electively remove lymph nodes by neck dissection or to remove the sentinel lymph node at such tumor infiltration depths. In future this strategy may change if, for instance, genetic analysis could provide clinicians with a tool that can reliably predict the presence or exclude the presence of metastasis. For PDT case selection, most clinicians probably would select tumor cases of maximal 4 mm thick to avoid treating the neck, while systemically a photosensitizer has been injected. Estimation of thickness of a lesion can be reliably performed with

MRI [61] or with ultrasound [62]. MRI analysis and tumor thickness correlated well on histological specimens. In fact tumor thickness on MRI corresponded well with the presence of lymph node metastasis [63]. Ultrasound can be applied intraorally and shows good correlation with tumor thickness. It was reported that maneuvering the ultrasound probe in the oral cavity works well and was only hampered in case of limited mouth opening [62].

Patient factors can determine whether PDT is suitable as treatment. It is obvious that patients should have some understanding of PDT and the effect a systemically administered photosensitizer can have on tissue which has been exposed to light. Therefore, the patient should be able to understand and willing to cooperate on how to avoid excessive exposure of (day)light. Next to that, the patient should have the opportunity to be able to stay out of daylight for the required time and to continue to live at home. This means that all aspects of daily live that require going outside should be covered by informal care (spouse, family, neighbors, etc.). Patients are given instructions for the allowed light exposure and a light metering device for measuring the light at home and someone at home should be able to use this.

Instructions to Patients and Possible Adverse Events

When a tumor is suitable for treatment with PDT, the patient should be informed on the difference between surgery and PDT treatment. Since photofrin and mTHPC do not have a registration yet for the primary treatment of early oral squamous cell carcinoma, it should be made clear to the patient that it is an off label use of the drug. Contrary to the popular notion, it is legal in the United States, Europe, and in many other countries to use drugs off-label. Up to one-fifth of all drugs are prescribed off-label [64]. This should be part of the informed consent which should be based upon a clear appreciation and understanding of the facts, implications, and future consequences. Treatment options for tumor cases are usually discussed within a hospital's multidisciplinary tumor board. It is advisable to obtain the consent of the tumor board before suggesting PDT treatment to the patient. The information on the difference between surgery and PDT as a primary treatment and should balance the short-term and long-term morbidities. For PDT the information to the patient should include the diminished-light protocol, possible consequences of breaking the protocol, the expected clinical course of PDT and healing process, and postillumination pain and swelling. A general miscomprehension of the light protocol can be that patients should stay in the dark for the complete period after i.v. administration of a photosensitizer. In case of mTHPC patients should stay out of daylight for 2 weeks but by no means in the complete dark. Photofrin requires a longer time indoors which is reported to be 1 month. The light protocol applicable to mTHPC prescribes a daily increase of exposure to light of 100 lux. That means that 1 week after the administration of mTHPC the patient can be exposed to 700 lux, which is close to normal indoor ambient light with closed curtains. After 2 weeks, the patient gradually can increase exposure to daylight, avoiding sunbathing. For mTHPC the injection site, usually the medial cubital vein in the cubical fossa of the arm, contains a relatively high concentration of sensitizer because it is poorly water soluble and precipitates at the injection site at which it slowly dissolves or bleaches. This makes the injection site prolonged photosensitive and this should explicitly be explained to the patient that this site should be covered when going outdoors. For photofrin the advised duration for staying out of direct daylight is 30 days, but again this does not mean that the patient should stay indoors in the dark. Since photofrin is water soluble the injection site is not specifically at risk. Within the first weeks of photosensitivity the patient is allowed to go outside after sunset with protective clothing and sunglasses. Adverse events that have been reported are mainly related to unintended light exposure [49]. For mTHPC blistering and burns can occur on the skin, especially at the injection site (Fig. 4a, b). Hyperpigmentation has been reported as well. The blisters and burns have been reported to heal well with proper care.

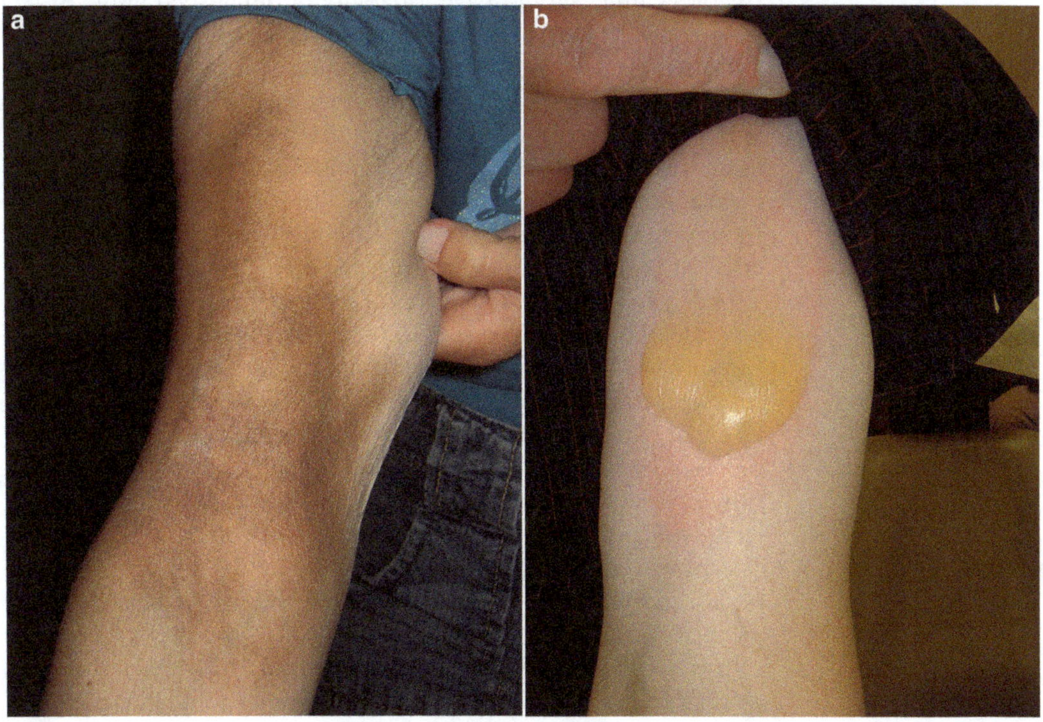

Fig. 4 Main side effects of intravenously administered photosensitizers. When light protocols are not strictly followed, hyperpigmentation (**a**) or blisters (**b**) can occur. Usually these resolve completely in time

Lipodystrophia has been reported after use of mTHPC but this rarely occurs. For photofrin, adverse events are reported to be skin reactions (edema, blisters) and ocular reactions.

Clinical Aspects of PDT

Although the science behind PDT is complex, performing the treatment is not. It requires less technical skills than performing surgery in the oral cavity. It does require knowledge on how to use photosensitizers and how to guide the incident light onto the target area. Next to that the clinician should instruct coworkers, anesthetists and nurses on the do's and don'ts.

The photosensitizer is injected in a darkened room with a small light bulb (60 W) after which the patient can leave for home after sunset. The darkened room should effectively shield daylight and have controllable light switches. Injection rate should be slow for mTHPC because it can be painful. mTHPC is dissolved in a solution that contains ethanol which yields pain upon administration which is immediately resolved when administration is completed. Illumination is often performed under general anesthesia. This is necessary because the patient should lay still and should allow shielding in the oral cavity to prevent unwanted illumination of the surrounding tissues. The OR and pre and postoperative care unit (recovery unit) should have capability of diminished light. At day 4 for mTHPC 400 lux is allowed which is already a level of ambient light that allows nurses to do their regular procedures. Intubation of the patient can be performed with a regular laryngoscope provided that the procedure does not need minutes of exposure to the light. Experienced anesthetists should perform the endotracheal intubation. During general anesthesia the pulse oximeter, used for monitoring the patients' oxygen saturation level, can create a PDT effect at the nail at which it is placed [65]. Therefore it should be switched from nail to nail at regular intervals of maximal 10 min, or preferably, put on at regular intervals for a short moment to measure the blood oxygen saturation.

Separating the target tissue from the surrounding tissue is an essential part of PDT, especially when mTHPC is used. This can be done by using wet surgical cloths that are draped around the tumor/target area. To prevent shifting, these cloths can be sutured to the mucosa. PDT can have dual selectivity, that is, selectivity by selective tumor uptake of the drug or selecting the area that will be illuminated. Some authors describe the use of black wax for protecting the normal tissue while a gap in the wax exposes the tumor and required normal tissue margin [53]. Separating the target tissue and performing the illumination should be performed by one person, while operating the light source should be done by a second person.

Pain is especially present after mTHPC PDT in the oral cavity. In contrast, pain after mTHPC PDT in other anatomical areas such as skin or skull base is not painful and seldom requires opioids. Pain after PDT in the oral cavity can be well controlled by using proper medication. Before ending the procedure under general anesthesia the patient should be given proper amount of morphine which should be continued postillumination by means of oral or transdermally applied opioid prescriptions as long as necessary. Swelling usually occurs within a few hours after PDT. It depends on the anatomical area if the airway will be compromised. PDT with superficial illumination seldom leads to airway obstruction in the oral cavity [66]. Edema with risk of airway obstruction occurs mainly when interstitial illumination is performed. The tongue base area is the site at risk for postillumination edema with airway obstruction. Therefore performing a tracheotomy should be considered in those specific cases. Intraoral swelling after superficial PDT seldom leads to feeding problems. Occasionally, a nasogastric feeding tube is necessary for the first day. Postillumination swelling can be influenced by administering prednisone/dexamethasone.

The normal clinical course shows edema and sloughing of the mucosa of the treated area at the first 24 h. This is followed by tissue necrosis which will be present for weeks. Slowly the necrotic tissue will be discharged, usually in small pieces. Within 8–12 weeks the tissue will be healed. Occasionally, an infection of the necrotic area will occur which can be easily treated with penicillin.

Patients usually can be discharged quite shortly after illumination. Since general anesthesia is short and no surgical procedure is involved the burden of the procedure is low for the patient. Some patients can be discharged from the hospital the same or next day. Longer admissions may be necessary in cases of insufficient informal care at home. Follow up can easily be organized by regular phone calls by nurse practitioners.

Conclusion

PDT should be considered as one of the modalities to treat potentially malignant disorders and early oral and accessible oropharyngeal squamous cell carcinoma. It is minimally invasive and has clear potential where other modalities are contraindicated or may lead to high morbidity while the tumor burden is low. 5-ALA can be administered topically in case of PMD and mTHPC and photofrin systemically in case of early cancers. The efficacy of PDT of early squamous cell carcinoma is comparable to surgery. There is no cumulative toxicity and can be repeated when necessary.

References

1. Wile AG, Dahlman A, Burns RG, Berns MW. Laser photoradiation therapy of cancer following hematoporphyrin sensitization. Lasers Surg Med. 1982;2(2):163–8.
2. Dougherty TJ, Kaufman JE, Goldfarb A, Weishaupt KR, Boyle D, Mittleman A. Photoradiation therapy for the treatment of malignant tumors. Cancer Res. 1978;38(8): 2628–35.
3. Warnakulasuriya S, Johnson NW, van der Waal I. Nomenclature and classification of potentially malignant disorders of the oral mucosa. J Oral Pathol Med. 2007;36(10):575–80.
4. Warnakulasuriya S, Kovacevic T, Madden P, et al. Factors predicting malignant transformation in oral potentially malignant disorders among patients accrued over a 10-year period in South East England. J Oral Pathol Med. 2011;40(9):677–83.
5. Ho PS, Chen PL, Warnakulasuriya S, Shieh TY, Chen YK, Huang IY. Malignant transformation of oral potentially malignant disorders in males: a retrospective cohort study. BMC Cancer. 2009;9:260. doi:10.1186/1471-2407-9-260.
6. Lee CH, Ko AM, Yen CF, et al. Betel-quid dependence and oral potentially malignant disorders in six Asian countries. Br J Psychiatry. 2012;201(5):383–91.
7. Schepman KP, van der Meij EH, Smeele LE, van der Waal I. Malignant transformation of oral leukoplakia: a follow-up study of a hospital-based population of 166 patients with oral leukoplakia from The Netherlands. Oral Oncol. 1998;34(4):270–5.
8. Brennan M, Migliorati CA, Lockhart PB, et al. Management of oral epithelial dysplasia: a review. Oral Surg Oral Med Oral Pathol Oral Radiol Endod. 2007;103(Suppl):S19.e1–12.
9. Ho MW, Field EA, Field JK, et al. Outcomes of oral squamous cell carcinoma arising from oral epithelial dysplasia: rationale for monitoring premalignant oral lesions in a multidisciplinary clinic. Br J Oral Maxillofac Surg. 2013; 51(7):594–9.
10. Nayan S, Gupta MK, Strychowsky JE, Sommer DD. Smoking cessation interventions and cessation rates in the oncology population: an updated systematic review and meta-analysis. Otolaryngol Head Neck Surg. 2013;149(2):200–11.
11. van der Hem PS, Nauta JM, van der Wal JE, Roodenburg JL. The results of CO2 laser surgery in patients with oral leukoplakia: a 25 year follow up. Oral Oncol. 2005;41(1):31–7.
12. Braakhuis BJ, Bloemena E, Leemans CR, Brakenhoff RH. Molecular analysis of surgical margins in head and neck cancer: more than a marginal issue. Oral Oncol. 2010;46(7): 485–91.
13. Jerjes W, Hamdoon Z, Hopper C. Photodynamic therapy in the management of potentially malignant and malignant oral disorders. Head Neck Oncol. 2012;4:16.
14. Amit M, Yen TC, Liao CT, et al. Clinical nodal stage is a significant predictor of outcome in patients with oral cavity squamous cell carcinoma and pathologically negative neck metastases: results of the international consortium for outcome research. Ann Surg Oncol. 2013;20(11):3575–81.
15. Amit M, Yen TC, Liao CT, et al. Improvement in survival of patients with oral cavity squamous cell carcinoma: an international collaborative study. Cancer. 2013;119(24):4242–8.
16. Liu JC, Shah JP. Surgical technique refinements in head and neck oncologic surgery. J Surg Oncol. 2010;101(8):661–8.
17. Shah JP, Gil Z. Current concepts in management of oral cancer—surgery. Oral Oncol. 2009;45(4–5):394–401.
18. Eisbruch A, Foote RL, O'Sullivan B, Beitler JJ, Vikram B. Intensity-modulated radiation therapy for head and neck cancer: emphasis on the selection and delineation of the targets. Semin Radiat Oncol. 2002;12(3):238–49.
19. Melchers LJ, Schuuring E, van Dijk BA, et al. Tumour infiltration depth ≥4 mm is an indication for an elective neck dissection in pT1cN0 oral squamous cell carcinoma. Oral Oncol. 2012;48(4):337–42.
20. Vissink A, Jansma J, Spijkervet FK, Burlage FR, Coppes RP. Oral sequelae of head and neck radiotherapy. Crit Rev Oral Biol Med. 2003;14(3):199–212.
21. Saini R, Poh CF. Photodynamic therapy: a review and its prospective role in the management of oral potentially malignant disorders. Oral Dis. 2013;19(5):440–51.
22. de Vijlder HC, Sterenborg HJ, Neumann HA, Robinson DJ, de Haas ER. Light fractionation significantly improves the response of superficial basal cell carcinoma to aminolaevulinic acid photodynamic therapy: five-year follow-up of a randomized, prospective trial. Acta Derm Venereol. 2012;92(6):641–7.
23. Kubler A, Haase T, Rheinwald M, Barth T, Muhling J. Treatment of oral leukoplakia by topical application of 5-aminolevulinic acid. Int J Oral Maxillofac Surg. 1998;27(6):466–9.
24. Kawczyk-Krupka A, Waskowska J, Raczkowska-Siostrzonek A, et al. Comparison of cryotherapy and photodynamic therapy in treatment of

oral leukoplakia. Photodiagnosis Photodyn Ther. 2012;9(2):148–55.

25. Jerjes W, Upile T, Hamdoon Z, Mosse CA, Akram S, Hopper C. Photodynamic therapy outcome for oral dysplasia. Lasers Surg Med. 2011;43(3):192–9.
26. Fan KF, Hopper C, Speight PM, Buonaccorsi G, MacRobert AJ, Bown SG. Photodynamic therapy using 5-aminolevulinic acid for premalignant and malignant lesions of the oral cavity. Cancer. 1996;78(7):1374–83.
27. Sieron A, Kosciarz-Grzesiok A, Kawczyk-Krupka A, Sieron-Stoltny K, Misiak A. Application of photodynamic therapy in the treatment of premalignant and malignant changes of head and neck. Wiad Lek. 2008;61(10–12):283–7.
28. Sieron A, Adamek M, Kawczyk-Krupka A, Mazur S, Ilewicz L. Photodynamic therapy (PDT) using topically applied delta-aminolevulinic acid (ALA) for the treatment of oral leukoplakia. J Oral Pathol Med. 2003;32(6):330–6.
29. Lin HP, Chen HM, Yu CH, Yang H, Wang YP, Chiang CP. Topical photodynamic therapy is very effective for oral verrucous hyperplasia and oral erythroleukoplakia. J Oral Pathol Med. 2010;39(8):624–30.
30. Wang CY, Tsai T, Chiang CP, Chen HM, Chen CT. Improved diagnosis of oral premalignant lesions in submucous fibrosis patients with 5-aminolevulinic acid induced PpIX fluorescence. J Biomed Opt. 2009;14(4):044026.
31. Yu CH, Lin HP, Chen HM, Yang H, Wang YP, Chiang CP. Comparison of clinical outcomes of oral erythroleukoplakia treated with photodynamic therapy using either light-emitting diode or laser light. Lasers Surg Med. 2009;41(9):628–33.
32. Yu CH, Chen HM, Hung HY, Cheng SJ, Tsai T, Chiang CP. Photodynamic therapy outcome for oral verrucous hyperplasia depends on the clinical appearance, size, color, epithelial dysplasia, and surface keratin thickness of the lesion. Oral Oncol. 2008;44(6):595–600.
33. Chen HM, Chen CT, Yang H, et al. Successful treatment of an extensive verrucous carcinoma with topical 5-aminolevulinic acid-mediated photodynamic therapy. J Oral Pathol Med. 2005;34(4):253–6.
34. Chen HM, Yu CH, Tu PC, Yeh CY, Tsai T, Chiang CP. Successful treatment of oral verrucous hyperplasia and oral leukoplakia with topical 5-aminolevulinic acid-mediated photodynamic therapy. Lasers Surg Med. 2005; 37(2):114–22.
35. Chen HM, Chen CT, Yang H, et al. Successful treatment of oral verrucous hyperplasia with topical 5-aminolevulinic acid-mediated photodynamic therapy. Oral Oncol. 2004; 40(6):630–7.
36. Tsai JC, Chiang CP, Chen HM, et al. Photodynamic therapy of oral dysplasia with topical 5-aminolevulinic acid and light-emitting diode array. Lasers Surg Med. 2004;34(1): 18–24.
37. Chen K, Chang BZ, Ju M, Zhang XH, Gu H. Comparative study of photodynamic therapy vs CO2 laser vaporization in treatment of condylomata acuminata: a randomized clinical trial. Br J Dermatol. 2007;156(3):516–20.
38. Rigual NR, Thankappan K, Cooper M, et al. Photodynamic therapy for head and neck dysplasia and cancer. Arch Otolaryngol Head Neck Surg. 2009;135(8):784–8.
39. Biel MA. Photodynamic therapy of head and neck cancers. Methods Mol Biol. 2010; 635:281–93.
40. Rigual N, Shafirstein G, Cooper MT, et al. Photodynamic therapy with 3-(1′-hexyloxy-ethyl) pyropheophorbide a for cancer of the oral cavity. Clin Cancer Res. 2013;19(23): 6605–13.
41. de Visscher SA, Dijkstra PU, Tan IB, Roodenburg JL, Witjes MJ. mTHPC mediated photodynamic therapy (PDT) of squamous cell carcinoma in the head and neck: a systematic review. Oral Oncol. 2013;49(3):192–210.
42. Woolgar JA. Histopathological prognosticators in oral and oropharyngeal squamous cell carcinoma. Oral Oncol. 2006;42(3):229–39.
43. Biel M. Advances in photodynamic therapy for the treatment of head and neck cancers. Lasers Surg Med. 2006;38(5):349–55.
44. Ikeda H, Tobita T, Ohba S, Uehara M, Asahina I. Treatment outcome of photofrin-based photodynamic therapy for T1 and T2 oral squamous cell carcinoma and dysplasia. Photodiagnosis Photodyn Ther. 2013;10(3): 229–35.
45. Schweitzer VG, Somers ML. PHOTOFRIN-mediated photodynamic therapy for treatment of early stage (tis-T2N0M0) SqCCa of oral cavity and oropharynx. Lasers Surg Med. 2010;42(1):1–8.
46. Dilkes MG, DeJode ML, Gardiner Q, Kenyon GS, McKelvie P. Treatment of head and neck cancer with photodynamic therapy: results after one year. J Laryngol Otol. 1995; 109(11):1072–6.
47. Ris HB, Altermatt HJ, Inderbitzi R, et al. Photodynamic therapy with chlorins for diffuse malignant mesothelioma: initial clinical results. Br J Cancer. 1991;64(6):1116–20.
48. D'Cruz AK, Robinson MH, Biel MA. mTHPC-mediated photodynamic therapy in

patients with advanced, incurable head and neck cancer: a multicenter study of 128 patients. Head Neck. 2004;26(3):232–40.

49. Hopper C, Kubler A, Lewis H, Tan IB, Putnam G. mTHPC-mediated photodynamic therapy for early oral squamous cell carcinoma. Int J Cancer. 2004;111(1):138–46.
50. Lou PJ, Jager HR, Jones L, Theodossy T, Bown SG, Hopper C. Interstitial photodynamic therapy as salvage treatment for recurrent head and neck cancer. Br J Cancer. 2004;91(3):441–6.
51. Betz CS, Rauschning W, Stranadko EP, et al. Optimization of treatment parameters for foscan-PDT of basal cell carcinomas. Lasers Surg Med. 2008;40(5):300–11.
52. Wildeman MA, Fles R, Herdini C, et al. Primary treatment results of nasopharyngeal carcinoma (NPC) in Yogyakarta, Indonesia. PLoS One. 2013;8(5):e63706.
53. Copper MP, Triesscheijn M, Tan IB, Ruevekamp MC, Stewart FA. Photodynamic therapy in the treatment of multiple primary tumours in the head and neck, located to the oral cavity and oropharynx. Clin Otolaryngol. 2007;32(3):185–9.
54. Copper MP, Tan IB, Oppelaar H, Ruevekamp MC, Stewart FA. Meta-tetra(hydroxyphenyl) chlorin photodynamic therapy in early-stage squamous cell carcinoma of the head and neck. Arch Otolaryngol Head Neck Surg. 2003; 129(7):709–11.
55. Kubler AC, de Carpentier J, Hopper C, Leonard AG, Putnam G. Treatment of squamous cell carcinoma of the lip using foscan-mediated photodynamic therapy. Int J Oral Maxillofac Surg. 2001;30(6):504–9.
56. Karakullukcu B, van Oudenaarde K, Copper MP, et al. Photodynamic therapy of early stage oral cavity and oropharynx neoplasms: an outcome analysis of 170 patients. Eur Arch Otorhinolaryngol. 2011;268(2):281–8.
57. Jerjes W, Upile T, Hamdoon Z, Alexander Mosse C, Morcos M, Hopper C. Photodynamic therapy outcome for T1/T2 N0 oral squamous cell carcinoma. Lasers Surg Med. 2011; 43(6):463–9.
58. van Benthem HE, Sterenborg HJ, van der Meulen FW, van Gemert MJ. Performance of a light applicator for photodynamic therapy in the oral cavity: calculations and measurements. Phys Med Biol. 1997;42(9):1689–700.
59. de Visscher SA, Melchers LJ, Dijkstra PU, et al. mTHPC-mediated photodynamic therapy of early stage oral squamous cell carcinoma: a comparison to surgical treatment. Ann Surg Oncol. 2013;20(9):3076–82.
60. Karakullukcu B, Stoker SD, Wildeman AP, Copper MP, Wildeman MA, Tan IB. A matched cohort comparison of mTHPC-mediated photodynamic therapy and trans-oral surgery of early stage oral cavity squamous cell cancer. Eur Arch Otorhinolaryngol. 2013;270(3): 1093–7.
61. Lam P, Au-Yeung KM, Cheng PW, et al. Correlating MRI and histologic tumor thickness in the assessment of oral tongue cancer. AJR Am J Roentgenol. 2004;182(3):803–8.
62. Lodder WL, Teertstra HJ, Tan IB, et al. Tumour thickness in oral cancer using an intra-oral ultrasound probe. Eur Radiol. 2011; 21(1):98–106.
63. Boland PW, Watt-Smith SR, Hopper C, Golding SJ. Magnetic resonance imaging predicts survival and occult metastasis in oral cancer: a dual-centre, retrospective study. Br J Oral Maxillofac Surg. 2013;51(8):696–701.
64. Radley DC, Finkelstein SN, Stafford RS. Off-label prescribing among office-based physicians. Arch Intern Med. 2006;166(9): 1021–6.
65. Theodossy T, Chapman M, Mitchell V, Hopper C. Anaesthetic considerations for patients receiving photodynamic therapy in head and neck surgery. Eur J Anaesthesiol. 2007;24(3):225–9.
66. Story W, Sultan AA, Bottini G, Vaz F, Lee G, Hopper C. Strategies of airway management for head and neck photo-dynamic therapy. Lasers Surg Med. 2013;45(6):370–6.

Chapter 22

Photodynamic Therapy of Oropharyngeal Malignancies

M. Barış Karakullukcu

Multidiscipline Involvement and Informed Consent

The oropharynx is a section of the upper aerodigestive tract which includes a variety of structures located between the soft palate superiorly and the hyoid bone inferiorly. It consists of the base of the tongue, which includes the pharyngoepiglottic folds and the glossoepiglottic folds; tonsillar region, which includes the fossa and the anterior and posterior pillars; soft palate, which includes the uvula; and posterior and lateral pharyngeal walls. There are no anatomic barriers separating the oropharynx from the oral cavity anteriorly, the nasopharynx superiorly, and the supraglottic larynx and hypopharynx inferiorly. The overwhelming majority of oropharyngeal cancers are squamous cell carcinomas. A substantial part of oropharyngeal cancers are human papilloma virus (HPV) associated, which have somewhat different clinical presentation, and are more radiosensitive and have better prognosis than non-HPV-associated oropharyngeal cancers. Oropharyngeal tumors have a considerable risk of metastasizing to the lymph nodes of the neck and retropharyngeal region. The variety of structures and the absence of anatomic borders make it difficult to come up with a "one size fits all" treatment strategy.

The primary treatment for oropharyngeal cancer is either surgery and/or radiation therapy, either with or without accompanying chemotherapy. These conventional treatments can have undesired effects, especially when applied to recurrent tumors. There is a place for photodynamic therapy (PDT) to treat superficial tumors as primary treatment and deeper recurrent tumors,

Brian J.-F. Wong and Justus Ilgner (eds.), *Biomedical Optics in Otorhinolaryngology: Head and Neck Surgery*,
DOI 10.1007/978-1-4939-1758-7_22, © Springer Science+Business Media New York 2016

when conventional treatments cannot be given or would cause too much morbidity.

A thorough workup and multidisciplinary approach is essential to consider a tumor treatable with PDT. The most important consideration is involvement of lymphatic nodes. Lymph node metastasis screening, including imaging and fine-needle aspiration cytology (FNAC) of suspected lymph nodes, should be carried out. PDT is a local treatment, having none to slight indirect effect on lymph node metastasis. Therefore in the presence of lymphatic metastasis, alternative treatments would be a better option. Since the penetration of light is a limiting factor for PDT, the depth of the tumor should be assessed with imaging. The next step in the workup is comparing the possible undesired effect of different treatment strategies, such as problems with reconstruction, swallowing, and articulation.

For example, PDT of a superficial tumor involving both sides of the soft palate would provide adequate treatment in one session, with minimal to no tissue loss, has advantages over surgery which would require reconstruction, or radiation treatment which requires several sessions.

Another good example is the treatment of base of tongue tumors, recurrent after (chemo)radiation treatment. Many of these lesions require total glossectomy, rendering the patient unable to swallow and articulate. A good number of patients refuse such a surgery. Interstitial photodynamic therapy (iPDT) can be applied with some success, which will be explained later in this chapter.

Superficial Tumors

PDT can be indicated for the treatment of superficial primary tumors as well as secondary or recurrent tumors.

Patient selection and workup: The accurate selection of PDT candidate lesions is essential for success. The workup should include screening for metastasis. It is well known that even small tumors of the oropharynx have a considerable risk of lymph node metastasis, not only to the neck nodes but to the retropharyngeal nodes as well. In our institute the workup consists of ultrasonography of both sides of the neck with eventual FNAC of suspicious nodes and MRI of the region [1].

The depth, or better expressed the thickness, should be assessed as accurately as possible, before deeming a lesion a PDT candidate. PDT is limited by penetration of light in the tumor tissue. The penetration of treatment light is dependent on many factors, such as the wavelength, fluence, fluence rate, and optical properties of the treatment volume. These properties are explained in detail elsewhere in this book. The wavelength of the treatment light is chosen according to the activation properties of photosensitizers (PS). The most commonly used PSs for the oropharynx are photofrin activated by 630 nm wavelength and temoporfin (mTHPC) by 652 nm wavelength light. In our institute we use temoporfin as our preferred PS. The observed treatment effect is around 8–10 mm [2, 3]. We would like to include a safety and inaccuracy margin of at least 4 mm. Therefore we accept a cut-off of 4 mm thickness for PDT. The thickness is evaluated with a combination of ultrasound and MRI. The ultrasound appears to be more accurate in determining the depth, compared to MRI [4], however, not all lesions of the oropharynx are easily accessible with ultrasound. If there is controversy between the two imaging methods the deeper measurement is accepted to be on the safe side.

Once the candidacy is established, the treatment options are considered and compared by a multidisciplinary tumor board. PDT has the advantage of minimal tissue loss and scarring, no need for reconstruction, and very frequently single stage treatment over conventional methods for the well selected superficial tumors.

The photosensitivity caused by systemic photosensitizers requires that the patients receive adequate counseling. The period of photosensitivity is dependent on the photosensitizer and can range from a few hours to 6 weeks. Temoporfin causes a photosensitivity of 2 weeks. In our institute a dedicated nurse practitioner informs and thereafter follows the patients. Patients should be provided with printed light avoidance guidelines and a light meter to measure ambient light in the living quarters. Every day, the patient can be exposed to more light according to the guidelines provided to the patient. The patients also receive information about airway management, feeding, and other aspects of the postoperative course.

Treatment Technique The PS is administered a certain time before the procedure, depending on the optimal drug light interval of the type of PS used. In case of temoporfin, this drug light interval is 4 days.

The selection of light delivery technique is dependent on the location of the tumor. Essentially two different light diffuser types are usually used: linear diffuser providing a cylinder of light over a length of the diffuser or a microlens providing a spot of light. Tumors of the soft palate, tonsillar pillars and sometimes the pharyngeal back wall can be approached transorally and treated with a spot of light by using an optical fiber with a microlens tip. A linear diffuser inserted via the nose can provide light coverage of lesions located in the vallecula, side wall, or back wall of the oropharynx. The normal structures should be protected from the PDT effect by using a black shielding wax. Figure 1 demonstrates the approaches

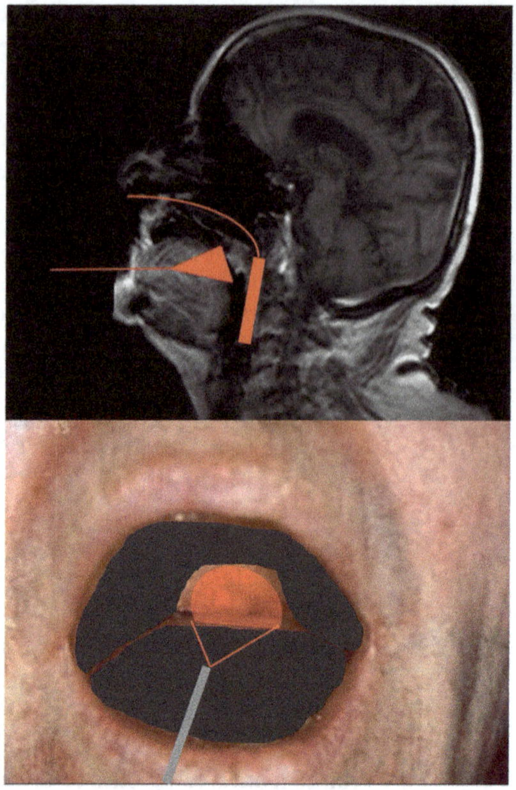

Fig. 1 While superficial tumors located on the soft palate can be treated with a spot of light from a microlens diffuser, extended surface tumors of the back, front, or side wall of the oropharynx can be treated with a linear diffuser inserted via the nose (*top*). The normal tissues should be protected with black wax (*bottom*)

and the shielding of normal tissues. In our institute, we give 20 J/cm^2 fluence, with a fluence rate of 100 mW/cm^2. The treatment takes 200 s/light spot. If the tumor cannot be covered with one spot several spots can be used. The tumor and 5–10 mm mucosal margin should be treated.

Postprocedure course is marked by edema and local pain. We routinely administer systemic dexamethasone and taper over 2 weeks. The pain management is with fentanyl transdermal patches, paracetamol (acetaminophen), and locally applied lidocaine gel.

The airway management and feeding should be carefully considered. PDT of smaller lesions of the soft palate or tonsil area does not cause airway or feeding problems. Treatment of widespread lesions of the posterior or lateral pharynx wall or the tongue base might necessitate an elective temporary tracheotomy and tempo-

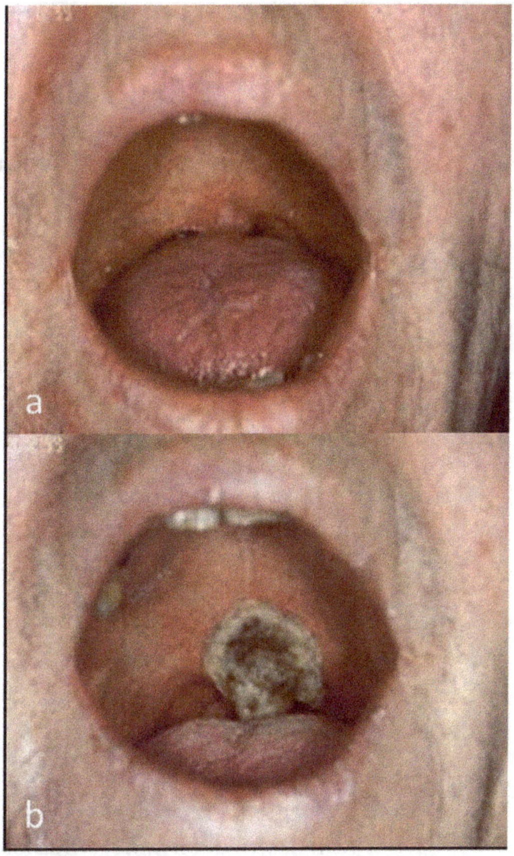

Fig. 2 **A** superficial tumor located on the soft palate before (**a**) and 2 weeks after (**b**) PDT. The treatment response is marked by necrosis

rary tube feeding. Once the edema subsides tracheotomy can be closed and oral intake can be started.

The tissue response to PDT is mainly necrosis. Figure 2 demonstrates an uvula squamous cell cancer treated with PDT and the necrosis 2 weeks after the treatment. The necrosis disappears and gets replaced by mucosa 4–6 weeks after PDT. If larger areas are treated, this period may take longer, sometimes up to 6 months.

Clinical Outcomes PDT of the oropharynx is not separately reported in the literature. In a series of 170 patients of oral cavity and oropharyngeal cancer we have published [5], we reported 26 patients with oropharynx cancer treated with surface PDT. The overall complete response was 66 %. All of the primary lesions (seven lesions) had complete response. Second primary or recurrent lesions had lower complete response rate (53 %). Other published series with temoporfin or photofrin include oropharyngeal cancers but do not report separate results [6–24].

Deep-Seated Tumors

Many of the recurrent tumors in the base of tongue and tonsillar region are deep tumors. One of the limitations of PDT is the depth of penetration of light. When tumors are illuminated from the surface, the therapeutic effect is observed 8–10 mm deep with temoporfin mediated PDT [2, 3]. This depth may vary with the variations in optical properties of the tumor. Other photosentizers may have different depth of therapeutic effect based on the activation wavelength. Therefore, deeper tumors should be treated with implanting light sources in the tumor, e.g., interstitial PhotoDynamic Therapy (iPDT) [25–30].

There is not enough evidence yet to propose iPDT as a curative treatment for the primary cancers. The current indication is recurrent or multiple primary cancers. The most common treatment for base of tongue and tonsil cancers is radiation treatment. Transoral robotic surgery (TORS) is gaining popularity in the treatment of smaller tumors. If the tumor recurs locally, curative treatment option, more often than not, involves total glossectomy. A considerable number of patients refuse total glossectomy because of the associated morbidity. Some centers define such tumors as functionally inoperable [31]. iPDT can be an alternative to total glossectomy.

Treatment Technique The main purpose of preoperative evaluation is to determine whether the entire tumor volume can be treated with PDT. Therefore, the recurrent residual disease should be locoregional without distant metastasis. In our clinic we use PET scan to rule out distant metastasis.

We believe it is essential to establish a treatment plan before actually undertaking the treatment. In our clinic we use a brachytherapy based approach and brachytherapy planning software to simulate the treatment. There are centers which prefer intraoperative decision-making and implantation based on ultrasound imaging. The rest of this chapter is a description of brachytherapy based temoporfin mediated iPDT method.

Magnetic resonance imaging (MRI) is the imaging tool of choice for oropharynx tumors providing the clearest delineation of the neoplastic tissues. We find it important that the entire gross tumor volume (GTV) plus at least 5 mm margins around the tumor are adequately treated. The relationship of the tumor to the carotid arteries and mandibular should be determined to avoid complications. Tumors invading the bone are harder to treat because of penetration and reflection of light. Customized brachytherapy software is used to plan iPDT. The planning is very similar to that of ionizing brachytherapy. The point sources of radiation are replaced by linear array of light emitting point sources produced by

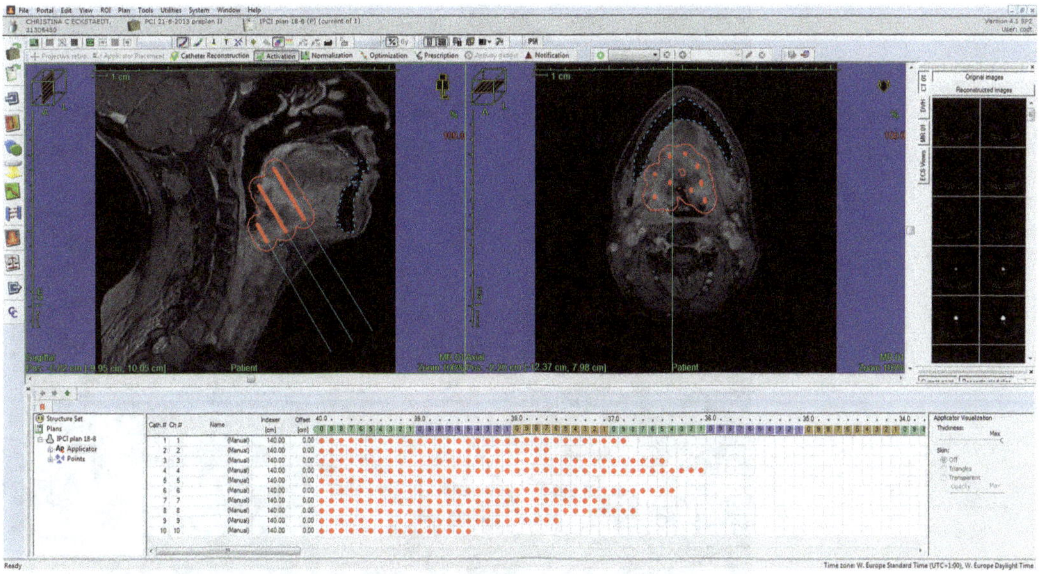

Fig. 3 **A** screenshot of treatment simulation as seen on a brachytherapy software. Such a simulation allows viewing possible insertion angles and arrangements. The length of diffusers can be observed at the *lower part* of the screen

a linear diffuser. The light sources are planned to lie parallel to each other, at a distance of not greater than 15 mm, to account for the treatment effect depth of 8 mm. The planning provides us with an adequate idea of the number of light sources necessary to be implanted and insertion angle. The illumination phase can be simulated, in other words the light sources can virtually be turned on, to see if there is any geographic miss, which can thereafter be corrected by modifying the planning. Figure 3 is a screenshot of the actual simulation of a patient with recurrent base of tongue tumor. Figure 4 shows a 3-dimensional reconstruction of a simulated iPDT of the same tumor. The planned angle of light source implantation is visible in relation to the mandible and hyoid bone.

Implantation of light sources is usually performed under general anesthesia. The tumors located in the base of the tongue are better implanted with brachytherapy loop catheters that penetrate from the skin surface to the oropharyngeal lumen and are fixed both on the mucosa and the skin surface to eliminate shifting artifacts. Perfect parallel and straight placement of catheters is usually not possible. Therefore the placement should be checked with intra-operative CT scan. The air containing catheters are easily visible on CT scan. The brachytherapy software can automatically load the catheters with light sources and run the simulation again. Figure 5 demonstrates this confirmation simulation. If there are areas not receiving light an additional catheter can be placed.

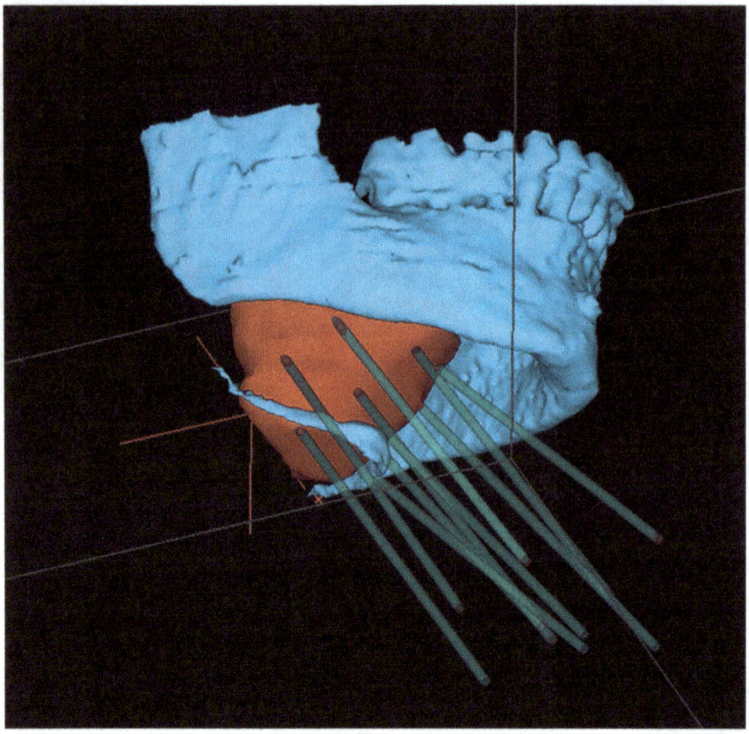

Fig. 4 **A** 3-dimensional reconstruction of the iPDT simulation. The planned light sources in relation to the mandible and hyoid bone can be observed

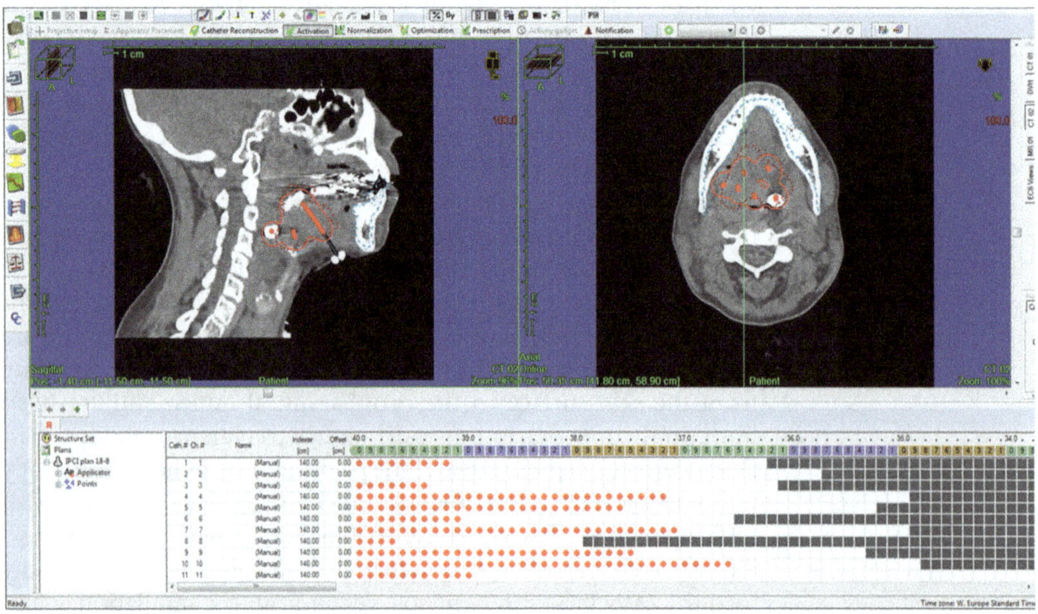

Fig. 5 **A** simulation on an intraoperative confirmation CT. The actual places of the air containing catheters can be easily seen. The software recognizes the catheters and fills in the light sources automatically

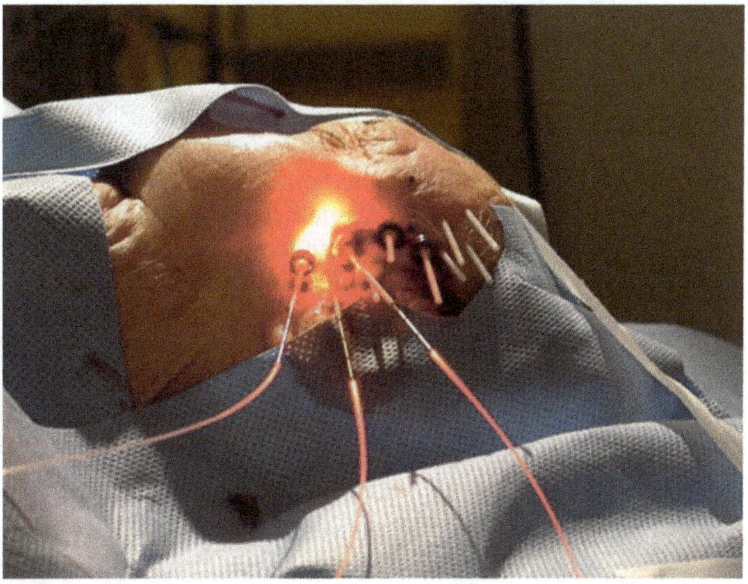

Fig. 6 Light delivery to a base of tongue tumor by linear diffusers introduced through brachytherapy loop catheters

We use 4–6 linear diffusers simultaneously to deliver light can be connected to the laser and used simultaneously to deliver light (Fig. 6). The length of the diffusers light-emitting section is determined by the pretreatment planning. The length can be fine tuned by introducing metal shielding tubes over the diffusers. The diffusers are introduced into the placed catheters. It is very important that the catheters do not have blood in them since hemoglobin is an important light absorber at this wavelength and works like a filter. Preferred illumination fluence is 30 J/cm of diffuser length. So a 4 cm diffuser would deliver 120 J. The illumination takes 300 s with a fixed fluence rate. Multiple diffusers can be used simultaneously (Fig. 6). Once the illumination is complete the catheters can be removed.

Periprocedure Course

Many of the patients who are candidates for iPDT have received extensive treatment to the upper aerodigestive tract. Therefore, many patients already have impaired swallowing and/or airway functions. When iPDT is applied to a cancer located in the upper aerodigestive tract, substantial edema follows impairing the airway patency and swallowing function. It is advisable to perform a tracheostomy and introduce a feeding tube.

The edema and pain peak at the first post-treatment day and subside gradually. In many cases the tracheostomy tube can be removed 7 days after treatment. Some patients might remain tracheostomy and/or feeding tube dependent which is related to the extent of the treatment and previous treatments. We routinely administer systemic dexamethasone and taper over 2 weeks. The pain management is with fentanyl transdermal patches, paracetamol (acetaminophen), and locally applied lidocaine gel.

In 2–3 weeks following iPDT, the tumor can be observed to turn pale and start to become necrotic. In the following 2–3 months, necrosis of the tumor becomes obvious with pieces of necrotic tissue becoming detached. This process is dependent on the size of the treated cancer and can take up to 6 months. The response is determined with MRI at 3 and 6-month post-treatment time points. Communication with the radiologist is crucial, as necrosis at 3-month post-treatment can easily be confused with residual cancer and even some cases interpreted as cancer progression. At 6 months, the effect of the treatment is more obvious, presenting as tissue defects where the cancer previously existed.

Clinical Outcomes There is not much published data over iPDT of oropharyngeal tumors. We have reported iPDT of 20 bases of tongue tumors, with complete response in 9 patients and long-term disease control in 4 patients. Jerjes et al. reported ultrasound guided PDT of 21 patients with base of tongue tumors [30].

Adverse Events If any part of the skin gets exposed to sunlight for an extended time, within the first 3 weeks following photosensitizer administration, the patient will get a second or third degree burn. As necrotic tissue detaches, it can rarely be accompanied by bleeding. In case of major bleeding intra-arterial embolization can be considered. The most common adverse event with iPDT is tissue defects. In some cases there can be through-and-through defects between the skin and the oropharynx. Therefore, it is crucial to protect the uninvolved tissue from the treatment light.

References

1. Nieuwenhuis EJ, Castelijns JA, Pijpers R, van den Brekel MW, Brakenhof RH, van der Waal I, Snow GB. Leemans CR Wait-and-see policy for the N0 neck in early-stage oral and oropharyngeal squamous cell carcinoma using ultrasonography-guided cytology: is there a role for identification of the sentinel node? Head Neck. 2002;24(3):282–9.
2. Ris HB, Altermatt HJ, Nachbur B, Stewart JC, Wang Q, Lim CK, Bonnett R, Althaus U. Effect of drug-light interval on photodynamic therapy with meta-tetrahydroxyphenylchlorin in malignant mesothelioma. Int J Cancer. 1993;53(1):141–6.
3. Chang SC, Buonaccorsi G, MacRobert A, Bown SG. Interstitial and transurethral photodynamic therapy of the canine prostate using meso-tetra-(m-hydroxyphenyl) chlorin. Int J Cancer. 1996;67:555–62.
4. Lodder WL, Teertstra HJ, Tan IB, Pameijer FA, Smeele LE, van Velthuysen ML, van den Brekel MW. Tumour thickness in oral cancer using an intra-oral ultrasound probe. Eur Radiol. 2011;21(1):98–106.
5. Karakullukcu B, van Oudenaarde K, Copper MP, Klop WM, van Veen R, Wildeman M, Bing TI. Photodynamic therapy of early stage oral cavity and oropharynx neoplasms: an outcome

analysis of 170 patients. Eur Arch Otorhinolaryngol. 2011;268(2):281–8.
6. Biel M. Advances in photodynamic therapy for the treatment of head and neck cancers. Lasers Surg Med. 2006;38:349–55.
7. Biel MA. Photodynamic therapy of head and neck cancers. Methods Mol Biol. 2010;635: 281–93.
8. Andrejevic-Blant S, Hadjur C, Ballini JP, Wagnières G, Fontolliet C, van den Bergh H, Monnier P. Photodynamic therapy of early squamous cell carcinoma with tetra(m-hydroxyphenyl)chlorin: optimal drug-light interval. Br J Cancer. 1997;76(8):1021–8.
9. Keller GS, Doiron DR, Fisher CU. Photodynamic therapy in otolaryngology-head and neck surgery. Arch Otolaryngol. 1985;111:758–61.
10. Feyh J, Goetz A, Muller W, Konigsberger R, Kastenbauer E. Photodynamic therapy in head and neck surgery. J Photochem Photobiol B. 1990;7:353–8.
11. Feyh J, Gutmann A, Leunig A. A photodynamic therapy in head and neck surgery. Laryngol Rhinol Otol. 1993;72:273–8.
12. Wenig BL, Kurtzman DM, Grossweiner L, Mafee JF, Harris DM, Lobraico RV, Prycz RA, Appelbaum EL. Photodynamic therapy in the treatment of squamous cell carcinoma of the head and neck. Arch Otolaryngol Head Neck Surg. 1990;116:1267–70.
13. Grossweiner LI, Hill JH, Lobraico RV. Photodynamic therapy of head and neck squamous cell carcinoma: optical dosimetry and clinical trial. Photochem Photobiol. 1987;46:911–7.
14. Schweitzer VG. Photodynamic therapy for treatment of head and neck cancer. Otolaryngol Head Neck Surg. 1990;102:225–32.
15. Gluckman JL. Hematoporphyrin photodynamic therapy: is there truly a future in head and neck oncology? Reflections on a 5-year experience. Laryngoscope. 1991;101:36–42.
16. Grant WE, Hopper C, Speight PM, Macrobert AD, Bown SC. Photodynamic therapy of malignant and premalignant lesions in patients with "field cancerization" of the oral cavity. J Laryngol Otol. 1993;107(12):1140–5.
17. Biel MA. Photodynamic therapy and the treatment of head and neck neoplasia. Laryngoscope. 1998;108:1259–68.
18. Poate TW, Dilkes MG, Kenyon GS. Use of photodynamic therapy for the treatment of squamous cell carcinoma of the soft palate. Br J Oral Maxillofac Surg. 1996;34:66–8.
19. Grosjean P, Savary JF, Wagnieres G, Mizeret J, Woodtli A, Fontolliet C, et al. Phototherapy of pharyngeal, oesophageal and bronchial early squamous cell carcinomas after sensitisation by tetra (m-hydroxyphenyl) chlorin (mTHPC). Med Chir Dig. 1996;25:411–3.
20. Copper MP, Tan IB, Oppelaar H, Ruevekamp MC, Stewart FA. Meta-tetra(hydroxyphenyl) chlorin photodynamic therapy in early-stage squamous cell carcinoma of the head and neck. Arch Otolaryngol Head Neck Surg. 2003;129:709–11.
21. D'Cruz AK, Robinson MH, Biel MA. mTHPC-mediated photodynamic therapy in patients with advanced, incurable head and neck cancer: a multicenter study of 128 patients. Head Neck. 2004;26:232–40.
22. Lorenz KJ, Maier H. Photodynamic therapy with meta-tetrahydroxyphenylchlorin (Foscan®) in the management of squamous cell carcinoma of the head and neck: experience with 35 patients. Eur Arch Otorhinolaryngol. 2009;266(12):1937–44.
23. Copper MP, Triesscheijn M, Tan IB, Ruevekamp MC, Stewart FA. Photodynamic therapy in the treatment of multiple primary tumours in the head and neck, located to the oral cavity and oropharynx. Clin Otolaryngol. 2007;32:185–9.
24. Tan IB, Dolivet G, Ceruse P, Vander Poorten V, Roest G, Rauschning W. Temoporfin-mediated photodynamic therapy in patients with advanced, incurable head and neck cancer: a multicenter study. Head Neck. 2010;32:1597–604.
25. Lou PJ, Jager HR, Jones L, Theodossy T, Bown SG, Hopper C. Interstitial photodynamic therapy as salvage treatment for recurrent head and neck cancer. Br J Cancer. 2004;91:441–6.
26. Karakullukcu B, Nyst HJ, van Veen RL, Hoebers FJ, Hamming-Vrieze O, Witjes MJ, de Visscher SA, Burlage FR, Levendag PC, Sterenborg HJ, Tan IB. mTHPC mediated interstitial photodynamic therapy of recurrent nonmetastatic base of tongue cancers: development of a new method. Head Neck. 2012;34(11):1597–606.
27. Karakullukcu B, van Veen RL, Aans JB, Hamming-Vrieze O, Navran A, Teertstra HJ, van den Boom F, Niatsetski Y, Sterenborg HJ, Tan IB. MR and CT based treatment planning for mTHPC mediated interstitial photodynamic therapy of head and neck cancer: description of the method. Lasers Surg Med. 2013;45(8):517–23.
28. Jerjes W, Upile T, Hamdoon Z, Nhembe F, Bhandari R, Mackay S, et al. Ultrasound-guided photodynamic therapy for deep seated pathologies: prospective study. Lasers Surg Med. 2009;41:612–21.
29. Jerjes W, Upile T, Alexander Mosse C, Hamdoon Z, Morcos M, Morley S, et al.

Prospective evaluation of 110 patients following ultrasound-guided photodynamic therapy for deep seated pathologies. Photodiagn Photodyn Ther. 2011;8:297–306.

30. Jerjes W, Upile T, Hamdoon Z, Abbas S, Akram S, Mosse CA, et al. Photodynamic therapy: the minimally invasive surgical intervention for advanced and/or recurrent tongue base carcinoma. Lasers Surg Med. 2011;43:283–92.

31. Kreeft A, Tan IB, van den Brekel MW, Hilgers FJ, Balm AJ. The surgical dilemma of 'functional inoperability' in oral and oropharyngeal cancer: current consensus on operability with regard to functional results. Clin Otolaryngol. 2009;34(2):140–6.

Chapter 23

Photodynamic Therapy for the Management of Laryngeal Malignancies

Merrill A. Biel

Photodynamic Therapy for the Management of Laryngeal Malignancies

Carcinoma of the larynx accounts for 25–30 % of all carcinomas of the head and neck [1]. Early carcinomas of the larynx (Cis, T1, T2) and severe dysplasia are presently treated with either radiation therapy or surgery alone. Five-year cure rates achieved with this therapy is 75–90 %. Radiation therapy has the advantage of preserving the physical integrity of the larynx, thereby preserving the voice. Radiation therapy, however, has significant disadvantages even when small laryngeal fields of radiation are used. These disadvantages include discomfort and mucositis during and for potential prolonged periods after therapy, permanently altered voice quality, dysphagia, chondroradionecrosis of the larynx and trachea, and the extensive length of therapy (6–7 weeks) [2, 3]. Surgical therapy for early carcinomas, that is, T1 and T2, of the larynx includes performing a partial cordectomy or hemilaryngectomy. Although cure rates are high, surgical removal of portions of the vocal cord or hemilarynx results in significant alteration of the quality of voice [4].

Severe dysplasia and Cis may also be treated with either radiation or limited surgery with either microsurgical techniques or laser excision. Le reported on 82 patients with Cis of which 15 were treated with vocal cord stripping with a 56 % local control rate, 13 treated with extensive laser resection/hemilaryngectomy with a 71 % local control rate, and 54 treated with radiotherapy with a 79 % local control rate. Anterior commissure involvement was a significant negative prognostic factor. Subjective voice quality was good

Brian J.-F. Wong and Justus Ilgner (eds.), *Biomedical Optics in Otorhinolaryngology: Head and Neck Surgery*, DOI 10.1007/978-1-4939-1758-7_23, © Springer Science+Business Media New York 2016

to excellent in 73 % of patients who underwent vocal cord stripping, 40 % of those who underwent extensive resection, and 68 % who underwent radiation therapy [5]. Zeitels reported on seven patients with Cis undergoing microsurgical resection. Two patients developed subsequent microinvasive cancer requiring more aggressive treatment [6]. Smith reported on 25 patients with Cis treated with surgical resection with an 88 % cure rate [7]. Sittel reported on laser excision of vocal cord cancers and noted significant effect on voice with anterior commissure resections even when done in a staged fashion [8]. Chone reported on 48 patients with early glottis cancer treated with laser microsurgical resection. He noted a 79 % local control rate and a 96 % laryngeal preservation rate [9]. Rucci presented the results of 81 patients treated with CO_2 laser therapy for Cis and T1 glottic cancers and noted a 35 % recurrence rate [10].

Garcia-Serra reported on 30 patients with Cis treated with radiotherapy with an 88 % local control rate. Review of literature for radiotherapy of Cis demonstrated an 87.4 % weighted local control rate at 5 years on 705 patients in 22 published reports. Review of ten reports of laser excision treatments of Cis demonstrated an 82.5 % control rate in 177 patients. Many required multiple laser excisions [11].

Damm reported on 29 patients with Cis treated with laser excision. Seventy-six percent (22/29) required more than one laser excision for persistence of disease, nine of which were in the anterior commissure. Two-year disease-free survival rate was 86 %. Dysphonia was reported in all patients and none had improved voice over the pretreatment state [12]. A literature review of control rates of various treatments for Cis were as follows: laser excision (104 patients), 20 % initial failure rate and 1 % larynx lost; vocal cord stripping (235 patients), 34 % failure rate and 12 % larynx lost; and radiotherapy (481 patients), 16 % failure rate and 7 % larynx lost [12]. The literature therefore demonstrates that surgical techniques to treat Cis are best limited to those patients where the Cis does not involve the anterior commissure or the bilateral vocal cords. Khan reported a 20-year experience of definitive radiotherapy for early glottic cancers on 141 patients. The 5-year local control rate was 94 % for T1a, 83 % for T1b, 87 % for T2a, and 65 % for T2b. Of those patients with impaired voice, 73 % noted significant voice improvement after radiotherapy [13]. Hafidh presented the results of 150 patients treated with radiotherapy for T1/T2 glottic cancers. Seventy-one percent of T1 and 63.3 % of T2 carcinomas were controlled with radiotherapy with an average follow-up of 37 months [14]. Hartl presented a review of treatment options for glottis cancer and noted using primary radiotherapy a 43–91 % control rate for T1 carcinomas and a 50–85 % control rate for T2 carcinomas [15]. Lee reported on the oncologic outcomes of 118 patients with T1 and T2 glottic cancer treated with one-stage transoral laser microsurgery. The 5-year disease-free survival rate was 87.9 % and local control rate with laser alone, including multiple treatments for recurrence, was 94.2 % [16]. Batella performed a voice quality study of patients who underwent endoscopic laser surgery and radiotherapy for T1 glottic carcinomas and noted that voice quality was affected both by surgery and radiotherapy, although there was a reduced impact on the patient's perception of voice quality after radiotherapy [17].

The optimal treatment for severe dysplasia and early carcinomas of the larynx would be one that is effective, safe, repeatable, minimally invasive, nonsurgical, and a less time-consuming therapy than radiotherapy. Photodynamic therapy is potentially such a treatment for severe dysplasia and early carcinomas of the larynx.

Photodynamic Therapy

Photodynamic therapy (PDT) is a minimally invasive treatment involving the use of a photosensitizing drug and laser light for the treatment of a variety of cancers. When administered, these compounds are accumulated and retained to a greater degree in malignant tissues than normal tissues. The drugs remain inactive until exposed to a specific wavelength of light. The light, usually from a laser, is transmitted through specially modified fiber optics and activates the drug. The resulting photochemical reaction results in the production of oxygen radicals thereby destroying diseased cells with little effect on normal tissues. To date, PDT has been used to treat carcinomas in many organs, and Photofrin-based PDT has been approved by the US FDA to treat early- and end-stage endobronchial and esophageal squamous cell carcinomas and Barrett's dysplasia. In particular, the use of PDT to treat early carcinomas of the head and neck has been promising [18–26].

The generally accepted mechanism of action of PDT is that there is an energy transfer process from the light-activated or light-excited triplet state of the photosensitizer to oxygen producing singlet oxygen which in turn causes irreversible oxidation of some essential cellular component. It has also been shown that the vasculature changes within the tumor necrosis subsequent to PDT result in ischemia that is responsible for tumor necrosis. Either or both are sufficient to explain the remarkable necrosis of tumors within 2–5 days following PDT with Photofrin.

Photofrin^{R} (porfimer sodium) concentrates in malignant tissue, is activated by penetrating light (630 + 3 nm), produces fluorescence, and is photochemically efficient. Photofrin^{R} has produced only one major side effect as a result of its use: light sensitivity.

Photodynamic therapy has been demonstrated to be effective in the treatment of early carcinomas of the head and neck [18–26]. Furthermore, preliminary studies on the treatment of benign laryngeal papillomatosis with PDT have demonstrated this treatment to be safe and effective [27, 28].

The advantage of PDT therapy for early carcinomas of the larynx is the ability to preserve normal endolaryngeal tissue while effectively treating the carcinomas. This results in improved laryngeal function and voice quality [29]. Furthermore, PDT requires a short duration of therapy as compared to radiation therapy, is repeatable and carries less risk than surgical therapy, and is performed as an outpatient noninvasive treatment. Importantly, the use of PDT does not preclude the use of radiotherapy or surgery in the future for new primary or recurrent disease. The following is a retrospective review of the author's 144 patients treated with Photofrin-based photodynamic therapy for early laryngeal cancers between 1990 and 2010.

Materials and Methods

The author's clinical experience with PDT for the treatment of laryngeal carcinomas spans 23 years. One hundred forty-four patients with focal Cis, T1, T2, T3, and T4 glottic carcinomas of the larynx with N0 necks, of which 120 were Cis and T1 and 17 were T2, were treated with PDT from February 1990 to September 2010. All patients were treated according to specific protocols in accordance with FDA and local IRB approvals. Pretreatment evaluation included a history and physical examination, endoscopic examination with tumor mapping and biopsy, routine laboratory evaluation, and photographic documentation. CT or MRI scanning was performed for all patients with tumor stage greater than T1N0. All treatments were performed using the photosensitizer PHOTOFRIN (Pinnacle Biologics, Bannockburn, IL) as an off-label use indication. The male-to-female ratio was 109:35, with an age range of 24–92 years.

Photofrin was injected intravenously at a dose of 2.0 mg/kg over a 5 min period as an outpatient procedure. Approximately 48 h after the injection, the patients underwent treatment with light from an Nd:Yag-pumped dye laser (Laserscope) or a 630 nm diode laser (AngioDynamics, Latham, NY) at a 630 nm wavelength. Light was delivered to the tissue bed with a 400 μm fused silica optical microlens fiber (LaserGuide, Inc., Buellton, CA). A microlens treatment was used for all tumors with a depth of less than 3 mm. These light treatments were performed at 80 J/cm^2 and 150 mw/cm^2. For T2 or greater laryngeal tumors, cylindrical diffusers 0.5–2.5 cm in length were placed in the tumor bed using an

18-gauge catheter under laryngoscopic guidance. These light treatments were performed at 100 J/cm fiber length and 400 mw/cm fiber length. All treatments were performed on an outpatient basis under general anesthesia with standard laryngoscopy.

On completion of treatment, each patient received Decadron 10 mg intravenously for one dose to reduce tissue edema and was discharged on oral pain medications. All patients were instructed to avoid daylight for 30 days. Tumor response was evaluated at 1 week, 1 month, and then monthly thereafter for 1 year and every 3 months thereafter. Multiple biopsy specimens of the treated area were obtained for most patients 1 month after treatment to evaluate a complete histopathologic response.

Results

One hundred thirty-seven patients with recurrent or primary Cis, T1N0, and T2N0 laryngeal tumors were treated with PDT for cure. Four patients had recurrent Cis, 116 patients had T1N0 carcinomas of the true vocal cord of which 27 were radiation failures, and 17 patients had T2N0 carcinomas of the true vocal cord of which 9 were radiation failures. All patients underwent a single microlens light treatment and most T2 tumors also underwent cylindrical diffuser implants into the paraglottic space. All treatments were performed under general anesthesia with standard laryngoscopy and all patients were discharged to home the same day of PDT treatment. All patients obtained a complete histopathologic response after a single light treatment (Figs. 1 and 2). With a follow-up of up to 60 months (mean 57 months), there were 14

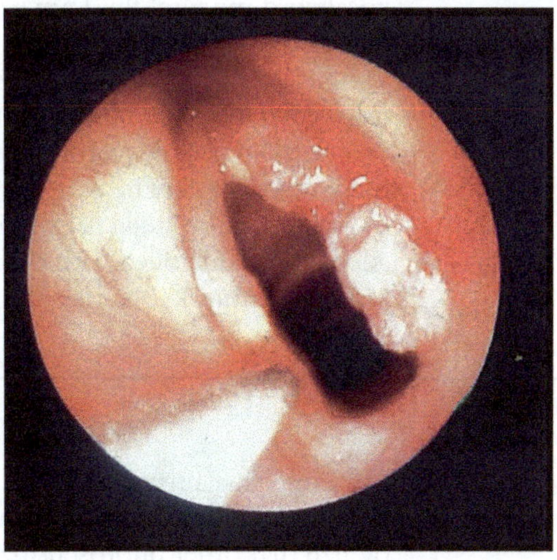

Fig. 1 Recurrent right vocal cord cancer as a failure of radiotherapy

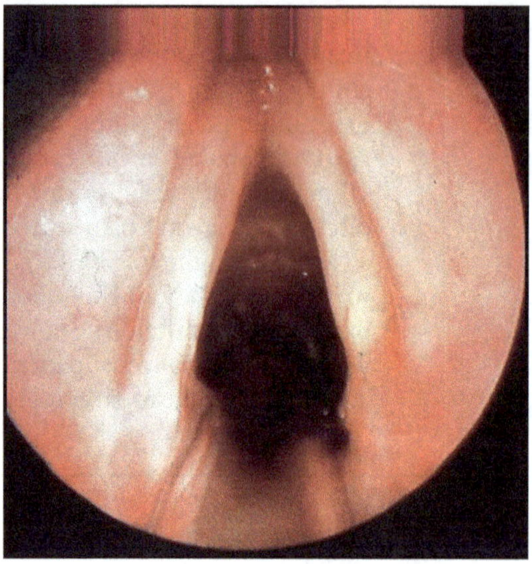

Fig. 2 Six weeks after PDT treatment of recurrent right vocal cord cancer with resolution of disease

recurrences for a 5-year cure rate of 90 %. Importantly, all the recurrences were salvaged using either PDT, surgery, or radiation for a total 5-year cure rate of 100 %. In the entire treatment group there were no episodes of airway compromise and the degree of postoperative pain was minimal and easily controlled with oral analgesics. No patients required a tracheostomy before or after PDT treatment. All patients after treatment developed an immediate breathy voice that persisted for 2–3 weeks. At 4–6 weeks after treatment, the quality of voice was universally much improved over the pretreatment state. In addition, videostroboscopy 6 weeks post PDT treatment performed on ten patients demonstrated a normal vocal cord mucosal fluid wave on the treated vocal cord.

In the entire series of 144 patients, no patient developed a significant sun-induced photosensitivity reaction, i.e., significant facial edema or skin blistering. In all patients the treated area demonstrated maximal necrosis by 7 days after light treatment, and there was complete healing by 4 weeks after treatment. The degree of treatment-related pain was minimal and limited and was adequately controlled with oral analgesics. The pain was uniformly resolved within 2–3 weeks of treatment.

Discussion

Although this author has presented the results of Photofrin-based PDT for the treatment of laryngeal cancers, it is important to recognize that other photosensitizers have been used and continue to be investigated for the treatment of head and neck cancers with very similar results [25, 26].

Table 1
Summary of published results with Photofrin PDT of early squamous cell cancer of the larynx

Study	Patients	Lesion and site	Drug, dose (mg/kg)	Response (*n*)		
				Complete	Partial	None
Feyh et al. [19]	12	T1 and T2, larynx	Photosan III	11	1	0
Freche et al. [18]	32	T1, larynx	HPD, 3	25	7	0
Schweitzer [21]	10	T1, larynx	Photofrin, 2	8	2	0
Gluckman [20]	2	T1, larynx	Photofrin, 2	2	0	2
Biel [22, 23]	110	Cis, T1 and T2 larynx	Photofrin, 2	110	10	0
Rigual [24]	6	Severe dysplasia and T1 larynx	Photofrin, 2	5	0	1

Patients with early-stage cancers or early recurrences of the larynx (Cis, Tl, T2) tend to have an excellent response to PDT. Of 172 patients in this group, all patients obtained a durable complete response rate of 88 % with up to a 16-year follow-up.

Multiple centers have reported phase II study data on the use of Photofrin-based PDT to treat Cis-T2 carcinomas of the larynx [18–24] (Table 1). Freche (1990) reported on 32 patients with T1 vocal cord carcinomas treated primarily with PDT. Twenty-five of 32 patients obtained a complete response for a complete response rate of 78 % [18]. Feyh (1996) treated 12 patients with Tis-T2 laryngeal carcinomas. Eleven of 12 patients obtained a complete response for a complete response rate of 91 % [19]. Gluckman (1991) treated two patients with T1 carcinomas of the larynx, both of which obtained a complete response [20]. Schweitzer (2000) treated ten patients with Tis-T2 carcinomas of the larynx of which eight obtained a complete response for an 80 % complete response rate [21]. Biel (2006) treated 110 patients with early laryngeal tumors (Tis, T1, T2), 32 of which were radiation failures, treated with Photofrin 2 mg/kg using a microlens fiber at 80 J/cm^2, 48 h after Photofrin injection. All but ten patients (91 %) obtained a durable complete response after a single PDT treatment (100 % salvage) with a follow-up of up to 201 months (mean 91 mos.) [23]. Rigual (2009) treated six patients with severe dysplasia and T1 glottic carcinomas. Five of six patients obtained a complete response [24].

Dilkes treated five patients with T1-2 laryngeal tumors with Foscan PDT. Only one of the five patients had no recurrence of disease [25].

Grossman reported on the treatment of one patient with the use of oral Levulan PDT to treat a patient with multiple recurrent glottis severe dysplasia despite CO_2 laser excisions and vocal fold strippings. They demonstrated a complete response after one treatment and the patient remains free of disease for 6 months [26].

Cis, T1, and T2 carcinomas of the larynx appear to be particularly effectively treated with PDT. A literature review of control rates of various treatments for Cis of the vocal cord was as follows: laser excision (104 patients), 20 % initial failure rate requiring further therapy and 1 % larynx lost; vocal cord stripping (235 patients), 34 % failure rate and 12 % larynx lost; and radiotherapy (481 patients), 16 % failure rate and 7 % larynx lost [12]. The literature demonstrated that surgical techniques to treat Cis are best limited to those patients where the Cis does not involve the anterior commissure or the bilateral vocal cords. Hartl presented a review of treatment options for glottis cancer and noted using primary radiotherapy a 43–91 % control rate for T1 carcinomas and a 50–85 % control rate for T2 carcinomas [15]. Rucci presented the results of 81 patients treated with CO_2 laser therapy for Cis and T1 glottic cancers and noted a 35 % recurrence rate [10].

The present clinical series demonstrates the efficacy of Photofrin-mediated photodynamic therapy as a curative treatment for Cis, T1 (85–91 %), and T2 (72 %) primary or recurrent squamous cell carcinomas of the larynx. PDT for laryngeal carcinomas results in no glottic scarring as compared to conventional laser or surgical excision or vocal cord stripping. For recurrent carcinomas of the larynx that have failed conventional radiation therapy, PDT allows excellent voice preservation and may eliminate the need for partial or total laryngectomy. Also, PDT can be repeated without additional functional laryngeal compromise that can occur from repeated conventional laser surgery or cordectomy. Importantly, PDT treatment of primary T1 and T2 laryngeal carcinomas reserves radiation therapy for treatment of recurrences or of second head and neck primaries that may occur in these high-risk patients.

The side effects of PDT treatment of laryngeal carcinomas are quite minimal as compared to that of conventional radiotherapy or surgery. PDT treatment is performed as a single outpatient procedure as compared to 6–7 weeks of radiotherapy or the hospitalization associated with a partial or total laryngectomy. The photosensitivity of Photofrin is a temporary inconvenience not associated with systemic toxicity and is minimized by patient education and temporary changes in daily outdoor activities. The photosensitivity does however last for approximately 4 weeks.

Conclusion

Photodynamic therapy for treatment of Cis, T1, and T2 laryngeal carcinomas in the present series has cure rates that are comparable to if not better than that of conventional therapies with less morbidity of treatment. PDT should be considered as a reasonable option for the treatment of primary and recurrent Cis, T1, and T2 squamous cell carcinomas of the larynx.

References

1. Shah JP, Karnell LH, Hoffman HT, et al. Patterns of care for cancer of the larynx in the United States. Arch Otolaryngol Head Neck Surg. 1997;123:475–83.
2. VonEssen CF. Larynx and pyriform sinus. In: Fletcher GH, editor. Textbook of radiotherapy. Philadelphia: Lea & Febiger; 1982. p. 330–64.
3. Morris MR, Canonico D, Blank C. A critical review of radiotherapy in the management of T1 glottic carcinoma. Am J Otolaryngol. 1994;15(4):276–80.
4. Bailey BJ, Biller HF. Glottic carcinomas. In: Biller BJ, editor. Surgery of the Larynx. Philadelphia: W. B. Saunders; 1985. p. 257–77.
5. Le Q, Takamiya R, Shu H, et al. Treatment results of carcinoma in situ of the glottis. Arch Otolaryngol Head Neck Surg. 2000;126:1305–12.
6. Zeitels SM. Phonomicrosurgical treatment of early glottic cancer and carcinoma in situ. Am J Surg. 1996;172:704–9.
7. Smith JC, Johnson JT, Myers EN. Management and outcome of early glottic carcinoma. Otolaryngol Head Neck Surg. 2002;126(4):356–64.
8. Sittel C, Eckel H, Eschenburg C. Phonatory results after laser surgery for glottic carcinoma. Otolaryngol Head Neck Surg. 1998;119(4):418–24.
9. Chone CT, Yonehara E, Martins JEF, Altemani A, Crespo AN. Importance of anterior commissure in recurrence of early glottic cancer after laser endoscopic resection. Arch Otolaryngol Head Neck Surg. 2007;133(9):882–7.
10. Rucci L, Romagnoli P, Scala J. CO_2 laser therapy in Tis and T1 glottic cancer: indications and results. Head Neck. 2010;32:392–8.
11. Garcia-Serra A, Hinerman RW, Amdur RJ, Morris CG, Mendenhall WM. Radiotherapy for carcinoma in situ of the true vocal cords. Head Neck. 2002;24:390–4.
12. Damm M, Sittel C, Streppel M, Eckel HE. Transoral CO2 laser surgical management of glottic carcinoma in situ. Laryngoscope. 2002;110:1215–21.
13. Khan MK, Koyfman SA, Hunter GK, Reddy CA, Saxton JP. Definitive radiotherapy for early (T1-2) glottic squamous cell carcinoma: a 20 year Cleveland clinic experience. Radiat Oncol. 2012;7:193.
14. Hafidh M, Tibbo J, Trites J, Corsten G, Hart RD, Nasser J, Wilke D, Taylor SM. Radiotherapy for T1 and T2 laryngeal cancer: the Dalhousie University experience. J Otolaryngol Head Neck Surg. 2009;38(4):434–9.
15. Hartl DM, Ferlito A, Brasnu DR, Langendijk JA, Rinaldo A, Silver CE, Wolf GT. Evidence-based review of treatment options for patients with glottic cancer. Head Neck. 2011;33:1638–48.
16. Lee HS, Chun B, Kim SW, Kim ST, Oh JH, Hong JC, Lee KD. Transoral laser microsurgery for early glottic cancer as a one-stage single-modality therapy. Laryngoscope. 2013;123:2670–4.
17. Batella FN, Cueva MJC, Gonzalez BS, Pendas JLL, Gil G, Llames AL, Pantiga RA, Nieto CS. Voice quality after endoscopic laser surgery and radiotherapy for early glottis cancer: objective measurements emphasizing the Voice Handicap Index. Eur Arch Otorhinolaryngol. 2008;265:543–8.
18. Freche C, DeCorbiere S. Use of photodynamic therapy in the treatment of vocal cord carcinoma. J Photochem Photobiol B. 1990;6:291–6.
19. Feyh J, Goetz A, Muller W, et al. Photodynamic therapy in head and neck surgery. J Photochem Photobiol B. 1990;7:353–8.
20. Gluckman JL. Hematoporphyrin photodynamic therapy: is there truly a future in head and neck oncology? Reflections on a 5-year experience. Laryngoscope. 1991;101:36–42.
21. Schweitzer V. Photofrin-mediated photodynamic therapy for treatment of early stage oral cavity and laryngeal malignancies. Lasers Surg Med. 2001;29(4):305–13.
22. Biel MA. Photodynamic therapy and the treatment of head and neck neoplasia. Laryngoscope. 1998;108:1259–68.
23. Biel MA. Advances in photodynamic therapy for the treatment of head and neck cancer. Lasers Surg Med. 2006;38:349–55.
24. Rigual NR, Thankappan K, Cooper M, Sullivan MA, Dougherty T, Popat SR, Loree TR, Biel MA, Henderson B. Photodynamic therapy for

head and neck dysplasia and cancer. Arch Otolaryngol Head Neck Surg. 2009;135(8): 784–8.

25. Dilkes MG, DeJode ML. m-THPC photodynamic therapy for head and neck cancer. Lasers Med Sci. 1996;11(1):23–9.
26. Grossman C, Zhu T, Finlay J, Dimofte A, Malloy K, O'Malley BO, Weinstein G, Busch TM, Quon H. Targeted laryngeal photodynamic therapy with a balloon diffusing light source. Photodiagn Photodyn Ther. 2010;7:158–61.
27. Abramson AL, Shikowitz MJ, Mullooly VM, Steinberg BM, Hyman RB. Variable light-dose effect on photodynamic therapy for laryngeal papillomas. Arch Otolaryngol Head Neck Surg. 1994;120(8):852–5.
28. Shikowitz MJ, Abramson AL, Steinberg BM, DeVoti J, Bonagura VR, Mullooly V, Nouri M, Ronn AM, Inglis A, McClay J, Freeman K. Clinical trial of photodynamic therapy with meso-tetra (hydroxyphenyl) chlorin for respiratory papillomas. Arch Otolaryngol Head Neck Surg. 2005;131(2):99–105.
29. Silbergleit AK, Somers ML, Schweitzer VG, Gardner GM, Peterson E. Vocal fold vibration after photofrin-mediated photodynamic therapy for treatment of early-stage laryngeal malignancies. J Voice. 2013;27(6):762–4.

Chapter 24

Photodynamic Therapy for Advanced Malignancies and Palliation

Waseem Jerjes and Colin Hopper

Photodynamic therapy (PDT) has proved its usefulness in the management of deep-seated head and neck malignancies, with the aim to provide local control or for palliation purposes. The principles of this minimally invasive surgical intervention (PDT) depend on three factors: (1) systemic administration of a photosensitiser and its accumulation in the target tissue (i.e. pathology), (2) light (of a specific wavelength) delivery to the target tissue and (3) the resultant photochemical reaction from the interaction between the photosensitiser, the oxygen in the target tissue and the light (Fig. 1). This reaction, which lasts for few hours, results in selective injury to the target tissue with some collateral tissue damage. The extent of this selective tissue injury is influenced by many factors, including the photosensitiser (type and concentration), the delivered light (dose and dose rate) and the target tissue (oxygen availability and cellular localisation) [1–12].

Photosensitisers

Until now, two generations of photosensitisers are used in interventional oncology in head and neck. First generation photosensitisers include Profimer Sodium (Photofrin) which has been successfully used in Barrett's high-grade dysplasia, oesophageal and endobronchial carcinomas. To achieve maximal absorption and high effectivity, the following parameters must be applied: light wavelength 630 nm, drug dose 2 mg/kg, drug/light interval 48–72 h, fluence 100–200 J/cm^2 and fluence rate 100 mW/cm^2 [1–12].

Brian J.-F. Wong and Justus Ilgner (eds.), *Biomedical Optics in Otorhinolaryngology: Head and Neck Surgery*,
DOI 10.1007/978-1-4939-1758-7_24, © Springer Science+Business Media New York 2016

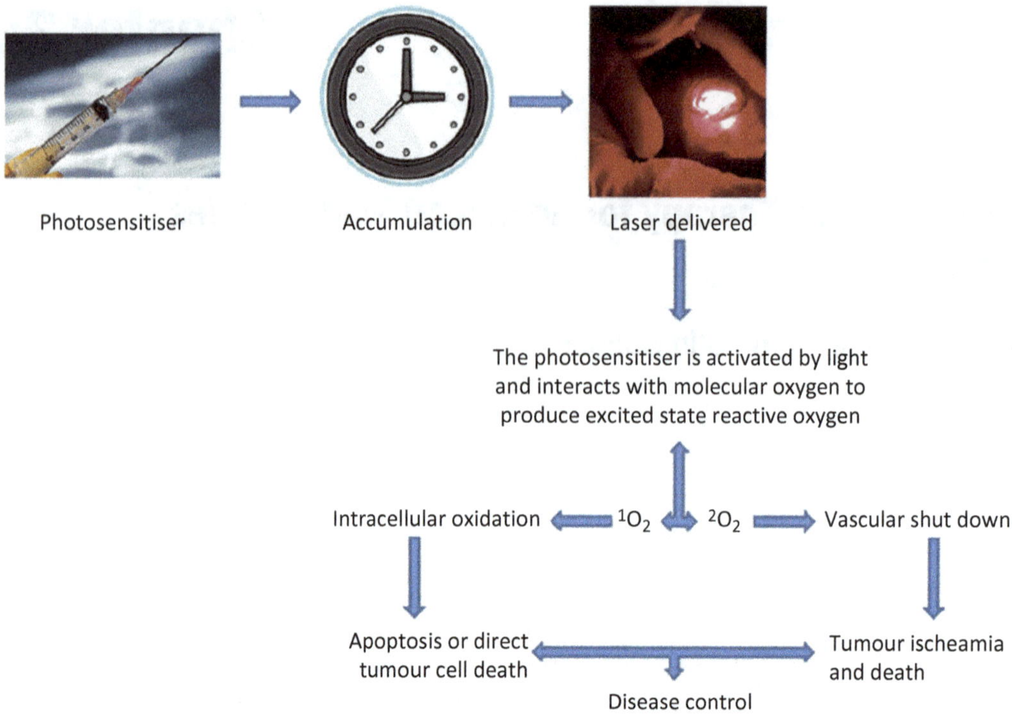

Fig. 1 Principal of photodynamic therapy. The figure is adapted from authors' own article: Jerjes W, Upile T, Akram S, Hopper C. The surgical palliation of advanced head and neck cancer using photodynamic therapy. Clin Oncol (R Coll Radiol). 2010 Nov;22(9):785–91

Second generation photosensitisers include 5-aminolevulinic acid which has been successfully used in basal cell carcinoma, actinic keratosis and oral dysplasia. To achieve maximal absorption and high effectivity, the following parameters must be applied: light wavelength 635 nm, drug dose (20 % paste or systemically "oral 60 mg/kg" or "intravenous 30 mg/kg"), drug/light interval 3–6 h, fluence 100 J/cm^2 and fluence rate 100–150 mW/cm^2 [1–12].

mTHPC (Meso-tetrahydroxyphenyl chlorin, Foscan) is another second generation photosensitiser which has been extensively used in the management of deep-seated pathologies in the head and neck, including carcinomas, some sarcomas and vascular anomalies. To achieve maximal absorption and high effectivity, the following parameters must be applied: light wavelength 652 nm, drug dose 0.15 mg/kg, drug/light interval 96 h, fluence 10–20 J/cm^2 and fluence rate 100 mW/cm^2 [1–12].

Third generation photosensitisers are still being assessed through clinical trials and yet to be introduced for use in clinical practice. The aim of the third generation photosensitisers will be to offer better tumour specificity with less collateral tissue damage and shorter period of generalised body photosensitivity [1–12].

Delivery of Light

This depends entirely on the target tissue (i.e. pathology) location and size. Surface illumination probes are used to deliver the laser light to the superficial target tissue. Depth of penetration and effect varies per photosensitiser, delivered light and target tissue, as discussed earlier. For example, surface illumination of a diseased area in the head and neck using mTHPC formula (light wavelength 652 nm, drug dose 0.15 mg/kg, drug/light interval 96 h, fluence 10–20 J/cm^2 and fluence rate 100 mW/cm^2) can lead to tissue damage of up to 10 mm in depth. Obviously deep-seated pathologies require special delivery and guiding systems [1–12] (Fig. 2).

Spinal needles are inserted in deeper target tissues and bare tip fibre optic probes are passed through them to deliver the light. First these spinal needles require guidance to provide appropriate positioning in the target tissue allowing the delivery of light to the suspect tissue centre and margins. This was initially achieved by using multi-hole grids; since then many guiding modalities have been used successfully, including two-dimensional ultrasound (US), magnetic resonance imaging (MRI), computed tomography (CT), nasoendoscopy, laryngoscopy and bronchoscopy. The delivery of light to the margins is essential in order to achieve local control and prevent disease recurrence. Superficial bulky pathologies can always be reduced surgically, and then remaining tissue and its margins can be subjected to photodynamic therapy [1–12] (Fig. 2).

Target Tissue Reaction

Two pathways have been described as a consequence of the photochemical interaction. Direct targeting of the target tissue (i.e. tumour) cells by initiating a sequence leading to necrosis and/or apoptosis; this is resulted from singlet oxygen generation. The indirect targeting, second pathway, sequence affects the target tissue vessels, causing intimal hyperplasia leading to cell ischemia and death [1–12].

Following this, it is postulated that a series of inflammatory and immunology processes continue to work on the target tissue and leads to disintegration (tissue necrosis) and resorption (which

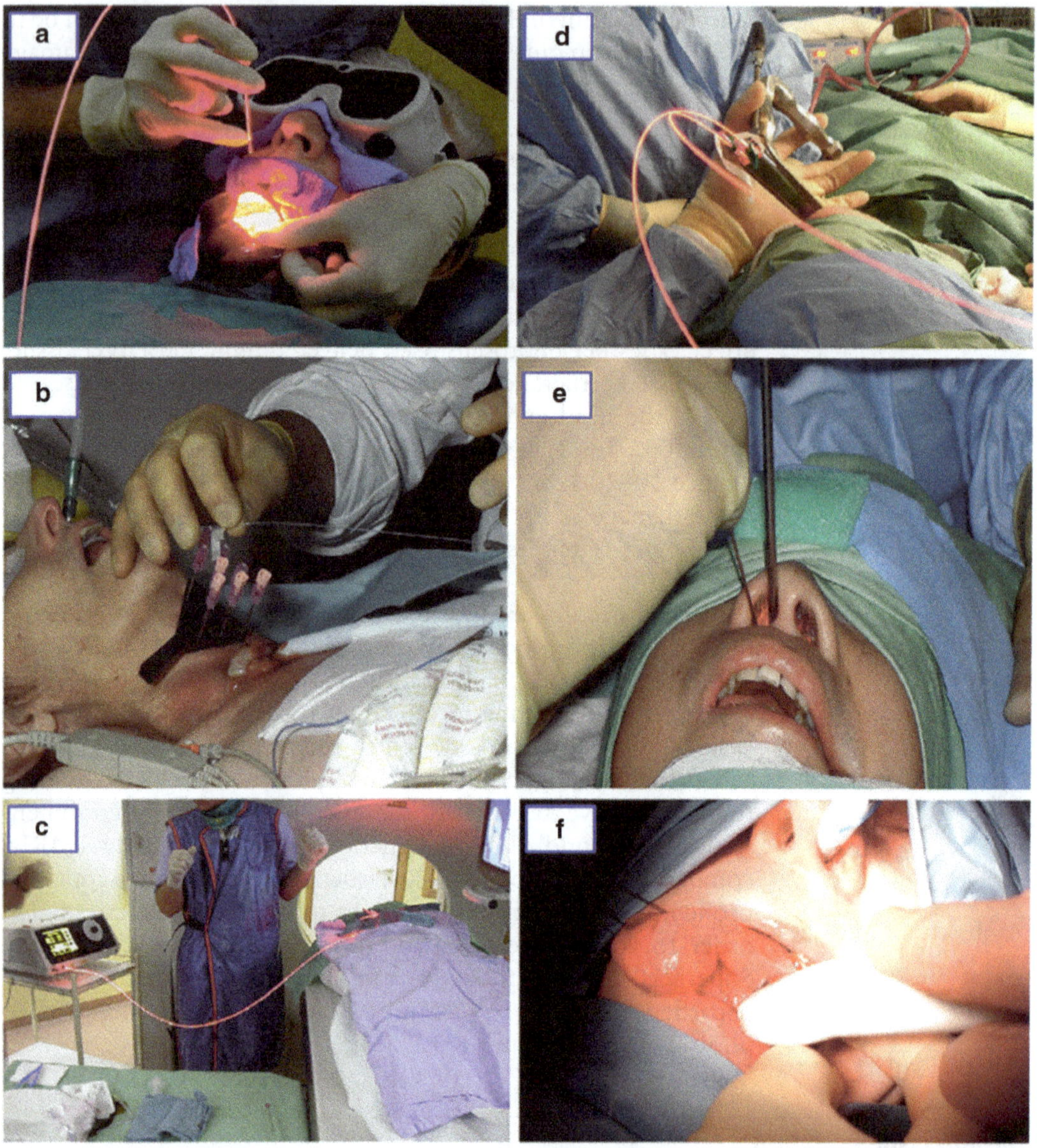

Fig. 2 Mode of light delivery. (**a**) Surface illumination; (**b**) prefabricated grid guided; (**c**) magnetic resonance imaging guided; (**d**) laryngoscope guided; (**e**) nasendoscope guided; (**f**) ultrasound guided. The figure is adapted from authors' own article: Jerjes W, Upile T, Akram S, Hopper C. The surgical palliation of advanced head and neck cancer using photodynamic therapy. Clin Oncol (R Coll Radiol). 2010 Nov;22(9):785–91

may take few weeks) (Fig. 3) and followed by generation of healthy tissue. There is minimal damage to the tissue architecture which facilitates the regeneration process without scarring. The nerves tend to be preserved or sustain minimal damage due to the non-thermal (cold) nature of this reaction. The photosensitiser and the photochemical process cause minimal accumulative toxicity allowing treatment repetition [1–12].

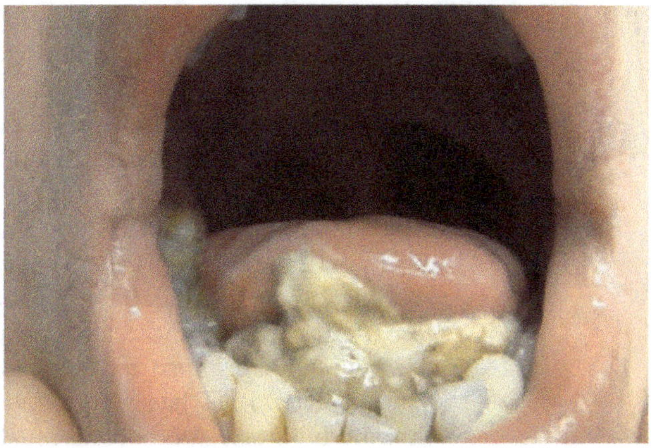

Fig. 3 Clinical image showing tissue changes and sloughing post-PDT. The figure is adapted from authors' own article: Jerjes W, Upile T, Hamdoon Z, Alexander Mosse C, Morcos M, Hopper C. Photodynamic therapy outcome for T1/T2 N0 oral squamous cell carcinoma. Lasers Surg Med. 2011 Aug;43(6):463–9

Head and Neck Cancer

The incidence of this disease remains high and known to increase with age. The majority of patients, at time of diagnosis, are above the age of 50 years and a significant number of them present with advanced disease. Patients diagnosed with squamous cell carcinoma, the most common malignancy in this area, have modest survival figures at 3 and 5 years. The overall survival is just above 50 % and the prognosis usually depends on the primary tumour size and nodal disease. The conventional treatment modalities include surgery, radiotherapy and/or chemotherapy. Despite these interventions, recurrent rate is high and is usually associated with poor outcome. It is reasonable to suggest that there is no "magic bullet" to patients presenting with advanced and/or recurrent head and neck cancer. However, clinicians and scientists continue to develop new techniques and/or invent new therapies that can lead to improved local control and better prognosis [1–12].

Surgery remains the gold standard for this unforgiving disease. The general aim here is to completely remove the primary tumour (with clear margins) and any involved cervical lymphatic chain. If this procedure generates a defect, then reconstruction is required by using local or regional flap or free tissue transfer with the aim to preserve form and function. In case of poor disease control (i.e. positive margins, metastasis), radiotherapy with/out chemotherapy can be used as the only remaining option.

Radiotherapy and/or chemotherapy have been used independent of surgery to treat head and neck cancer with variable success rates. Overall, these modalities have been very helpful in inducing long-term remission in many head and neck cancer patients. Unfortunately, side effects may arise and can be very debilitating and have a negative impact on the quality of life (i.e. mucositis, radiotherapy-induced tumours, osteoradionecrosis, flap failure, etc.) [1–12].

Photodynamic therapy (PDT) has been developed as an option to patients with advanced and/or recurrent head and neck cancer who failed one or more of the conventional modalities and as a palliative option. PDT has been found to be very helpful in reducing tumour bulk size (compromising breathing, swallowing and/or speech mechanisms or causing significant pain), controlling tumour invasion of neurovascular structures (causing significant pain), dealing with problems where tumours invade the walls of small or intermediate size vessels (causing bleeding), as well as dealing with many complex tumour-related issues (i.e. visual disturbances in retrobulbar tumours and bony invasions) with minimal or reduced side effects [1–12].

Forty-five patients with persistent or recurrent head and neck cancer were subjected to 0.15 mg/kg mTHPC-PDT. The results showed that nine patients achieved a complete response and five are alive and free of disease 10–60 months later. The median survival was 16 months for the 33 responders, but only 2 months for the 12 nonresponders. The only serious complication was one patient who had a disease-related carotid artery rupture [13]. Jäger et al. reported the use of an open interventional magnetic resonance system to guide interstitial PDT for advanced head and neck tumours and found this technique to be accurate and safe. Initial results were encouraging, with minimal procedural morbidity, successful palliation of symptoms and prolongation of expected survival time [14].

A study by Jerjes et al. prospectively evaluated the outcome after ultrasound-guided interstitial PDT of deep-seated advanced pathologies. Sixty-eight patients were treated using 0.15 mg/kg mTHPC as the photosensitising agent. All three patients who presented with visual problems reported improvement after treatment. Fourteen out of 17 patients reported improvement in breathing. Improvement in swallowing was reported by 25/30 patients; whereas speaking improvement was evident in 16/22 patients and 33/44 reported reduction in the disfigurement caused by their pathology. A clinical assessment showed that half of the patients had a "good response" to the treatment and a third reported a "moderate response," with two patients in remission. Radiological assessment comparing imaging 6 weeks post-

PDT with the baseline showed stable pathology with no change in size in 13 patients, a minimal response in 18 patients, a moderate response in 23 patients and a significant response in 11 patients [3]. A further study confirmed the previous findings that photodynamic therapy is a very effective treatment in patients with advanced and/or recurrent head and neck carcinomas and sarcomas [7].

PDT was identified as successful palliative modality in the treatment of advanced and/or recurrent tongue base carcinoma. Twenty-one consecutive patients with this disease were subjected to US-guided mTHPC-PDT under general anaesthesia. Nine of the 11 patients who presented with breathing problems reported improvement after treatment. Also, 19 of the 21 patients reported improvement of swallowing. Improvement of speech was reported by 11 of 13 patients. Clinical assessment showed that more than half of the patients had "good response" to the treatment and about a third reported "moderate response." Radiological assessment comparing imaging 6 week post-PDT to the baseline showed stable pathology with no change in size in four patients, minimal response in seven patients, moderate response in six patients, and significant response in two patients [6]. A further follow-up study confirmed the findings and the palliative benefits of PDT in advanced tongue base carcinomas [8]. Photodynamic therapy was a very successful palliative therapy for a group of patients with advanced recurrent nasopharyngeal carcinomas [10].

The current evidence suggests that photodynamic therapy is an appropriate treatment for patients with advanced and/or recurrent head and neck cancer. PDT can control disease growth, control pain and bleeding. Unfortunately, the curative intent of PDT in this cohort of patients is very difficult to achieve. Generally this cohort, at the time or presentation, have already failed one or more conventional treatment and have a significantly reduced life span. The medical literature has highlighted one concerning issue related to the effect of PDT on the tumour margins. Currently, there is a suggestion that this intervention can eliminate all tumour cells in the centre but have a lesser effect on the peripheries (margins) [15]. In a systematic review, de Visscher et al. concluded that mTHPC-PDT, the curative intent of PDT is still not fully shown in the current literature and as a result high quality comparative, randomised studies are needed. de Visscher et al. postulated that palliative treatment with PDT seems to increase the quality of life in otherwise untreatable patients [16]. Rigual et al. suggested that the adjuvant use of HPPH-photodynamic therapy and surgery for head and neck squamous cell carcinoma seems safe and deserves further study [17].

The London Procedure to Treat Advanced or Recurrent Head and Neck Cancer

The patient is usually discussed at the head and neck multidisciplinary team meeting. It has to be agreed that photodynamic therapy is, at the time of assessment, the most suitable intervention to the patient. The patient is informed of the discussion and outcome of the meeting, as well as the pros and cons of the offered intervention. The patient makes an informed decision to receive PDT for his head and neck disease. The patient is educated about this unique therapy and the steps of the treatment and what to expect in the peri-PDT and post-PDT periods to reduce anxiety and psychological trauma. This includes brief period of localised pain while administering the photosensitiser, pain (treatment area) in the first 24–72 h, inflammatory reaction in the first 24–72 h leading to local tissue swelling that may acutely compromise airway, swallowing or speech, other tissue changes leading to changes in color and size and generation of mal odour (as a result of tissue necrosis) and photosensitivity in the post-PDT period and risk of skin burn [1–12, 15, 18].

On day 4 (96 h before light delivery), mTHPC (0.15 mg/kg, the photosensitiser) is administered intravenously into the midcubital vein. This would allow the photosensitiser to accumulate in the pathological (target) area. The patient is kept in a dim-light side room to avoid systemic photosensitisation. On day 0 (light deliver day), the patient is taken to theatre and special PDT precautions is applied to theatre and staff to prevent any accidental injury to the patient or staff. The patient is prepped and draped as with any standard surgical procedure. A head and neck radiologist, using 2D ultrasound (with high resolution), examines the pathological tissue (centre and periphery) with the probe to assess tumour volume, depth, invasion of vascular structures, hollow organs or hard tissue. Then 18 gauge 70 mm long spinal needles are inserted under ultrasound guidance into the target tissue. Needles are (generally) inserted parallel to each other with 1 cm distance in between to ensure no overlapping fields. If the treatment field is close to a major blood vessel (i.e. carotid artery), a safety distance of 1 cm between the needle and the vessel is implemented to avoid causing damage to the vessel wall in case it contained tumour. A four-channel 652 nm diode laser is used for illumination. Bare polished tip laser light delivery fibres with a core diameter of 400 mm are introduced through the spinal needles into the suspect. The fibres are allowed to protrude by 2–3 mm from the needle tip into tissue to ensure maximal tissue illumination. Light is then delivered from the fibres at 20 J/cm^2 per site (200 s/treatment). Each bare tip fibre delivers an output power of about 0.5 W (Fig. 4) [1–12, 15, 18].

Histopathological specimens acquired from the previous studies in our centre showed that illumination from one bare tip fibre

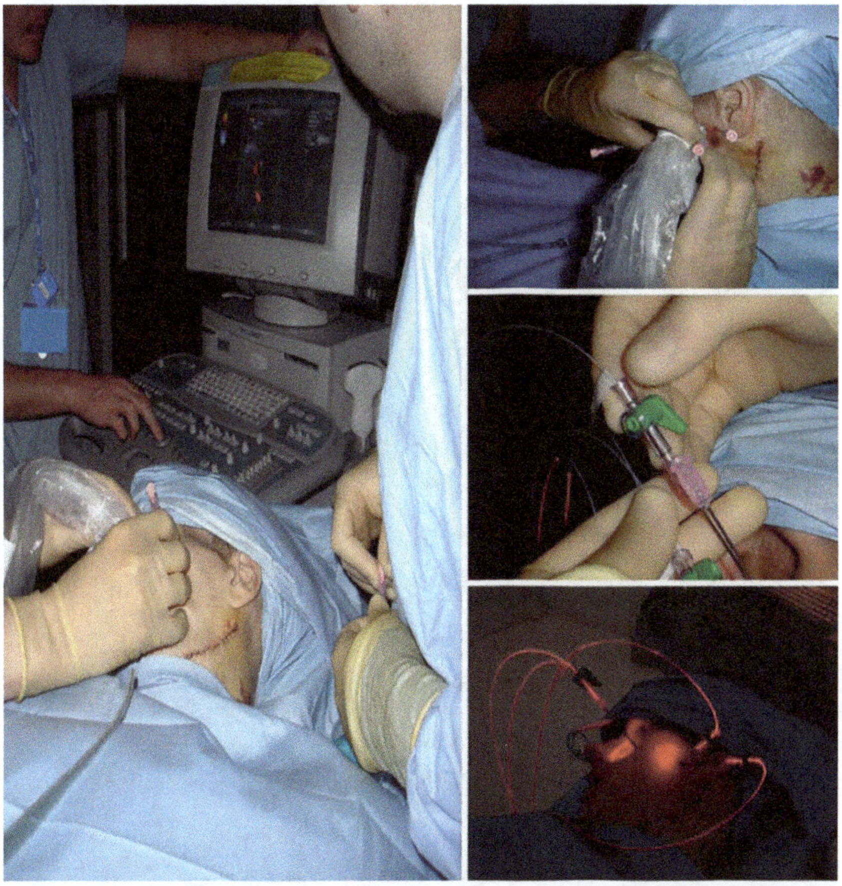

Fig. 4 Ultrasound-guided interstitial photodynamic therapy. Note needle insertion, optical fibres feeding into the needle, and tissue illumination. The figure is adapted from authors' own article: Jerjes W, Upile T, Vincent A, Abbas S, Shah P, Mosse CA, McCarthy E, El-Maaytah M, Topping W, Morley S, Hopper C. Management of deep-seated malformations with photodynamic therapy: a new guiding imaging modality. Lasers Med Sci. 2009 Sep;24(5):769–75

results in a 1 cm in diameter pathological tissue necrosis, when using mTHPC (meso-tetrahydroxyphenyl chlorin, Foscan). Hence, fibres are placed 1 cm away from each other to cover all the volume of the suspect area. Any residual pathological tissue in between the necrotic areas is also expected to die following oxygen deprivation. Overlapping treatment fields is clinically insignificant, as 200 s illumination of the area is adequate to activate the non-thermal photochemical process. Thick tumours are treated with 1 cm pull back at each time to ensure illumination of the whole tumour volume. Diffuser fibres are used when treating vascular tumours, together with the bare polished tip fibres. The structure of the vascular tumours allows maximal tissue illumination when using those types of fibres (Fig. 5) [1–12, 15, 18].

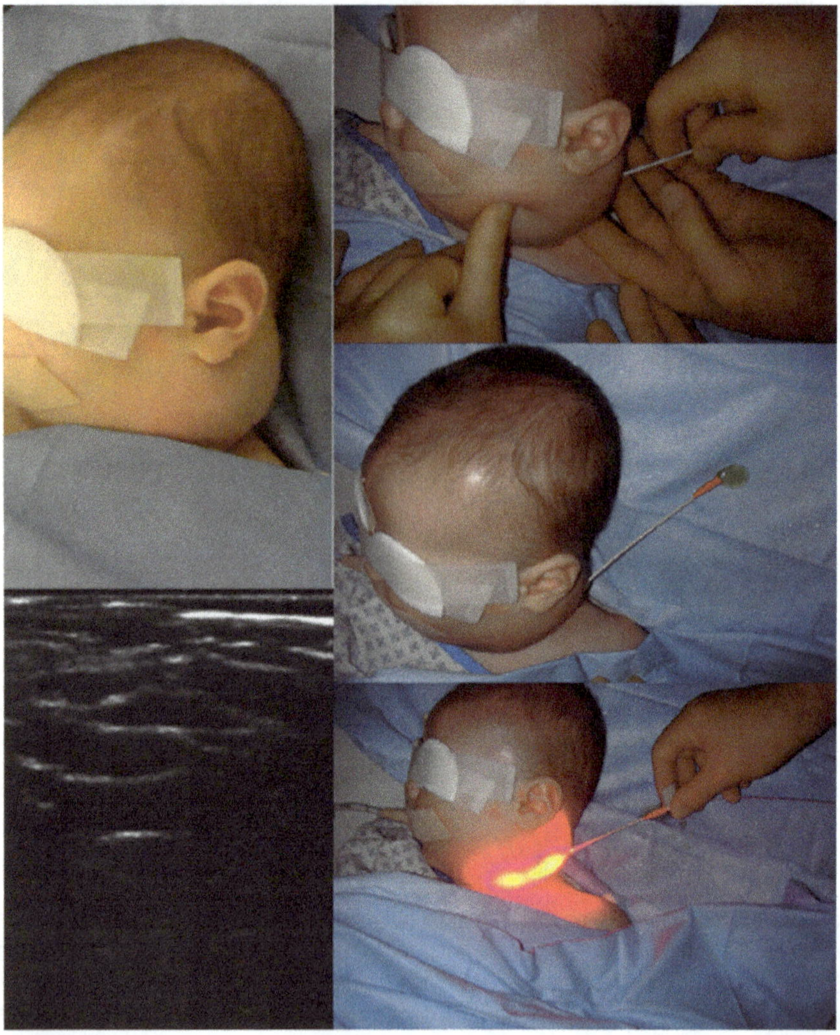

Fig. 5 *Top left*: clinical image showing the 5-month-old infant in surgical drapes prior to the minimally invasive procedure. The marked swelling of the *left* side of face and neck indicate the cystic hygroma. *Bottom left*: Intraoperative ultrasound image showing the cystic hygroma. Right side images: showing needle insertion under US-guidance, lymph fluid drainage and illumination of the cystic hygroma. The figure is adapted from authors' own article: Hamdoon Z, Jerjes W, Upile T, Akram S, Hopper C. Cystic hygroma treated with ultrasound-guided interstitial photodynamic therapy: case study. Photodiagnosis Photodyn Ther. 2010 Sep;7(3):179–82

Difficulties arise when the tumour metastasises via the lymphatic system. In this case it is not feasible to induce a therapeutic photochemical reaction in a whole area of the body (e.g. neck). Photochemical reaction can be induced in single or multiple lymph nodes under image guidance, but this is sometimes difficult to perform where there is a complex lymphatic chain as in the neck (Fig. 6). An iso-illumination treatment plan is carefully implemented and supervised by a senior physicist to ensure adequate

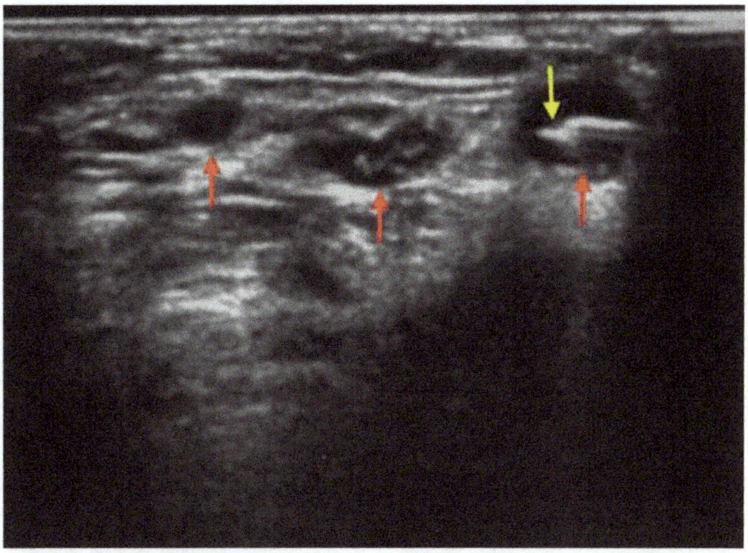

Fig. 6 Ultrasound image showing three level II metastatic cervical lymph nodes (*red arrows*). Note needle insertion in the node on the *right hand* side prior to PDT treatment (*yellow arrow*). The figure is adapted from authors' own article: Jerjes W, Upile T, Hamdoon Z, Nhembe F, Bhandari R, Mackay S, Shah P, Mosse CA, Brookes JA, Morley S, Hopper C. Ultrasound-guided photodynamic therapy for deep-seated pathologies: prospective study. Lasers Surg Med. 2009 Nov;41(9): 612–21

light delivery to all suspect areas with minimal overlapping between the fields of treatment using a grid system. No measurements are made with regard to the distribution of the light fluence rate, the optical properties, the drug concentration and the tissue oxygenation for PDT, as these factors had already been quantified in previous studies carried out in our centre [1–12, 15, 18].

The position of the pulse oximeter is changed every 30 min to avoid any skin burn or nail damage that would result from photochemical reaction by the red light (660 nm). Patients are discharged from hospital care 5–7 days postoperatively. Post-PDT, patients experience a considerable amount of pain in the treated area. The pain usually peaks at 48–72 h from illumination. Special PDT pain protocols are followed. The standard regimen involves a fentanyl transdermal patch 72HR 12 mg/h with morphine sulphate (immediate release) as needed for breakthrough pain. Dose escalating the patient's own pain medication or prescribing patient-controlled analgesics is implemented when indicated. Usually different specialist centres have different PDT pain control protocols depending on experience and the areas treated. Airway control is a priority, as compromise can occur as part of the local inflammatory reaction. Elective tracheostomy before interstitial PDT is implemented when managing advanced tumours in

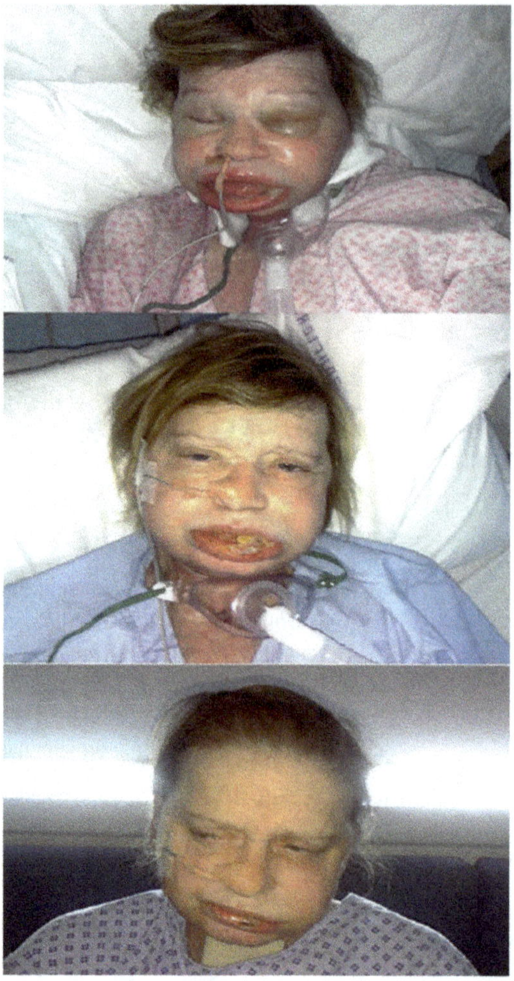

Fig. 7 Significant facial swelling after surface illumination PDT; day 2 (*top*), day 4 (*middle*) and day 6 (*bottom*). The figure is adapted from authors' own article: 12. Jerjes W, Upile T, Abbas S, Vincent A, Hopper C. The developing role of photodynamic therapy in multidisciplinary oncological care. Oncol News 2008;3(3): 12–15

the oropharyngeal/laryngeal region (Fig. 7). For example, a tracheostomy tube is inserted intra-operatively and kept for 3–5 days postoperatively; intravenous steroids are also given for 3 days to reduce local inflammatory responses [1–12, 15, 18].

A common finding is that adjacent macroscopically normal appearing tissue can become photosensitised and undergo necrosis or apoptosis, causing ulceration of the mucosa or skin. The best way of reducing these effects is by shielding macroscopically normal adjacent tissues. Healing usually occurs with little or no scarring and the procedure can be repeated with only a small amount of cumulative toxicity. There is sparing of tissue architecture, providing a matrix for regeneration of normal tissue [1–12, 15, 18].

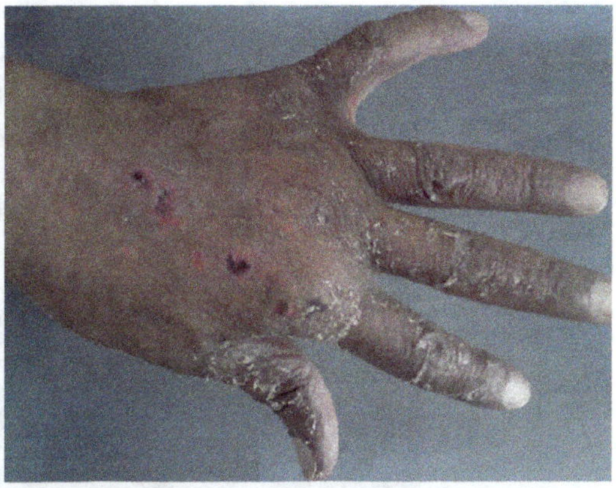

Fig. 8 Accidental sun exposure 2 weeks after photodynamic therapy led to skin burn of the dorsal hand associated with ulceration and peeling of the skin. The figure is adapted from authors' own article: Jerjes W, Upile T, Akram S, Hopper C. The surgical palliation of advanced head and neck cancer using photodynamic therapy. Clin Oncol (R Coll Radiol). 2010 Nov;22(9):785–91

Photosensitivity represents a problem as the skin continues to be sensitive to light for up to 8 weeks; sometimes for 13 weeks with some photosensitisers. Gradual light re-exposure at an incremental rate of 100 lux/day is implemented. Every patient is instructed on the need to avoid direct sun exposure for up to 2 weeks after injection and is given light exposure guidelines. Sometimes patients fail to achieve a gradual re-exposure to sunlight and as a result they develop skin burn, first or second degree, when they are exposed for the first time to direct sunlight after 3–4 weeks of treatment (Fig. 8). Also, the skin over the injection site (especially the arm area) is more sensitive to light, and skin burn has been reported to occur up to 10 weeks after the photosensitisation in this area [1–12, 15, 18].

Six weeks postoperatively, re-staging magnetic resonance imaging or computed tomography views, where appropriate, are acquired to assess outcome (Fig. 9). Patients are asked to report on the outcome of their therapy if there is any improvement, no change or worsening of symptoms by completing a special questionnaire developed for patients receiving PDT of the head and neck (modified from the University of Washington Quality of Life Questionnaire for head and neck cancer patients). A postoperative clinical assessment is reported by the treating clinician at the first post-PDT review (at 4–6 weeks). A postoperative radiological assessment is reported by the same interventional radiologist [1–12, 15, 18].

Many studies have shown that head and neck cancer responds favourably to PDT (Fig. 10). Advanced/recurrent tumours can also be treated with salvage/palliative therapy, with the aim of

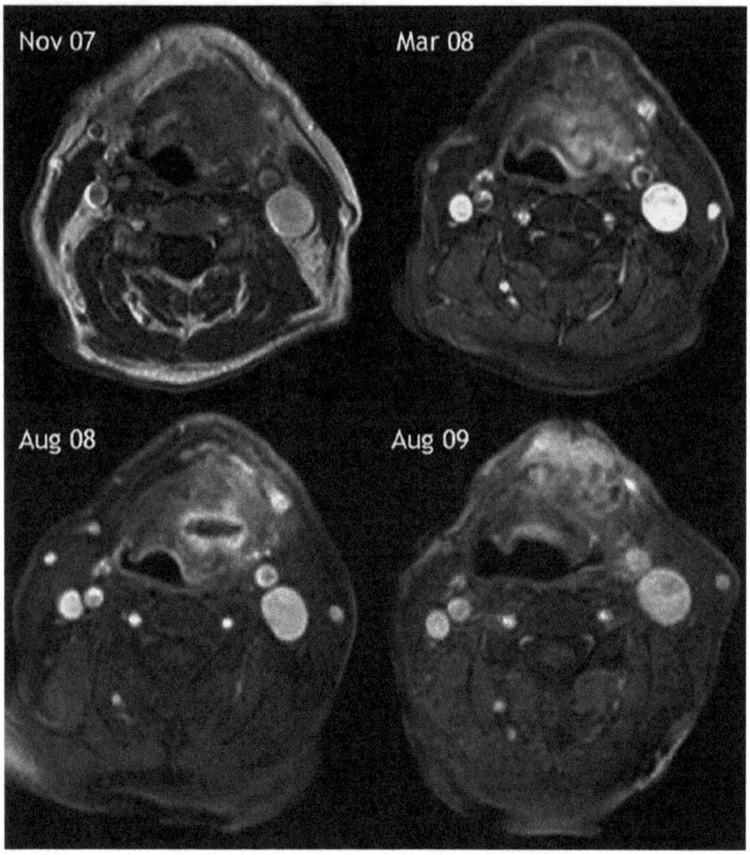

Fig. 9 *Top left* (Nov 07): pre-PDT noncontrast enhancing axial MRI showing extensive chondrosarcoma of the hyoid bone causing narrowing of the airway. *Top right* (Mar 08): 2 months post-first round of PDT contrast enhancing MRI showing extensive necrosis, tissue changes and peritumour inflammation. Bottom left (Aug 08): 7 months post-first round of PDT contrast enhancing MRI showing central necrotic area and architectural changes. The scan was acquired following an infection episode which was associated with pus discharge from the previously treated area. Bottom right (Aug 09): 8 months post-second round of PDT contrast enhancing MRI showing tumour shrinkage, tissue regeneration and improvement in airway. Residual tumour can be seen in the subcutaneous tissue but nowhere near the hyoid. The images are the best exact match that could be achieved. The figure is adapted from authors' own article: Nhembe F, Jerjes W, Upile T, Hamdoon Z, Hopper C. Chondrosarcoma of the hyoid treated with interstitial photodynamic therapy: case study. Photodiagnosis Photodyn Ther. 2009 Sep–Dec;6(3–4):235–7

reducing the tumour bulk to improve function and also to reduce bleeding and to control pain (Fig. 11). The only curative treatment option remains surgery, but this is frequently not feasible. Photodynamic therapy can achieve significant palliation in a minimally invasive fashion. Photodynamic therapy can now be very accurately directed by radiological imaging to document and

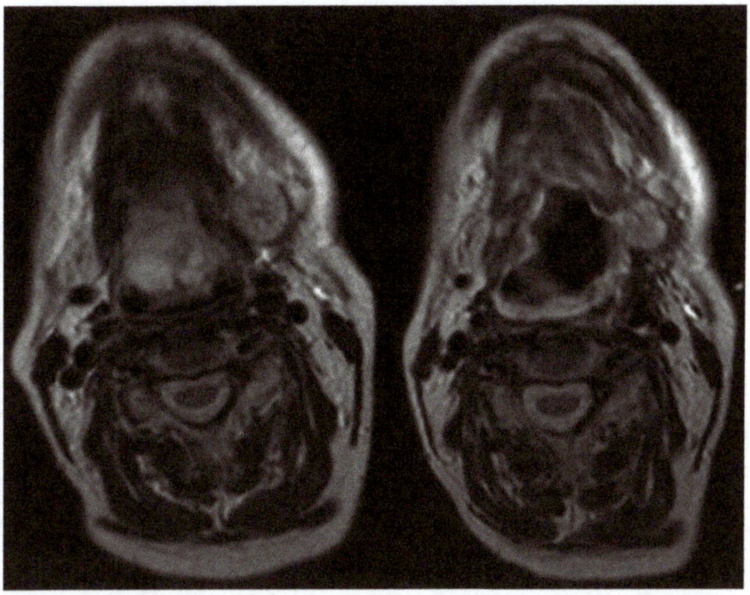

Fig. 10 Pre- and post-PDT MRI of tongue base adenoid cystic carcinoma. The patient showed radiological significant response. The figure is adapted from authors' own article: Jerjes W, Upile T, Hamdoon Z, Abbas S, Akram S, Mosse CA, Morley S, Hopper C. Photodynamic therapy: The minimally invasive surgical intervention for advanced and/or recurrent tongue base carcinoma. Lasers Surg Med. 2011 Apr;43(4):283–92

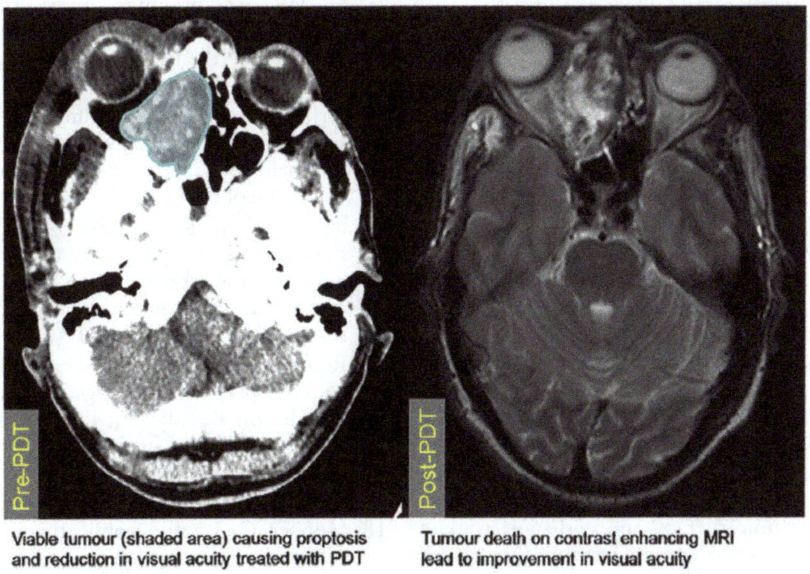

Fig. 11 **Pre-PDT** CT showing a soft tissue mass occupying the sinonasal area with retrobulbar extension causing proptosis and visual symptoms. Post-PDT MRI showing tumour shrinkage and death and reduction of retrobulbar tumour mass leading to improvement in visual symptoms. The figure is adapted from authors' own article: Hamdoon Z, Jerjes W, Upile T, Akram S, Hopper C. Metastatic renal cell carcinoma to the orofacial region: A novel method to alleviate symptoms and control disease progression. Photodiagnosis Photodyn Ther. 2010 Dec;7(4):246–50

optimise laser-guided photo-activation of the chemo-sensitiser. Rapid local tumour control often results, enabling the patient to benefit from both a higher quality and length of life [1–12, 15, 18].

References

1. Sharwani A, Jerjes W, Hopper C, Lewis MP, El-Maaytah M, Khalil HS, Macrobert AJ, Upile T, Salih V. Photodynamic therapy down-regulates the invasion promoting factors in human oral cancer. Arch Oral Biol. 2006;51(12):1104–11.
2. Jerjes W, Upile T, Betz CS, El Maaytah M, Abbas S, Wright A, Hopper C. The application of photodynamic therapy in the head and neck. Dent Update. 2007;34(8):478–80, 483–4, 486.
3. Jerjes W, Upile T, Hamdoon Z, Nhembe F, Bhandari R, Mackay S, Shah P, Mosse CA, Brookes JA, Morley S, Hopper C. Ultrasound-guided photodynamic therapy for deep seated pathologies: prospective study. Lasers Surg Med. 2009;41(9):612–21.
4. Jerjes W, Upile T, Petrie A, Riskalla A, Hamdoon Z, Vourvachis M, Karavidas K, Jay A, Sandison A, Thomas GJ, Kalavrezos N, Hopper C. Clinicopathological parameters, recurrence, locoregional and distant metastasis in 115 T1-T2 oral squamous cell carcinoma patients. Head Neck Oncol. 2010;2:9.
5. Jerjes W, Upile T, Akram S, Hopper C. The surgical palliation of advanced head and neck cancer using photodynamic therapy. Clin Oncol (R Coll Radiol). 2010;22(9):785–91.
6. Jerjes W, Upile T, Hamdoon Z, Abbas S, Akram S, Mosse CA, Morley S, Hopper C. Photodynamic therapy: the minimally invasive surgical intervention for advanced and/or recurrent tongue base carcinoma. Lasers Surg Med. 2011;43(4):283–92.
7. Jerjes W, Upile T, Alexander Mosse C, Hamdoon Z, Morcos M, Morley S, Hopper C. Prospective evaluation of 110 patients following ultrasound-guided photodynamic therapy for deep seated pathologies. Photodiagnosis Photodyn Ther. 2011;8(4):297–306.
8. Jerjes W, Upile T, Radhi H, Hopper C. Photodynamic therapy and end-stage tongue base cancer: short communication. Head Neck Oncol. 2011;3:49.
9. Jerjes W, Hamdoon Z, Hopper C. Photodynamic therapy in the management of potentially malignant and malignant oral disorders. Head Neck Oncol. 2012;4:16.
10. Abbas S, Jerjes W, Upile T, Vaz F, Hopper C. The palliative role of PDT in recurrent advanced nasopharyngeal carcinoma: case series. Photodiagnosis Photodyn Ther. 2012;9(2):142–7.
11. Jerjes W, Upile T, Abbas S, Hopper C. Photodynamic therapy role in the premalignancy/malignancy of the head and neck. Oncol News. 2008;2(5):8–10.
12. Jerjes W, Upile T, Abbas S, Vincent A, Hopper C. The developing role of photodynamic therapy in multidisciplinary oncological care. Oncol News. 2008;3(3):12–5.
13. Lou PJ, Jäger HR, Jones L, Theodossy T, Bown SG, Hopper C. Interstitial photodynamic therapy as salvage treatment for recurrent head and neck cancer. Br J Cancer. 2004;91(3):441–6.
14. Jäger HR, Taylor MN, Theodossy T, Hopper C. MR imaging-guided interstitial photodynamic laser therapy for advanced head and neck tumors. AJNR Am J Neuroradiol. 2005;26(5):1193–200.
15. Jerjes W, Upile T, Radhi H, Hopper C. Photodynamic therapy vs. photochemical internalization: the surgical margin. Head Neck Oncol. 2011;3:53.
16. de Visscher SA, Dijkstra PU, Tan IB, Roodenburg JL, Witjes MJ. mTHPC mediated photodynamic therapy (PDT) of squamous cell carcinoma in the head and neck: a systematic review. Oral Oncol. 2013;49(3):192–210.
17. Rigual NR, Shafirstein G, Frustino J, Seshadri M, Cooper M, Wilding G, Sullivan MA, Henderson B. Adjuvant intraoperative photodynamic therapy in head and neck cancer. JAMA Otolaryngol Head Neck Surg. 2013;139(7):706–11.
18. Hopper C. Photodynamic therapy: a clinical reality in the treatment of cancer. Lancet Oncol. 2000;1:212–9.

Chapter 25

Photodynamic Therapy of Malignancies of the Nasopharynx, the Nasal Cavity, and the Paranasal Sinuses

M. Barış Karakullukcu

PDT of the Nasopharyngeal Carcinoma

Nasopharyngeal carcinoma (NPC) is endemic in certain parts of South East Asia and to a lesser degree in the Mediterranean basin [1]. Treatment for primary NPC is radiotherapy (RT) with or without chemotherapy depending on the stage. NPC, especially if Epstein–Barr Virus (EBV) related is very responsive to RT [2–8]. However, there is still 20–30 % risk of local recurrence [2–8]. Usual treatment options for early stage recurrent or persistent NPC are brachytherapy, external re-radiation therapy, stereotactic radiosurgery, and salvage nasopharyngectomy [8–22]. Despite promising responses, re-RT causes a high incidence of major late complications, such as brain necrosis, cranial nerve palsies, and catastrophic hemorrhages [8–19]. The newer RT strategies such as stereotactic radiation and IMRT have decreased complication rate. However, the indication for re-RT is limited by the cumulative dose and the interval between the initial RT and the recurrence. In persistent disease, since the time elapsed after primary RT is minimal, there is no role for re-RT. Photodynamic therapy (PDT) can be a useful treatment tool in treating locally persistent/recurrent NPC.

PDT has been studied in the past to treat locally recurrent/persistent NPC [23–27]. Sun et al. [23] reported hematoporphyrin derivative (HpD) mediated PDT of 137 patients with recurrent or residual NPC. He reported complete response in 55 % of the patients. Other centers reported smaller series of HpD mediated

Brian J.-F. Wong and Justus Ilgner (eds.), *Biomedical Optics in Otorhinolaryngology: Head and Neck Surgery*, DOI 10.1007/978-1-4939-1758-7_25, © Springer Science+Business Media New York 2016

PDT of NPC with similar results [24–26]. Our group performed a feasibility study in Indonesia with temoporfin (mTHPC) mediated PDT of recurrent and persistent NPC [27]. Temoporfin has a longer activation wavelength than HpD and therefore a deeper treatment effect. Twenty-two patients were treated in three different combinations of photosensitizer dose and drug light intervals. The combination of temoporfin 0.15 mg/kg and 96 h of drug light interval provided better overall survival than other regimens tested. Ten of 22 patients treated in this trial were alive at the time of publication, with a mean follow-up of 58 months. Recently, Succo et al. published promising results with temoporfin mediated PDT of recurrent/persistent NPC [28].

Multidiscipline Involvement and Informed Consent

A thorough evaluation of the patient is essential. NPC is a tumor that metastasizes readily and not only to neck nodes but also to retropharyngeal lymph nodes. Since PDT is a local treatment regional and distant metastasis should be ruled out by using imaging techniques such as positron emission tomography (PET) and ultrasound (US) combined with fine needle aspiration cytology (FNAC). The local spread of the disease can best be appreciated by magnetic resonance imaging (MRI). The depth of infiltration of the tumor is very important to determine the PDT method to be used. Computed tomography (CT) gives valuable information about bony structures of the skull base. CT is useful if intraoperative navigation devices are to be used.

Once the recurrent/persistent tumor is adequately evaluated, treatment options should be considered at a multidisciplinary tumor board. Small tumors can be candidates for surgical removal, either with an open or endoscopic approach. Re-RT can be considered for recurrent tumors. The potential complications should be carefully evaluated by the radiotherapist. PDT is a viable option for local persistent/recurrent NPC. The depth of infiltration should be carefully evaluated to determine if intracavitary light delivery is sufficient or light sources should be implanted in the tissues. MRI, CT, and PET-CT are tools that can be used to evaluate the spread of the tumor. In some cases, PDT can be given to provide palliation. We have reported a case of recurrent T4N0M0 NPC with intracranial extension, treated with PDT [29]. The patient had diplopia before the treatment which resolved after PDT.

Once the candidacy is established, the possible complications of PDT should be discussed with the patient. The most common adverse events are headache and otitis media [27]. Although not observed before potentially PDT of the nasopharynx can cause damage to prevertebral muscles. Tumors with intracranial extensions were treated and no cerebrospinal fluid leak or meningitis was observed [27].

Additionally, the patient should receive adequate counseling over light sensitivity. At our institute a dedicated nurse practitioner is responsible for counseling the patients. The period of photosensitivity is dependent on the photosensitizer and can range from a few hours to 6 weeks. Temoporfin causes a photosensitivity of 2–3 weeks. Patients should be provided with printed light avoidance guidelines and a light meter to measure ambient light in the living quarters. Every day, the patient can be exposed to more light according to the guidelines provided to the patient.

Treatment Technique The extent of the tumor determines the treatment technique. Tumors that are thinner than 5–10 mm can be treated with intracavitary illumination (Fig. 1). This means that the light source can be placed in the nasopharynx and the whole nasopharynx cavity can be illuminated. Tumors extending deeper can be treated by implanting light sources in the tissues [interstitial PDT (iPDT)]. Many times a combination of two techniques is necessary.

The PS Photodynamic therapy (PDT) NPC PS is administered at a certain time before the procedure, depending on the optimal drug light interval of the type of PS used. In case of temoporfin this drug light interval is 4 days.

Our group has developed an applicator for PDT of the nasopharynx. The applicator is based on a brachytherapy applicator and adapted to provide equal distribution of light in the nasopharynx [30]. The applicator has a black silicone flange that protects

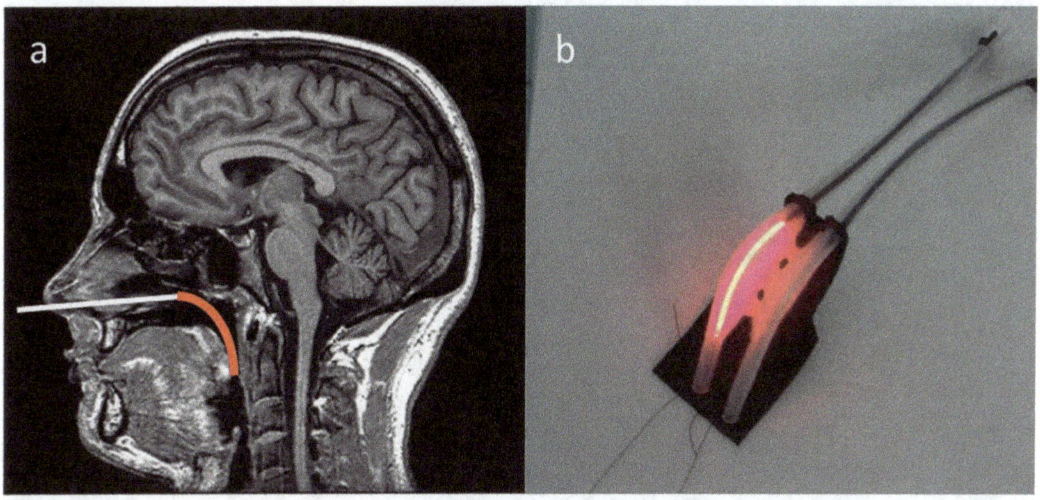

Fig. 1 The PDT of the nasopharynx is carried out by placing linear diffusers in the nasopharynx (**a**). The whole cavity is treated. The applicator can be seen on the *right* (**b**). The *black* silicone flange protects the soft palate. Two treatment channels can be used to introduce linear diffusers in the nasopharynx

the posterior surface of the soft palate (Fig. 1). This applicator can be placed under local anesthesia in the form of xylocaine spray. Two suction catheters are introduced nasally and recovered from the mouth. The applicator is attached to the catheters and gently pulled via the oral cavity into the nasopharynx. Two linear diffusers are introduced to the channels of the applicator. Black shielding tubes are introduced over the light diffusers to adapt the effective length of the diffusers and protect the nasal cavity from PDT. The light delivery is tolerated by the patients and takes two times 200 s. We prefer to give a fluence of 20 J/cm diffuser length at a fluence rate of 100 mW/cm. The applicator can be removed after light delivery.

NPC has the tendency to grow deep along the Eustachian tubes. Linear diffusers can be introduced to Eustachian tubes under endoscope guidance and light can be delivered (Fig. 2). Any other deep extension of the tumor can be accessed by using clear silicone sharp-pointed brachytherapy catheters. Intraoperative navigation devices are very useful in determining the placement of these catheters. Linear diffusers or bulb fibers can be introduced into the brachytherapy catheters to perform iPDT. iPDT should preferably be performed under general anesthesia, as it involves endoscopic manipulation of the nasopharynx.

Postprocedure Course Patients can be discharged the same day after PDT. Light precautions should strictly be followed by the patients. The postprocedure period is marked by headache radiat-

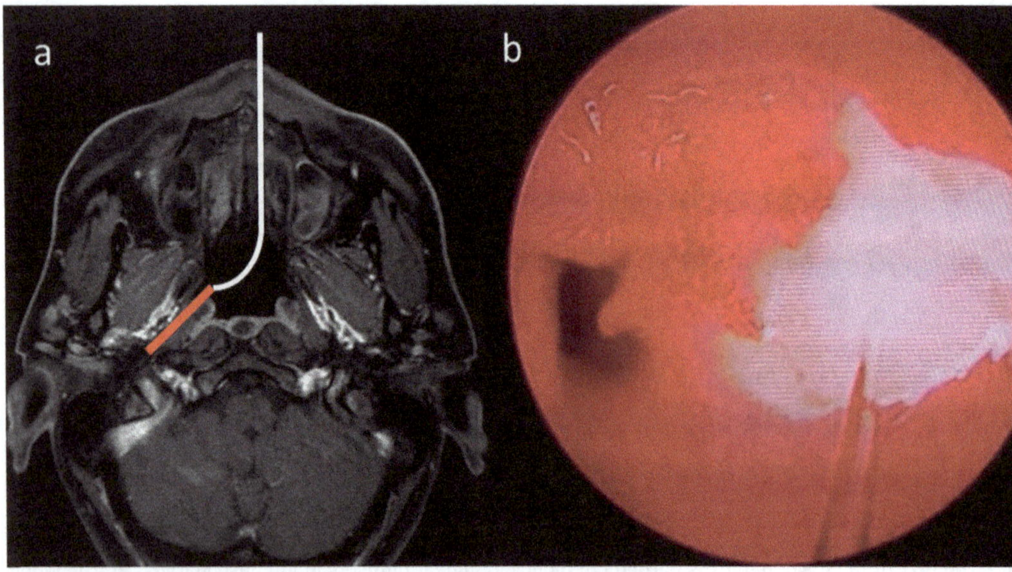

Fig. 2 Linear diffusers can be introduced in the Eustachian tubes, which is a common way nasopharynx cancer spreads. On the *left* the approach route can be seen (**a**). On the *right* is the endoscopic view of the nasopharynx during the light delivery to the *left* Eustachian tube (**b**)

ing to the neck in about half of the patients. Systemic corticosteroids and opioids are used to control the pain and edema. Patients are called by the dedicated nurse practitioner weekly. On week 3 the patient comes to outpatient clinic for debridement.

Photodynamic Therapy of Nasal Cavity and Paranasal Sinuses

The term "cancer of the nasal cavity (NC) and the paranasal sinuses (PNS)" or sinonasal cancers includes a variety of tumors with very different biological characteristics and variable prognosis. While squamous cell carcinoma can progress rapidly, adenoid cystic carcinoma can stay indolent for years. These tumors are quiet rare [31] and therefore are frequently pooled together when reporting treatment results. Depending on the histopathology of the tumor, combinations of surgery, radiotherapy (RT), and chemotherapy are the established treatment modalities. The mainstay treatment is radical surgery combined with radiation therapy [32–37]. However, radical surgery and high dose radiotherapy are challenging because of the proximity of important structures, such as the skull base, orbits, and internal carotid arteries [36]. Despite the advancement in diagnostic techniques and treatment modalities, the tumor will recur in 50–60 % of patients with locally advanced disease and long-term survival rates are disappointing [32, 33, 35, 37]. When these tumors recur, curative options are limited. Salvage surgery is the conventional treatment, but not always possible because of the risk of severe postoperative dysfunction and a high risk of leaving residual tumor behind [38]. Chemotherapy can be an option as a palliation [39]. Re-RT in the form of brachytherapy, intensity modulated radiation therapy (IMRT), cyber-knife radiation, and proton beam radiotherapy are reported with some success but also with serious adverse events such as osteonecrosis, cataract, visual acuity impairment, brain edema, and brain abscess [38, 40–47].

The main limitation of salvage surgery of the sinonasal tumors is achieving adequate surgical margins. The combination of photodynamic therapy (PDT) and surgery can provide additional treatment margins where surgery cannot be performed [48].

Multidiscipline Involvement and Informed Consent

At our institution, our multidisciplinary board considers combination of maximal surgery and adjuvant photodynamic therapy as a treatment option in cases of recurrent sinonasal tumors. The first option is always radical salvage surgery. If radical surgery is not possible, re-RT is considered. Very frequently re-RT is not possible because of cumulative toxicity to important structures in the vicinity. For such recurrent tumors we try to use maximal resection, with preservation of important structures and PDT. Even if in the presence of limited distant metastasis the combination treatment can be considered to control local disease and prevent progression of the tumor to adjacent structures.

There is no published data on the application of PDT at this location. In our experience temoporfin (mTHPC) mediated PDT can be safely used even for tumors extending intracranially (data submitted for publication). However, due to the absence of extensive experience, PDT of the sinonasal tumors should be considered as experimental and the patients have to be informed about possible catastrophic adverse events such as cerebrospinal fluid (CSF) leak, meningitis, and bleeding. Our unpublished data of 12 patients demonstrate long-term local disease control in about half of the patients. The concept has to be tested more to report over clinical success.

Treatment Technique The workup in our institute includes a magnetic resonance imaging (MRI) and a computed tomography (CT) of the NC and PNS and positron emission tomography (PET-CT) to rule out distant metastasis. MRI gives very clear images of extension of the tumor and helps us determine the treatment strategy. The treatment strategy involves maximal removal of the tumor. Maximal removal can mean removing all macroscopic tumors, but it can also mean removing the tumor where possible and leaving thin tumor tissue behind where resection is technically not possible or there is danger of damaging an important structure. From other treatment sites, we know that the treatment depth of temoporfin mediated PDT is 8–10 mm [49]. Therefore, it is strongly desirable not to leave tumor tissue thicker than 8–10 mm. The surgical resection should facilitate PDT by removing the structures that might impair light distribution. We have found it useful to open all sinuses, remove the turbinates, possibly the nasal septum, and create large cavities. Depending on the location of the tumor the resection can be carried out endoscopically or by open procedures such as transoral maxillectomy.

It is logistically better to stage the treatment into surgical resection and PDT 2–3 weeks later. There are several reasons for this suggestion. If the photosensitizer (PS) is administered before the operation, the patient would be light sensitive during the operation. The lights of the endoscope or operation room lights would activate the PS causing uncontrolled PDT effect. The second reason is: hemoglobin absorbs light very close to the wavelength that is used to activate the PS. If there is bleeding during PDT, the blood will act as a filter against treatment light and limit activation of the PS in the targeted tissues. The 2–3 week interval allows adequate hemostasis and with rigorous nasal showers the crusts in the nasal cavity can be removed.

The PS is administered a certain time before the procedure, depending on the optimal drug light interval of the type of PS used. In case of temoporfin this drug light interval is 4 days.

The preferred light delivery method depends on the targeted area. If the sphenoid sinus or back wall of the maxillary sinuses are targeted a microlens diffuser emitting a circular spot of light can be used. The spot can be observed if the light of the endoscope is turned off (Fig. 3). The microlens diffuser provides a relatively uniform distribution of treatment light.

If direct approach is not possible like the anterior portions of the ethmoid cavity or frontal sinuses linear diffusers emitting light along a length of the fiber can be used. Figure 4 demonstrates the use of a linear diffuser combined with a saline filled spacer to treat

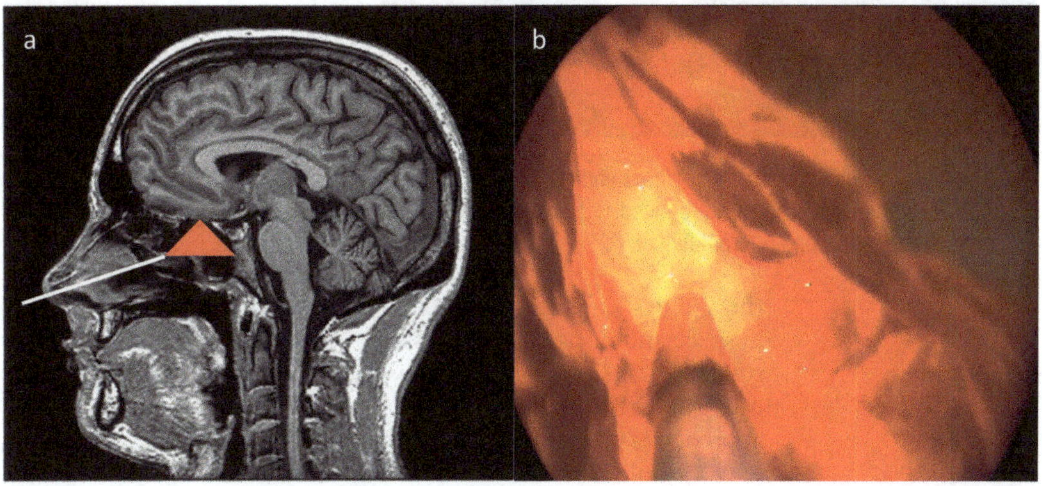

Fig. 3 PDT of the back wall of the sinonasal cavity can be carried out using a microlens diffuser. On the *left* the approach route to the back wall of the sinonasal cavity is represented (**a**). On the *right* the spot of treatment light can be observed through the endoscope (**b**)

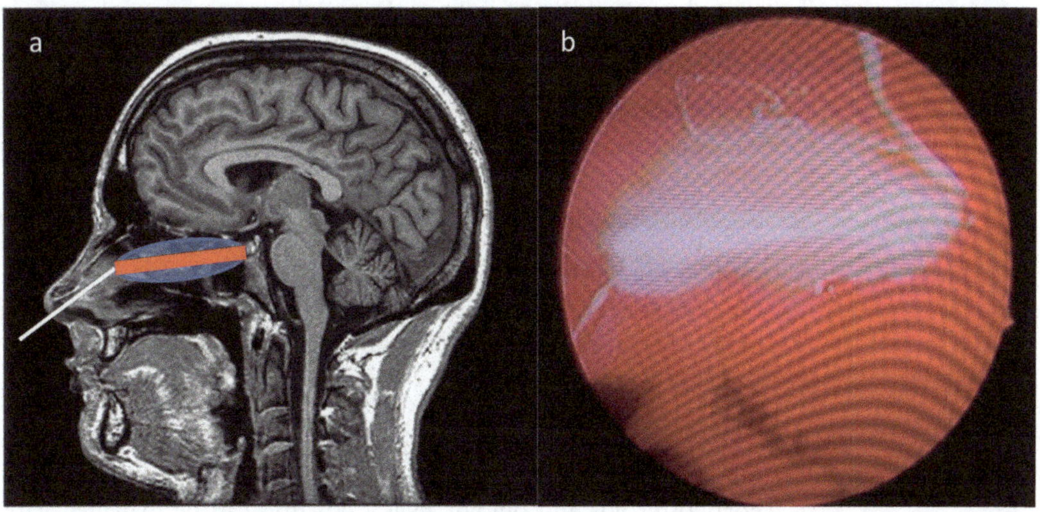

Fig. 4 The whole length of the anterior skull base can be illuminated by introducing spacers filled with saline and linear diffusers. On the *left* is a schematic representation of the approach route (**a**). On the *right* is the endoscopic view of such a treatment (**b**)

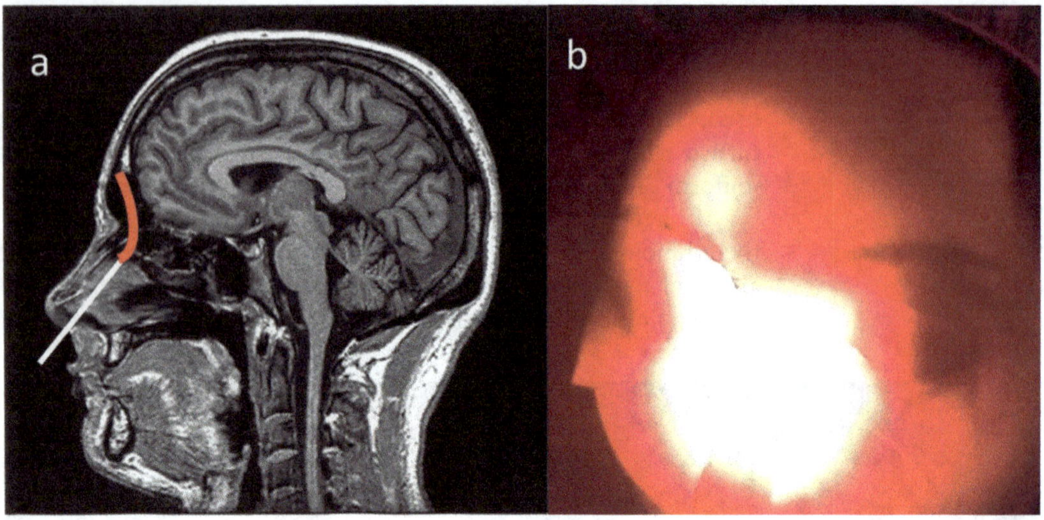

Fig. 5 The frontal sinus can be approached endoscopically or by open approach. Once the natural ostium is enlarged linear diffusers can be introduced in to the frontal sinus (**a**). The illumination of the sinus can be observed through the skin and frontal bone (**b**)

the anterior skull base. The spacer provides that the diffuser is fixed in space and not against the tissues. Figure 5 demonstrates PDT of right frontal sinus. Frontal sinuses can be approached endoscopically or externally through a fenestration approach. If a fenestration approach is preferred the spacer can be fixed during the operation, which would facilitate the PDT stage of the treatment.

Although PDT of the sinonasal tumors can be carried out under topical anesthesia, general anesthesia is usually necessary. We prefer to apply 20 J/cm^2, at a fluence rate of 100 mW/cm^2. Naturally, the presence of scattering from bony structures and, therefore, buildup of light and optical properties of the target tissues cause variability in the delivered light dose.

Postprocedure Course Even though PDT was applied to the skull base and in some cases to tumors extending intracranial, none of the patients treated developed cerebrospinal fluid (CSF) leakage or short-term meningitis. There were no cases of major bleeding even though the internal carotid artery was exposed in the sphenoid sinus in two patients. The most common adverse event is temporary diplopia due to edema of the orbital medial rectus muscle. The diplopia can be managed by administering systemic corticosteroids. PDT causes necrosis of the treated tissues which might require debridement.

All patients experienced facial edema and pain of different degrees until 4–6 weeks after PDT, which was controllable by corticosteroids and opioids. Nasal crusting can be managed with frequent nasal rinsing and cleaning at the office. The patients will experience an unpleasant odor due to the necrosis.

References

1. Yu MC, Yuan JM. Epidemiology of nasopharyngeal carcinoma. Semin Cancer Biol. 2002; 12:421–9.
2. Wei WI, Sham JST. Nasopharyngeal carcinoma. Lancet. 2005;365:2041–54.
3. Lin JC, Jan JS. Locally advanced nasopharyngeal cancer: long-term outcomes of radiation therapy. Radiology. 1999;211(2):513–8.
4. Al Sarraf M, LeBlanc M, Giri PG, Fu KK, Cooper J, Vuong T, Forastiere AA, Adams G, Sakr WA, Schuller DE, et al. Chemoradiotherapy versus radiotherapy in patients with advanced nasopharyngeal cancer: phase III randomized Intergroup study 0099. J Clin Oncol. 1998;16:1310–7.
5. Wee J, Tan EH, Tai BC, Wong HB, Leong SS, Tan T, Chua ET, Yang E, Lee KM, Fong KW, et al. Randomized trial of radiotherapy versus concurrent chemoradiotherapy followed by adjuvant chemotherapy in patients with American Joint Committee on Cancer/ International Union against cancer stage III and IV nasopharyngeal cancer of the endemic variety. J Clin Oncol. 2005;23:6730–8.
6. Leung TW, Wong VY, Sze WK, Lui CM, Tung SY. High-dose-rate intracavitary brachytherapy boost for early T stage nasopharyngeal carcinoma{private}. Int J Radiat Oncol Biol Phys. 2008;70:361–7.
7. Palazzi M, Orlandi E, Bossi P, Pignoli E, Potepan P, Guzzo M, Franceschini M, Scaramellini G, Cantu G, Licitra L, et al. Further improvement in outcomes of nasopharyngeal carcinoma with optimized radiotherapy and induction plus concomitant chemotherapy: an update of the Milan experience. Int J Radiat Oncol Biol Phys. 2009;74:774–80.
8. Zhang L, Zhao C, Ghimire B, Hong MH, Liu Q, Zhang Y, Guo Y, Huang YJ, Guan ZZ. The role of concurrent chemoradiotherapy in the treatment of locoregionally advanced nasopharyngeal carcinoma among endemic population: a meta-analysis of the phase III randomized trials. BMC Cancer. 2010;10:558.
9. Chang JTC, See LC, Liao CT, Ng SH, Wang CH, Chen IH, Tsang NM, Tseng CK, Tang SG, Hong JH. Locally recurrent nasopharyngeal carcinoma. Radiother Oncol. 2000;54:135–42.
10. Suarez C, Rodrigo JP, Rinaldo A, Langendijk JA, Shaha AR, Ferlito A. Current treatment options for recurrent nasopharyngeal cancer. Eur Arch Otorhinolaryngol. 2010;267:1811–24.
11. Lee AW, Law SC, Foo W, Poon YF, Cheung FK, Chan DK, Tung SY, Thaw M, Ho JH. Retrospective analysis of patients with nasopharyngeal carcinoma treated during 1976–1985: survival after local recurrence. Int J Radiat Oncol Biol Phys. 1993;26:773–82.
12. Law SC, Lam WK, Ng MF, Au SK, Mak WT, Lau WH. Reirradiation of nasopharyngeal carcinoma with intracavitary mold brachytherapy: an effective means of local salvage. Int J Radiat Oncol Biol Phys. 2002;54:1095–113.
13. Kwong DL, Wei WI, Cheng AC, Choy DT, Lo AT, Wu PM, Sham JS. Long term results of radioactive gold grain implantation for the treatment of persistent and recurrent nasopharyngeal carcinoma. Cancer. 2001;91:1105–13.
14. Leung TW, Tung SY, Sze WK, Sze WM, Wong VY, Wong CS, O SK. Salvage radiation therapy for locally recurrent nasopharyngeal carcinoma. Int J Radiat Oncol Biol Phys. 2000;48:1331–8.
15. Leung TW, Tung SY, Sze WK, Sze WM, Wong VY, O SK. Salvage brachytherapy for patients with locally persistent nasopharyngeal carcinoma. Int J Radiat Oncol Biol Phys. 2000; 47:405–12.
16. Teo PM, Kwan WH, Chan AT, Lee WY, King WW, Mok CO. How successful is high-dose (> or = 60 Gy) reirradiation using mainly external beams in salvaging local failures of nasopharyngeal carcinoma? Int J Radiat Oncol Biol Phys. 1998;40:897–913.
17. Lee AW, Foo W, Law SC, Poon YF, Sze WM, O SK, Tung SY, Chappell R, Lau WH, Ho JH. Recurrent nasopharyngeal carcinoma: the puzzles of long latency. Int J Radiat Oncol Biol Phys. 1999;44:149–56.
18. Hwang JM, Fu KK, Phillips TL. Results and prognostic factors in the retreatment of locally recurrent nasopharyngeal carcinoma. Int J Radiat Oncol Biol Phys. 1998;41:1099–111.
19. Chua DT, Sham JS, Kwong PW, Hung KN, Leung LH. Linear accelerator-based stereotactic radiosurgery for limited, locally persistent, and recurrent nasopharyngeal carcinoma: efficacy and complications. Int J Radiat Oncol Biol Phys. 2003;56:177–83.
20. Stoker SD, van Diessen JN, de Boer JP, Karakullukcu B, Leemans CR, Tan IB. Current treatment options for local residual nasopharyngeal carcinoma. Curr Treat Options Oncol. 2013;14(4):475–91.
21. Chen MK, Lai JC, Chang CC, Liu MT. Minimally invasive endoscopic nasopharyngectomy in the treatment of recurrent T1-2a nasopharyngeal carcinoma. Laryngoscope. 2007;117:894–6.
22. Wei WI, Chan JY, Ng RW, Ho WK. Surgical salvage of persistent or recurrent nasopharyngeal

carcinoma with maxillary swing approach—critical appraisal after 2 decades. Head Neck. 2011;33(7):969–75.

23. Sun ZQ. Photodynamic therapy of nasopharyngeal carcinoma by argon or dye laser—an analysis of 137 cases. Zhonghua Zhong Liu Za Zhi. 1992;14:290–2.
24. Kulapaditharom B, Boonkitticharoen V. Photodynamic therapy in management of head and neck cancers and precancerous lesions. J Med Assoc Thai. 2000;83:249–58.
25. Tong MC, van Hasselt CA, Woo JK. Preliminary results of photodynamic therapy for recurrent nasopharyngeal carcinoma. Eur Arch Otorhinolaryngol. 1996;253:189–92.
26. Lofgren LA, Hallgren S, Nilsson E, Westerborn A, Nilsson C, Reizenstein J. Photodynamic therapy for recurrent nasopharyngeal cancer. Arch Otolaryngol Head Neck Surg. 1995; 121:997–1002.
27. Nyst HJ, Wildeman MA, Indrasari SR, Karakullukcu B, van Veen RL, Adham M, Stewart FA, Levendag PC, Sterenborg HJ, Tan IB. Temoporfin mediated photodynamic therapy in patients with local persistent and recurrent nasopharyngeal carcinoma after curative radiotherapy: a feasibility study. Photodiagnosis Photodyn Ther. 2012;9(3):274–81.
28. Succo G, Rosso S, Fadda GL, Fantini M, Crosetti E. Salvage photodynamic therapy for recurrent nasopharyngeal carcinoma. Photodiagnosis Photodyn Ther. 2014;11(2):63–70.
29. Indrasari SR, Timmermans AJ, Wildeman MA, Karakullukcu MB, Herdini C, Hariwiyanto B, Tan IB. Remarkable response to photodynamic therapy in residual T4N0M0 nasopharyngeal carcinoma: a case report. Photodiagnosis Photodyn Ther. 2012;9(4):319–20.
30. Nyst HJ, van Veen RL, Tan IB, Peters R, Spaniol S, Robinson DJ, Stewart FA, Levendag PC, Sterenborg HJ. Performance of a dedicated light delivery and dosimetry device for photodynamic therapy of nasopharyngeal carcinoma: phantom and volunteer experiments. Lasers Surg Med. 2007;39(8):647–53.
31. Jemal A, Thomas A, Murray T, Thun M. Cancer statistics. CA Cancer J Clin. 2002; 52:23–47.
32. Boyle JO, Shah KC, Shah JP. Craniofacial resection for malignant neoplasms of the skull base: an overview. J Surg Oncol. 1998;69:275–84.
33. Ganly I, Patel SG, et al. Craniofacial resection for malignant paranasal sinus tumors: report of an international collaborative study. Head Neck. 2005;27(7):575–84.
34. Woertgen C, Rothoerl RD, Hosemann W, Strutz J. Quality of life following surgery for malignancies of anterior skull base. Skull Base. 2007;17(2):119–23.
35. Castelnuovo PG, Belli E, Bignami M, Battaglia P, Sberze F, Tomei G. Endoscopic nasal and anterior craniotomy resection for malignant nasoethmoid tumors involving the anterior skull base. Skull Base. 2006;16(1):15–8.
36. Jansen EP, Keus RB, Hilgers FJ, Haas RL, Tan IB, Bartelink H. Does the combination of radiotherapy and debulking surgery favor survival in paranasal sinus carcinoma? Int J Radiat Oncol Biol Phys. 2000;48(1):27–35.
37. Hoppe BS, Stegman LD, Zelefsky MJ, et al. Treatment of nasal cavity and paranasal sinus cancer with modern radiotherapy techniques in the postoperative setting—the MSKCC experience. Int J Radiat Oncol Biol Phys. 2007;67:691–702.
38. Iwata H, Tatewaki K, Inoue M, Yokota N, Sato K, Shibamato Y. Salvage stereotactic reirradiation using the Cyberknife for the local recurrence of nasal or paranasal carcinoma. Radiother Oncol. 2012;104(3):355–60.
39. Wong SJ, Machtay M, Li Y. Locally recurrent, previously irradiated head and neck cancer: concurrent re-irradiation and chemotherapy, or chemotherapy alone? J Clin Oncol. 2006;24:2653–8.
40. Hoebers F, Heemsbergen W, Moor S, et al. Reirradiation for head and neck cancer: delicate balance between effectiveness and toxicity. Int J Radiat Oncol Biol Phys. 2011;81:e111–8.
41. Lee N, Chan K, Bekelman JE, Zhung J, Mechalakos J, Narayana A, Wolden S, Venkatraman ES, Pfister D, Kraus D, Shah J, Zelefsky MJ. Salvage reirradiation for recurrent head and neck cancer. Int J Radiat Oncol Biol Phys. 2007;68(3):731–40.
42. Strege RJ, Kovacs G, Maune S, Holland D, Niehoff P, Eichmann T, Mehdorn HM. Feasibility of combined operation and perioperative intensity—modulated brachytherapy of advanced/recurrent malignancies involving the skull base. Strahlenther Onkol. 2005; 181:97–107.
43. Tortochaux J, Tao Y, Tournay E, Lapeyre M, Lesaunier F, Bardet E, Janot F, Lusinchi A, Benhemou E, Bontemps P, Maignon P, Calais G, Daly-Schveitzer N, Verrelle P, Bourhis J. Randomized phase III trial (GORTEC 98-03) comparing re-irradiation plus chemotherapy versus methotrexate in patients with recurrent or a second primary head and neck squamous cell carcinoma, treated with a palliative intent. Radiother Oncol. 2011;100:70–5.
44. Zenda S, Kohno R, Kawashima M, Arahira S, Nishio T, Tahara M, Hayashi R, Kishimoto S,

Ogino T. Proton beam therapy for unresectable malignancies of the nasal cavity and paranasal sinuses. Int J Radiat Oncol Biol Phys. 2011;81(5):1473–8.

45. Glatzel M, Büntzel J, Schröder D, Küttner K, Fröhlich D. High-dose-rate brachytherapy in the treatment of recurrent and residual head and neck cancer. Laryngoscope. 2002;112(8 Pt 1):1366–71.

46. Fontanesi J, Hetzler D, Ross J. Effect of dose rate on local control and complications in the re-irradiation of head -and-neck tumors with interstitial iridium-192. Int J Radiat Oncol Biol Phys. 1989;17:365–9.

47. Chen AM, Daly ME, El-Sayed I, Garcia J, Lee NY, Bucci MK, Kaplan MK. Patterns of failure after combined modality approaches incorporating radiotherapy for sinonasal undifferentiated carcinoma of the head and neck. Int J Radiat Oncol Biol Phys. 2008;70:338–43.

48. Karakullukcu B, van Oudenaarde K, Copper MP, Klop WM, van Veen R, Wildeman M, Bing TI. Photodynamic therapy of early stage oral cavity and oropharynx neoplasms: an outcome analysis of 170 patients. Eur Arch Otorhinolaryngol. 2011;268(2):281–8.

49. Karakullukcu B, Nyst HJ, van Veen RL, Hoebers FJ, Hamming-Vrieze O, Witjes MJ, de Visscher SA, Burlage FR, Levendag PC, Sterenborg HJ, Tan IB. mTHPC mediated interstitial photodynamic therapy of recurrent nonmetastatic base of tongue cancers: development of a new method. Head Neck. 2012;34(11):1597–606.

Part IV

Optical Diagnostics: Introduction

Waseem Jerjes and Colin Hopper

Abstract

Optical diagnosis of abnormal processes in tissue is a new branch of science that expects to grow and develop over the next few years. The non-invasive nature of this technology accompanied with its ability to provide instant cost-effective diagnosis of disease will form the basis of clinical diagnosis in dentistry, medicine and surgery in the future. Current evidence from ongoing lab-based and clinical studies support the notion that many cellular and subcellular changes occurring in tissue can be detected using this technology. The introduction of this technology in every day clinical practice is being achieved but at a slow rate due to many technical factors. Ultimately, the aim of this technology is to be the gold standard of disease diagnosis, which until now is being achieved by histopathology.

Key words Optical diagnosis, Optical diagnostics, Optical biopsy, Tissue disease, Dysplasia, Cancer, Tumour, Diagnosis

Early detection of head and neck pre-malignant and malignant lesions can, in theory, lead to early intervention and overall reduction in mortality and improvement of quality of life. The "gold standard" intervention is surgery and the outcome, usually, depends on achieving clear surgical margins. Failure to do so leads to residual disease and increases the risk of recurrence and the need for adjuvant therapies. The identification of the pathological processes in the suspect lesion (at the time of diagnosis or monitoring) or in the surgical margin (at the time of surgery) requires accurate assessment of the microscopic changes and avoid any errors that can result from non-representative biopsy or pathologies with similar clinical characteristics [1–6].

The use of optical technology in clinical medicine has advanced our understanding of many physiological and pathophysiological processes occurring at cellular and subcellular levels. The term "optical biopsy" has been widely used over the past two decades to describe the use of optical technology in assessing tissue state, by acquiring a specific optical signature of the examined area. The majority of optical processes are still being assessed in clinical trials and have not been introduced as "independent" tools in clinical practice. All acquired optical signatures generated from these tools are, currently, compared to the tissue histopathology which continues to be the "gold standard" [1–6].

Standard diagnosis of tissue disease is achieved by visual inspection and a surgical biopsy, when required. It is impractical to biopsy everyone and the clinical guidelines for taking a biopsy continue to change based on our experience and clinical governance issues. Many adjuvant diagnostic tools (i.e. brush biopsy, vital staining, molecular markers, cytology and chemiluminescence) have been developed to aid the clinician in the decision-making process, but unfortunately many have suffered from variable degrees of accuracy due to many clinician-related and patient-related factors. Despite that, researchers continue to examine many non-invasive real-time diagnostic tools with the aim to identify the ultimate diagnostic utility [1–6].

It is postulated that an ideal diagnostic tool in the head and neck should provide real-time diagnosis and be handheld or mounted on endoscopes, easy to use especially in outpatients setting, cost-effective, operator independent and can provide photo-documentation of the examined area. The tool should have already been validated against the gold standard with high sensitivity and specificity and be of minimally invasive nature. Other functions for a diagnostic tool include: monitoring lesions at risk of malignant transformation, monitoring of haemoglobin tissue perfusion in free flaps and therapeutic drug levels during chemo- and photodynamic therapy, guiding consent and sampling, guiding treatment and guiding other treatment modalities (i.e. photodynamic therapy) the assessment of surgical margins and have a beneficial use in sentinel node biopsy [1–6].

The development of optical diagnostics is a current necessity. Optical biopsies can be acquired through different modalities; each has its own mechanism of action and requires different modes of data analysis. Their use will help reduce tissue trauma, reduce the workload on pathology departments and reduce the time the anxious patient has to wait for a diagnosis. With histopathology, the processing of biopsy material and the interpretation of the results inevitably lead to diagnostic delay and the added possibility of taking an unrepresentative sample. With optical biopsy, a light of a specific wavelength is fired into tissue, and the reflected light is measured in such a way that a specific optical signature can be generated (i.e. cellular and subcellular changes in elastic scattering spectroscopy, molecular vibration in Raman spectroscopy, surface morphology by microendoscopy, biochemical changes from tissue fluorescence or the use of interferometric (superimposing or interfering waves) tomographic technology in the case of optical coherence tomography) [1–6].

The anatomy of the head and neck is unique and complex. As the oral cavity and the aero-digestive tracts are easily accessible to examination (direct or endoscopic visualisation), it is feasible that disease process can be assessed by using optical diagnostic tools. This will enable diagnosis at an early stage and can potentially improve prognosis and quality of life. The outlook will improve even further if optical tools were available for surveillance and early detection of malignant transformation and recurrence, following an intervention. The ultimate aim is to be able to differentiate areas of similar clinical characteristics (i.e. dysplasia and carcinoma in situ), rather than just differentiating between normal and abnormal tissues. Several pathological lesions can be interrogated using optical diagnostics including: hyperkeratosis, inflammation, dysplasia, carcinoma in situ and neoplasia [1–6].

The current lesional assessment/monitoring in outpatients are influenced by many factors, including: patient-related, clinician-related (i.e. documentation adequacy, grade, experience…etc.) and clinical environment-related (i.e. workload, funding…etc.). As such, a decision making of "regression" or "progression" of the lesion may not be straight forward and may not even reflect the real case. Hence, the use of an "optical diagnostics" tool may help to eliminate all these variations and make the line between the two scenarios less blurry. If appropriately applied in clinical field, these tools can increase the clinicians' confidence in decision-making and ensure faster processing of patients in the clinic, reducing waiting times and improving outcome. Furthermore, the optical signatures acquired from the outpatient setting can be saved in the patient's records and be used as a guide in the subsequent reviews. These signatures can also be used to undertake selective biopsy procedure in non-homogenous lesions in order to achieve the most accurate diagnosis of the tissue state. This will allow an appropriate disease treatment which will potentially reduce the recurrent rate as well as the risk of residual disease. Theoretically, safe margins will be easier to achieve when using these optical tools, and this will reduce the need for any adjuvant therapy which will give an enhanced prognosis, associated with reduction in morbidity and mortality [1–6].

The use of optical diagnostics can potentially improve our evidence-based dental and medical practice and its accurate image documentation allowing improved auditing and clinical governance leading to better choices for the clinician when assessing a suspect tissue, making a diagnosis and guiding therapy. Training and education will improve and evolve leading to less clinical errors and more appropriate confident decisions. The current pre-clinical and clinical studies in the optical technology field are generating a library of normative and pathological signatures which will act as a standard reference. There is still much work to be done, but ultimately it is anticipated that the clinician will be able to use these validated technologies in every day practice when dealing with any suspicious lesion in the head and neck area.

Optical diagnosis of the head and neck is a rapidly evolving area of clinical research that can be readily translated to improve patient care and overall quality of life. The results from the immediate ex vivo and the in vivo studies are very promising and suggest that it is possible for these tools to replace histopathology when it comes to certain pathologies in the near future [1–6].

References

1. Swinson B, Jerjes W, El-Maaytah M, Norris P, Hopper C. Optical techniques in diagnosis of head and neck malignancy. Oral Oncol. 2006;42(3):221–8.
2. Upile T, Jerjes W, Betz CS, El Maaytah M, Wright A, Hopper C. Optical diagnostic techniques in the head and neck. Dent Update. 2007;34(7):410–2, 415–6, 419–20 passim.
3. Upile T, Jerjes W, Sterenborg HJ, El-Naggar AK, Sandison A, Witjes MJ, Biel MA, Bigio I, Wong BJ, Gillenwater A, MacRobert AJ, Robinson DJ, Betz CS, Stepp H, Bolotine L, McKenzie G, Mosse CA, Barr H, Chen Z, Berg K, D'Cruz AK, Stone N, Kendall C, Fisher S, Leunig A, Olivo M, Richards-Kortum R, Soo KC, Bagnato V, Choo-Smith LP, Svanberg K, Tan IB, Wilson BC, Wolfsen H, Yodh AG, Hopper C. Head & neck optical diagnostics: vision of the future of surgery. Head Neck Oncol. 2009;1:25.
4. Upile T, Jerjes WK, Sterenborg HJ, Wong BJ, El-Naggar AK, Ilgner JF, Sandison A, Witjes MJ, Biel MA, van Veen R, Hamdoon Z, Gillenwater A, Mosse CA, Robinson DJ, Betz CS, Stepp H, Bolotine L, McKenzie G, Barr H, Chen Z, Berg K, D'Cruz AK, Sudhoff H, Stone N, Kendall C, Fisher S, MacRobert AJ, Leunig A, Olivo M, Richards-Kortum R, Soo KC, Bagnato V, Choo-Smith LP, Svanberg K, Tan IB, Wilson BC, Wolfsen H, Bigio I, Yodh AG, Hopper C. At the frontiers of surgery: review. Head Neck Oncol. 2011;3(1):7.
5. Jerjes WK, Upile T, Wong BJ, Betz CS, Sterenborg HJ, Witjes MJ, Berg K, van Veen R, Biel MA, El-Naggar AK, Mosse CA, Olivo M, Richards-Kortum R, Robinson DJ, Rosen J, Yodh AG, Kendall C, Ilgner JF, Amelink A, Bagnato V, Barr H, Bolotine L, Bigio I, Chen Z, Choo-Smith LP, D'Cruz AK, Gillenwater A, Leunig A, MacRobert AJ, McKenzie G, Sandison A, Soo KC, Stepp H, Stone N, Svanberg K, Tan IB, Wilson BC, Wolfsen H, Hopper C. The future of medical diagnostics: review paper. Head Neck Oncol. 2011;3:38.
6. Upile T, Jerjes W, Radhi H, Mahil J, Rao A, Hopper C. Elastic scattering spectroscopy in assessing skin lesions: an "in vivo" study. Photodiagnosis Photodyn Ther. 2012;9(2):132–41.

Chapter 26

Fluorescence and Reflectance Spectroscopy for Detection of Oral Dysplasia and Cancer

Richard A. Schwarz, Rebecca R. Richards-Kortum, and Ann M. Gillenwater

Introduction

Oral cancer is a serious health problem in many regions of the world. An estimated 263,000 new cases and 127,000 deaths due to oral cancer occur annually worldwide, including 24,000 new cases and 5500 deaths in the United States [1, 2]. The primary treatment method remains surgical resection, which may be followed by postoperative radiation therapy [3, 4]. Despite significant advances in treatment methods for oral cancer, patient survival rates have not shown substantial improvement. Failure to improve patient outcomes is likely secondary to delays in diagnosis until disease is at advanced stages, when treatment is more difficult, more morbid, and less successful than interventions for early oral cancers [5, 6]. Delayed diagnosis of patients with oral cancer is due in part to the lack of effective screening tools, insufficient education, difficulty in evaluating the risk of malignant transformation in oral potentially malignant lesions (OPMLs), and the high rate of recurrence following treatment [7–10].

The development and progression of neoplastic changes in the oral cavity lead to measurable changes in the optical properties of oral tissue. Malignant transformation results in alterations in metabolic activity and tissue architecture, that in turn cause changes in the natural autofluorescence of oral tissue derived from endogenous fluorophores in the epithelial and stromal layers [11, 12]. Microvascularization and reduced oxygen saturation cause

Brian J.-F. Wong and Justus Ilgner (eds.), Biomedical Optics in Otorhinolaryngology: Head and Neck Surgery,
DOI 10.1007/978-1-4939-1758-7_26, © Springer Science+Business Media New York 2016

changes in light absorption due to oxyhemoglobin and deoxyhemoglobin [13, 14]. Increased nuclear size, pleomorphism, and architectural changes alter the light scattering properties of tissue [15, 16].

These changes in optical properties during neoplastic progression can be detected using noninvasive optical techniques, potentially aiding in early detection and diagnosis. Observations of autofluorescence from tumor tissue in animals were reported as early as the 1920s [17]. Building on the extensive use of fluorescence to characterize cellular metabolism in the 1950s and 1960s [18, 19], optical spectroscopy emerged as a potential tool for clinical diagnostics in the 1980s [20, 21]. The rapid expansion of spectroscopic diagnostic methods at this time was facilitated by the availability of a wide variety of lasers for high-spectral intensity excitation and high-quality fiber optics for clinical probe development.

Various spectroscopic methods have been reported for the detection of dysplasia and cancer in the oral cavity and other organ sites, including fluorescence spectroscopy, elastic scattering spectroscopy, diffuse reflectance spectroscopy, Raman scattering spectroscopy, and time-resolved fluorescence spectroscopy, to name a few [22–24]. Each of these techniques involves the noninvasive interrogation of tissue using illumination light with selected characteristics and detection of the wavelength-dependent (spectral) characteristics of light emitted from the tissue to provide diagnostically relevant information. This chapter focuses on fluorescence spectroscopy, in which narrowband illumination light is used to excite endogenous fluorophores, and reflectance spectroscopy, in which broadband (white) illumination light is used to interrogate the elastic scattering properties and absorption properties of tissue.

Endogenous Fluorophores, Absorbers, and Scatterers in the Oral Mucosa

Light energy (photons) incident upon tissue can be absorbed by molecules naturally present within the tissue, either within cells or in the extracellular matrix. Certain types of these molecules can subsequently undergo a radiative relaxation process in which a photon with lower energy (longer wavelength) is emitted. This process is termed fluorescence. Autofluorescence refers to fluorescence from fluorophores naturally present in tissue. Sources of autofluorescence in oral tissue are shown in Table 1 [11]. These include the amino acids tryptophan, tyrosine, and phenylalanine; structural proteins including collagen, collagen crosslinks, and elastin; the coenzymes reduced nicotinamide adenine

Table 1
Endogenous tissue fluorophores

Fluorophore	Excitation maxima (nm)	Emission maxima (nm)
NADH	290,340	440,450
FAD	450	515
Collagen crosslinks	325	400
Elastin crosslinks	325	400
Collagen powder	280,265,330,450	310,385,390,530
Elastin powder	350,410,450	420,500,520
Tryptophan	280	350
Tyrosine	Not determined	300
Phenylalanine	Not determined	280
Pyridoxine	332	400
Lipofuscin	340–395	430–460,540
Eosinophils	370,500	440,550

NADH nicotinamide adenine dinucleotide, *FAD* flavine adenine dinucleotide, *nm* nanometers

Adapted with permission from Richards-Kortum R, Sevick-Muraca E. Ann Rev Phys Chem. 1996;47:555–606

dinucleotide (NADH) and flavin adenine dinucleotide (FAD); keratin; and porphyrins [25, 26]. The spatial distribution of these fluorophores is depth-dependent, with substantial differences between the epithelium and the supporting stroma [27]. Autofluorescence originating in the epithelium is primarily due to NADH, FAD, and a superficial keratin layer, which may be present depending on the anatomic site. In the stroma, collagen fibers, collagen crosslinks, and elastin fibers produce a strong fluorescence signal (Fig. 1).

Not all molecules that absorb light subsequently emit fluorescence. Hemoglobin, for example, undergoes a fast nonradiative relaxation and therefore does not exhibit measurable fluorescence except by highly specialized techniques; yet it is an important absorber of light in tissue [28, 29]. Oxy and deoxyhemoglobin have characteristic absorption spectra that may be readily observed in spectroscopic measurements of tissue using broadband illumination. The presence and relative concentration of oxy and deoxyhemoglobin may be detected through spectroscopic measurements.

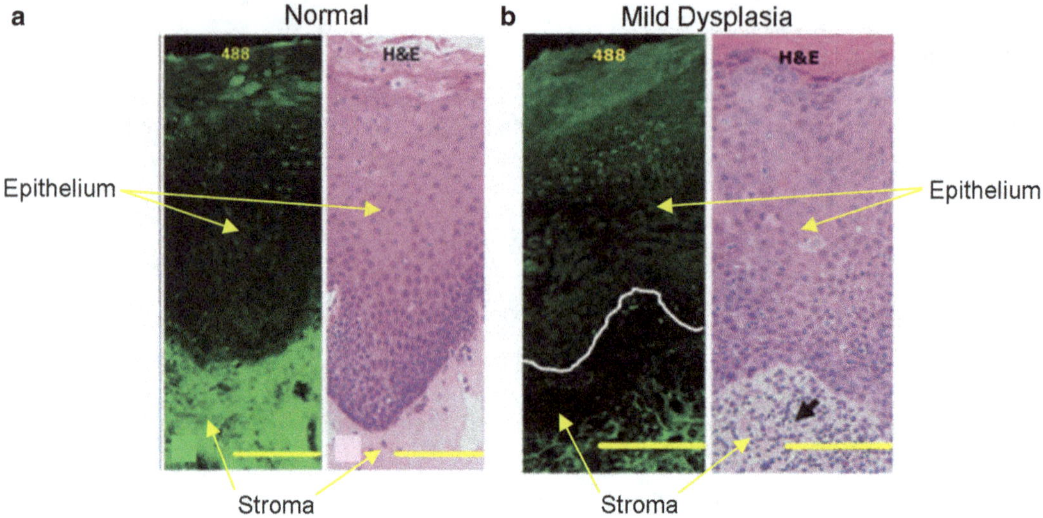

Fig. 1 Fluorescence confocal images of fresh oral tissue slices at 488 nm excitation, with corresponding hematoxylin and eosin (H&E) stained pathology sections. (**a**) Normal oral tissue without inflammation. (**b**) Oral tissue with mild dysplasia and mild/moderate inflammation, with the location of the basement membrane indicated by a *white line* in the confocal image. Note that the confocal images show intense stromal autofluorescence in (**a**) and reduced stromal autofluorescence in (**b**). Scale bars: 200 μm in the confocal images; 125 μm in the H&E images. *Black arrow*: lymphocytic infiltration. Adapted with permission from Pavlova I, Williams M, El-Naggar A, Richards-Kortum R, Gillenwater A. Clin Cancer Res. 2008;14(8):2396–2404

Tissue is a turbid medium in which light propagation is strongly affected by scattering as well as absorption. Photons that scatter elastically from cell nuclei, mitochondria, and other organelles undergo changes in propagation direction. Multiple scattering events may occur before a photon is absorbed or re-emitted from the tissue. Light scattering is sensitive to the size, shape, and distribution of the scatterers and is therefore affected by changes in nuclear/cytoplasm ratio and pleomorphism in cell nuclei.

With neoplastic progression the epithelium may display increased metabolic activity, increased nuclear size, increased nuclear/cytoplasm ratio, and pleomorphism, while the stroma may display enhanced microvascularization, influx of inflammatory cells, and breakdown of collagen crosslinks. Reduced blue-green stromal autofluorescence intensity and increased nuclear size and crowding within the epithelium are typically observed at dysplastic and cancerous sites. Thus spectroscopic measurements of tissue autofluorescence, absorption, and scattering may be used to characterize the disease state of tissue.

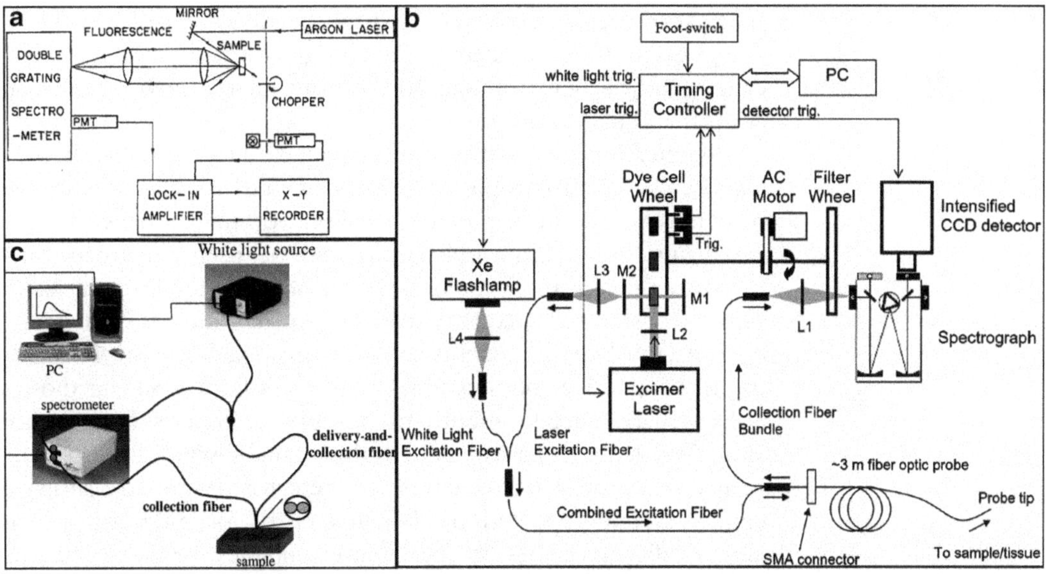

Fig. 2 Examples of spectroscopic instrumentation. (**a**) An early system used for laser-induced fluorescence spectroscopy of normal and cancerous animal tissue ex vivo. (**b**) A clinical system capable of laser-induced fluorescence spectroscopy at a range of excitation wavelengths, as well as reflectance spectroscopy. (**c**) A clinical system for differential path length reflectance spectroscopy. (**a**) Adapted with permission from Alfano RR, Tata DB, Cordero J, et al. *IEEE J Quant Electron.* 1984;QE-20(12):1507–1511. (**b**) Adapted with permission from Tunnell JW, Desjardins AE, Galindo L, et al. "Instrumentation for multi-modal spectroscopic diagnosis of epithelial dysplasia," *Technol Cancer Res Treat.* (http://www.tcrt.org), Adenine Press, 2003;2(6):505–514. (**c**) Adapted with permission from Amelink A, Kaspers OP, Sterenborg HJCM, et al. *Oral Oncol.* 2008;44:65–71

Instrumentation

The development of spectroscopic instrumentation for the detection of oral neoplasia over the past three decades has been driven primarily by technological advances in light sources, probes, spectrometers, and detectors; and secondarily by the demands of the clinical environment as these research devices have seen increasing clinical use. Figure 2a shows an early system used by Alfano et al. to perform laser-induced fluorescence spectroscopy of normal and cancerous animal tissue ex vivo [20]. The system included an argon laser source, a double grating spectrometer, photomultiplier tubes, and an x–y recorder. Advances in laser sources, fiber optics, and detectors soon led to the development of complex instruments capable of measuring a wide range of spectroscopic parameters in patients in vivo. Figure 2b shows a clinical spectroscopy system reported by Tunnell et al., capable of both laser-induced fluorescence spectroscopy at a range of excitation wavelengths (enabled by the tunable excimer-pumped dye laser) and reflectance spectroscopy (enabled by the Xenon flashlamp) [30]. The system uses an intensified charge-coupled device (CCD) camera as the detector and features automated instrumentation control and data acquisition.

While complex systems of this type have allowed researchers to explore the spectroscopic properties of oral tissue in detail, the recent trend has been towards smaller, portable devices that are easy to use in the clinic and require minimal user adjustment during daily operation. These devices are often designed to measure only a few selected spectra whose diagnostic value has been previously established. This trend has been accelerated by the availability of inexpensive, high spectral brightness light-emitting diodes (LEDs), which are frequently used in place of laser sources or arc lamp/flashlamp sources and by the availability of high-performance miniature spectrometers and detectors. Figure 2c shows a clinical system reported by Amelink et al. for differential path length reflectance spectroscopy that exemplifies the trend towards simple, miniaturized devices that measure only selected spectra of interest [31].

A key component of most clinical spectroscopic instruments is the fiber optic probe, which transmits the excitation light to the tissue and returns the collected light to the detection system. A multitude of probe designs and configurations have been reported in the literature as reviewed by Utzinger [32]. The geometric arrangement of excitation and collection fibers can be used to maximize the desired spectral signal or interrogate the tissue in a specific manner (Fig. 3). Angled or side-looking probes are common [33]. Different depths in tissue may be interrogated through the use of different source–detector fiber separations, designs that incorporate miniature lenses, or differential path length configurations [31, 34–36]. The fiber optic probe is typically (though not always) designed to be placed in contact with the tissue at the measurement site. This implies that there should be some method for guiding the selection of sites to be measured with the spectroscopic probe. This may be either the clinician's judgment or some type of macroscopic imaging or scanning technique that can rapidly identify high-risk regions within the oral cavity [37].

Fig. 3 (continued) reflection (θ_{crit} = critical angle); (**g**) illumination and collection using the same fiber; (**h**) illumination and collection using adjacent fibers; (**i–j**) illumination and collection using adjacent fibers, with beveled fibers to improve collection efficiency; (**k**) hexagonal fiber configuration for submersion; (**l**) hexagonal fiber configuration for measurement of surfaces; (**m**) single excitation fiber and multiple collection fibers at different source–detector separations to sample different depths within tissue. Adapted with permission from Utzinger U and Richards-Kortum RR, *J Biomed Opt.* 2003;8(1):121–147

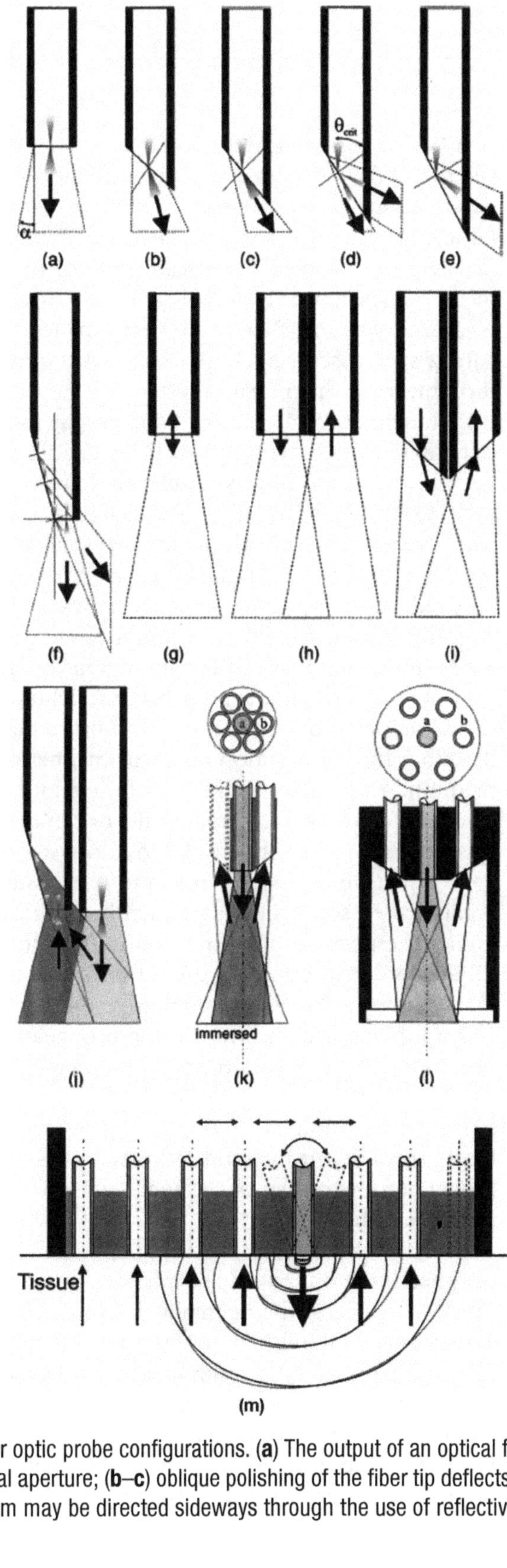

Fig. 3 Examples of fiber optic probe configurations. (**a**) The output of an optical fiber is described by the half angle α or the numerical aperture; (**b–c**) oblique polishing of the fiber tip deflects the output beam; (**d–f**) part or all of the output beam may be directed sideways through the use of reflective coatings or total internal

Analysis Methods

Analysis of clinical spectroscopic data from oral tissue has generally focused on two areas: (1) determination of biological properties of tissue, such as concentration and distribution of specific fluorophores and absorbers, based on the measured spectra; and (2) determination of the disease state of the tissue based on the measured spectra and/or biological properties calculated from the measured spectra. Diagnostic performance is evaluated by comparing spectroscopic results to a gold standard, such as histopathology, from the measured site.

Mathematical models of light propagation in tissue are typically used as the starting point for data analysis. These models are beyond the scope of this chapter and are only mentioned briefly here; extensive information is available in the literature [38–41]. The models describe tissue in terms of wavelength-dependent optical properties including absorption, scattering, anisotropy, reduced scattering, and refractive index [42]. These definitions typically require simplifying assumptions in which parameter values are assigned uniformly to certain regions or layers of tissue.

The most general approach to modeling light propagation in tissue involves the radiative transport equation (RTE), which describes the propagation of electromagnetic radiation through a medium in which absorption, scattering, and emission occur [43]. The RTE can be solved numerically or can be simplified by further approximations to obtain closed form solutions. The diffusion approximation, in which absorption is assumed to be minimal compared to scattering, is frequently used; but its applicability is limited, especially at short source–detector separations [44]. Higher-order solutions to the RTE such as the P_3 approximation may also be used [39]. An alternative approach is the use of Monte Carlo models, which simulate the propagation of large numbers (millions) of photons through computer-based virtual models of tissue, with the trajectory of each photon governed by probabilities for absorption, scattering, and emission events based on the local properties of the modeled tissue [45–47]. The Monte Carlo model output consists of the aggregate results from these millions of tracked photons.

Whatever particular modeling approach is selected, the model parameters are optimized and adjusted based on comparison of the model output to experimentally measured spectra. Once sufficient agreement is established between the model and measured data, further experimental measurements may be used to calculate tissue properties and biological parameters. Spectral features, calculated tissue properties, and/or calculated biological parameters are then used to predict the disease state of the tissue. Mathematical techniques such as principal component analysis may be used to reduce the dimensionality of the data. Diagnostic prediction algorithms may involve classification techniques such as linear discriminant analysis, logistic regression, cluster analysis, neural networks, decision trees, and other methods [48–50].

Clinical Studies

Studies by Alfano et al. in animal tissue and nonoral human tissues established the potential for spectroscopic diagnosis of dysplasia and cancer [20, 21]. Kolli et al. performed early spectroscopic studies of oral lesions in vivo, measuring 31 patients with primary intraepithelial neoplasia or invasive squamous cell carcinoma of the oral cavity and pharynx using a Xenon flashlamp-based spectroscopy system [51]. Using a portable spectrofluorimeter with a nitrogen-pumped dye laser source, Dhingra et al. observed reduced autofluorescence intensity in neoplastic lesions compared to normal tissue in broad emission peaks centered at 450 nm (at 370 nm excitation) and 490 nm (at 410 nm excitation) [52]. In a study of 49 patients, Betz et al. similarly reported reduced autofluorescence emission intensity from neoplastic oral mucosa compared to normal tissue in the 500-nm wavelength region [53]. Interestingly, these measurements were performed in a noncontact configuration using an endoscope with a Xenon arc lamp, a CCD camera, and a spectrometer.

As successive clinical studies showed alterations in autofluorescence emission in diseased tissue relative to healthy tissue (typically reduced blue–green autofluorescence intensity, and sometimes increased red autofluorescence associated with porphyrins), researchers began to systematically explore the optimal excitation and emission wavelengths for detecting these disease-related spectroscopic changes. Heintzelman et al. identified optimal excitation wavelengths for detection of oral neoplasia as 350, 380, and 400 nm, paired with an emission wavelength of 472 nm [54]. They reported 90 % sensitivity and 88 % specificity in a training set of 20 subjects, and 100 % sensitivity and 98 % specificity in a validation set of 56 subjects, for distinguishing normal oral tissue from dysplasia and cancer. Figure 4 shows fluorescence excitation-emission matrices (EEMs) from cancerous and normal tissue measured in this study, collected using a Xenon arc lamp-based spectroscopy system. Van Staveren et al. reported the use of artificial neural network classification methods to distinguish abnormal from normal oral tissue with 86 % sensitivity and 100 % specificity in a study of 23 subjects, based on 420 nm excitation and 465–650 nm emission [48].

Autofluorescence spectra measured from tissue may be substantially affected by absorption of excitation and/or emission

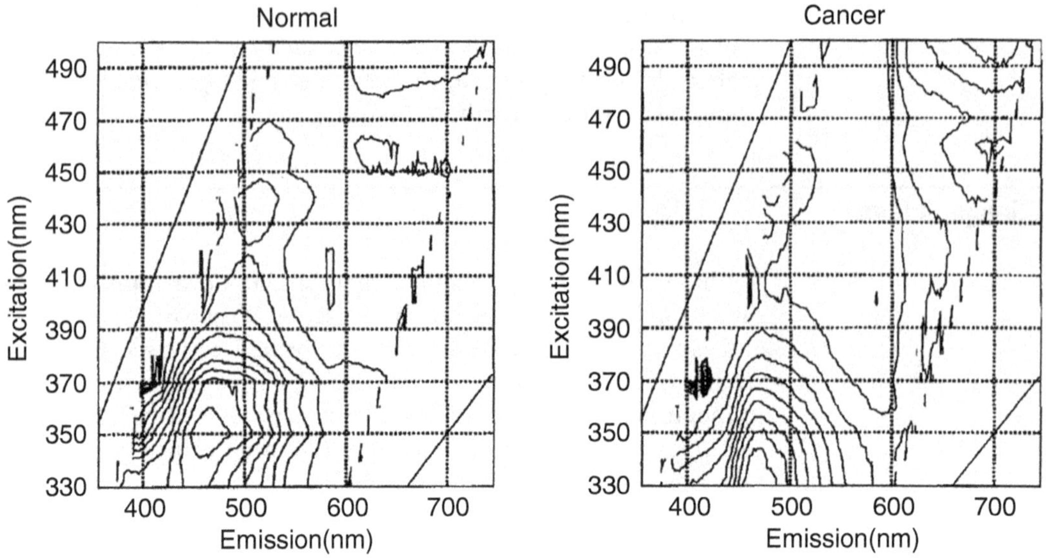

Fig. 4 Fluorescence excitation emission matrices (EEMs) from normal and cancerous oral tissue. *nm* nanometers. Reprinted with permission from Heintzelman DL, Utzinger U, Fuchs H, et al. *Photochem Photobiol.* 2000;72(1):103–113

light by oxy and deoxyhemoglobin present in the blood within intact tissue. Modeling and analysis of these effects are further complicated by the fact that blood is located within the vessels of varying diameter, rather than uniformly distributed throughout the tissue [55]. Müller et al. demonstrated the use of information from reflectance spectra to correct for the effects of hemoglobin absorption on fluorescence spectra, resulting in "intrinsic" fluorescence spectra [56] (Fig. 5). In the same study, the authors extracted biological parameters from the measured spectra (contributions to the intrinsic fluorescence spectra from NADH and collagen) and used them to classify tissue in binary decision plots [56] (Fig. 6). De Veld et al. also implemented a mathematical method for correcting autofluorescence spectra for the effects of blood absorption based on diffuse reflectance measurements [57]. In a study of 155 patients and 70 healthy volunteers, they reported excellent discrimination of cancer from healthy tissue [area under receiver operator characteristic curve (AUC) = 0.98] and successful discrimination of lesions from healthy mucosa (AUC = 0.90). However, they found that discrimination of benign lesions from dysplastic and malignant lesions was less successful (AUC = 0.77) [57].

In recent clinical studies, researchers have explored new measurement configurations, implemented probe designs that target the epithelial layer where early precancerous changes occur, examined the effects of different oral sites on spectral measurements,

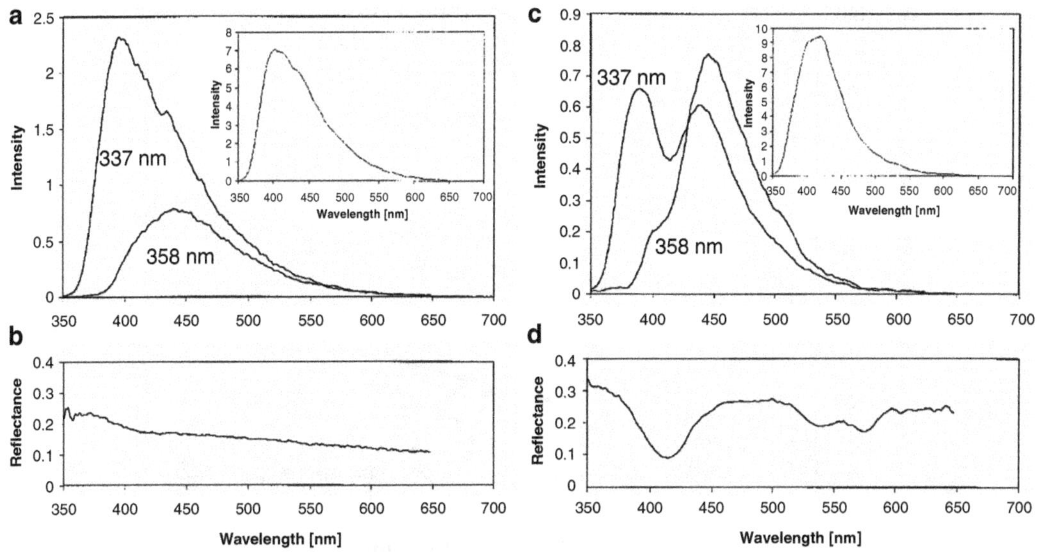

Fig. 5 Fluorescence spectra (**a**, **c**) measured at two oral sites, each excited at 337 nm and 358 nm, respectively, and corresponding reflectance spectra (**b**, **d**) at the same sites. Differences in fluorescence line shape between (**a**) and (**c**) are for the most part due to hemoglobin variations, which can also be observed in the corresponding reflectance spectra (**b**, **d**). The insets show the calculated 337-nm excited intrinsic fluorescence. *nm* nanometers. Reprinted with permission from Müller MG, Valdez TA, Georgakoudi I, et al. *Cancer.* 2003;97:1681–1692

and investigated the challenge of distinguishing benign lesions such as inflammation from dysplastic and cancerous lesions. Nieman et al. reported a study of 27 patients using oblique polarized reflectance spectroscopy [58]. Schwarz et al. measured 60 patients and 64 healthy volunteers using Xenon arc lamp-based spectroscopy system with a ball lens coupled fiber optic probe, which permits depth-sensitive targeting of epithelial or stromal regions [59] (Fig. 7). In this study, normal/benign lesions and mild dysplasia were distinguished from moderate/severe dysplasia and cancer with an AUC of 0.96 in the training set and 0.93 in the validation set. McGee et al. reported anatomy-based algorithms for spectroscopic diagnosis based on the properties of different anatomic sites within the oral cavity [60]. Amelink et al. developed a configuration for differential path length spectroscopy and used it to distinguish dysplastic from nondysplastic leukoplakias with an AUC of 0.87 in a study of 18 patients [31, 61].

Multimodal Diagnostics

In addition to point-probe spectroscopy, other noninvasive optical modalities for in vivo detection of oral dysplasia and cancer include macroscopic autofluorescence imaging and high-resolution

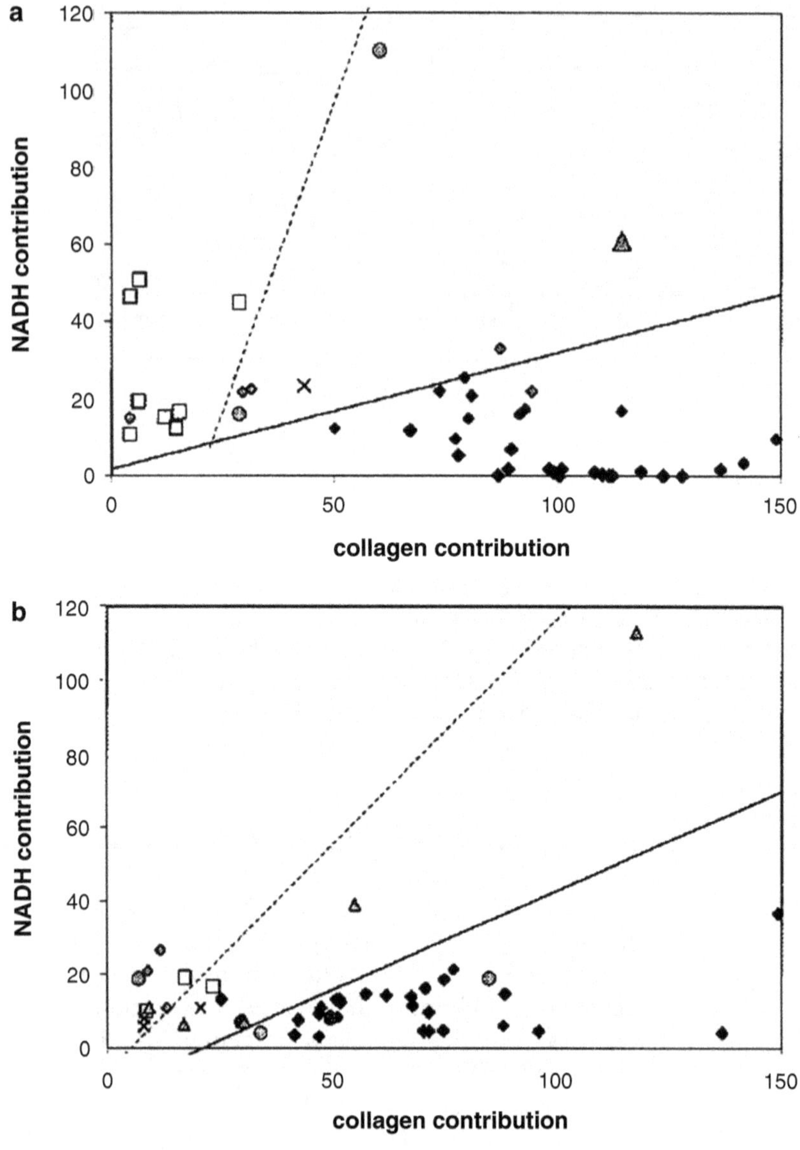

Fig. 6 Binary decision plots demonstrating the contributions of collagen and NADH to the intrinsic fluorescence tissue spectra at 337 nm and 358 nm excitation. (**a**) Nonkeratinized epithelium. (**b**) Keratinized epithelium. Note that the collagen contribution decreases and the NADH contribution increases with progression towards malignancy. The *solid line* separates normal from abnormal tissue and the *dotted line* separates dysplastic from cancerous tissue. *Darkly shaded* diamond: normal. *Darkly shaded* triangle: mild dysplasia. *Shaded circle*: moderate dysplasia. *Lightly shaded* diamond: severe dysplasia. *Open square*: cancer. *Solid circle*: inflammation. X: hyperkeratosis. *NADH* nicotinamide adenine dinucleotide, *nm* nanometers. Reprinted with permission from Müller MG, Valdez TA, Georgakoudi I, et al. *Cancer*. 2003;97:1681–1692

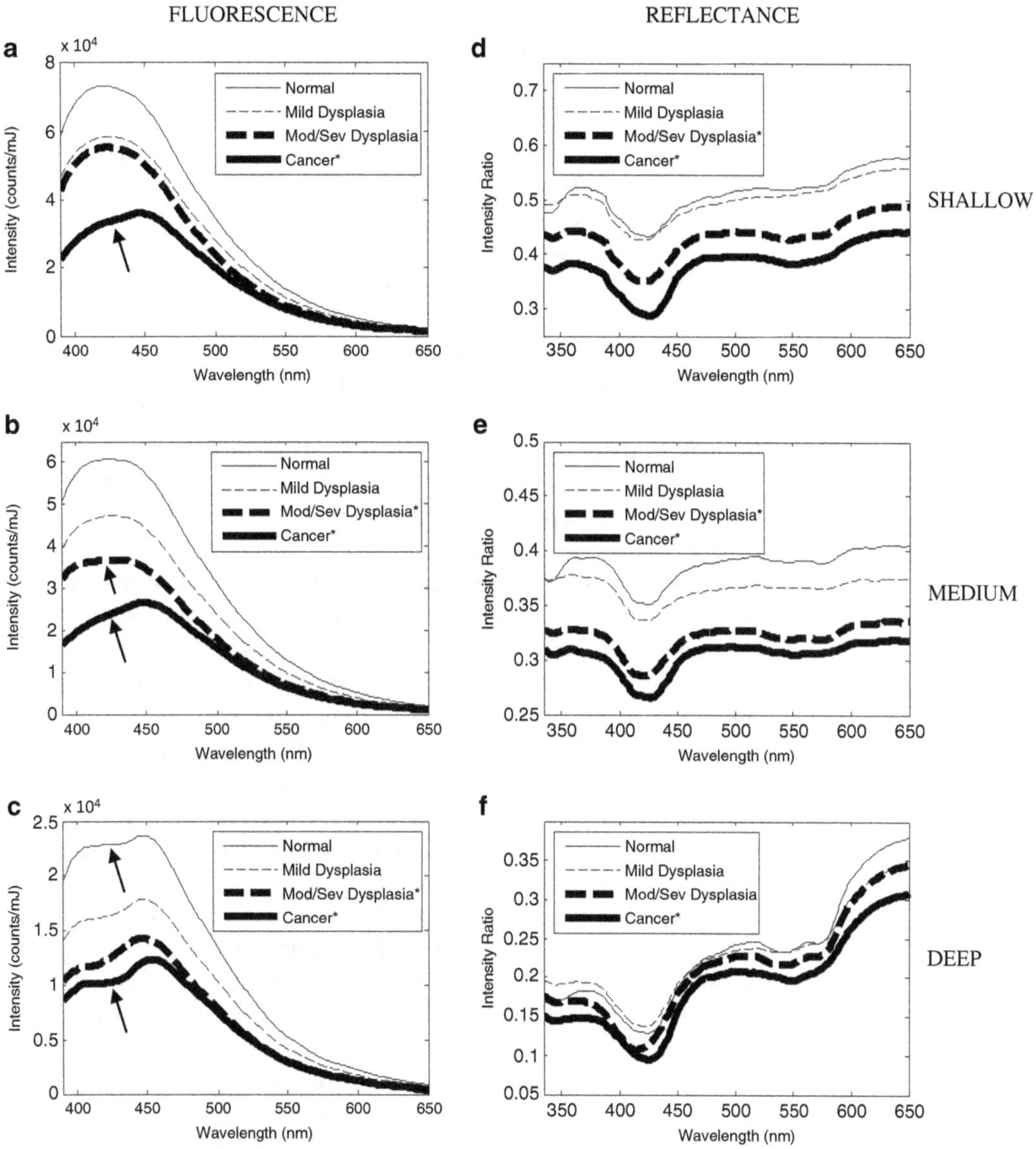

Fig. 7 Average spectra of nonkeratinized oral tissue by diagnosis, illustrating differences in data obtained at different depths. *Left column*: Fluorescence spectra at 350 nm excitation; *arrows* indicate absorption of fluorescent light by hemoglobin. *Right column*: Reflectance spectra with *white* light illumination. *Top*, *middle*, and *bottom*: Shallow, medium, and deep target depths (epithelium, basal epithelium/shallow stroma, and stroma, respectively). An *asterisk* (*) next to a diagnostic category indicates a statistically significant difference with respect to normal tissue. *Mod/Sev* moderate/severe, *mJ* millijoule, *nm* nanometers. Reprinted with permission from Schwarz RA, Gao W, Weber CR, et al. *Cancer*. 2009;115:1669–1679

imaging [62, 63]. These methods operate on different spatial scales from spectroscopy and are sensitive to different tissue parameters. Macroscopic autofluorescence imaging is sensitive to loss of autofluorescence in the stroma; spectroscopy is sensitive to metabolic changes, architectural changes, and angiogenesis; and high-resolution imaging is sensitive to nuclear morphology in the superficial epithelium. The combination of fluorescence and reflectance spectroscopy with optical imaging modalities offers certain advantages. Macroscopic autofluorescence imaging can be used to quickly identify high-risk regions within the oral cavity and guide the placement of the spectroscopic probe. Data from autofluorescence imaging, spectroscopy, and/or high-resolution imaging may be combined to provide a more complete analysis of the tissue and improved diagnostic specificity. Two-step diagnostic algorithms may be constructed based on different modalities, with the threshold in the first step set for high sensitivity and the threshold in the second step set for high specificity.

There are several commercially available macroscopic autofluorescence imaging devices that may be used in combination with spectroscopy. One such device is the VELscope® (LED Dental Ltd., Atlanta, Georgia), which is a handheld instrument that allows direct visualization of tissue fluorescence [64, 65]. An independent study suggests that it has a high sensitivity for detecting oral mucosal disorders, but a low specificity for dysplasia [66]. The VELscope may be used to guide placement of the spectroscopic probe, thus taking advantage of the VELscope's sensitivity while potentially improving diagnostic specificity.

An early example of the multimodal combination of imaging and spectroscopy is the work of Onizawa et al., who combined fluorescence film photography with measurements of autofluorescence using a chroma meter [67]. A second example is the previously mentioned study by Betz et al., in which a beamsplitter was used to direct a small portion of the light from the center of the endoscopic fluorescence image to an optical multichannel analyzer for spectral analysis [53]. More recently, Bedard et al. reported a pilot clinical study using a hyperspectral imaging device called a snapshot spectral imaging spectrometer [68]. This device collects image data with a complete spectrum associated with each pixel in the image (Fig. 8).

Discussion

A large and growing body of research indicates that fluorescence and reflectance spectroscopy can be useful tools to aid clinicians in detecting oral dysplasia and cancer. Optical spectroscopy has certain advantages. It is a straightforward method to implement in a clinical setting and clinical devices can be made small and portable.

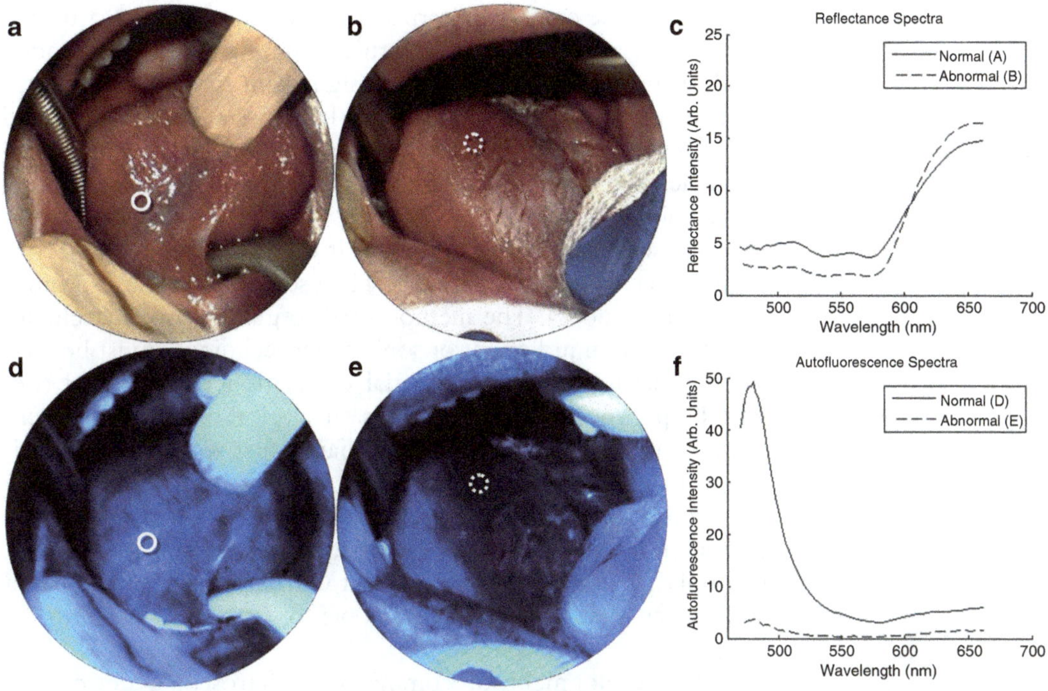

Fig. 8 Hyperspectral imaging using the snapshot spectral imaging spectrometer. (**a**, **d**) *Right ventral tongue* (clinical description: normal) in reflectance and autofluorescence modes, respectively. A biopsy (*solid circle*) indicated normal epithelium. (**b**, **e**) *Right dorsal tongue* (clinical description: erythroplakia) in reflectance and autofluorescence modes, respectively. A biopsy (*dotted circle*) indicated squamous cell carcinoma. Reflectance spectra (C) display characteristic oxyhemoglobin peaks. Autofluorescence images and spectra (F) show loss of *blue-green* autofluorescence at the abnormal site. Reprinted with permission from Bedard N, Schwarz RA, Hu A, et al. *Biomed Opt Express.* 2013;4(6):938–949

A variety of spectroscopic techniques, illumination and collection wavelengths, and probe designs can be tailored for specific applications. Spectral measurements provide quantitative data that can be rapidly analyzed at the point of care to provide information about tissue composition, tissue structure, and disease status. Spectral data from point probe measurements can readily be analyzed in an objective, quantitative manner without some of the concerns involved in quantitative image analysis, such as how to select appropriate regions of interest within an image. It is relatively easy to create a set of physical reference standards that can be measured frequently to monitor system performance over time during clinical studies [69].

Spectroscopy does, however, have a number of important limitations for in vivo screening and diagnosis, as summarized in a useful review by de Veld et al. [70]. In order to relate the measured spectra to biological characteristics of tissue it is necessary to account for the complex interplay of autofluorescence, scattering, absorption, and tissue architecture. The mathematical models used for the analysis often require significant simplifying assumptions or prior knowledge regarding local tissue composition and structure [71]. Variations are often observed in spectra measured from healthy tissue in different patients or from different oral sites. Point-probe spectroscopy only provides information about the sites selected for measurement; it can therefore be subject to sampling error and it cannot easily be used to screen large regions of the oral mucosa. The method used to guide probe placement, whether clinical judgment or some other technique, must be considered carefully. Accurate spatial correlation of measured sites with biopsy specimens or locations on surgical specimens is essential and may be more challenging than it first appears. While evidence in the literature shows that spectroscopy can accurately distinguish healthy tissue from dysplasia and cancer, the presence of benign lesions can complicate diagnostic classification. Finally, spectral data may not have the direct visual appeal of image-based techniques that display macroscopic or microscopic views of tissue.

The development of commercial spectroscopic devices for diagnosis of oral neoplasia has lagged behind the development of commercial imaging devices such as the VELscope. Even so, the potential for clinical use of spectroscopy remains high. It is most likely to be clinically implemented in combination with macroscopic imaging methods to guide probe placement, or in multimodal devices such as the snapshot spectral imaging spectrometer [68]. If spectroscopy can consistently help reduce the false positive rate associated with autofluorescence imaging, it will be a valuable diagnostic tool. Rapid, noninvasive optical techniques including spectroscopy are particularly well suited for use in low-resource settings, where laboratory facilities and expertise for conventional diagnosis may not be available [72].

In the future, the role of clinical spectroscopy and imaging may be transformed as molecular specific contrast agents for the identification of dysplasia and cancer become available for in vivo clinical use. The combination of molecular specific labeling with high spectral- and spatial-resolution optical methods could open up new opportunities for screening and diagnosis of dysplasia and cancer, as well as assessment of surgical margins. In our own research with resected tissue specimens labeled ex vivo using molecular specific contrast agents, we have found spectroscopy to be a useful tool to determine the penetration and localization of the contrast agent within the tissue. With the rapid growth in molecular imaging and the increasing availability of molecular probes for targeting specific biomarkers, spectroscopic measurement techniques for interrogating these probes will continue to be of interest.

References

1. Ferlay J, Shin HR, Bray F, Forman D, Mathers C, Parkin DM. Estimates of worldwide burden of cancer in 2008: GLOBOCAN 2008. Int J Cancer. 2010;127:2893–917.
2. Jemal A, Siegel R, Xu J, Ward E. Cancer statistics, 2010. CA Cancer J Clin. 2010;60:277–300.
3. Kalavrezos N, Bhandari R. Current trends and future perspectives in the surgical management of oral cancer. Oral Oncol. 2010;46: 429–32.
4. Ow TJ, Myers JN. Current management of advanced resectable oral cavity squamous cell carcinoma. Clin Exp Otorhinolaryngol. 2011;4(1): 1–10.
5. Rapidis AD, Gullane P, Langdon JD, Lefebvre JL, Scully C, Shah JP. Major advances in the knowledge and understanding of the epidemiology, aetiopathogenesis, diagnosis, management and prognosis of oral cancer. Oral Oncol. 2009;45:299–300.
6. Petersen PE. Oral cancer prevention and control—the approach of the World Health Organization. Oral Oncol. 2009;45:454–60.
7. Lingen MW, Kalmar JR, Karrison T, Speight PM. Critical evaluation of diagnostic aids for the detection of oral cancer. Oral Oncol. 2008;44:10–22.
8. Fedele S. Diagnostic aids in the screening of oral cancer. Head Neck Oncol. 2009;1:5.
9. Ho MW, Risk JM, Woolgar JA, et al. The clinical determinants of malignant transformation in oral epithelial dysplasia. Oral Oncol. 2012;48:969–76.
10. Eckardt A, Barth EL, Kokemueller H, Wegener G. Recurrent carcinoma of the head and neck: treatment strategies and survival analysis in a 20-year period. Oral Oncol. 2004;40:427–32.
11. Richards-Kortum R, Sevick-Muraca E. Quantitative optical spectroscopy for tissue diagnosis. Annu Rev Phys Chem. 1996;47: 555–606.
12. Fryen A, Glanz H, Lohmann W, Dreyer T, Bohle RM. Significance of autofluorescence for the optical demarcation of field cancerisation in the upper aerodigestive tract. Acta Otolaryngol. 1997;117:316–9.
13. Takatani S, Graham MD. Theoretical analysis of diffuse reflectance from a two-layer tissue model. IEEE Trans Biomed Eng. 1979;26(12): 656–64.
14. Amelink A, Christiaanse T, Sterenborg HJCM. Effect of hemoglobin extinction spectra on optical spectroscopic measurements of blood oxygen saturation. Opt Lett. 2009;34(10): 1525–7.
15. Mourant JR, Canpolat M, Brocker C, et al. Light scattering from cells: the contribution of the nucleus and the effects of proliferative status. J Biomed Opt. 2000;5(2):131–7.
16. Backman V, Gopal V, Kalashnikov M, et al. Measuring cellular structure at submicrometer scale with light scattering spectroscopy. IEEE J Sel Top Quantum Electron. 2001;7(6):887–93.
17. Policard A. Etude sur les aspects offerts par des tumeurs expérimentales examinées à la lumière de Wood. C R Soc Biol (Paris). 1924;91:1423–4.
18. Chance B, Thorell B. Localization and kinetics of reduced pyridine nucleotide in living cells by microfluorometry. J Biol Chem. 1959;234: 3044–50.
19. Chance B, Cohen P, Jobsis F, Schoener B. Intracellular oxidation-reduction states in vivo. Science. 1962;137(3529):499–508.
20. Alfano RR, Tata DB, Cordero J, Tomashefsky P, Longo FW, Alfano MA. Laser induced fluorescence spectroscopy from native cancerous and normal tissue. IEEE J Quantum Electron. 1984;20(12):1507–11.
21. Alfano RR, Tang GC, Pradhan A, Lam W, Choy DSJ, Opher E. Fluorescence spectra from cancerous and normal human breast and lung tissues. IEEE J Quantum Electron. 1987;23(10):1806–11.
22. Bigio IJ, Bown SG. Spectroscopic sensing of cancer and cancer therapy. Cancer Biol Ther. 2004;3(3):259–67.
23. Mahadevan-Jansen A, Richards-Kortum R. Raman spectroscopy for the detection of cancers and precancers. J Biomed Opt. 1996;1(1): 31–70.
24. Marcu L. Fluorescence lifetime techniques in medical applications. Ann Biomed Eng. 2012; 40(2):304–31.
25. Gillenwater A, Jacob R, Richards-Kortum R. Fluorescence spectroscopy: a technique with potential to improve the early detection of aerodigestive tract neoplasia. Head Neck. 1998;20(6):556–62.
26. Inaguma M, Hashimoto K. Porphyrin-like fluorescence in oral cancer. Cancer. 1999;86: 2201–11.
27. Pavlova I, Williams M, El-Naggar A, Richards-Kortum R, Gillenwater A. Understanding the biological basis of autofluorescence imaging for oral cancer detection: high-resolution fluorescence microscopy in viable tissue. Clin Cancer Res. 2008;14(8):2396–404.
28. Prahl SA (2013) Optical absorption of hemoglobin. Available at: http://omlc.ogi.edu/spectra/hemoglobin. Accessibility verified 12 Dec 2013.

29. Zheng W, Li D, Zeng Y, Luo Y, Qu JY. Two-photon excited hemoglobin fluorescence. Biomed Opt Express. 2010;2(1):71–9.
30. Tunnell JW, Desjardins AE, Galindo L, et al. Instrumentation for multi-modal spectroscopic diagnosis of epithelial dysplasia. Technol Cancer Res Treat. 2003;2(6):505–14.
31. Amelink A, Kaspers OP, Sterenborg HJCM, van der Wal JE, Roodenburg JLN, Witjes MJH. Non-invasive measurement of the morphology and physiology of oral mucosa by use of optical spectroscopy. Oral Oncol. 2008;44:65–71.
32. Utzinger U, Richards-Kortum RR. Fiber optic probes for biomedical optical spectroscopy. J Biomed Opt. 2003;8(1):121–47.
33. Baran TM, Fenn MC, Foster TH. Determination of optical properties by interstitial white light spectroscopy using a custom fiber optic probe. J Biomed Opt. 2013;18(10):107007.
34. Pfefer TJ, Schomacker KT, Ediger MN, Nishioka NS. Multiple-fiber probe design for fluorescence spectroscopy in tissue. Appl Opt. 2002;41(22):4712–21.
35. Pfefer TJ, Agrawal A, Drezek RA. Oblique-incidence illumination and collection for depth-selective fluorescence spectroscopy. J Biomed Opt. 2005;10(4):044016.
36. Schwarz RA, Gao W, Daye D, Williams MD, Richards-Kortum R, Gillenwater AM. Autofluorescence and diffuse reflectance spectroscopy of oral epithelial tissue using a depth-sensitive fiber-optic probe. Appl Opt. 2008;47(6):825–34.
37. Roblyer D, Kurachi C, Stepanek V, et al. Objective detection and delineation of oral neoplasia using autofluorescence imaging. Cancer Prev Res (Phila). 2009;2(5):423–31.
38. Hielscher AH, Kim HK, Klose AD. Forward models of light transport in biological tissue. In: Boas DA, Pitris C, Ramanujam N, editors. Handbook of biomedical optics. Boca Raton, FL: CRC Press; 2011. p. 319–36.
39. Hull EL, Foster TH. Steady-state reflectance spectroscopy in the P_3 approximation. J Opt Soc Am A. 2001;18(3):584–99.
40. Jacques SL, Pogue BW. Tutorial on diffuse light transport. J Biomed Opt. 2008;13(4):041302.
41. Patterson MS, Chance B, Wilson BC. Time resolved reflectance and transmittance for the non-invasive measurement of tissue optical properties. Appl Opt. 1989;28(12):2331–6.
42. Jacques SL. Optical properties of biological tissues: a review. Phys Med Biol. 2013;58:R37–61.
43. Arridge SR. Optical tomography in medical imaging. Inverse Prob. 1999;15:R41–93.
44. Hielscher AH, Alcouffe RE, Barbour RL. Comparison of finite-difference transport and diffusion calculations for photon migration in homogeneous and heterogeneous tissues. Phys Med Biol. 1998;43:1285–302.
45. Flock ST, Patterson MS, Wilson BC, Wyman DR. Monte Carlo modeling of light propagation in highly scattering tissues—I: model predictions and comparison with diffusion theory. IEEE Trans Biomed Eng. 1989;36(12):1162–8.
46. Zhu C, Liu Q. Review of Monte Carlo modeling of light transport in tissues. J Biomed Opt. 2013;18(5):050902.
47. Pavlova I, Weber CR, Schwarz RA, Williams M, El-Naggar A, Gillenwater A, Richards-Kortum R. Monte Carlo model to describe depth selective fluorescence spectra of epithelial tissue: applications for diagnosis of oral precancer. J Biomed Opt. 2008;13(6):064012.
48. van Staveren HJ, van Veen RLP, Speelman OC, Witjes MJH, Star WM, Roodenburg JLN. Classification of clinical autofluorescence spectra of oral leukoplakia using an artificial neural network: a pilot study. Oral Oncol. 2000;36:286–93.
49. de Veld DCG, Skurichina M, Witjes MJH, Duin RPW, Sterenborg HJCM, Roodenburg JLN. Clinical study for classification of benign, dysplastic, and malignant oral lesions using autofluorescence spectroscopy. J Biomed Opt. 2004;9(5):940–50.
50. Majumder SK, Gupta A, Gupta S, Ghosh N, Gupta PK. Multi-class classification algorithm for optical diagnosis of oral cancer. J Photochem Photobiol B. 2006;85:109–17.
51. Kolli VR, Savage HE, Yao TJ, Schantz SP. Native cellular fluorescence of neoplastic upper aerodigestive mucosa. Arch Otolaryngol Head Neck Surg. 1995;121(11):1287–92.
52. Dhingra JK, Perrault DF, McMillan K, et al. Early diagnosis of upper aerodigestive tract cancer by autofluorescence. Arch Otolaryngol Head Neck Surg. 1996;122(11):1181–6.
53. Betz CS, Mehlmann M, Rick K, et al. Autofluorescence imaging and spectroscopy of normal and malignant mucosa in patients with head and neck cancer. Lasers Surg Med. 1999;25:323–34.
54. Heintzelman DL, Utzinger U, Fuchs H, et al. Optimal excitation wavelengths for in vivo detection of oral neoplasia using fluorescence spectroscopy. Photochem Photobiol. 2000;72(1):103–13.

55. Lau C, Šćepanović O, Mirkovic J, et al. Re-evaluation of model-based light-scattering spectroscopy for tissue spectroscopy. J Biomed Opt. 2009;14(2):024031.
56. Müller MG, Valdez TA, Georgakoudi I, et al. Spectroscopic detection and evaluation of morphologic and biochemical changes in early human oral carcinoma. Cancer. 2003;97:1681–92.
57. de Veld DCG, Skurichina M, Witjes MJH, Duin RPW, Sterenborg HJCM, Roodenburg JLN. Autofluorescence and diffuse reflectance spectroscopy for oral oncology. Lasers Surg Med. 2005;36:356–64.
58. Nieman LT, Kan CW, Gillenwater A, Markey MK, Sokolov K. Probing local tissue changes in the oral cavity for early detection of cancer using oblique polarized reflectance spectroscopy: a pilot clinical trial. J Biomed Opt. 2008;13(2):024011.
59. Schwarz RA, Gao W, Weber CR, et al. Noninvasive evaluation of oral lesions using depth-sensitive optical spectroscopy. Cancer. 2009;115:1669–79.
60. McGee S, Mardirossian V, Elackattu A, et al. Anatomy-based algorithms for detecting oral cancer using reflectance and fluorescence spectroscopy. Ann Otol Rhinol Laryngol. 2009; 118(11):817–26.
61. Amelink A, Sterenborg HJCM, Roodenburg JLN, Witjes MJH. Non-invasive measurement of the microvascular properties of non-dysplastic and dysplastic oral leukoplakias by use of optical spectroscopy. Oral Oncol. 2011;47: 1165–70.
62. Roblyer D, Richards-Kortum R, Sokolov K, et al. Multispectral optical imaging device for in vivo detection of oral neoplasia. J Biomed Opt. 2008;13(2):024019.
63. Pierce M, Yu D, Richards-Kortum R. High-resolution fiber-optic microendoscopy for in situ cellular imaging. J Vis Exp. 2011;47:e2306. doi:10.3791/2306.
64. Lane PM, Gilhuly T, Whitehead P, et al. Simple device for the direct visualization of oral-cavity tissue fluorescence. J Biomed Opt. 2006; 11(2):024006.
65. Poh CF, Ng SP, Williams PM, et al. Direct fluorescence visualization of clinically occult high-risk oral premalignant disease using a simple hand-held device. Head Neck. 2007; 29:71–6.
66. Awan KH, Morgan PR, Warnakulasuriya S. Evaluation of an autofluorescence based imaging system (VELscope™) in the detection of oral potentially malignant disorders and benign keratoses. Oral Oncol. 2011;47:274–7.
67. Onizawa K, Yoshida H, Saginoya H. Chromatic analysis of autofluorescence emitted from squamous cell carcinomas arising in the oral cavity: a preliminary study. Int J Oral Maxillofac Surg. 2000;29:42–6.
68. Bedard N, Schwarz RA, Hu A, et al. Multimodal snapshot spectral imaging for oral cancer diagnostics: a pilot study. Biomed Opt Express. 2013;4(6):938–49.
69. Marín NM, MacKinnon N, MacAulay C, et al. Calibration standards for multicenter clinical trials of fluorescence spectroscopy for in vivo diagnosis. J Biomed Opt. 2006;11(1): 014010.
70. de Veld DCG, Witjes MJH, Sterenborg HJCM, Roodenburg JLN. The status of in vivo autofluorescence spectroscopy and imaging for oral oncology. Oral Oncol. 2005;41:117–31.
71. Pavlova I, Weber CR, Schwarz RA, Williams MD, Gillenwater AM, Richards-Kortum R. Fluorescence spectroscopy of oral tissue: Monte Carlo modeling with site-specific tissue properties. J Biomed Opt. 2009;14(1): 014009.
72. Gray LV, Schwarz RA, Richards-Kortum R. Imaging as a tool for global cancer control. Comput Med Imaging Graph. 2013;37: 195–6.

Chapter 27

Elastic Scattering Spectroscopy for Thyroid Disease

Jennifer E. Rosen and Nicholas J. Giordano

Abbreviations

μm	Micrometers
ATC	Anaplastic thyroid cancer
BMC	Boston Medical Center
BUSM	Boston University School of Medicine
ESS	Elastic light-scattering spectroscopy
DTC	Differentiated thyroid cancer
FNA	Fine needle aspiration
FNAB	Fine needle aspiration biopsy
FTC	Follicular thyroid cancer
IRB	Institutional Review Board
MTC	Medullary thyroid cancer
NIH	National Institutes of Health
nm	Nanometers
NPV	Negative predictive value
PCA	Principal component analysis
PPV	Positive predictive value
PTC	Papillary thyroid cancer
SVM	Support vector mechanisms
T3	Triiodothyronine
T4	Thyroxine
TSH	Thyroid stimulating hormone

Introduction

The Normal Function of the Thyroid Gland

The thyroid gland is anatomically located in the neck, just below the laryngeal prominence, or what's more commonly referred to as the "Adam's apple." The thyroid is a bilobed, butterfly-shaped organ that is connected by an isthmus that wraps around the larynx. The cells of the thyroid gland are arranged in round follicles,

Brian J.-F. Wong and Justus Ilgner (eds.), *Biomedical Optics in Otorhinolaryngology: Head and Neck Surgery*,
DOI 10.1007/978-1-4939-1758-7_27, © Springer Science+Business Media New York 2016

surrounding a central core of colloid material and are themselves surrounded by perifollicular c-cells which secrete calcitonin.

The thyroid has a wide range of functions in the human body and is one of the largest endocrine glands. Thyroid function is critical because thyroid hormone regulates metabolic rates, protein synthesis, and organ function. The main products of the follicular cells of the thyroid gland are two hormones: triiodothyronine (T_3) and thyroxine (T_4). These hormones principally affect the regulation of metabolism within the body.

The production of T_3 and T_4 is regulated by another hormone in the body, thyroid stimulating hormone (TSH) released by the pituitary gland. There is a negative-feedback loop between the amounts of TSH and T_4 production to regulate normal body functions.

Thyroid Disorders

There are three main thyroid disorders.

1) Hyperthyroidism—an overactive thyroid
2) Hypothyroidism—an underactive thyroid
3) Thyroid Nodule—a thyroid neoplasm

Hyperthyroidism is primarily caused from an overproduction of the main thyroid hormones, T_3 and T_4. There is a lack of the negative feedback mechanism which would normally inhibit the production of thyroid hormones. Hypothyroidism usually occurs when not enough T_3 or T_4 is naturally produced by the body. All three of these thyroid disorders may present with an enlarged thyroid gland, also referred to as a goiter. Our discussion here will primarily focus on thyroid nodules and the use of spectroscopy, in particular elastic scattering spectroscopy, for diagnosis and treatment.

Thyroid Nodules

Thyroid nodules are common. At 60 years of age, approximately 50 % of the population has at least one thyroid nodule [1, 2]. The clinical spectrum of a presenting thyroid nodule can range from a small, singular incidental nodule or a large, symptomatic, pressure-inducing mass that can take up the near entirety of a thyroid lobe. Thyroid nodules can be single or multiple. It is important to evaluate the function of the thyroid gland in patients with thyroid nodules, best done by drawing a serum TSH level, to determine if the patient is euthyroid, hyperthyroid, or hypothyroid as this alters the differential diagnosis and subsequent management.

Thyroid Cancer

Approximately, 5 % of thyroid nodules are found to be malignant [3]. There are four main histologic types of thyroid cancer. (1) Papillary thyroid cancer, (2) follicular thyroid cancer, (3) medullary thyroid cancer, and (4) anaplastic thyroid cancer.

Papillary thyroid cancer (PTC) is by far the most common of all thyroid cancers, occurring in approximately 80 % of the cases [4, 5]. Females are three times as likely to be diagnosed with PTC and it is usually not an aggressive cancer. Diagnosis of this particular form of cancer typically occurs between the ages of 30 and 50 years of age. Nearly 22 % of patients with PTC are found to have evidence of metastatic spread to the surrounding lymph nodes at the time of diagnosis [6–10].

Follicular thyroid cancer (FTC) makes up approximately 15 % of all thyroid cancers and also arises from the follicular cells of the thyroid gland [11, 12]. Similar to PTC, females are three times more likely to be diagnosed with this particular cancer. This particular type of cancer can be more aggressive, especially in older patients. FTC is typically diagnosed in individuals from 40 to 60 years of age. FTC more commonly spreads hematogenously (through the bloodstream) to areas such as bone, brain, or lung.

Papillary and follicular thyroid cancers arise from the follicular cells themselves which make up the thyroid gland. They are usually grouped as "differentiated thyroid cancer" or DTC.

Medullary thyroid cancer (MTC) occurs in approximately 10 % of all thyroid cancers [13]. This form of thyroid cancer is found to have an incidence equal in the female and male population and is found to have a 50 % 5-year survival rate for stage IV cancer. MTC is often diagnosed in patients between 40 and 50 years of age. Medullary thyroid cancer arises from the perifollicular "c" cells and can often be found in patients with the RET gene mutation, in patients with familial thyroid cancer, or in the setting of an abnormal calcitonin level.

Anaplastic thyroid cancer (ATC) is rare, occurring in less than 5 % of thyroid nodules [14, 15]. It is found to have a higher occurrence in females and is the most invasive and aggressive form of thyroid cancer. The 5-year survival rate with ATC is approximately 7 % and is typically diagnosed in patients of the age of 65. The cells of origin are not clearly identified, but most likely are dedifferentiated follicular cells.

Thyroid cancer is the most common form of endocrine malignancy in the United States. An estimated 60,000 new cases of thyroid cancer will be diagnosed in 2013 [4, 5]. Incidence rates of thyroid cancer have been growing by 7 % each year [16–18]. These growing rates of thyroid cancer may be in part due to advancements in imaging techniques such as neck ultrasonography [19, 20], but a concomitant increase in thyroid neoplasms of all sizes has occurred

[16]. Despite an increase in incidence, there is a stable mortality rate from thyroid cancer [4, 16].

Evaluating Thyroid Nodules to Determine Malignancy

Patients found to have a thyroid nodule, either by palpation or by radiologic studies, should undergo evaluation by a trained physician [2, 21]. A complete history and physical exam including the thyroid gland and adjacent cervical lymph nodes should be performed, as this will alter the diagnosis and treatment of the patient. Serum TSH should be measured in the initial evaluation. Patients should undergo ultrasound evaluation of their thyroid gland [19, 20]. Patients when appropriate should undergo ultrasound-guided fine needle aspiration biopsy of their suspicious thyroid nodule. This allows for the removal of cells/tissue that then undergoes evaluation by cytopathology. A FNA is comprised of a nonsterile procedure in which a patient has a series of biopsy needles, usually 23 gauge or greater, inserted through the skin into their thyroid gland and directed to the worrisome nodule with ultrasound guidance. Each needle is used to collect cells from the thyroid, and those cells are then either smeared on a slide or placed in preservation fluid and evaluated by pathology. Specimens are first determined to be diagnostic or nondiagnostic based on the number of cells and clusters which are criteria for adequacy [22]. The benign category of cytology is by far the most common.

The diagnostic accuracy of a FNA not only depends on the clinical sensitivity of the test but also on the operator (i.e., the person performing the FNAB). Patients with nondiagnostic aspirates may either undergo close observation and subsequent rebiopsy or may undergo surgery for the purpose of diagnosis.

In 2009, the National Institutes of Health Consensus Conference published their reference statement on the Bethesda System for Reporting Thyroid Cytopathology [22–24]. The purpose of this was to allow for synoptic reporting and commonality of language across thyroid cytopathology. Until this time the language used in reporting out cytology widely varied and practitioners had to determine their individual institutions' likelihood of malignancy in these categories.

Aspirates determined to be "adequate" or "diagnostic" then are reported as malignant, benign or "indeterminate." About 5 % of thyroid FNAB cytology are read as "malignant." Patients with malignant nodules are usually recommended to undergo surgery for treatment of their cancer. Patients with a "malignant" thyroid FNAB cytology are usually found to have papillary thyroid cancer. Determination of follicular cancer or Hũrthle cell cancer is made on the final postoperative surgical pathology, as the capsular lining of the nodule needs to be entirely examined for any areas of spread to make this diagnosis. Cytology alone cannot determine follicular cancer or Hũrthle cell cancer for this reason. Patients with benign nodules may also undergo surgery for symptomatic reasons, if there are other worrisome nodules, or if the nodule is large in size and sampling error may be a concern.

The category of "indeterminate" was further broken down based on increasing risk of malignancy: in order, this is atypia of uncertain significance, follicular lesion of uncertain significance, follicular neoplasm/suspicious for follicular neoplasm, Hurthle cell neoplasm and suspicious for malignancy. It now may appear that the category "atypia of uncertain significance" may have a higher rate of malignancy than previously recognized. Patients with "indeterminate" biopsies often undergo surgery for the purpose of diagnosis alone. FNA biopsy is, therefore a good screening test for cancer, but its predictive value is low in that the technique has a high rate of false positives (indeterminates) which leads to a high number of diagnostic operations.

Patients who are known to have the diagnosis of thyroid cancer before surgery usually undergo ultrasound evaluation of the central and lateral neck and may undergo a central neck lymph node dissection at the time of their thyroidectomy [19, 20]. Patients who are not known to have a certain diagnosis, i.e., the patients with "indeterminate" biopsies undergoing surgery for diagnostic purposes, do not usually have central node dissections. Since about 35 % of patients with "indeterminate" biopsies are found to actually have a malignancy when their thyroid gland is examined postoperatively, they have in essence been undertreated and potentially understaged [25]. For the 65 % of patients with "indeterminate" biopsies who are found to have benign disease, they have had to take on the potential risks of the operation and may necessitate lifelong thyroid hormone replacement. Clearly, an adjunct to improve preoperative diagnosis is needed to reduce costs and improve quality of life.

A number of adjunctive modalities have been evaluated, including radiologic imaging, ultrasound elastography [26, 27], and a series of different types of molecular markers [25, 28, 29]. Although many of these are commercially available, none have 100 % accuracy, often require a send-away test that may take weeks to return and delay treatment and are operator dependent. For that reason, we and others have turned to the use of spectral guidance and diagnostic capabilities to improve on-site, point-of-care determination of malignancy of patients with thyroid nodules.

Elastic Scattering Spectroscopy

Elastic scattering spectroscopy (ESS) is an optical imaging technique which uses broadband light to take measurements [30]. The broadband light is from 300 to 800 nm wavelengths including regions of ultraviolet, visible, and infrared light. Broadband light is nonionizing with no known negative side effects [31, 32]. ESS has been used to aid in diagnosis in other organs and tissues in the body including the esophagus [33–35], oral cavity lesions [36], breast tissue [37–41], and colonic polyps [42, 43]. In all of these studies, ESS was found to distinguish benign from malignant spectra with a high degree of accuracy.

ESS works by emitting photons to make a point measurement. A cartoon graphic below depicts the basic functions of ESS in a dual fiber (source–detector) setup (Fig. 1).

The photon carries with it information about its traveled path, and when compiled and displayed on a computer, this displays a spectrum. The spectrum is a visual representation of the matter that the photon traveled through. This spectrum represents that point measurements that ESS took and is directly affected by the size and density of the organelle with which the photon interacted.

ESS is capable of performing an "optical biopsy" because this optical method is sensitive to most of the features that pathologists look for under the microscope [44]. Cellular and subcellular components like the nucleus, nucleolus, and mitochondria are represented and accounted for in the ESS optical spectrum. Through studying ESS in other organs and tissues it has been found that ESS is sensitive to both cellular and subcellular morphological features and therefore features associated with malignant transformation are detected by ESS [42].

US-guided FNAB is a good screening tool for malignant nodules in the thyroid and has a high negative predictive value for malignant thyroid tissue [45, 46]. However, US-guided thyroid FNAB

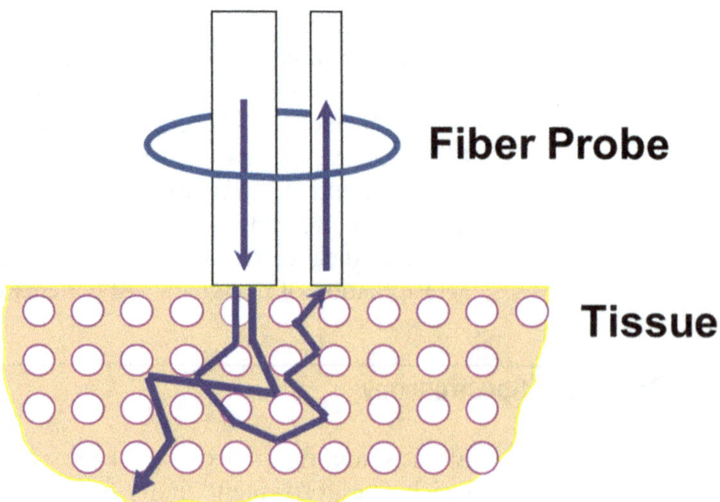

Fig. 1 A cartoon graphic demonstrating the scattering of light upon interaction with a tissue of interest

has a low specificity and low positive predictive value [47]. With the established sensitivity of ESS and its ability to detect morphological changes in tissue beyond the spectra currently visible to pathologists, ESS may provide a unique optical solution to diagnosing thyroid cancer.

Background on Elastic Scattering Spectroscopy

Photonics can be used to identify thyroid tissue based on several optical properties, most of which are wavelength dependent. These include absorption, anisotropy factor, elastic scattering, fluorescence, inelastic scattering, phase function, and reduced scattering coefficient.

Refractive index elastic scattering spectroscopy (ESS) works through analyzing the interaction of electromagnetic radiation with miniaturized optical resonators found in the tissue of interest. For biomedical applications, the targets of ESS are often cellular or subcellular in size placing the interaction of light on the microscopic scale. The spectrum attained with ESS has four main variables based upon the tissue with which it interacts: (1) size, (2) shape, (3) optical properties, and (4) wavelength of incident light. Combined, these four variables make up the majority of differentiation between spectra attained in biological tissue. The clinical utility of ESS is only starting to emerge as biomedicine is adopting and recognizing the clinical utility of this technology. Near-instant feedback and nonionizing radiation make this imaging technique an attractive candidate in the rapidly changing field of biomedicine.

ESS works off of differentiating tissues based on the scattering properties of different mediums, which is defined by the scattering coefficient (μ_s). The scattering coefficient defines the probability a photon has of being scattered per a unit length. When a tissue scatters light, there are multiple possible paths through the tissue and, therefore, a variety of possible distances photons can travel on their path from the source to the detector. Distances traveled by photons will depend upon the tissue of interests' scattering angle probability and how many scattering events occurred upon the path from the source to detector. This finding provides a method to obtain information about the tissue with which the light interacts.

Biological Applications of ESS

For ESS, tissue is treated as a turbid medium. Measurements of optical properties are done on a bulk scale within tissues. This is important because multiple particles, often of varying size will be measured together. One of the inherit properties of ESS is that it can characterize particles beyond the diffraction limit of the optical system [48–50]. These types of scattering involve no loss or gain of energy by radiation, but may produce multiple scattering events by having a single scatterer interact with a scattering center. This event of multiple scattering is analogous to diffusion.

One of the first investigations of the structure of living cells that used light scattering spectroscopy came from the work of Brunsting et al. in 1974 [51, 52]. The complex structure of a cell makes it a difficult object to identify with spectroscopy. Components of a cell range in size from a few nanometers to the size of the cell itself, approximately 100 μm. Each component within a cell may have a wide variety of refractive indices. To the contrary, some studies have indicated that several cell structures have similar indices of refraction and therefore can be viewed as a single object.

ESS is defined by Rayleigh and Mie scattering [53, 54]. Rayleigh scattering occurs when the particle measured is much smaller than the wavelength of the incident light. Therefore, Rayleigh scattering is strongly dependent on size. Mie scattering occurs over a broader spectrum of light and explains scattering events which occur with particles that have a diameter which is slightly smaller, equal to, or larger than the wavelength of the incident light. Approximations of Mie theory allow for solutions to particles of a variety of shapes. Mie theory is sensitive to particle size, but not shape.

Signals of light scattering spectroscopy (LSS) from the micro to the nanoscale structures of cells present unique structure-dependent patterns in wavelength. It has been proven that LSS is sensitive enough to detect slight changes in tissue architecture [55].

Typically, with ESS several millimeters of a tissue is illuminated with broadband light, and the spectra obtained from the scattering particles represents information on the average-sized particles within the several millimeter field of view. However, this application of ESS is not always ideal, as in cancer diagnostics. Numerous investigators have developed optical techniques to link local microstructures with scattering features. Recently, an optical method for ESS has been developed to detect distinct and localized scattering features of a single particle [56].

ESS has recently been studied for its ability to diagnose thyroid cancer. In 2011, we reported on our findings from an ex vivo trial that ESS could discriminate benign from malignant thyroid nodules with a high degree of accuracy [45]. We then developed a miniaturized version of the ESS tool to fit through the center of a 23-gauge needle. This would enable ESS readings to be collected at the same time as fine needle aspiration biopsy without changing clinician practice in a significant fashion. The smaller optical geometry of the probe made measurements more sensitive to Rayleigh scattering and allowed for the insertion of the device into a biopsy needle [46]. Done in conjunction with cytology, results of this demonstrated that applications of ESS can very well be applied as an efficient, nonionizing imaging technique to provide cancer diagnostics in real time.

The question remains as to the biological underpinnings of the ESS spectra. A small portion can be accounted for by hemoglobin absorption, as the thyroid gland is a highly vascular organ and thyroid cancer is a vascular entity. In most forms of thyroid cancer, the normal follicular morphology with a ring of cells around a center of reflective colloid material is lost and the cells become more densely packed. The nuclei become irregular with nuclear inclusions, grooves and psammoma bodies, all of which are likely to change the reflective and absorptive capacity of the gland. The ESS appearance of different components including calcifications and cystic material also becomes clearly abnormal (Fig. 2).

As the field of translational biomedical photonics steadily advances over the next several years, ESS may be employed in clinical settings to aid as a diagnostic tool for cancer. In vivo spectroscopy appears to have the sensitivity to identify individual cell types, the ability to provide data in real time, and proven ability to differentiate between benign and malignant thyroid tissue with a high degree of accuracy. With further validation, ESS shows promise of

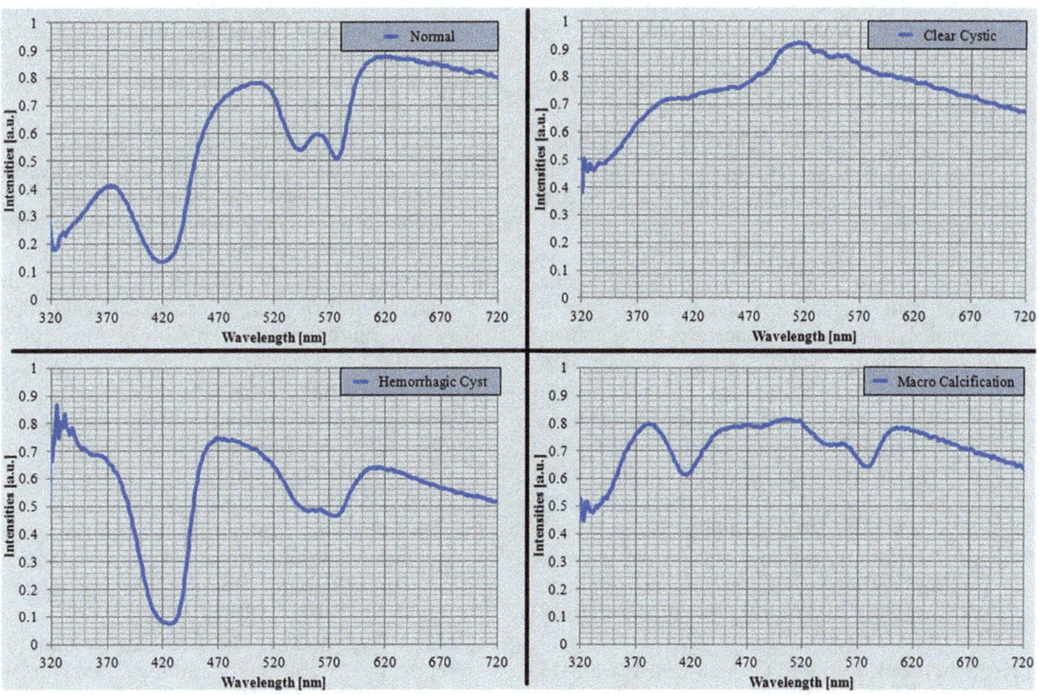

Fig. 2 Spectral pattern of ESS data collected during thyroid ultrasound-guided fine needle aspiration using integrated ESS-biopsy syringe demonstrates a distinctly different appearance of (**a**) normal, (**b**) cystic, (**c**) hemorrhagic cyst, and (**d**) microcalcifications

becoming an important tool for diagnosing thyroid cancer and aiding in the management of patients with thyroid nodules. Because of the use of preoperative needle-guided cytology, the potential exists to test and use additional forms of miniaturized spectroscopy as well.

References

1. Tunbridge WM, Evered DC, Hall R, et al. The spectrum of thyroid disease in a community: the Whickham survey. Clin Endocrinol. 1977;7:481–93.
2. Cooper DS, Doherty GM, Haugen BR, et al. Revised American Thyroid Association management guidelines for patients with thyroid nodules and differentiated thyroid cancer. Thyroid. 2009;19:1167–214.
3. Hegedus L. Clinical practice. The thyroid nodule. N Engl J Med. 2004;351:1764–71.
4. Siegel R, Ma J, Zou Z, Jemal A. Cancer statistics, 2014. CA Cancer J Clin. 2014;64:9–29.
5. Jemal A, Simard EP, Dorell C, et al. Annual report to the nation on the status of cancer, 1975–2009, featuring the burden and trends in human papillomavirus (HPV)-associated cancers and HPV vaccination coverage levels. J Natl Cancer Inst. 2013;105(10):749–50.
6. Qubain SW, Nakano S, Baba M, Takao S, Aikou T. Distribution of lymph node micrometastasis in pN0 well-differentiated thyroid carcinoma. Surgery. 2002;131:249–56.
7. Grebe SK, Hay ID. Thyroid cancer nodal metastases: biologic significance and therapeutic considerations. Surg Oncol Clin N Am. 1996;5:43–63.
8. Scheumann GF, Gimm O, Wegener G, Hundeshagen H, Dralle H. Prognostic significance and surgical management of locoregional lymph node metastases in papillary thyroid cancer. World J Surg. 1994;18:559–67. Discussion 67-8.
9. Hay ID, Grant CS, van Heerden JA, Goellner JR, Ebersold JR, Bergstralh EJ. Papillary thyroid microcarcinoma: a study of 535 cases observed in a 50-year period. Surgery. 1992;112:1139–46. Discussion 46-7.
10. Ito Y, Uruno T, Nakano K, et al. An observation trial without surgical treatment in patients with papillary microcarcinoma of the thyroid. Thyroid. 2003;13:381–7.
11. Aschebrook-Kilfoy B, Grogan RH, Ward MH, Kaplan E, Devesa SS. Follicular thyroid cancer incidence patterns in the United States, 1980–2009. Thyroid. 2013;23:1015–21.
12. Ban EJ, Andrabi A, Grodski S, Yeung M, McLean C, Serpell J. Follicular thyroid cancer: minimally invasive tumours can give rise to metastases. ANZ J Surg. 2012;82:136–9.
13. American Thyroid Association Guidelines Task Force, Kloos RT, Eng C, et al. Medullary thyroid cancer: management guidelines of the American Thyroid Association. Thyroid. 2009;19:565–612.
14. Aldehaim M, Mahmood R, Hussain F, et al. Anaplastic thyroid cancer: a retrospective analysis of 120 cases. Gulf J Oncol. 2014;1:32–7.
15. Haymart MR, Banerjee M, Yin H, Worden F, Griggs JJ. Marginal treatment benefit in anaplastic thyroid cancer. Cancer. 2013;119:3133–9.
16. Davies L, Welch HG. Current thyroid cancer trends in the United States. JAMA Otolaryngol Head Neck Surg. 2014;140:317–22.
17. Ito Y, Nikiforov YE, Schlumberger M, Vigneri R. Increasing incidence of thyroid cancer: controversies explored. Nat Rev Endocrinol. 2013;9:178–84.
18. Sosa JA, Hanna JW, Robinson KA, Lanman RB. Increases in thyroid nodule fine-needle aspirations, operations, and diagnoses of thyroid cancer in the United States. Surgery. 2013;154:1420–6. Discussion 6-7.
19. Fish SA, Langer JE, Mandel SJ. Sonographic imaging of thyroid nodules and cervical lymph nodes. Endocrinol Metab Clin N Am. 2008; 37:401–17, ix.
20. Frates MC, Benson CB, Charboneau JW, et al. Management of thyroid nodules detected at US: society of radiologists in ultrasound consensus conference statement. Ultrasound Q. 2006;22:231–8. Discussion 9-40.
21. Alexander EK, Cooper D. The importance, and important limitations, of ultrasound imaging for evaluating thyroid nodules. JAMA Intern Med. 2013;173:1796–7.
22. Cibas ES, Ali SZ. The Bethesda system for reporting thyroid cytopathology. Am J Clin Pathol. 2009;132:658–65.
23. Cibas ES, Baloch ZW, Fellegara G, et al. A prospective assessment defining the limitations

of thyroid nodule pathologic evaluation. Ann Intern Med. 2013;159:325–32.

24. Cibas ES, Sanchez MA. The National Cancer Institute thyroid fine-needle aspiration state-of-the-science conference: inspiration for a uniform terminology linked to management guidelines. Cancer. 2008;114:71–3.
25. Alexander EK, Kennedy GC, Baloch ZW, et al. Preoperative diagnosis of benign thyroid nodules with indeterminate cytology. N Engl J Med. 2012;367:705–15.
26. Lyshchik A, Higashi T, Asato R, et al. Thyroid gland tumor diagnosis at US elastography. Radiology. 2005;237:202–11.
27. Rago T, Santini F, Scutari M, Pinchera A, Vitti P. Elastography: new developments in ultrasound for predicting malignancy in thyroid nodules. J Clin Endocrinol Metab. 2007;92:2917–22.
28. Nikiforov YE, Ohori NP, Hodak SP, et al. Impact of mutational testing on the diagnosis and management of patients with cytologically indeterminate thyroid nodules: a prospective analysis of 1056 FNA samples. J Clin Endocrinol Metab. 2011;96:3390–7.
29. Nikiforova MN, Wald AI, Roy S, Durso MB, Nikiforov YE. Targeted next-generation sequencing panel (ThyroSeq) for detection of mutations in thyroid cancer. J Clin Endocrinol Metab. 2013;98:E1852–60.
30. Joshi S, Singh-Moon RP, Wang M, et al. Transient cerebral hypoperfusion assisted intraarterial cationic liposome delivery to brain tissue. J Neuro-Oncol. 2014;118:73–82.
31. Mourant JR, Fuselier T, Boyer J, Johnson TM, Bigio IJ. Predictions and measurements of scattering and absorption over broad wavelength ranges in tissue phantoms. Appl Opt. 1997;36:949–57.
32. Mourant JR, Johnson TM, Los G, Bigio IJ. Non-invasive measurement of chemotherapy drug concentrations in tissue: preliminary demonstrations of in vivo measurements. Phys Med Biol. 1999;44:1397–417.
33. Lovat LB, Johnson K, Mackenzie GD, et al. Elastic scattering spectroscopy accurately detects high grade dysplasia and cancer in Barrett's oesophagus. Gut. 2006;55:1078–83.
34. Zhu Y, Fearn T, Mackenzie G, et al. Elastic scattering spectroscopy for detection of cancer risk in Barrett's esophagus: experimental and clinical validation of error removal by orthogonal subtraction for increasing accuracy. J Biomed Opt. 2009;14:044022.
35. Rodriguez-Diaz E, Bigio IJ, Singh SK. Integrated optical tools for minimally invasive diagnosis and treatment at gastrointestinal endoscopy. Robot Comput Integr Manuf. 2011;27:249–56.
36. Sharwani A, Jerjes W, Salih V, et al. Assessment of oral premalignancy using elastic scattering spectroscopy. Oral Oncol. 2006;42:343–9.
37. Bigio IJ, Bown SG, Briggs G, et al. Diagnosis of breast cancer using elastic-scattering spectroscopy: preliminary clinical results. J Biomed Opt. 2000;5:221–8.
38. Johnson KS, Chicken DW, Pickard DC, et al. Elastic scattering spectroscopy for intraoperative determination of sentinel lymph node status in the breast. J Biomed Opt. 2004;9:1122–8.
39. Austwick MR, Clark B, Mosse CA, et al. Scanning elastic scattering spectroscopy detects metastatic breast cancer in sentinel lymph nodes. J Biomed Opt. 2010;15:047001.
40. Keshtgar MR, Chicken DW, Austwick MR, et al. Optical scanning for rapid intraoperative diagnosis of sentinel node metastases in breast cancer. Br J Surg. 2010;97:1232–9.
41. Bigio IJ. Real-time pathology to guide breast surgery: seeing alone is not believing. Clin Cancer Res. 2012;18:6083–5.
42. Dhar A, Johnson KS, Novelli MR, et al. Elastic scattering spectroscopy for the diagnosis of colonic lesions: initial results of a novel optical biopsy technique. Gastrointest Endosc. 2006;63:257–61.
43. Rodriguez-Diaz E, Castanon DA, Singh SK, Bigio IJ. Spectral classifier design with ensemble classifiers and misclassification-rejection: application to elastic-scattering spectroscopy for detection of colonic neoplasia. J Biomed Opt. 2011;16:067009.
44. Mourant JR, Boyer J, Hielscher AH, Bigio IJ. Influence of the scattering phase function on light transport measurements in turbid media performed with small source-detector separations. Opt Lett. 1996;21:546–8.
45. Suh H, A'Amar O, Rodriguez-Diaz E, Lee S, Bigio I, Rosen JE. Elastic light-scattering spectroscopy for discrimination of benign from malignant disease in thyroid nodules. Ann Surg Oncol. 2011;18:1300–5.
46. Rosen J, Suh H, Giordano N, et al. Preoperative discrimination of benign from malignant disease in thyroid nodules with indeterminate cytology using elastic light-scattering spectroscopy. IEEE Trans Biomed Eng. 2013;61:2336–40.

47. Yip L. Molecular diagnostic testing and the indeterminate thyroid nodule. Curr Opin Oncol. 2014;26:8–13.
48. Boustany NN, Boppart SA, Backman V. Microscopic imaging and spectroscopy with scattered light. Annu Rev Biomed Eng. 2010;12:285–314.
49. Itzkan I, Qiu L, Fang H, et al. Confocal light absorption and scattering spectroscopic microscopy monitors organelles in live cells with no exogenous labels. Proc Natl Acad Sci U S A. 2007;104:17255–60.
50. Fang H, Qiu L, Vitkin E, et al. Confocal light absorption and scattering spectroscopic microscopy. Appl Opt. 2007;46:1760–9.
51. Brunsting A. Can light-scattering techniques be applied to flow-through cell analysis? J Histochem Cytochem. 1974;22:607–15.
52. Brunsting A, Mullaney PF. Differential light scattering from spherical mammalian cells. Biophys J. 1974;14:439–53.
53. Castagner JL, Bigio IJ. Particle sizing with a fast polar nephelometer. Appl Opt. 2007;46:527–32.
54. Mulvey CS, Sherwood CA, Bigio IJ. Wavelength-dependent backscattering measurements for quantitative real-time monitoring of apoptosis in living cells. J Biomed Opt. 2009;14:064013.
55. Li X, Chen Z, Taflove A, Backman V. Optical analysis of nanoparticles via enhanced backscattering facilitated by 3-D photonic nanojets. Opt Express. 2005;13:526–33.
56. Liu Y, Li X, Kim YL, Backman V. Elastic backscattering spectroscopic microscopy. Opt Lett. 2005;30:2445–7.

Chapter 28

Fluorescence Imaging (Auto and Enhanced)

Christian Stephan Betz, Anna Englhard, Veronika Volgger, and Andreas Leunig

Reasons for Optical Screening

The earlier a tumor of the upper aerodigestive tract (UADT) gets diagnosed and treated, the better the prognosis. Unfortunately, however, early lesions tend to remain silent for a long period, which often delays the first presentation to a medical professional, so about two-thirds of UADT cancers are first detected at an advanced tumor stage. Extensive screening programs of patients at risk might be helpful to ameliorate the situation. However, even if those individuals with premalignant or early invasive lesions do see a medical doctor or other trained care worker, misdiagnosis is still possible due to the following reasons:

- Being typical precancerous conditions, leuko- and erythroplakias are usually easily detectable by visual inspection, and it is generally understood that upon detection one or more representative tissue biopsies are taken in order to establish a histopathological diagnosis. If no dysplasia or early invasive growth is found, the lesion is either removed in a minimally invasive fashion or just followed up closely without any intervention. If a more severe pathology is confirmed, the lesion is resected according to common guidelines with a safety margin of 0.5 cm. As different pathologies can be present within the same lesions, however, mis-sampling can lead to an underestimation of the severity of the condition and thus to a delay of adequate treatment.

Brian J.-F. Wong and Justus Ilgner (eds.), *Biomedical Optics in Otorhinolaryngology: Head and Neck Surgery*,
DOI 10.1007/978-1-4939-1758-7_28, © Springer Science+Business Media New York 2016

- Other mucosal cancers arise directly from macroscopically innocuous mucosa and might—at least in early stages—appear as an ulcer, erosion, or even only slightly roughened healthy mucosa and do not yet display typical morphologic features of malignant tumors. Therefore, they may easily be mistaken for some chronic inflammatory condition or go by unnoticed altogether.

In order to improve the situation outlined above, high sensitivity screening tools have lately attracted considerable scientific attention, and implementation of some of these methods (such as fluorescence imaging) into clinical routine has recently been made possible by medically licensed and commercially available systems.

Basics of Fluorescence Imaging

Auto-fluorescence Imaging

Following adequate excitation, certain molecules within the tissue emit fluorescence to the surface that can be picked up using specialized equipment. The characteristics of the most important tissue "autofluorophores" are listed in Table 1.

As depicted, visible violet-blue excitation leads to the emission of fluorescence in the violet to green visible spectrum. Additionally, there are intermediate products of heme biosynthesis (porphyrins) that produce a bright red fluorescence. For the sake of completeness it should be mentioned that the amino acid tryptophan is another autofluorophore with excitation in the ultraviolet range, but has been omitted in the table and further text as it is not excited by commercially available fluorescence imaging systems.

While the porphyrins display a very narrow range of excitation and emission properties, FAD and NADH as well as the fluorescent structural proteins collagen, elastin, and keratin have relatively broad excitation and emission bands. Therefore, all of these molecules are excited by exposure to short-wave visible light, which is used in all of the commercially available autofluorescence imaging (AFI) systems.

A simplified schematic diagram of the complex principles that underlie the autofluorescence diagnosis of malignant tumors is displayed in Fig. 1. The green autofluorescence is thereby regularly diminished in cancerous tissue if compared to regular mucosa.

The main causes for this are thought to be threefold.

1. Most importantly, the structural proteins collagen and elastin as the main contributors to tissue autofluorescence are localized in the submucosal layer only, so the regular thickening of the epithelial layer in (pre)malignant mucosal lesions leads to a shielding of the discernable fluorescence.

Table 1
Excitation and emission peaks of the most important endogenous fluorophores (adapted from Wagnieres [1] and Chang [2])

Fluorophore	Cytological occurrence	Histological occurrence	Presence	Excitation peaks (nm)	Emission peaks (nm)
NADH	Intracellular	All layers	Always	260 + 350	440 + 450
FAD	Intracellular	All layers	Always	450	515
Collagen	Extracellular	Submucosa	Always	330	390
Elastin	Extracellular	Submucosa	Always	350	420
Keratin	Intra/ extracellular	Upper mucosa	In the presence of hyperkeratinization	340	430
Porphyrins	Intracellular	Superficial	In the presence of bacterial colonization	405	635

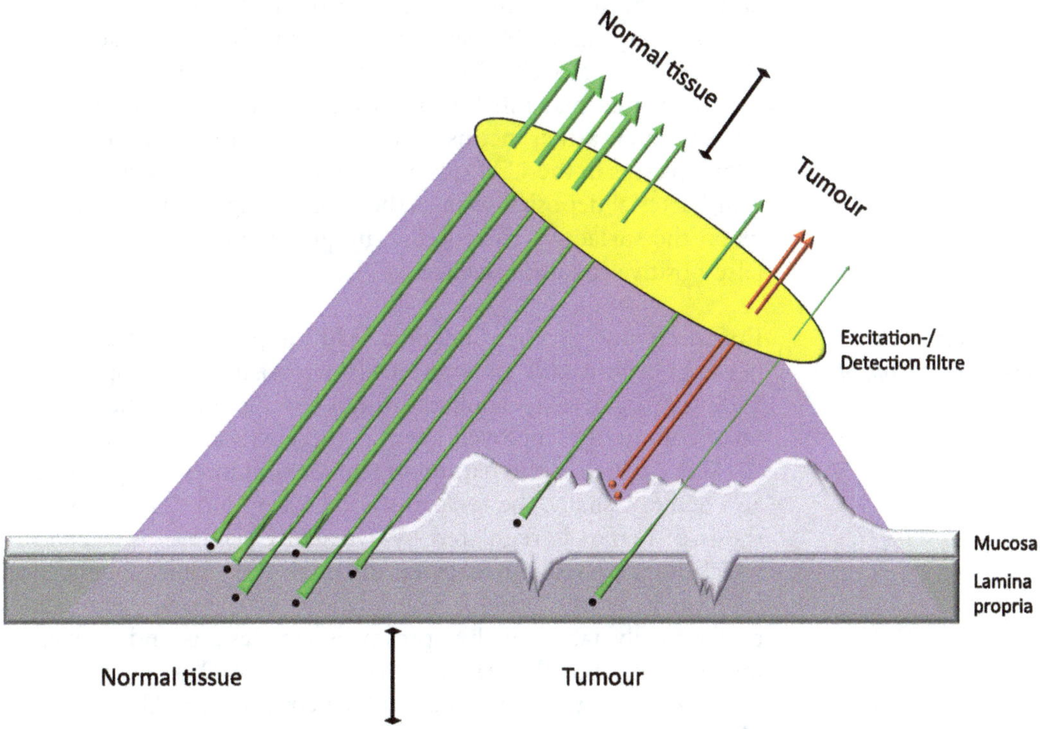

Fig. 1 Schematic representation of AFI based on the excitation of endogenous fluorophores in different tissue layers. Tumor tissue (*right*) differs from normal tissue in the following respects: (1) It contains smaller amounts of *green-fluorescent* fluorophores. (2) The intensity of the fluorescence is decreased by the thickened epithelial layer. (3) There is a variable amount of porphyrin-containing bacterial deposits that produce a *red fluorescence*

2. Furthermore, neoplastic tissue in the UADT has been shown to contain smaller concentrations of the intracellular, fluorescing enzymes NADH and FAD than normal tissue. Additionally, tumor tissue seems to have greater mitochondrial activity at its disposal than normal tissue; this shifts the balance from fluorescing NADH and FAD to the nonfluorescent compounds NAD and FADH.
3. A third factor that might also attribute to a reduction of autofluorescence signals over neoplastic mucosal lesions to a certain extent is an increased absorption of the excitation light by hemoglobin.

In clinical autofluorescence examinations, malignant lesions are therefore demarcated by a darker shade of green than their healthy surroundings.

The remaining two fluorescent molecules, which are present under certain circumstances only, are a common source of error in the interpretation of imaging results (Table 1). Keratin as a structural protein in cases of mucosal hyperkeratinization emits a pale green to whitish fluorescence when excited, but its occurrence is rather unspecific. Porphyrins show a bright red fluorescence, but they are of questionable value in the diagnosis of upper aerodigestive neoplasms as well. They are mainly produced by certain bacterial strains that may inhabit the surface of ulcerating tumors, so its distribution is rather inconsistent and nonhomogeneous on mucosal neoplasms in the UADT. In addition, other nonspecific fluorescent bacterial deposits, such as those occurring at gingival margins or on the surface of the tongue, frequently produce a confusing, false-positive red fluorescence.

Enhanced Fluorescence Imaging

Enhanced fluorescence imaging (EFI) implies that the contrast between healthy and (pre)cancerous mucosa in AFI is improved by adding exogenously applied, tumor-specific fluorophores. The most commonly employed agent is thereby 5-aminolevulinic acid (5-ALA), which is the natural precursor of fluorescent porphyrins and heme. Usually, the formation of 5-ALA (and thus the biosynthesis of heme) is regulated by a negative feedback mechanism, which is surpassed if it is given directly. After topical application (e.g., as a mouthwash for examinations of the oral cavity), it is preferentially taken up by (pre)malignant lesions and converted into strongly red fluorescent Protoporphyrin IX (PPIX). This is most likely due to (1) an enhanced penetration of 5-ALA into neoplastic tissue due to an impaired superficial lipid barrier, (2) an augmented conversion of 5-ALA into PPIX in malignant cells due to increased enzyme activities and (3) a retention of PPIX in malignant cells due to a reduced conversion into heme.

Figure 2 schematically illustrates EFI using exogenously applied 5-ALA-induced PPIX. Cancerous tissue is thereby not demarcated by a darker shade of green, but by bright red. This red-to-green contrast has been compared to a streetlight before (red: cancer, green: normal tissue).

Implementation of Fluorescence Imaging

To date, there are six commercially available systems on the market that can be used for clinical fluorescence imaging in the head and neck field: the D-Light C/AF System (KARL STORZ GmbH, Tuttlingen, Germany), the DAFE System (Richard Wolf, Knittlingen, Germany), the SAFE-3000 System (PENTAX Europe GmbH, Hamburg, Germany), the AFI-Lucera System (Olympus Deutschland GmbH, Hamburg, Germany), the VELScope Vx (Visually Enhanced Lesion Scope, LED Dental, White Rock, British Columbia, Canada), and the Identafi System (StarDental, DentalEZ Group, Malvern, PA, USA). The first four

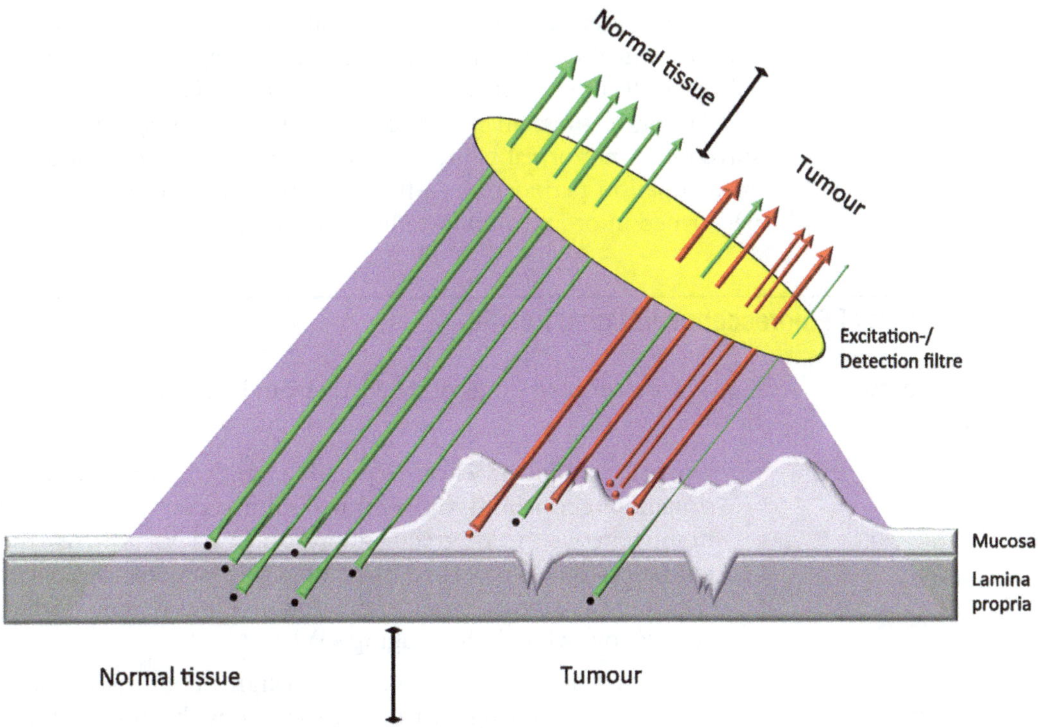

Fig. 2 Schematic representation of EFI using 5-ALA-induced PPIX. In addition to the principles described and illustrated for AFI in Fig. 5, which are also true for EFI, the right-sided cancerous tissue contains a much red-fluorescing PPIX than the left-sided healthy tissue

of those are endoscopic systems that are marketed for use in the UADT (especially the STORZ system) and the tracheobronchial tree (all four); the latter two are small, handheld devices that are advertised for oral examinations in dental offices. All six systems provide white light illumination and fluorescence excitation in the blue/near-UV.

The D-Light C/AF System is the only one marketed for AFI as well as EFI—the remaining five systems are designed for AFI only. Whereas the systems by STORZ, PENTAX, LED Dental, and StarDental perform a direct visualization of the detected fluorescence signals, the output of the Wolf system is a superimposed display of two separate detection ranges (500–590 nm and 600–700 nm) in false colors, and the Olympus system combines two reflectance images (at 550 nm and 610 nm) with the autofluorescence information in a combined display. The main properties of the four systems are presented in Table 2.

Both AFI and EFI can be performed under general anesthesia (e.g., if an invasive tissue biopsy of the lower pharynx or larynx is anticipated) as well as in awake patients, and the systems can easily be switched from white light into fluorescence mode and back.

For AFI, no special preparation is necessary, whereas EFI is performed after application and incubation of 5-ALA. For oral and oropharyngeal examinations, the substance is applied as a rinsing solution (200 mg 5-ALA dissolved in 50 ml of H_2O) for 15 min. For laryngeal sites, an inhalation of 5-ALA (30 mg 5-ALA dissolved in 5 ml normal saline) is performed. Following application, an incubation period of 1–2 h is kept before the examination is performed in order to achieve the best possible results.

Interpretation of Fluorescence Imaging Results

Auto-fluorescence Imaging

Autofluorescence findings of the UADT can be classified into three distinct groups:

- Normal autofluorescence: Regularly stratified, nonkeratinized squamous epithelium with a normal submucosa shows a typical homogeneous, pale green fluorescence (Fig. 3). As the excitation light is absorbed by hemoglobin, superficial capillaries show a greater contrast to the surroundings than in normal endoscopy (white light imaging = WLI).
- Decreased autofluorescence: (Pre)malignant mucosal lesions as well as other changes that are associated with a thickening of the mucosal layer are usually highlighted by a circumscribed area of diminished autofluorescence (Fig. 4). Thereby, tumor precursors cannot be distinguished from invasive cancers based on their autofluorescent properties. Inflammatory thickenings of the mucosa and other changes such as benign neoplasms,

Table 2
Comparison of commercially available systems for fluorescence imaging of the UADT

System	Suitable for	Excitation	Detection	Marketed for	Display	Setup
D-Light C/ AF System	AFI + EFI	375–440 nm	>475 nm	UADT + lung	Direct display of fluorescence	Endoscopic system (fiberoptic)
DAFE System	AFI	390–460 nm	500–590 + 600–700 nm	(UADT+) lung	False color image	Endoscopic system (fiberoptic)
SAFE-3000 System	AFI	408 nm	430–700 nm	(UADT+) lung	Direct display of fluorescence	Endoscopic system (chip on the tip)
AFI-Lucera Elite System	AFI	390–470 nm + 540–560 nm	490–700 nm	(UADT+) lung	Combined display (AFI and reflectance)	Endoscopic system (chip on the tip)
VELscope Vx	AFI	400–460 nm	>475 nm	Oral cavity	Direct display of fluorescence	Handheld device (excitation light and detection filters integrated)
Identafi System	AFI	405 nm (+545 nm)	?	Oral cavity	Direct display of fluorescence	Handheld device (excitation light integrated; special eyewear equipped with detection filters)

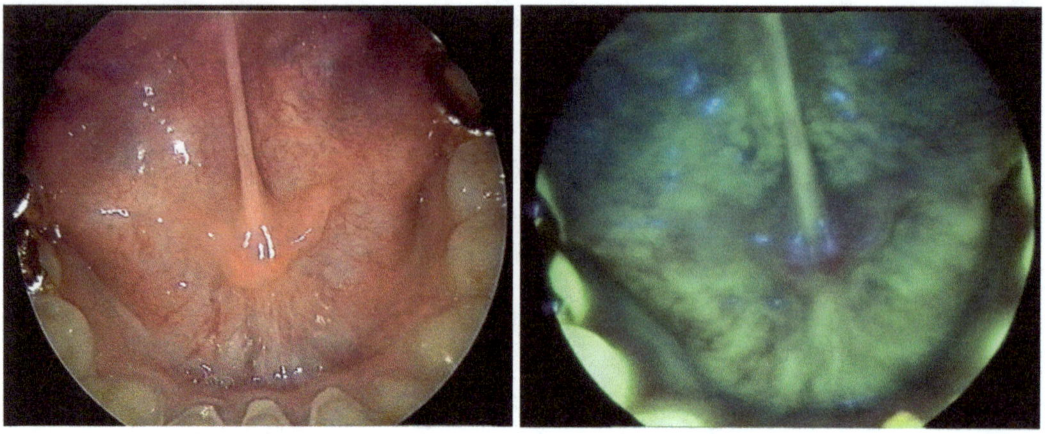

Fig. 3 Example for a finding with normal tissue autofluorescence from a healthy floor of mouth on the *right* and corresponding *white light image* on the *left*

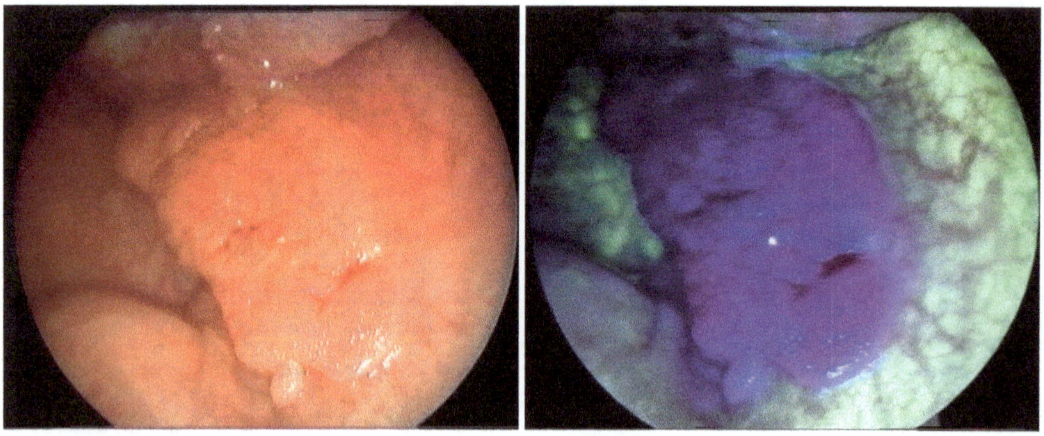

Fig. 4 Transoral view of a T2 squamous cell carcinoma of the *right* soft palate under *white light* on the *left* and in AFI on the *right*

submucous hemorrhages, and fibrotic changes due to previous surgery may also result in a decreased autofluorescence (Fig. 5). However, especially inflammatory lesions usually cause less well-defined areas of decreased autofluorescence than neoplastic changes, so that a differentiation is feasible in the hands of an experienced investigator.

- Increased autofluorescence: In cases of pathological, superficial mucosal keratinization, the strong green to white fluorescence of keratin becomes increasingly apparent, and is "masking" the fluorescence from underneath (Fig. 6). Therefore, heavily keratinized lesions (which may range from hyperkeratinized

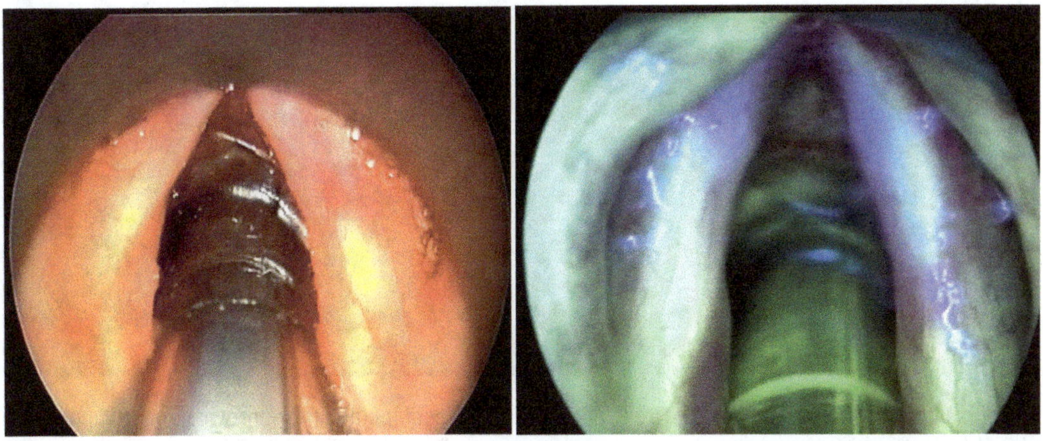

Fig. 5 Example for a "false-positive" reduction in autofluorescence intensities on the *right* side and corresponding WLI on the *left* side in a patient with chronic laryngitis

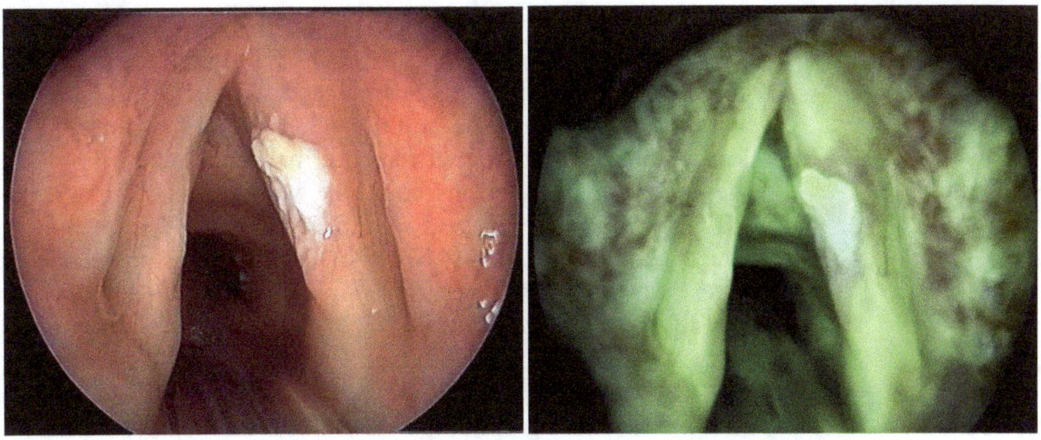

Fig. 6 Hyperkeratotic, highly dysplastic lesion of the right vocal cord (*left*: WLI, *right*: AFI)

normal epithelium all the way to invasive cancer in histopathology) cannot be further differentiated using AFI.

Enhanced Fluorescence Imaging

After adequate application and incubation of 5-ALA, normal tissue usually remains green (i.e., showing normal autofluorescence), whereas neoplastic tissue boasts a strong, red fluorescence based on the accumulation of PPIX (Fig. 7). The red-to-green "streetlight" contrast is thereby easily visible. Similar to AFI, the exact type and severity of the pathology cannot be differentiated, and inflammatory or other benign mucosal lesions tend to induce false-positive results. In addition, areas with a high grade of bacterial colonization (e.g., gingival margins, dorsum of tongue, etc.) often show "false-positive" red fluorescence, as does pre-irradiated tissue.

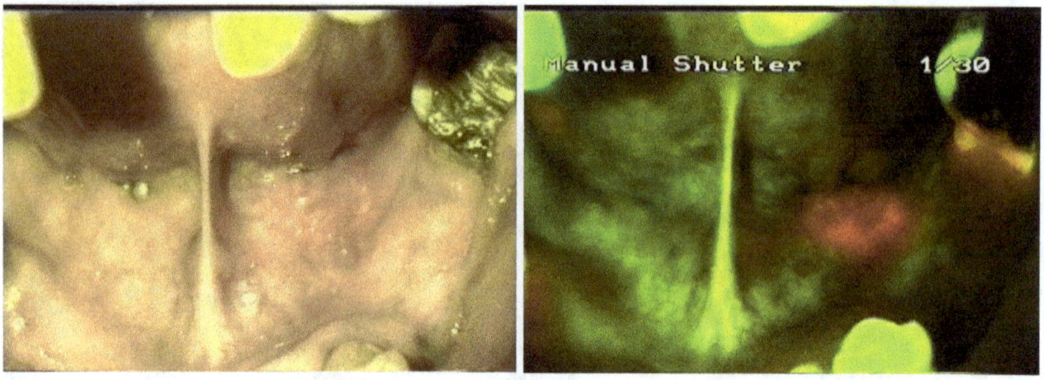

Fig. 7 Example of a T1 squamous cell carcinoma of the *left floor* of mouth. In EFI following topical application of 5-ALA, the tumor contrasts sharply with its normal surroundings (*left*: WLI; *right*: EFI)

Personal Experience

A: Oral and Oropharyngeal Lesions

Autofluorescence Imaging

In our own experience using the STORZ D-Light C/AF System on 128 patients with suspicious or cancerous lesions of the oral cavity or oropharynx, the additional use of AFI enabled us to clearly identify an additional ten (pre)malignant mucosal lesions. The (pre)malignant lesions could be well identified in 89.5 % (WLI) vs. 84.2 % (AFI) and superficially delimited from normal tissue in 37.9 % (WLI) vs. 57.9 % (AFI). The histopathological correlation of tissue biopsies from suspicious areas ($n=236$) yielded a sensitivity of 95.8 % (WLI) vs. 93.3 % (AFI). As no random tissue biopsies were taken, a reliable specificity could not be determined, yet it felt fairly low. AFI was very easily performed in addition to WLI and did not significantly alter the duration times of examination per patient.

Enhanced Fluorescence Imaging

In a publication from our group on 68 patients with high suspicion for—or histologically proven—SCC of the oral cavity or oropharynx and using the STORZ D-Light C/AF System, an additional eight (pre)malignant lesions were identified only because EFI was used in conjunction with WLI [3]. The rate of lesions that were subjectively clearly identifiable was 89.7 % for both methods, whereas the rate of a good superficial demarcation of the lesions was 63.2 % for EFI and 35.3 % for WLI. The sensitivity for the histopathological correlation for $n=199$ tissue biopsies from suspicious areas was calculated as 99.2 % for WLI and 100 % for EFI. Again, reproducible numbers concerning the specificity of the method could not be calculated for the same reasons as mentioned above. Whereas the examination itself was performed as easily as for AFI, the patient preparation (application of 5-ALA and incubation) was sometimes proved to be quite a challenge for both the patients and the personnel involved.

B: Laryngeal Lesions

Autofluorescence Imaging

Just as for oral/oropharyngeal examinations, the additional AFI was well tolerated and easily performed. AFI to WLI was compared during direct and indirect laryngoscopy in 111 patients. With histopathologic diagnosis as standard, the diagnostic accuracies for indirect laryngoscopy were 78 % (WLI) and 90 % (AFI). The sensitivities for the detection of (pre)cancerous lesions were 85 % (WLI) vs. 91 % (AFI) and the specificities amounted to 69 % (WLI) and 87 % (AFI).

For direct visualization during microlaryngoscopy, the diagnostic accuracy of WLI was 89 % and that of AFI was 95 %. With histopathology as control, direct WLI of the larynx achieved a sensitivity of 92 % and a specificity of 86 %. The sensitivity of direct AFI laryngoscopy was 97 % and specificity 92 %.

In this study, a special focus was put onto the false results. Thereby, false-positive cases were mainly observed as secondary to scarring and chronic inflammation, whereas false-negative results were mainly caused by a (pathological) mucosal hyperkeratosis.

Enhanced Fluorescence Imaging

A total of 56 patients with suspicious, flat epithelial lesions ($n=7$ epithelial hyperplasias, $n=15$ mild epithelial dysplasias, $n=7$ moderate epithelial dysplasias, $n=10$ severe epithelial dysplasia, $n=17$ invasive carcinomas) were prospectively investigated using EFI following topical application of 5-ALA via inhalation in a previously published study [4]. Using the combined information obtained from WLI and EFI, a correct diagnosis could be obtained in 84 %, and the sensitivity was 97 % with a corresponding specificity of 64 %. Again, the EFI examinations were easily performed, but patient preparation (especially in direct laryngoscopy cases) proved to be challenging and time-consuming.

Review of Literature and Critical Discussion

General Points

Even though the advantages of screening for precancerous lesions as well as early UADT cancer especially in high-risk populations seem beyond all question, it is not yet clear by which means this is best achieved. The only thoroughly investigated technique with a proven benefit so far is regular oral screening by trained health workers [5]. More advanced methods such as toluidine blue staining, fluorescence imaging, or Narrow Band Imaging (NBI) might add additional information if used in conjunction with conventional white light examination. However, a recent Cochrane Review by Brocklehurst et al. from 2010 states that "no robust evidence was identified to support the use of … adjunctive technologies like toluidine blue, brush biopsy or fluorescence imaging within a primary care environment" [6]. The authors conclude that the data that are available on these methods so far need "to be supplemented by further randomized controlled trials to provide the highest level of evidence for practice."

Several recent reviews have looked at the different techniques (including AFI) that are currently tested and applied as an adjunct for UADT cancer diagnosis [7–9]. The common feeling is that—as RCTs concerning their effectiveness are still missing for all of them—all these methods seem promising in theory but that the "tantalizing implication that such technologies may improve detection of oral cancers and precancers beyond conventional oral examination alone has yet to be rigorously confirmed" [8]. Nevertheless, fluorescence imaging is generally felt to be a useful, easy to perform, and harmless diagnostic adjunct for UADT cancer screening.

Review of Literature on Fluorescence Imaging

When used in conjunction with white light inspection or endoscopy and supposedly rather independent of the system used and the areas of the UADT inspected, both AFI and EFI have yielded high sensitivities in various publications concerning the identification and delimitation of UADT lesions with values ranging between 83 and 99 % [3, 4, 10–27]. At the same time, these methods seem to be generally lacking specificity, so a further differentiation of areas that show alterations of normal mucosal autofluorescence (AFI) or increased PPIX fluorescence (EFI) does not seem possible. Not surprisingly, the outcome with regard to sensitivity and specificity was considerably worse when the method was evaluated as a stand-alone procedure [28–30], so the general recommendation would be to use both regular white light endoscopy and fluorescence imaging in conjunction at all times.

When comparing EFI and AFI, a comparative study of both methods from our group using a first-generation STORZ system found a slight advantage of EFI over AFI concerning identification of both tumor and borders [3]. When changing over to a newer system generation afterward, however, both methods were subjectively performing equally, so for the sake of practicality, we have mostly given up performing EFI altogether. In a recent meta-analysis including 16 studies and 1000 laryngeal lesions altogether, this trend toward a slight but statistically insignificant higher sensitivity of EFI over AFI (95 % vs. 91 %) in detecting (pre)cancerous lesions was confirmed, yet at the expense of specificity [29]. The authors recommend the general use of AFI, with EFI being reserved for the detection of recurrences following initial surgery.

Direct comparative studies concerning the clinical value of the different fluorescence imaging devices in the UADT are missing, but the available data suggest a similar performance with regard to statistical outcomes (see above). Obviously, the endoscopic systems are more expensive than the handheld dental devices, but on the other hand, they have a greatly expanded range of view. As the STORZ system is the only endoscopic device which is specifically marketed for the UADT, the range of available endoscopes (flexible and rigid) for this indication is much greater and better suited than for the other systems, making examinations in this complex anatomical region more comfortable. So far, none of the fluorescence imaging systems on the market is available with a high-definition resolution, but developments are under way at this moment.

Comparison of Fluorescence Imaging to Other Novel Screening Techniques

Traditionally, toluidine blue or acetowhite staining (or the combination of both) has been investigated and advertised for the identification and demarcation of superficial (pre)cancerous mucosal lesions of the UADT. The method has not been directly compared to fluorescence imaging, but if the published data on toluidine blue staining (reviewed by Gray et al. [31]) is taken into consideration, it seems that fluorescence imaging is slightly more sensitive to detect mucosal lesions especially in cases of dysplasia. Nevertheless, it would seem worthwhile to undertake a comparative study in order to better answer this question.

Another method that has recently drawn considerable attention with regard to an improved early diagnosis of (pre)cancerous lesions of the UADT and other epithelium-lined hollow organs is Narrow Band Imaging (NBI). This proprietary Olympus technology enhances the visualization of the mucosal and submucosal vasculature, which shows alterations in various pathological conditions. In combination with high-definition endoscopy, recent studies applying a classification system adapted from gastroenterology by Lin et al. [32] have hinted that it may be a useful adjunctive method to white light endoscopy for the detection of (pre)malignant mucosal lesions with sensitivities of 85–96 % and specificities of 79–100 % in the reported studies [33–35]. The method suffers from restrictions similar to those found for fluorescence imaging, namely its inability to provide useful information in the presence of hyperkeratinization and a fairly low specificity. Yet, it has been described that NBI might be helpful for a further differentiation of superficial mucosal lesions, which (if proven in larger studies) would mean a major advantage over fluorescence imaging. Triggered by publications from pulmonology and gastroenterology, which hint that "tri-modal imaging" (high-resolution endoscopy, AFI, and NBI) might improve diagnostic accuracy over each single or twin imaging method, respectively, one group has endeavored on the combined use of all three techniques in $n=73$ patients with head and neck lesions so far [36, 37]. They report on a comparable, high sensitivity for both AFI and NBI, whereas NBI showed a better specificity than AFI. In addition, they state that "there may be additive and discriminatory benefits" when both imaging methods are used in conjunction. Larger, confirmatory studies are required to look at these results in more depth and detail.

Outlook

We share the opinion of others [38] that—in order to stay competitive with other methods that are designed for an improvement of superficial mucosal lesions such as NBI—fluorescence imaging needs to be incorporated into wide range, high-definition (or even 4 K) endoscopic systems in the very near future. A combination of fluorescence imaging with other complementary, noninvasive methods such as NBI [36, 37], point spectroscopy [39], stroboscopy [40], red/green ratioing [41], optical coherence tomography [42], contact endoscopy [43], or confocal endomicroscopy [44] in order to increase the diagnostic performance seems promising in theory, but needs to be evaluated in larger trials concerning patient benefit and economical feasibility.

Summary and Conclusion

In conclusion, fluorescence imaging seems to be a helpful, sensitive, yet rather unspecific adjunctive tool for the detection and superficial delimitation of (pre)malignant lesions of the UADT. Especially, AFI seems recommendable for routine clinical use, as it is easy to perform and well accepted by the patients, whereas EFI should be reserved for special cases. In comparison, fluorescence imaging seems to perform similarly well as other adjunct methods for UADT cancer screening. Yet, more detailed statements concerning the true clinical value cannot be made at this point as direct comparative studies of different techniques and systems are mostly missing.

References

1. Wagnieres GA, Star WM, Wilson BC. In vivo fluorescence spectroscopy and imaging for oncological applications. Photochem Photobiol. 1998;68:603–32.
2. Chang SK. Understanding the variations in fluorescence spectra of gynecologic tissue. Dissertation at the University of Texas in Austin, USA; 2004.
3. Betz CS, Stepp H, Janda P, et al. A comparative study of normal inspection, autofluorescence and 5-ALA-induced PPIX fluorescence for oral cancer diagnosis. Int J Cancer. 2002;97:245–52.
4. Arens C, Dreyer T, Glanz H, Malzahn K. Indirect autofluorescence laryngoscopy in the diagnosis of laryngeal cancer and its precursor lesions. Eur Arch Otorhinolaryngol. 2004;261:71–6.
5. Sankaranarayanan R, Ramadas K, Thomas G, et al. Effect of screening on oral cancer mortality in Kerala, India: a cluster-randomised controlled trial. Lancet. 2005;365:1927–33.
6. Brocklehurst P, Kujan O, Glenny AM, et al. Screening programmes for the early detection and prevention of oral cancer. Cochrane Database Syst Rev. 2010;11:CD004150.
7. Driemel O, Kunkel M, Hullmann M, et al. Diagnosis of oral squamous cell carcinoma and its precursor lesions. J Dtsch Dermatol Ges. 2007;5:1095–100.
8. Lingen MW, Kalmar JR, Karrison T, Speight PM. Critical evaluation of diagnostic aids for the detection of oral cancer. Oral Oncol. 2008;44:10–22.
9. Patton LL, Epstein JB, Kerr AR. Adjunctive techniques for oral cancer examination and

lesion diagnosis: a systematic review of the literature. J Am Dent Assoc. 2008;139: 896–905.

10. Mehlmann M, Betz CS, Stepp H, et al. Fluorescence staining of laryngeal neoplasms after topical application of 5-aminolevulinic acid: preliminary results. Lasers Surg Med. 1999;25:414–20.
11. Leunig A, Betz CS, Mehlmann M, et al. Detection of squamous cell carcinoma of the oral cavity by imaging 5-aminolevulinic acid-induced protoporphyrin IX fluorescence. Laryngoscope. 2000;110:78–83.
12. Andersson-Engels S, Klinteberg C, Svanberg K, Svanberg S. In vivo fluorescence imaging for tissue diagnostics. Phys Med Biol. 1997;42:815–24.
13. Malzahn K, Dreyer T, Glanz H, Arens C. Autofluorescence endoscopy in the diagnosis of early laryngeal cancer and its precursor lesions. Laryngoscope. 2002;112:488–93.
14. Paczona R, Temam S, Janot F, Marandas P, Luboinski B. Autofluorescence videoendoscopy for photodiagnosis of head and neck squamous cell carcinoma. Eur Arch Otorhinolaryngol. 2003;260:544–8.
15. Sharwani A, Jerjes W, Salih V, et al. Fluorescence spectroscopy combined with 5-aminolevulinic acid-induced protoporphyrin IX fluorescence in detecting oral premalignancy. J Photochem Photobiol B. 2006;83:27–33.
16. Awan KH, Morgan PR, Warnakulasuriya S. Evaluation of an autofluorescence based imaging system (VELscope) in the detection of oral potentially malignant disorders and benign keratoses. Oral Oncol. 2011;47:274–7.
17. Rana M, Zapf A, Kuehle M, Gellrich NC, Eckardt AM. Clinical evaluation of an autofluorescence diagnostic device for oral cancer detection: a prospective randomized diagnostic study. Eur J Cancer Prev. 2012;21:460–6.
18. Lane P, Follen M, MacAulay C. Has fluorescence spectroscopy come of age? A case series of oral precancers and cancers using white light, fluorescent light at 405 nm, and reflected light at 545 nm using the Trimira identafi 3000. Gend Med. 2012;9:S25–35.
19. Koch FP, Kaemmerer PW, Biesterfeld S, Kunkel M, Wagner W. Effectiveness of autofluorescence to identify suspicious oral lesions—a prospective, blinded clinical trial. Clin Oral Investig. 2011;15:975–82.
20. Scheer M, Neugebauer J, Derman A, Fuss J, Drebber U, Zoeller JE. Autofluorescence imaging of potentially malignant mucosa lesions. Oral Surg Oral Med Oral Pathol Oral Radiol Endod. 2011;111:568–77.
21. Caffier PP, Schmidt B, Gross M, et al. A comparison of white light laryngostroboscopy versus autofluorescence endoscopy in the evaluation of vocal fold pathology. Laryngoscope. 2013;123:1729–34.
22. Hanken H, Kraatz J, Smeets R, et al. The detection of oral pre-malignant lesions with an autofluorescence based imaging system (VELscopeTM)—a single blinded clinical evaluation. Head Face Med. 2013;9:23.
23. Paderni C, Compilato D, Carinci F, et al. Direct visualization of oral-cavity tissue fluorescence as novel aid for early oral cancer diagnosis and potentially malignant disorders monitoring. Int J Immunopathol Pharmacol. 2011;24:121–8.
24. Jayaprakash V, Sullivan M, Merzianu M, et al. Autofluorescence-guided surveillance for oral cancer. Cancer Prev Res (Phila). 2009;2: 966–74.
25. Baletic N, Malicevic H, Petrovic Z, Marinkovic-Eric J, Peric A. Advantages and limitations of the autofluorescent diagnostics of the laryngeal cancer and precancerosis. Eur Arch Otorhinolaryngol. 2010;267:925–31.
26. Lane PM, Gilhuly T, Whitehead P, et al. Simple device for the direct visualization of oral-cavity tissue fluorescence. J Biomed Opt. 2006;11: 024006.
27. Poh CF, Zhang L, Anderson DW, et al. Fluorescence visualization detection of field alterations in tumor margins of oral cancer patients. Clin Cancer Res. 2006;12:6716–22.
28. Farah CS, Mcintosh L, Georgiou A, McCullough MJ. Efficacy of tissue autofluorescence imaging (VELscope) in the visualization of oral mucosal lesions. Head Neck. 2011;34:856–62.
29. Mehrotra R, Singh M, Thomas S, et al. A cross-sectional study evaluating chemiluminescence and autofluorescence in the detection of clinically innocuous precancerous and cancerous oral lesions. J Am Dent Assoc. 2010;141:151–6.
30. Sweeny L, Dean NR, Magnuson JS, Carroll WR, Clemons L, Rosenthal EL. Assessment of tissue autofluorescence and reflectance for oral cavity cancer screening. Otolaryngol Head Neck Surg. 2011;145:956–60.
31. Gray M, Gold L, Burls A, Elley K. The clinical effectiveness of toluidine blue dye as an adjunct to oral cancer screening in general dental practice. Report by the Department of Public Health and Epidemiology, University of Birmingham, UK; 2000.

32. Lin YC, Wang WH, Lee FK, Tsai WC, Weng HH. Value of narrow band imaging endoscopy in early mucosal head and neck cancer. Head Neck. 2012;34:1574–9.
33. Piazza C, Cocco D, Del Bon F, et al. Narrow band imaging and high definition television in evaluation of oral and oropharyngeal squamous cell cancer: a prospective study. Oral Oncol. 2010;46:307–10.
34. Chu PY, Tsai TL, Tai SK, Chang SY. Effectiveness of narrow band imaging in patients with oral squamous cell carcinoma after treatment. Head Neck. 2012;34:155–61.
35. Yang SW, Lee YS, Chang LC, Hwang CC, Chen TA. Diagnostic significance of narrow-band imaging for detecting high-grade dysplasia, carcinoma in situ, and carcinoma in oral leukoplakia. Laryngoscope. 2012;122:2754–61.
36. Nguyen PT, Salvado O, Masters IB, Farah CS, Fielding D. Combining autofluorescence and narrow band imaging with image analysis in the evaluation of preneoplastic lesions in the bronchus and larynx. J Bronchology Interv Pulmonol. 2010;17:109–16.
37. Nguyen P, Bashirzadeh F, Hodge R, et al. High specificity of combined narrow band imaging and autofluorescence mucosal assessment of patients with head and neck cancer. Head Neck. 2013;35:619–25.
38. Shin D, Vigneswaran N, Gillenwater A, Richards-Kortum R. Advances in fluorescence imaging techniques to detect oral cancer and its precursors. Future Oncol. 2010;6: 1143–54.
39. Lin K, Zheng W, Huang Z. Integrated autofluorescence endoscopic imaging and pointwise spectroscopy for real-time in vivo tissue measurements. J Biomed Opt. 2010;15: 040507.
40. Crosetti E, Pilotti F, Succo G. A new strategy for endoscopic staging of laryngeal carcinoma: multistep endoscopy. Acta Otorhinolaryngol Ital. 2012;32:175–81.
41. Roblyer D, Kurachi C, Stepanek V, et al. Objective detection and delineation of oral neoplasia using autofluorescence imaging. Cancer Prev Res (Phila). 2009;2:423–31.
42. Betz CS, Stepp H, Havel M, et al. A set of optical techniques for improving the diagnosis of early upper aerodigestive tract cancer. Med Laser Appl. 2008;23:175–85.
43. Arens C, Glanz H, Dreyer T, Malzahn K. Compact endoscopy of the larynx. Ann Otol Rhinol Laryngol. 2003;112:113–9.
44. Zheng W, Harris M, Kho KW, et al. Confocal endomicroscopic imaging of normal and neoplastic human tongue tissue using ALA-induced-PPIX fluorescence: a preliminary study. Oncol Rep. 2004;12:397–401.

Chapter 29

Confocal Endomicroscopy and Optical Coherence Tomography for Differentiation Between Low-Grade and High-Grade Lesions of the Larynx

Tino Just, Ellen Guder, Gabriele Witt, Atilla Ovari, Benjamin von Stülpnagel, Eva Lankenau, Friedrich Prall, Gereon Hüttmann, and Hans Wilhelm Pau

Introduction

Early diagnoses of high-grade lesions and early laryngeal cancer are most challenging. These findings need to be reliably differentiated from benign and low-grade lesions. Suspicious lesions may comprise various entities varying from hyperplasia with or without atypia and inflammation, low-grade and high-grade dysplasia, and carcinoma in situ to invasive carcinoma, respectively. A clinical survey demonstrated that even experienced laryngeal surgeons are not able to reliably assign similar clinical characteristics to low-grade or high-grade lesions [1]. The agreement between the surgeon's assessment and histopathology was fair. This misjudgment or limited precision of biopsy leads to the necessity for re-biopsy in cases of strong suspicion for early laryngeal cancer. To avoid unnecessary re-biopsies and to improve the precision of biopsy, imaging technologies may help to reliably identify cellular abnormalities or basement membrane violation. Over the last two decades, various imaging modalities were presented with a potential for in vivo diagnosis of laryngeal cancer. Among these, optical coherence tomography (OCT) [2, 3], narrow band imaging (NBI) [4], and confocal endomicroscopy (CEM) [5, 6] seem to be promising technologies.

Brian J.-F. Wong and Justus Ilgner (eds.), *Biomedical Optics in Otorhinolaryngology: Head and Neck Surgery*, DOI 10.1007/978-1-4939-1758-7_29, © Springer Science+Business Media New York 2016

OCT provides optical cross sections of the larynx and displays the various layers (stratified squamous epithelium and superficial and intermediate layer of the lamina propria). While the basement membrane itself is not detectable with OCT, the border between epithelium and lamina propria is defined as a basement membrane-like structure and is clearly displayed as gray graduation. Loss of integrity or violation of this structure is consistent with invasive carcinoma [2, 3].

NBI is an imaging technique that uses light of specific blue and green wavelength to enhance details of the surface of the epithelium, in particular, blood vessels. Activation of special filters leads to use of ambient light of wavelength between 440–460 nm and 540–560 nm [7]. Peak light absorption of hemoglobin at these wavelengths causes vessels to appear dark in color and leads to better identification of other surface structures and even small lesions. With the use of NBI-based classifications of blood vessels, changes in mucosal microvasculature were detected in premalignant and malignant lesions of the larynx [4]. However, NBI fails to detect cellular abnormalities and to display the basement membrane.

Confocal endomicroscopy (CEM) is a new technology that provides en-face images of the tissue and is mainly used for detection of high-grade dysplasia and adenocarcinoma of the esophagus. A meta-analysis was carried out to evaluate the diagnostic accuracy of CEM-based targeted biopsies [8]. In four out of seven studies per lesion, analysis for diagnosis of high-grade lesion and adenocarcinoma of the esophagus revealed a sensitivity and specificity of 68 % and 88 %, respectively. The authors concluded that in consequence of the low sensitivity and positive likelihood ratio, CEM may currently not replace standard histopathology.

So far, there are no data available from clinical studies that demonstrate in vivo a reliable differentiation between low-grade and high-grade lesions of the larynx. Biopsies of the larynx in patients with suspicious laryngeal lesions have significant sampling errors. The need for re-biopsies is time-consuming and is also associated with a potential risk of prolonged or persistent hoarseness. The aim of this clinicopathological study was to compare the OCT and CEM-based targeted biopsies with histopathology.

Materials and Methods

This prospective study was performed between January 2012 and December 2013 at the University of Rostock, Germany. OCT measurements were carried out in cooperation with the Institute for Biomedical Optics at the University of Lübeck, Germany. The studies (CEM study and CEM plus OCT study) were approved by the Ethics Committee of the General Medical Council of Mecklenburg, Western Pomerania. Informed consent was obtained from each patient before OCT and/or CEM measurements were carried out.

Patients

Patients with primary lesions of the true vocal cord suspicious for low-grade or high-grade lesions with an indication for microlaryngoscopy were recruited to participate in this study after informed consent was obtained and were included as soon as biopsies were taken for histopathology.

Exclusion criteria were no indication for biopsy or excision during microlaryngoscopy, patients found to have invasive laryngeal cancer clinically and by biopsy (T1-4), inability to provide informed consent, and age <18 years.

The CEM series consisted of a total of 67 patients (age 40–82 years, mean age 60.9 ± 11.2 years; 19 women and 48 men) recruited at the Department of Otorhinolaryngology and Department of the Clinic of Phoniatry and Paediatric Audiology of the University of Rostock. The OCT measurements started 3 months later. Out of the 67 patients, 39 patients were included in the CEM and OCT study (ten women and 29 men; age 44–82 years, mean age 62.4 ± 11 years).

Imaging Systems

For intraoperative OCT measurements, the OCT camera (Optomedical Technologies GmbH, Lübeck, Germany) was attached to the camera port of the surgical microscope Hi-R 1000 NIR (Haag-Streit Surgical GmbH, Wedel, Germany). The microscope is optimized for transmission in the near-infrared spectrum. Detailed information is presented elsewhere [9]. The microscope Hi-R 1000 NIR (Moeller Wedel GmbH, Wedel, Germany) is optimized for light transmission in the near-infrared spectral range (NIR). The OCT camera base device consists of four main components: an 840 nm broadband light source, a spectral domain OCT detector, motorized OCT reference optics, and an OCT scanner attached to the camera port. The motorized reference optics enables the surgeon to use OCT laryngoscopy at different working distances ranging from 220 to 500 mm. The OCT camera provides an optical window depth of 4.2 mm. The OCT picture shows 1024 pixels in depth. Therefore, the axial pixel distance is 4.1 μm in air and 3.1 μm inside tissue with an index of refraction of 1.34, respectively. The axial OCT resolution is about 10 μm in air and about 7.5 μm inside tissue. The lateral scan width depends on the magnification of the microscope and can be changed from 5 mm up to 30 mm. The lateral resolution of the OCT system depends on the central wavelength and the numerical aperture. The latter parameter changes with change of magnification and working distance. The best image quality is reached when the lateral resolution is about 23 μm at highest magnification and a working distance of 232 mm. For CEM measurements, a rigid endoscope was used with a length and diameter of 23 cm and 5 mm, respectively (Karl Storz GmbH & Co., KG; Tuttlingen, Germany). The endoscope is connected to the scanner of the Heidelberg Retina Tomograph II (HRTII, Heidelberg Engineering GmbH, Heidelberg, Germany). Detailed information is published elsewhere [10]. The scanning device provides images of 400 μm × 400 μm field of view. The average penetration depth is between 100 and 300 μm. The lateral and axial resolutions are about 1–2 and 2 μm, respectively. In contrast to OCT, CEM has to be used in contact mode.

Intraoperative Applications

The larynx was exposed using a Kleinsasser laryngoscope held by suspension (Karl Storz GmbH & Co. KG, Tuttlingen, Germany). All laryngeal lesions were photographed during microlaryngoscopy. Endoscopes (30° and 70°) were used to assess the laryngeal lesions whenever necessary. In vivo measurements started with OCT application. Using the operating microscope, a nominal working distance of between 224 and 280 mm was used (magnification of between ×4.0 and ×7.0). In the intraoperative setting, perpendicular OCT sections through the true vocal cords were performed, and the images and volume sections were digitally stored. The process was started manually, and cross-sectional and volume images were monitored on the dedicated screen. For orientation, a green pilot beam indicated the scanning field and enabled the surgeon to define the location of the biopsy and resection plane [11]. Next, a rigid endoscope was connected to the scanner of the HRTII and inserted through the laryngoscope. The endoscope was gently placed on the lesion. A contact gel was used (Vidisic® gel, Bausch & Lomb GmbH, Germany) to avoid strong reflections [10]. Three different modes were used for sampling (sections mode for images, sequence acquisition mode for a series of 100 images of a defined depth by moving the endoscope, and volume mode for a series of 40 images). Intraoperative CEM and OCT measurements increased the normal operating time for 10–12 min.

For comparison of CEM images and volume scans with OCT and histopathology at a later stage, the biopsy was taken as precisely as possible from the same region as scanned before.

Histopatho-logical Examination of Biopsies and Resection Specimens

Biopsies of regions examined with either CEM or CEM and OCT were fixed in 4 % formaldehyde solution, embedded in paraffin, and sectioned vertically. All specimens were submitted to the Institute of Pathology of the University of Rostock for histopathologic examination. Hematoxylin and eosin were used for staining. Dysplasia and squamous intraepithelial lesions were graded according to the World Health Organization guidelines [12].

Analysis of CEM and OCT Images and Correlation Analysis

For 47 biopsies/excisions of 39 patients (CEM and OCT series), OCT and CEM analyses were performed. Three investigators (E.G., B.S., and T. J.) reviewed the digitally stored OCT images of lesions for which corresponding histological sections were available.

The thickness measurements of the epithelium were performed blind and without histopathological knowledge. In biopsies and excisional biopsies, the OCT images of defined regions of the specimen (anterior, middle, posterior part of the true vocal cord) were compared with findings of the corresponding histopathological sections.

For OCT, the following criteria were used to classify epithelial lesions: thickness of the epithelium and identification and assessment of the integrity of the border between epithelial layer and the lamina propria as correlate of the basement membrane, which is clearly visible as gray graduation. In contrast to the published morphometric data of the thickness of the laryngeal epithelia [13, 14], cutoff between low-grade (mean 145 μm, 95 % CI of 121–169 μm) and high-grade lesion (mean 278 μm, 95 % CI of 242–314 μm) was defined as epithelium of about 180 μm thickness. In the literature, normal epithelium was defined as epithelium of about 150 μm [13]. Histopathological diagnoses comprising hyperkeratosis, hyperplasia with or without cell atypia, inflammation, and mild and moderate dysplasia were classified as low-grade lesions, while severe dysplasia and carcinoma in situ were classified as high-grade lesions.

All OCT raw data were imported and converted using Image J (Version 1.45s, NIH, USA). The measurement depth in air is 4.2 mm. Considering the refractive index of 1.34 in tissue, the measurement depth is reduced to 3.13 mm. This results in a pixel pitch of 3.13 μm. Descriptive statistics were applied to depict thickness of the epithelium. The software SPSS 21.0 (SPSS, Inc., Chicago, IL) was used for descriptive statistics. For all calculations, a p value of less than 0.05 was considered as statistically significant.

According to histopathology, CEM images were graded on a two-tiered scale as no or mild dysplasia (resembling low-grade SIL) or severe dysplasia/carcinoma in situ (resembling high-grade lesions).

Results

This clinicopathological study included a total of 67 patients, of whom 97 biopsies were taken. According to histopathology, 44 biopsies were non-dysplastic (mucosal inflammation with or without cell atypia, hyperkeratosis, epithelial hyperplasia), six biopsies showed mild dysplasia, and ten biopsies revealed moderate laryngeal dysplasia. In two biopsies, severe dysplasia was found, and in 35 biopsies, carcinoma in situ or microinvasive carcinoma was found.

A representative case of this study is demonstrated in Figs. 1 and 2. The right-sided lesion was biopsied for histopathology. The middle and lower part of the epithelium reveals dysplastic cells (Fig. 1b). The boundary between the epithelium (gray) and the

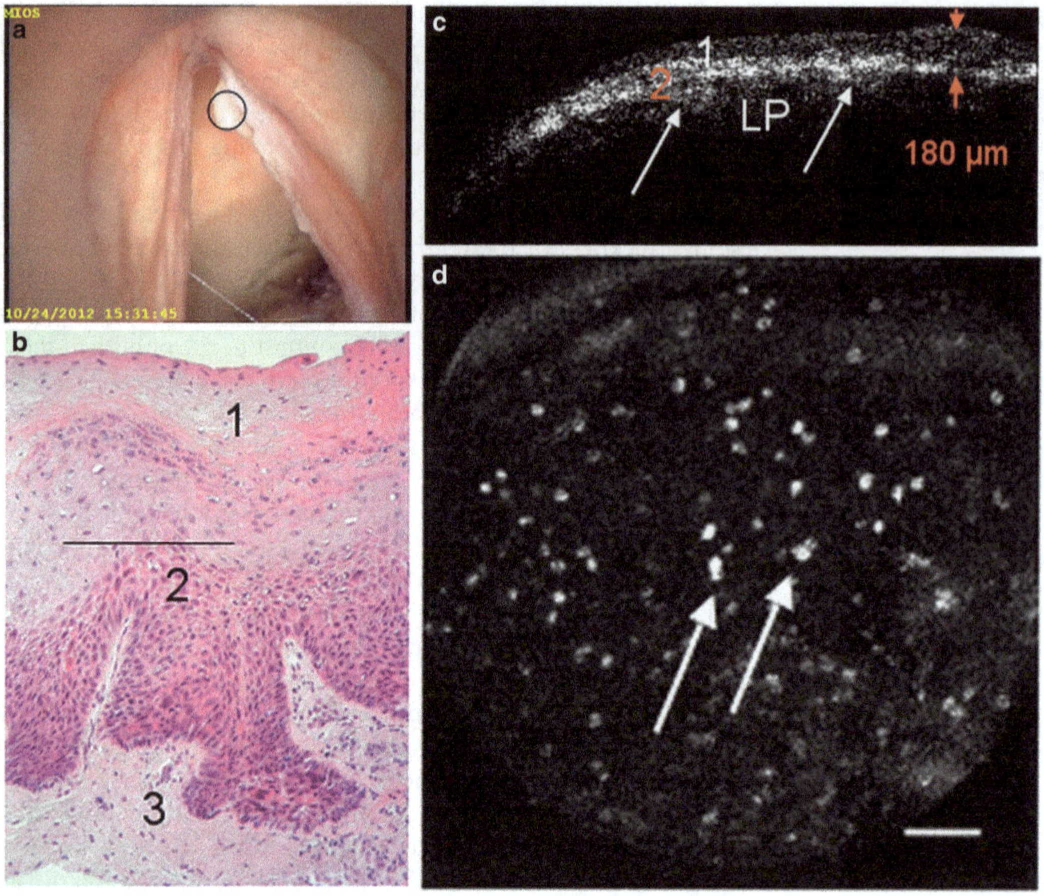

Fig. 1 **(a)** Photograph of a *right-sided* glottic lesion. *Circle* marks the biopsy taken for histopathology. (**b**) Histopathology (hematoxylin and eosin) reveals severe dysplasia with hyperkeratosis (1 = superficial and 2 = deep epithelial layer; 3 = lamina propria). (**c**) Optical coherence tomography of the *right* vocal cord. A representative cross section through the biopsied region reveals a thickened epithelial layer (1 = superficial and 2 = deep epithelial layer, LP = lamina propria) with an irregular but intact basal membrane (*arrows*). (**d**) Confocal microscopic image (en-face image) obtained from the *middle* layer of the biopsied region (about 150 μm, *black line* in B) demonstrates enlarged and irregular-shaped nuclei (*arrows*) and an irregular cell architecture (scale bar 50 μm)

lamina propria is clearly visible with OCT (Fig. 1c). There is an increased backscattering from the basement membrane region, suggesting a difference in optical properties between normal upper epithelium and epithelial dysplasia close to the basement membrane. The white irregular thickened line is defined as the basal membrane and dense cell layers above the basal membrane. Underneath the basement membrane, the lamina propria is detectable. Histology of the chordectomy specimen reveals a carcinoma in situ (Fig. 2b). In contrast to the preoperative OCT image, the epithelium appears thicker (about 220 μm). Both representative

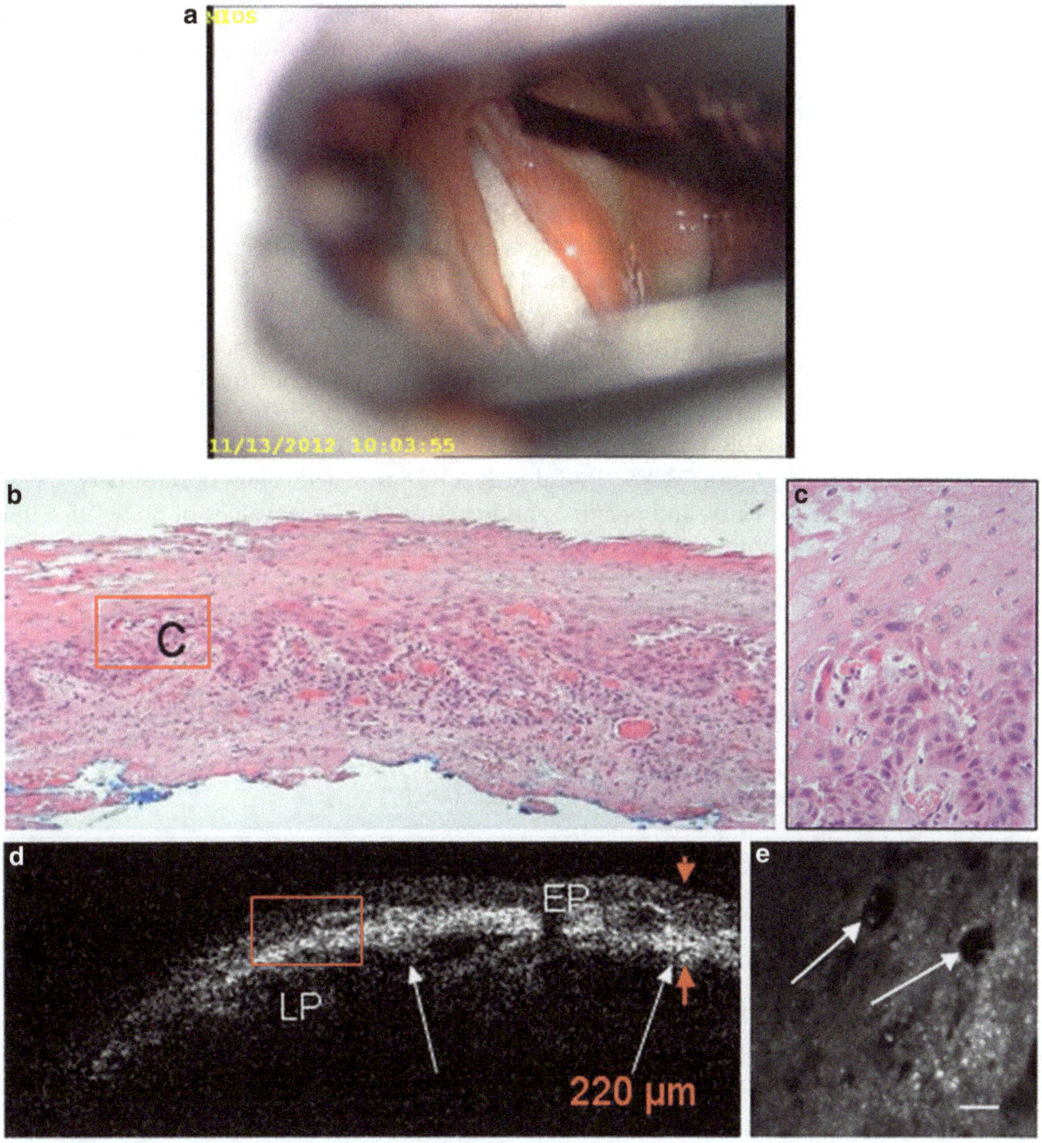

Fig. 2 **(a)** Photograph of the same *right-sided* glottic lesion. Keratotic mass was removed for diagnosis. (**b**) Histopathology of the subepithelial chordectomy specimen reveals a carcinoma in situ (hematoxylin & eosin). (**c**) Higher magnification of the red window. (**d**) Optical coherence tomography reveals a thickened epithelial layer (EP = epithelium) with an irregular (*arrows*) but intact basal membrane. Thickness of the epithelium exceeds 180 μm. (**e**) Confocal microscopic image (en-face image) obtained from the *middle* layer of the biopsied region (at about 150 μm in depths, *black line* in **b**) demonstrates enlarged cells and irregular-shaped nuclei (*arrows*) and an irregular cell architecture (scale bar 50 μm)

OCT images demonstrate a high-risk epithelium. The example CEM images (obtained from volume scans) demonstrate clearly changes of cell architecture (Figs. 1d and 2e).

In the CEM study ($N = 97$), consensus diagnoses of the laryngeal lesions were worked out and the CEM diagnoses were compared with histopathology (Table 1). Sensitivity, specificity, and positive and negative predictive values were calculated, and these were found to be 84 % (95 % confidence interval (CI) of 68–93 %), 91.5 % (95 % CI of 81–97 %), 86 % (95 % CI of 70–95 %), and 90 % (95 % CI of 79–96 %).

In the OCT and CEM study ($N = 47$), sensitivity, specificity, and positive and negative predictive values for CEM were calculated, and these were found to be 90 % (95 % CI of 68–98 %), 92 % (95 % CI of 73–99 %), 90 % (95 % CI of 68–98 %), and 92 % (95 % CI of 73–99 %) (Table 2). OCT revealed values of sensitivity, specificity, and positive and negative predictive values of 86 % (95 % CI of 63–96 %), 81 % (95 % CI of 60–93 %), 78 % (95 % CI of 56–92 %), and 87 % (95 % CI of 66–97 %) (Table 3). Inter-rater variability of CEM and OCT images was assessed using the digitally stored images and resulted in kappa = 0.75 ($P < 0.001$) for CEM and in kappa = 0.58 ($P < 0.001$) for OCT.

Table 1
Accuracy of confocal endomicroscopy (CEM) consensus ($N = 97$)

CEM	Histopathology		
No.		59	38
		Low-grade lesion	High-grade lesion
60	Low-grade lesion	54	6
37	High-grade lesion	5	32

Low-grade lesion = no dysplasia, mild and moderate dysplasia
High-grade lesion = severe dysplasia, carcinoma in situ/microinvasive carcinoma

Table 2
Accuracy of confocal endomicroscopy (CEM) consensus ($N = 47$)

CEM	Histopathology		
No.		26	21
		Low-grade lesion	High-grade lesion
26	Low-grade lesion	24	2
21	High-grade lesion	2	19

Low-grade lesion = no dysplasia, mild and moderate dysplasia
High-grade lesion = severe dysplasia, carcinoma in situ/microinvasive carcinoma

Table 3
Accuracy of optical coherence tomography (OCT) consensus (*N* = 47)

OCT	Histopathology		
No.		24	23
		Low-grade lesion	High-grade lesion
26	Low-grade lesion	21	5
21	High-grade lesion	3	18

Low-grade lesion = no dysplasia, mild and moderate dysplasia
High-grade lesion = severe dysplasia, carcinoma in situ/microinvasive carcinoma

Next, the test outcomes of the combination of OCT plus CEM were calculated. True positive and true negative were defined when CEM or OCT were positive and when CEM and OCT were negative, respectively. Compared with the test outcomes of OCT and CEM, sensitivity improved to 95 % (95 % CI of 74–99 %), while specificity decreased to 77 % (95 % CI of 56–90 %). Positive and negative predictive values were found to be 77 % (95 % CI of 56–90 %) and 95 % (95 % CI of 74–99 %), respectively.

Discussion

In this clinicopathological study, we demonstrated test outcomes for CEM and OCT to differentiate low-grade from high-grade laryngeal lesions. The following major results were found: (1) CEM revealed a higher sensitivity and higher positive predictive value than OCT when CEM and OCT were considered separately and (2) combination of CEM and OCT improves the sensitivity while the specificity decreases compared to test outcomes for CEM and OCT alone.

Diagnosis and management of laryngeal dysplasia were presented in 2010 [15]. 40 ENT surgeons and 40 pathologists attended a national workshop. As a result of this meeting, a consensus paper was published. In the presence of widespread laryngeal leukoplakia or confluent leukoplakia, histopathologic mapping of the laryngeal lesion with multiple biopsies was recommended, followed by staged resection if feasible. In addition, it was noted that laryngeal biopsies varied in size and surgeons should try to take larger biopsies when possible to make orientation and evaluation more reliable, particularly if there were previous difficulties in interpretation of the pathology. This poses the question whether it is feasible to improve the precision of biopsy using optical technologies to identify pathological regions within the epithelium and to get a reliable biopsy for diagnosis. A control group consisting of test outcomes without OCT and/or CEM-based targeted biopsies was not presented. Results of a pilot survey revealed a sensitivity, specificity, positive and negative predictive values, and predictive accuracy of 85, 56, 44, 90, and 65 % for agreement of histopathology and assessment of the laryngeal lesion to differentiate low-grade from high-grade lesions [1]. The survey included eight patients out of this histopathological study and can be addressed as a small sample. In both studies, only those laryngeal lesions were included which could not be easily assigned as benign or malign. Compared to the clinical survey, both CEM and OCT-targeted biopsies improved the test outcome considerably.

As a result of this study, the authors conclude that the management of persistent or recurrent squamous intraepithelial lesions as recommended, namely, complete excision of single and multiple lesions with severe dysplasia or carcinoma in situ, will not change [15]. However, the recommendation to excise recurrent focal mild dysplasia of the larynx rather than to observe it needs to be focused on by further studies. To monitor mild lesions of the larynx over time, a laryngoscope-based in vivo visualization of the laryngeal mucosa is needed. An OCT sampling device capable to monitor in vivo laryngeal cross sections during an office-based laryngoscopy was published in 2006 and 2013 [16, 17]. To introduce such an imaging modality in daily practice may further improve the presurgical diagnosis in patients with persistent hoarseness. In contrast to OCT, CEM is mainly used in contact mode via a single fiber or endoscope. Currently, CEM can only be applied during microlaryngoscopy under general anesthesia to get reliable information of the lesion. Therefore, OCT and CEM cannot currently be used as complementary imaging modalities via a microscope or laryngoscope.

In vivo diagnosis with optical technologies will not replace histopathology, but will improve the management of persistent or recurrent squamous intraepithelial lesions. It is conceivable that the use of high-speed technologies in the future will be capable to monitor in vivo laryngeal lesions over time in an office-based setting. The cost effectiveness to monitor laryngeal lesions over time rather than immediately biopsy mild dysplasia and to early diagnose high-grade lesions needs to be calculated. A meta-analysis on the management and follow-up of laryngeal dysplasia revealed an overall transformation rate from dysplasia to invasive carcinoma of about 17 %, while severe dysplasia/carcinoma in situ demonstrated a mean progression rate of about 30 % [18]. Therefore, the preferential aim in laryngology should be the early diagnosis of high-grade lesions. The present study demonstrated that optically targeted biopsies improve the test outcome. However, further developments and studies are needed to provide office-based technologies and then obtain results from multicenter studies.

Conclusions

On the basis of a prospective study, OCT and CEM with targeted biopsies demonstrate good diagnostic sensitivity and accuracy for detection of high-grade lesions. The test outcome in the study was much higher than it would be seen in clinical practice, and these results should be interpreted with caution due to the relatively low number of patients included in this study. However, further developments, namely, office-based imaging via laryngoscope and further studies, are needed.

Financial Support

There are no financial interests.

References

1. von Stülpnagel B, Hagen R, Olzowy B, Witt G, Pau HW, Just T. Comparative study between the surgeon's intraoperative evaluation and histopathology for diagnosis of laryngeal lesions. Int Sch Res Notices. 2014;2014:6. doi:10.1155/2014/63525. Article ID 635251.
2. Armstrong WB, Ridgway JM, Vokes DE, Guo S, Perez J, Jackson RP, Gu M, Su J, Crumley RL, Shibuya TY, Mahmood U, Chen Z, Wong BJ. Optical coherence tomography of laryngeal cancer. Laryngoscope. 2006;116:1107–13.
3. Just T, Lankenau E, Prall F, Hüttmann G, Pau HW, Sommer K. Optical coherence tomography allows for the reliable identification of laryngeal epithelial dysplasia and for precise biopsy: a clinicopathological study of 61 patients undergoing microlaryngoscopy. Laryngoscope. 2010;120:1964–70.
4. Bertino G, Cacciola S, Fernandes WB, Fernandes CM, Occhini A, Tinelli C, Benazzo M. Effectiveness of narrow band imaging in the detection of pre-malignant and malignant lesions of the larynx: validation of a new endoscopic clinical classification. Head Neck. 2014;37(2):215–22.
5. Pogorzelski B, Hanenkamp U, Goetz M, Kiesslich R, Gosepath J. Systematic intraoperative application of confocal endomicroscopy for early detection and resection of squamous cell carcinoma of the head and neck: a preliminary report. Arch Otolaryngol Head Neck Surg. 2012;138:404–11.
6. Just T, Stave J, Stachs O, Witt G, Guthoff R, Pau HW. Rigid confocal endoscopy of the larynx. In: Chau-Cang W, editor. Laser scanning, theory and applications. Rijeka: InTech; 2011.
7. Singh R, Mei SC, Sethi S. Advanced endoscopic imaging in Barrett's oesophagus: a review on current practice. World J Gastroenterol. 2011;17:4271–6.
8. Gupta A, Attar BM, Koduru P, Murali AR, Go BT, Agarwal R. Utility of confocal laser endomicroscopy in identifying high-grade dysplasia and adenocarcinoma in Barrett's esophagus: a systematic review and meta-analysis. Eur J Gastroenterol Hepatol. 2014;26:369–77.
9. Lankenau EM, Krug M, Oelckers S, Schrage N, Just T, Hüttmann G. iOCT with surgical microscopes: a new imaging during microsurgery. Adv Opt Technol. 2013;2:233–9.
10. Just T, Pau HW. Intra-operative application of confocal endomicroscopy using a rigid endoscope. J Laryngol Otol. 2013;127:599–604.
11. Just T, Lankenau E, Hüttmann G, Pau HW. Intra-operative application of optical coherence tomography with an operating microscope. J Laryngol Otol. 2009;123:1027–30.
12. Barnes L, Eveson JW, Reichart P, Sidransky D, editors. Pathology and genetics of head and neck tumours World Health Organization classification of tumours. Geneva: WHO press; 2005.
13. Kraft M, Glanz H, von Gerlach S, Wisweh H, Lubatschowski H, Arens C. Clinical value of optical coherence tomography in laryngology. Head Neck. 2008;30:1628–35.
14. Wong BJ, Jackson RP, Guo S, Ridgway JM, Mahmood U, Su J, Shibuya TY, Crumley RL,

Gu M, Armstrong WB, Chen Z. In vivo optical coherence tomography of the human larynx: normative and benign pathology in 82 patients. Laryngoscope. 2005;115:1904–11.
15. Mehanna H, Paleri V, Robson A, Wight R, Helliwell T. Consensus statement by otorhinolaryngologists and pathologists on the diagnosis and management of laryngeal dysplasia. Clin Otolaryngol. 2010;35:170–6.
16. Donner S, Deutsch S, Bleeker S, Ripken T, Krüger A. Concept for tremor compensation for a handheld OCT-laryngoscope. Proc. SPIE 8805, Head and Neck Optical Diagnosis. 2013:880503
17. Guo S, Hutchison R, Jackson RP, Kohli A, Sharp T, Orwin E, Haskell R, Chen Z, Wong BJ. Office-based optical coherence tomographic imaging of human vocal cords. J Biomed Opt. 2006;11:30501.
18. Weller MD, Nankivell PC, McConkey C, Paleri V, Mehanna HM. The risk and interval to malignancy of patients with laryngeal dysplasia; a systematic review of case series and meta-analysis. Clin Otolaryngol. 2010;35:364–72.

Chapter 30

Confocal Microscopy and Micro-endoscopy of the Larynx

Veronika Volgger, Anna Englhard, and Christian Stephan Betz

Introduction

The current gold standard in the evaluation of laryngeal lesions is white light examination followed by invasive tissue biopsy. This is a cost-intensive and time-consuming method, with a risk of over- or undertreatment in diffuse and widespread lesions. In the last decades, various optical techniques have been developed to noninvasively reveal in situ information about the histologic characteristics of tissues. Especially for the fine and fragile tissue of the larynx, a noninvasive tissue diagnosis seems to be of major importance, to reduce the risk of a function deficit after surgery.

There are, as mentioned above, different optical techniques to evaluate lesions of the larynx. Some of them only evaluate the surface of a lesion [such as autofluorescence imaging (AFI) and narrow band imaging (NBI)]; others are sectional imaging techniques [such as optical coherence tomography (OCT) and photoacoustic imaging (PAI)]. In this chapter confocal microscopy and confocal endomicroscopy are presented.

Confocal microscopy was first described in 1955 by Marvin Minsky. The first confocal microscopes became commercially available about 20 years later [1]. Confocal laser scanning microscopes (CLSMs) are mainly used in ophthalmology to evaluate the cornea, conjunctiva, and iris but can be used to evaluate tissue of various origins [2, 3].

In confocal laser endomicroscopy (CLE), the initial technique is brought to a miniaturized version. CLE is a noninvasive technique that allows visualization of tissue of the upper aerodi-

Brian J.-F. Wong and Justus Ilgner (eds.), *Biomedical Optics in Otorhinolaryngology: Head and Neck Surgery*, DOI 10.1007/978-1-4939-1758-7_30, © Springer Science+Business Media New York 2016

gestive tract (UADT). CLE has already found its way into clinical routine in gastroenterology and is tested in other fields, but it is still very new to the head and neck. CLE enables high-resolution, microanatomical analysis of targeted tissue ("optical biopsies") in vivo and in real time during endoscopy [4, 5]. By showing histologic characteristics of the mucosa and submucosa, it can differentiate different tissue types and gradings [6]. These findings could serve to reduce unnecessary biopsies and identify lesions needing further treatment. Moreover, by determining the exact margins of lesions, a more precise treatment can be rendered and unwanted effects from over- and under-resection minimized. Besides from better differentiating laryngeal lesions, there may be other indications where CLSM and CLE of the larynx could be useful.

Technical Background

In contrast to light microscopy, where the whole tissue sample is illuminated at the same time, in confocal laser scanning microscopy (CLSM), a laser focus is scanning laterally across a sample illuminating a single point in a certain depth at a time and providing high-resolution images. Then, induced fluorescence or reflectance is collected, while all out-of-focus light gets rejected by a pinhole in front of the detector (Fig. 1). With high numerical aperture objectives, submicron resolution can be achieved in all planes. Confocal laser endomicroscopy transfers this principle into a miniaturized endoscopic version. For the translation of confocal microscopy to in vivo CLE, the replacement of the traditional confocal pinhole by a single mode fiber is very important, because the optical fiber is acting as both the illumination point source and the detection pinhole, allowing the miniaturization required for endoscopy [7, 8].

CLSMs work at very high speed and produce high-resolution images of tissue up to depths between 100 and 500 μm within the oral cavity [9–11]. In CLE, due to the miniaturization, there are trade-offs between resolution, field of view, and penetration depth. In CLE two-dimensional tissue scanning is possible down to a (flexible or fixed) depth of approximately 250 μm. By stacking multiple scans recorded from different depths, even 3D imaging is possible. CLE images, in contrast to histopathological slides, are oriented parallel to the tissue surface ("en face" images). Lateral and axial resolutions down to 0.5 μm and 3 μm, respectively, fields of view as large as 800 × 450 μm, and probe diameters down to 1.0 mm have been achieved [7].

Because confocal imaging usually relies on tissue fluorescence (less common on reflectance), a fluorescent dye (applied topically

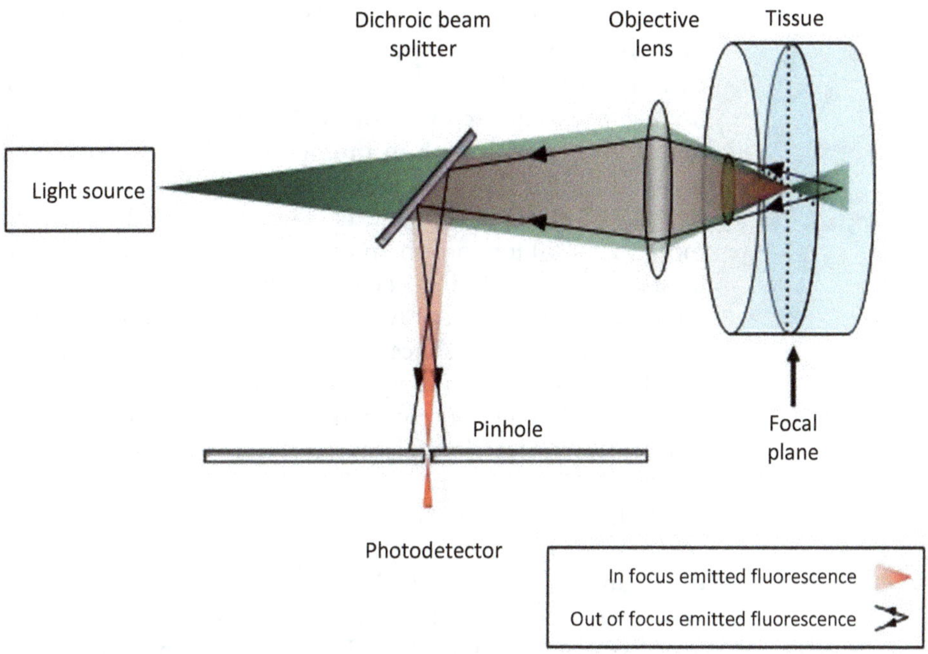

Fig. 1 Setup of a confocal (endo-) microscope (from Volgger et al. [15])

or intravenously) is necessary to make tissue visible. The brightness of the resulting image thereby corresponds to the intensity of detected fluorescence.

Fluorescent Stains for CLE

There are different fluorescent stains that have been used with CLE.

The only licensed contrast agent for being used with CLE in vivo in humans is intravenously applied fluorescein. The optimal dose for obtaining high-quality images (of the colon) seems to be 5 ml of a 10 % sodium fluorescein solution [12], but body weight adapted dosing is being discussed [13]. First studies of the UADT recommend an administration of 2.5–5 ml of a 10 % sodium fluorescein solution [14, 15]. The unbound contrast agent quickly diffuses across capillaries and highlights blood vessels and interstitial spaces for up to 30 min; however, the image quality deteriorates after 8 min [16]. First images can be taken 20–30 s after application of the contrast agent [17]. Fluorescein does not stain any intracellular structures, such as cell nuclei [7]. Fluorescein is known as an agent used in ophthalmology for retinal fluorescein angiography and is considered to be mostly safe. Serious adverse events such as acute hypotension or anaphylaxis are rare [18, 19]. A larger analysis on 2272 patients showed mild adverse reactions in 1.4 %, but no serious adverse events [20].

Intracellular as well as nuclear staining of the uppermost mucosa can be achieved by using topical contrast agents. None of them is officially licensed for in vivo use in humans, though their use has been reported previously. Nevertheless topical agents are regularly used with CLE in murine models or *ex vivo* on human tissue specimen. They are easy to apply and do not regularly carry the risk of systemic side effects. They typically do not penetrate more than 100 μm into the mucosa [6, 17]. The most commonly used agent is acriflavine [21–23], which stains the nuclei and is typically applied as acriflavine hydrochloride 0.05 %. However, there is considerable concern about a potential mutagenic effect, which has reduced its use in humans in vivo [24].

By combining fluorescein and topical acriflavine, it is possible to calculate nuclear/cytoplasm ratio, which is a useful indicator for cellular differentiation.

Other topical dyes (or precursors) that have been used for CLE are cresyl violet, hypericin, 5-aminolevulinic acid, topical fluorescein, and 2-NBDG (2-[*N*-(7-nitrobenz-2-oxa-1,3-diaxol-4-yl) amino]-2-deoxyglucose) [17, 25–28]. Potentially every fluorescent dye could be used for CLE—for the commercially available systems, only dyes with an absorption and emission maximum in the infrared spectrum are suitable.

Besides these unspecific stains, fluorescent probes directed against certain, disease-specific biomarkers are investigated in experimental settings [4]. Monoclonal antibodies targeted against the epidermal growth factor receptor (EGFR) or vascular endothelial growth factor (VEGF) have been successfully used in organ cultures, tissue samples, and human tumors grown in mice [29–31]. These specific markers might help to target lesions at risk during endoscopy and to predict response to targeted treatment [31].

Clinically Certified CLSM and CLE Systems

There are numerous clinically certified CLSM systems on the market. The four biggest producers of microscopes all have CLSMs in their assortment (Carl Zeiss, Leica Microsystems, Nikon, and Olympus). There are various other manufacturers producing CLSMs for special indications.

Currently, there are only two clinically certified, CE-marked, and FDA-approved CLE systems on the market for the in vivo use in humans.

One of them is the ISC 1000 endomicroscope (initially Pentax Life Care, Tokyo, Japan, and Optiscan Pty Ltd., Notting Hill,

Victoria, Australia, since 2008 Hoya Corporation, Tokyo, Japan, and Optiscan Pty Ltd., Notting Hill, Victoria, Australia). The CLE system is integrated into the distal tip of a conventional, large bore, flexible endoscope—this type of system is referred to as an endoscope-based confocal laser endomicroscope (eCLE). The Pentax system provides continuous scanning depths from 0 to 250 μm and has an excellent lateral resolution of 0.7 μm and a fixed field of view of 475 × 475 μm [7].

The other system is a probe-based confocal laser endomicroscopy (pCLE) system called Cellvizio (Mauna Kea Technologies, Paris, France). Various miniprobes with variable diameters and optical characteristics can be inserted through the working channel of any standard flexible or rigid endoscope. In contrast to the Pentax system, the focal plane of each confocal miniprobe is fixed.

The optical characteristics of both systems are compared in Table 1. Both work at an excitation wavelength of 488 nm and have a detection bandwidth in the upper visible range. Advantages of the Pentax system are a higher resolution and a variable and higher penetration depth. Disadvantages are the large diameter of the probe (rigid distal diameter 12.8 mm) and the limitation of bending of the distal tip, which weigh heavy in confined anatomical areas as the larynx [21]. The disadvantages of the probe-based system include a limited lifespan of 20 procedures per

Table 1
Commercially available confocal laser endomicroscopy systems and their optical characteristics

	Cellvizio system					**Pentax system**
	Gastro-/ Coloflex	Gastro-/ Coloflex UHD	Cholangioflex	AQ-Flex	Alveoflex	
Imaging rate (frames/s)	12					0.8 or 1.6
Depth of imaging (μm)	70–130 (fixed)	55–65 (fixed)	40–70 (fixed)	40–70 (fixed)	0–50 (fixed)	0–250 (flexible)
Lateral resolution (μm)	3.5	1	3.5	3.5	3.5	0.7
Field of view (μm)	Ø 600	Ø 240	Ø 325	Ø 325	Ø 600	475 × 475

miniprobe, which increases the maintenance costs. Advantages are the faster image acquisition rate (12 frames/s versus 0.8–1.6 frames/s) and the mosaic function, where single images are stitched together.

According to Optiscan, a third commercial CLE system is currently being developed in cooperation with Carl Zeiss Meditec AG (Jena, Germany) for the use in neurosurgery; ear, nose, and throat (ENT) surgery; and spinal surgery.

Implementation of Confocal Endomicroscopy Imaging

As mentioned above, to date, there are two commercially available systems on the market for clinical confocal endomicroscopy imaging in the head and neck field: the ISC 1000 endomicroscope (Hoya Corporation, Tokyo, Japan, and Optiscan Pty Ltd., Noting Hill, Victoria, Australia) and the Cellvizio system (Mauna Kea Technologies, Paris, France). They both work in fluorescence rather than in reflectance mode and have an excitation wavelength of 488 nm and a detection bandwidth in the upper visible range.

Confocal endomicroscopy can be performed both under general anesthesia (for examination of the lower pharynx and larynx) and in the awake patient. For imaging, a contrast agent is necessary. The only licensed stain for being used in vivo in humans with CLE is intravenously applied fluorescein. 2.5–5.0 ml of a 10 % fluorescein solution should be applied.

After intravenous injection fluorescein distributes in the vasculature and passes across the systemic capillaries to reach the tissues, highlighting extracellular matrix. Images can be generated a few seconds up to 30 min after application of the contrast agent, though image quality deteriorates significantly after approximately 8 min. To generate photographs or video files, the CLE probes need to be in direct contact with the mucosa. For the ISC 1000 endomicroscope, the large bore flexible endoscope with the integrated CLE system is directly placed on the tissue, which can be challenging for some areas (e.g., the larynx), while for the Cellvizio system, a miniprobe is inserted through a standard endoscope and then again placed onto the tissue. Our own experience showed the best images with the Gastroflex UHD miniprobe [15]. Usually CLE imaging requires two examiners—one has to place the endoscope on the lesion and the other one is needed to run the system. A CLE examination takes a few minutes. Figure 2 shows how the CLE probe is placed onto the vocal cord of a patient.

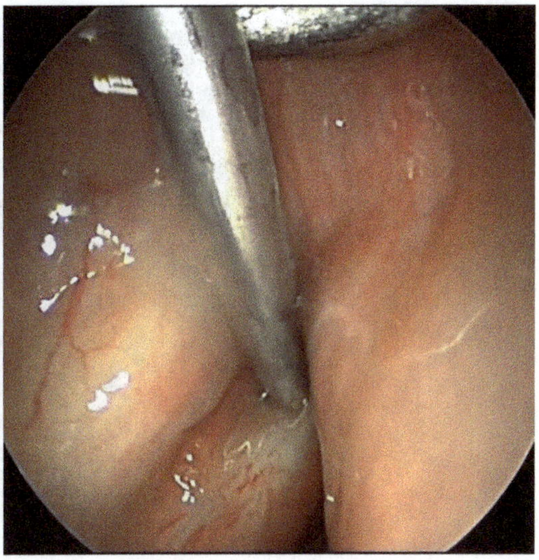

Fig. 2 Placement of the CLE probe onto the vocal cord

Interpretation of CLE Results

CLE, so far, has been mostly used in gastroenterology. Classification systems have been developed to help classify different lesions especially in the esophagus and colon.

As CLE is still very new to the head and neck, no official classification system exists. Nevertheless, certain characteristics of different lesions in the head and neck can be observed. Fluorescein does not allow for direct nuclear visualization, therefore nucleus/cytoplasm ratios cannot be used for diagnosis and grading of intraepithelial neoplasias.

In healthy mucosa a regular cellular size, shape, and architecture can be seen. Also capillaries can be seen. Figures 3, 4, and 5 show normal epithelium from different sites within the head and neck of patients and healthy volunteers.

In dysplasias cells vary in shape and size. An irregular cellular array can be found (Fig. 6).

Inflammatory lesions usually show enlarged intracellular spaces caused by edema.

In carcinomas CLE allows to visualize neo-angiogenesis, irregular cellular architecture, and poorly defined cell borders. Figures 7 and 8 show an early invasive carcinoma of the anterior commissure of the larynx and the corresponding pCLE image.

Highly hyperkeratotic lesions are very hard to investigate and interpret with CLE because light does not sufficiently penetrate the keratin layer.

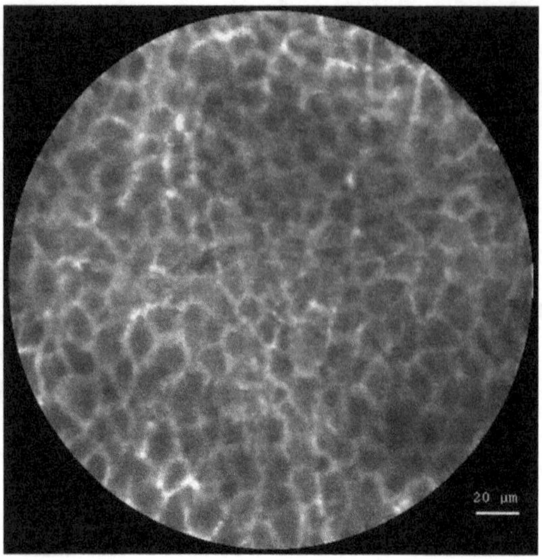

Fig. 3 pCLE image of healthy mucosa of the vocal cord in a patient showing regular cellular size, shape, and architecture

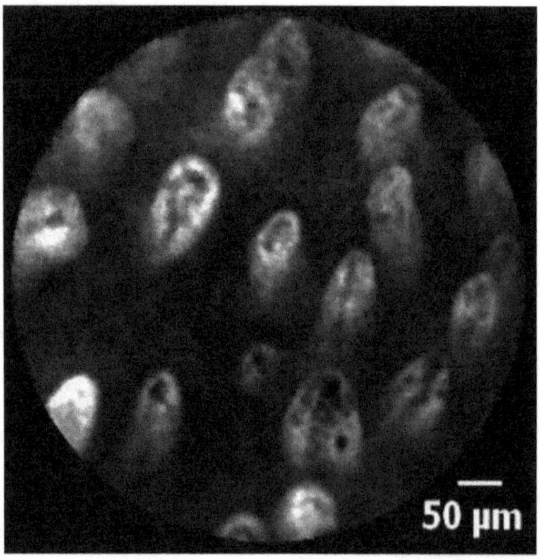

Fig. 4 pCLE image of healthy mucosa of the dorsum of tongue showing papillae in a healthy volunteer

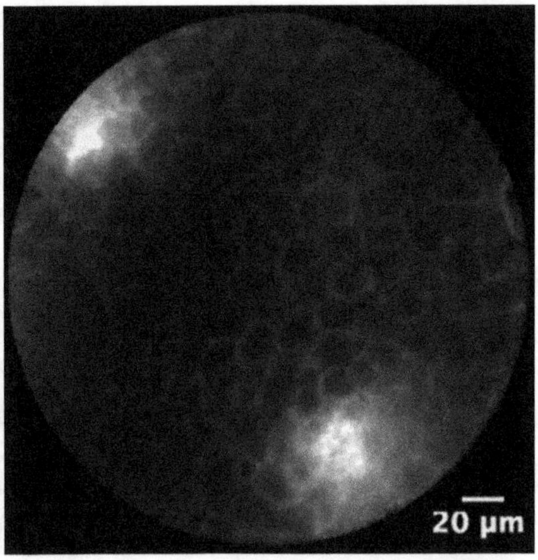

Fig. 5 pCLE image of the alveolar ridge in a healthy volunteer

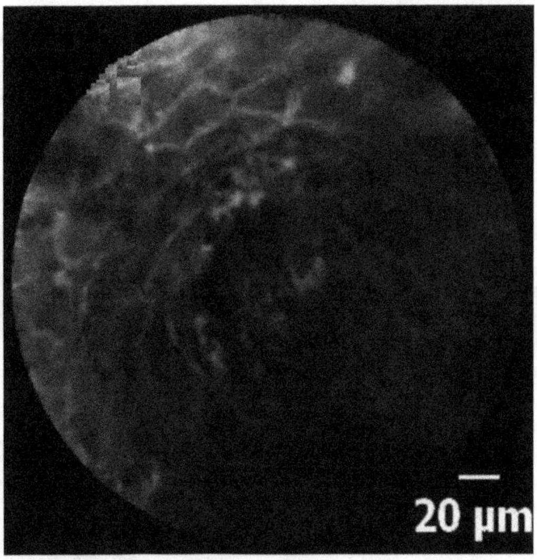

Fig. 6 pCLE image of a high-grade dysplasia of the vocal. Cells are irregular in size and shape and cellular borders are not clearly visible

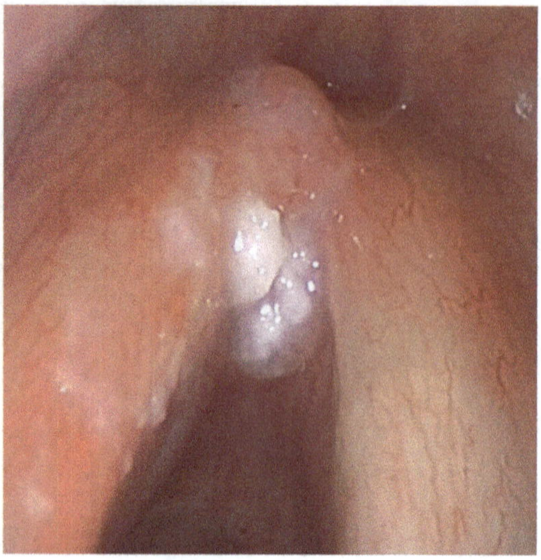

Fig. 7 Early invasive carcinoma of the anterior commissure in a 73-year-old male patient

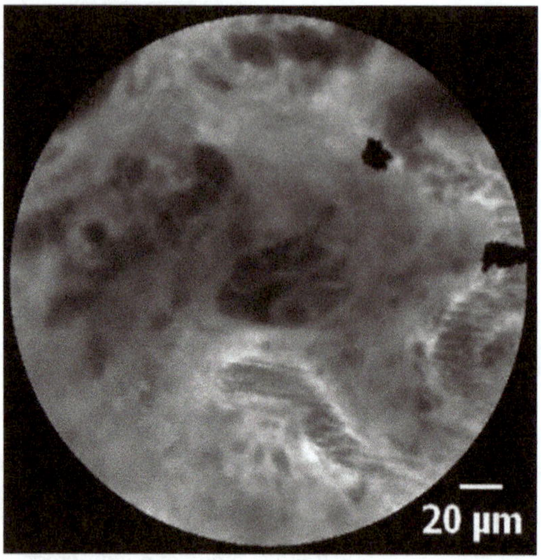

Fig. 8 pCLE image of an early invasive carcinoma of the anterior commissure in a 73-year-old male patient

Clinical Applications

In the 1980s and 1990s, animal and human tissue was first imaged in vivo with confocal microscopes. In vivo imaging was initially limited to easy accessible organs such as the eye, skin, and oral cavity [32, 33]). In order to increase accessibility to tissue, microscope modifications were made, such as building a mechanical arm and a rotatable head to image skin, lip, and tongue in vivo [11, 33–35]. In 2006 Just et al. were the first to use CLSM for the investigation of laryngeal tissue *ex vivo*, after applying it to other tissues of the UADT previously in the early 2000s [36, 37]. The authors tried to distinguish non-carcinoma (benign and premalignant lesions) from carcinoma (carcinoma in situ and invasive carcinoma) in 43 larynx specimen of 26 patients and reported about the findings in seven laryngectomy specimen. For the evaluation of tissue, they used the following criteria: nuclear size, nuclear density, number of nuclei, nucleus/cytoplasm ratio, regularity of the cell layers, morphology of cells of a cell layer, and occurrence of cellular junctions. Using these criteria for the differentiation between non-carcinoma and carcinoma, a sensitivity of 72.7 % and a specificity of 82.9 % were reached. They also described the appearance of healthy laryngeal mucosa and different pathologies in CLSM. Healthy mucosa could be visualized up to a depth of 200 μm. The layers of the lamina propria and the vocal ligament could be differentiated with CLSM. In healthy laryngeal mucosa, the superficial cell layer is characterized by a regular cell architecture. The cells near the basement membrane appear smaller and have a higher nucleus/cytoplasm ratio compared to the superficial cell layer. The border between superficial and basement cell layer is clearly visible, whereas the basement membrane itself cannot be identified. Additionally, elastic fibers of the subepithelial space and subepithelial vessels were detected. Inflammation is characterized by koilocytes—cells with a vacuolated cytoplasm and ballooned appearance. In dysplasias an irregular cell architecture and size can be found. In contrast to dysplasias, cellular junctions cannot be identified in carcinomas. Carcinomas also show atypical cells with an increased nucleus/cytoplasm ratio.

According to the authors, visualization of cells around the basement membrane is the precondition for in vivo diagnosis of precancerous lesions and seems possible in most laryngeal lesions. The main reason for low image quality or misinterpretation of images was severe hyperkeratosis and extensive hyperplasia.

Besides from evaluating laryngeal lesions, CLSM has been used to better understand pediatric laryngeal development [38, 39]. The current knowledge is limited by the lack of pediatric specimen availability. Preliminary imaging results with spectrally encoded confocal microscopy in porcine tissue and in pediatric laryngeal specimen demonstrate the potential for endomicroscopic imaging of the vocal folds. Images portraying epithelial cells, the basement membrane, and the lamina propria were obtained down to 375 μm/250 μm deep in the tissue, respectively. One patient was investigated in vivo with a prototype rigid handheld confocal endomicroscope and cellular details could be shown.

In vivo visualization of laryngeal tissue was only possible after confocal laser endomicroscopes were developed.

By far most clinical studies on CLE have been published in gastroenterology. Hallmark indications are (1) the differentiation of Barrett's dysplastic lesions from non-dysplastic mucosa in the esophagus [17] and (2) the detection of colorectal neoplasms especially in follow-up situations [40]. Classification systems have been developed to help classify those lesions. Furthermore, CLE has been used to evaluate hepatobiliary strictures, gastric cancer, celiac disease, and inflammatory bowel disease. The American Medical Association has recently approved three CPT (Current Procedural Terminology) codes to cover the use of CLE for the observation of intestinal mucosa during endoscopic procedures, which will facilitate the reimbursement process in the USA and might lead to a more frequent use and wider acceptance of this technology [15].

Further fields with significant scientific output on CLE are pulmonology, urology, and gynecology [23, 41–43].

Literature regarding the use of CLE in the context of head and neck pathologies has been sparse. Its use was first described in 2004 using topical 5-aminolevulinic acid (ALA)-induced protoporphyrin IX (PpIX) fluorescence in three patients with squamous cell carcinoma of the tongue and the findings were compared to mucosa of healthy volunteers [26]. Using a prototype rigid CLE system by Optiscan Pty Ltd., the authors could clearly notice changes in cellular size, regularity, and density in carcinomas when compared to healthy mucosa. Similarly, in 2007, Thong et al. used the same system and detailed their findings imaging normal oral mucosa and squamous cell carcinoma in humans and in a murine model [44]. They used topical PpIX and fluorescein as contrast agents and determined that CLE with both stains seems suitable to distinguish between normal, dysplastic, and cancerous tissue.

After several *ex vivo* studies using CLSM for the differentiation of UADT lesions, a group from Rice University, USA, published a preliminary report on the use of a prototype CLE system working in reflectance mode on eight patients with oral SCC in 2008 [45]. The authors used acetic acid for contrast enhancement and were able to show that nuclear morphology distinctly differed for normal mucosa and cancerous lesions.

From 2009, Abbaci et al. from the Institut Gustave Roussy in Villejuif, France, used the Cellvizio system in an *ex vivo* setting using various different morphological (fluorescein, acriflavine, cresyl violet, methylene blue, toluidine blue), functional (2-NBDG), and molecular (fluorescent EGFR antibody) stains. Based on >100 freshly obtained specimens from the head and neck, they were able to discern abnormal features in dysplastic and cancerous lesions when compared to normal controls. These features determining (pre)malignancy after morphological staining included changes in nuclear size and shape, changes in nuclear/cytoplasm ratio, and disorders of keratinization. However, the preliminary results of functional and molecular staining were more inconsistent. The authors also determined a high degree of correlation (sensitivities 92–97 %, specificities 85–97 %) when comparing CLE images (dually stained with fluorescein and acriflavine) and conventional H&E slides in blinded evaluations. This work still remains unpublished; however, it has been repeatedly presented at various international meetings.

In 2010, Haxel et al. published the results of a pilot study regarding the use of the Optiscan eCLE system for imaging of oral and oropharyngeal mucosa [46]. They were the first to describe the use of intravenous sodium fluorescein ($n=3$) in imaging of the upper aerodigestive tract. While imaging invasive squamous cell carcinoma, they were able to visualize neo-angiogenesis, irregular cellular architecture, and poorly defined cell borders. Additionally, they used topical acriflavine in *ex vivo* specimens and demonstrated differences in nuclear morphology and rates of mitoses in normal and dysplastic specimens. Despite these promising findings, they experienced difficulties in handling the large bore endoscope in confined anatomical areas of the UADT. In 2012, Pogorzelski et al. [14] published a case series describing the use of intraoperative CLE in squamous cell carcinoma of the head and neck. In vivo CLE of the larynx was reported for the first time. Their series consisted of 15 patients with SCC of the oral cavity ($n=4$), oropharynx ($n=7$), hypopharynx ($n=2$), and larynx ($n=2$). During resection of lesions, images were generated from the tumor site as well as from macroscopically normal mucosa. Neoplastic specimens showed nonhomogenous configuration of the superficial layers, irregular cellular and nuclear structures, blurry cellular definition, 3–4 capillaries per high-power field of view, and extended and irregular configuration of the capillaries.

In the early 2000s, Just et al. had published on the use of CLSM for different pathologic states of the UADT. To access more areas of the UADT, they have recently developed a prototype rigid CLE system and have applied it in a murine UADT cancer model and in human laryngeal pathologies in vivo [47, 48]. In $n=58$ mice with various states of dysplasia, they were able to differentiate low/moderate from high-grade dysplasia with a sensitivity of 73 % and a specificity of 88 % and a moderate interobserver agreement of $\kappa=0.59$. In volume scans of human vocal cords, they were able to show typical features of normal and pathologic states.

Later in 2012, Thong et al. expanded upon their prior study [44] and developed a prototype endomicroscope-embedded computing system for 3-D visualization of tissue [49]. This was applied first in a murine model and subsequently in vivo in healthy volunteers. In the human volunteers, they imaged the tongue, floor of mouth, buccal mucosa, and lip after topical application of hypericin or fluorescein. The results revealed impressive 3-D renderings of filiform papillae and cellular mucosal structures in video rate.

In an initial pilot study, our own group looked at dysplastic/early invasive lesions and normal mucosa (nine subsites of the UADT) in ten patients and five healthy volunteers using the Cellvizio system and intravenous fluorescein [15]. Visualization of tissue architecture at a subcellular level was possible, thus allowing us to differentiate normal and neoplastic mucosa. These distinctions were mostly based on changes in cellular sizes, shapes, and cellular arrangement. In normal mucosa we obtained the highest quality images with the most cellular detail when imaging was performed against a rigid backdrop such as in the hard palate and alveolar ridge.

Currently, we launched an *ex vivo* study on human tissue specimens comparing various stains, including morphological and molecular stains, as for their usefulness and applicability and an in vivo study to define the role of CLE in the differentiation between various noninvasive lesions of the UADT. The patients' recruitment for the in vivo study is almost complete and we expect interesting and clinically relevant results. Figures 9, 10, 11, and 12 show examples of lesions and healthy tissue within the UADT, and Table 2 gives an overview of the abovementioned studies on CLE in the head and neck.

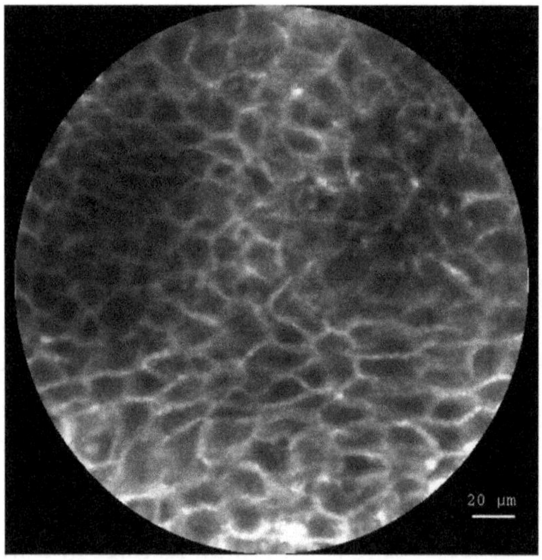

Fig. 9 pCLE image of normally appearing mucosa of the vocal cord in a 69-year-old patient

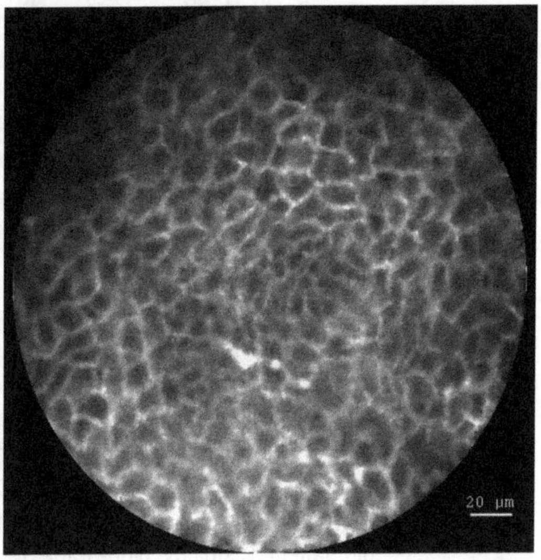

Fig. 10 pCLE image of a leukoplakia of the vocal cord in a 69-year-old patient. Histology: hyperplasia

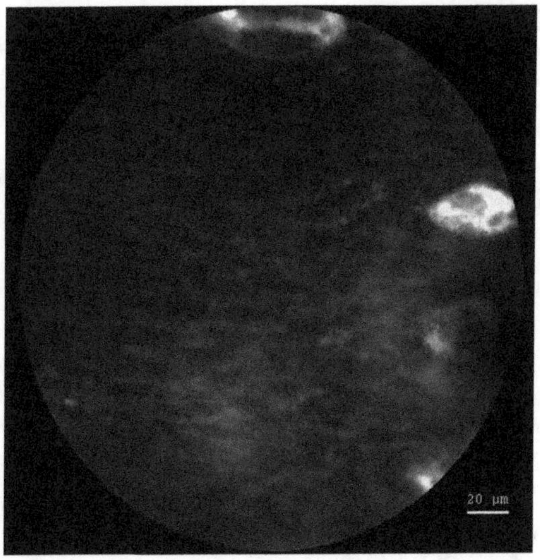

Fig. 11 pCLE image of normal mucosa of the ventral surface of tongue in a 73-year-old patient

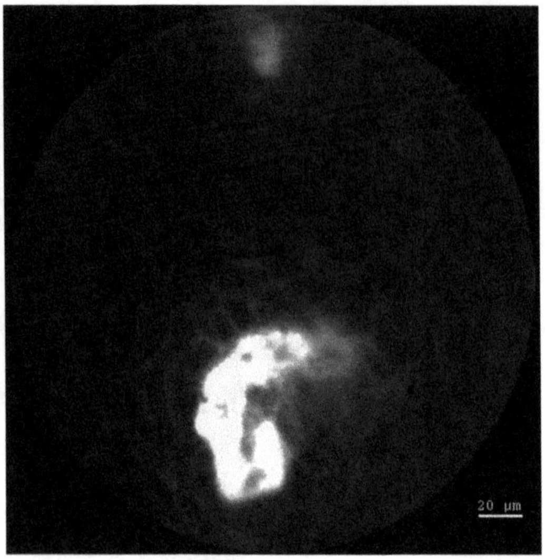

Fig. 12 pCLE image of a leukoplakia of the ventral surface of tongue in a 73-year-old patient. Histology: high-grade dysplasia

Table 2
Systems and fluorescent dyes used in CLE studies of the UADT

Study	Device used	Fluorescent dye
Zheng et al. [26]	Handheld, rigid Optiscan CLE probe	0.4 % of 5-ALA rinsing solution
Thong et al. [44]	Handheld, rigid Optiscan CLE probe	0.4 % 5-ALA rinsing solution in human model 0.4 % 5-ALA rinsing solution and 0.1 % topical fluorescein in murine model
Maitland et al. [45]	Handheld, rigid prototype CLE system (reflectance mode)	Topical acetic acid
Abbaci et al.	*Ex vivo*: Cellvizio Gastroflex flexible probe	*Ex vivo*: various morphological stains (fluorescein, acriflavine, cresyl violet, methylene blue, toluidine blue) and molecular stains
Haxel et al. [46]	In vivo: Optiscan eCLE system Ex vivo: handheld, rigid Optiscan CLE probe	In vivo: 5 ml 10 % IV fluorescein *Ex vivo*: 0.02 % topical acriflavine
Pogorzelski et al. [14]	Handheld, rigid Optiscan CLE probe	5 ml 10 % IV fluorescein
Farahati et al. [48]	*Ex vivo* murine model: prototype rigid CLE system	
Just et al. [47]	Prototype rigid CLE system	
Thong et al. [49]	Prototype endomicroscope-embedded computer based on Optiscan CLE system	0.004 % topical hypericin 0.1 % topical fluorescein
Own study	In vivo: Cellvizio Gastroflex UHD	2.5–5 ml 10 % IV fluorescein

Summary and Outlook

CLSM is a widely accepted technique for the microanatomical evaluation of various tissues. It has been shown to be suitable for the UADT, as its penetration depth exceeds the average thickness of the UADT epithelium and therefore allows to visualize the basement cell layer. CLE is a promising new, noninvasive diagnostic method providing microanatomical images of superficial tissue layers in vivo. The method has established itself in gastroenterology. In the UADT, CLE has shown promising results for the differentiation of normal mucosa and dysplastic/microinvasive lesions, but the described methods and the results are hardly comparable. The method has its limitations especially in the vertical assessment of tissue changes. There is a rather significant learning curve associated with image interpretation for the ENT specialist as well as for pathologists. Further studies are needed to better define the role of CLE in the UADT by standardizing diagnostic protocols concerning the type of system and contrast agent used and by deploying useful classification systems.

References

1. Minsky M. Memoir on inventing the confocal scanning microscope. Scanning. 1988;10: 128–38.
2. Petroll WM, Jester JV, Cavanagh HD. In vivo confocal imaging: general principles and applications. Scanning. 1994;16:131–49.
3. Stave J, Slowik C, Somodi S, Hahnel C, Grummer C, Guthoff R. Keratozytendichte der in vivo-Kornea: Automatische Messung mit einem modifiziertem konfokalen Mikroskop Microphthal. Klin Monatsbl Augenheilkd. 1998;213:38–44.
4. Paull PE, Hyatt BJ, Wassef W, Fischer AH. Confocal laser endomicroscopy: a primer for pathologists. Arch Pathol Lab Med. 2011;135:1343–8.
5. Goetz M, Watson A, Kiesslich R. Confocal laser endomicroscopy in gastrointestinal diseases. J Biophotonics. 2011;4:498–508.
6. Humphris J, Swartz D, Egan BJ, Leong RWL. Status of confocal laser endomicroscopy in gastrointestinal disease. Trop Gastroenterol. 2012;33:9–20.
7. Jabbour JM, Saldua MA, Bixler JN, Maitland KC. Confocal endomicroscopy: instrumentation and medical applications. Ann Biomed Eng. 2012;40:378–97.
8. Dickensheets DL, Kino GS. Scanned optical fiber confocal microscope. In: Proceedings of SPIE; 1994, p. 39–47.
9. White WM, Rajadhyaksha M, Gonzales S, Fabian RL, Anderson RR. Noninvasive imaging of human oral mucosa in vivo by confocal reflectance microscopy. Laryngoscope. 1999; 109:1709–17.
10. Just T, Pau HW, Bombor I, Guthoff R, Fietkau R, Hummel T. Confocal microscopy of the peripheral gustatory system: comparison between healthy subjects and patients suffering from taste disorders during radiochemotherapy. Laryngoscope. 2005;115:2178–82.
11. Just T, Stawe J, Pau HW, Guthoff R. In-vivo observation of papillae of the human tongue using confocal laser scanning microscopy. ORL J Otorhinolaryngol Relat Spec. 2005;67: 207–12.
12. Shahid MW, Crook JE, Meining A, et al. Exploring the optimal fluorescein dose in probe-based confocal laser endomicroscopy for colonic imaging. J Interv Gastroenterol. 2011;1:166–71.
13. Wallace MB, Sharma P, Lightdale C, et al. Preliminary accuracy and interobserver agreement for the detection of intraepithelial neoplasia in Barrett's esophagus with probe-based confocal laser endomicroscopy. Gastrointest Endosc. 2010;72:19–24.
14. Pogorzelski B, Hanenkamp U, Goetz M, et al. Systematic intraoperative application of confocal endomicroscopy for early detection and

resection of squamous cell carcinoma of the head and neck: a preliminary report. Arch Otolaryngol Head Neck Surg. 2012;138: 404–11.

15. Volgger V, Conderman C, Betz CS. Confocal laser endomicroscopy in head and neck cancer: steps forward? Curr Opin Otolaryngol Head Neck Surg. 2013;21(2):164–70.
16. Becker V, von Delius S, Bajbouj M, et al. Intravenous application of fluorescein for confocal laser scanning microscopy: evaluation of contrast dynamics and image quality with increasing injection-to-imaging time. Gastrointest Endosc. 2008;68(2):319–23.
17. Dunbar KB. Endomicroscopy in the evaluation of Barrett's esophagus. Curr Opin Gastroenterol. 2011;27(4):374–82.
18. Kwan AS, Barry C, McAllister IL, Constable I. Fluorescein angiography and adverse drug reactions revisited: the Lions Eye experience. Clin Experiment Ophthalmol. 2006;34:33–8.
19. O'goshi K, Serup J. Safety of sodium fluorescein for in vivo study of skin. Clin Experiment Ophthalmol. 2006;34:33–8.
20. Wallace MB, Meining A, Canto MI, et al. The safety of intravenous fluorescein for confocal laser endomicroscopy in the gastrointestinal tract. Aliment Pharmacol Ther. 2010;31:548–52.
21. Polglase A, McLaren WJ, Skinner SA, et al. A fluorescence confocal endomicroscope for in vivo microscopy of the upper and lower GI-tract. Gastrointest Endosc. 2005;62:686–95.
22. Kiesslich R, Burg J, Vieth M, et al. Confocal laser endoscopy for diagnosing intraepithelial neoplasias and colorectal cancer in vivo. Gastroenterology. 2004;127:706–13.
23. Fuchs FS, Zirlik S, Hildner K, et al. Confocal laser endomicroscopy for diagnosing lung cancer in vivo. Eur Respir J. 2013;41(6):1401–8.
24. ASGE Technology Committee, Kantsevoy SV, Adler DG, et al. Confocal laser endomicroscopy. Gastrointest Endosc. 2009;70:197–200.
25. Olivo M, Lau W, Manivasager V, et al. Macro-microscopic fluorescence of human bladder cancer using hypericin fluorescence cystoscopy and laser confocal microscopy. Int J Oncol. 2003;23:983–90.
26. Zheng W, Harris M, Kho KW, et al. Confocal endomicroscopic imaging of normal and neoplastic human tongue tissue using ALA-induced-PPIX fluorescence: a preliminary study. Oncol Rep. 2004;12:397–401.
27. Wang TD, Friedland S, Sahbaie P, et al. Functional imaging of colonic mucosa with a fibered confocal microscope for real time in vivo pathology. Clin Gastroenterol Hepatol. 2007;5:1300–5.
28. Gorospe EC, Leggett CL, Sun G, et al. Diagnostic performance of two confocal endomicroscopy systems in detecting Barrett's dysplasia: a pilot study using a novel bioprobe in ex vivo tissue. Gastrointest Endosc. 2012;76(5):933–8.
29. Hsu ER, Gillenwater AM, Hasan MQ, et al. Real-time detection of epidermal growth factor receptor expression in fresh oral cavity biopsies using a molecular-specific contrast agent. Int J Cancer. 2006;118:3062–71.
30. Goetz M, Ziebart A, Foersch S, et al. In vivo molecular imaging of colorectal cancer with confocal endomicroscopy by targeting epidermal growth factor receptor. Gastroenterology. 2010;138:435–46.
31. Foersch S, Kiesslich R, Waldner MJ, et al. Molecular imaging of VEGF in gastrointestinal cancer in vivo using confocal laser endomicroscopy. Gut. 2010;59:1046–55.
32. Rajadhyaksha M, Anderson RR, Webb RH. Video-rate confocal scanning laser microscope for imaging human tissues in vivo. Appl Opt. 1999;38:2105–15.
33. New KC, Petroll WM, Boyde A, Martin L, Corcuff P, Leveque JL, Lemp MA, Cavanagh HD, Jester JV. In vivo imaging of human teeth and skin using real-time confocal microscopy. Scanning. 1991;13:369–72.
34. Rajadhyaksha M, Gonzalez S, Zavislan JM, Anderson RR, Webb RH. In vivo confocal scanning laser microscopy of human skin II: advances in instrumentation and comparison with histology. J Invest Dermatol. 1999;113:293–303.
35. Just T, Zeisner C, Stave J, Pau HW. Konfokale Laser-Scanning Mikroskopie zur Beurteilung des Zungenepithels. Laryngo-Rhino-Otologie. 2004;83:108–12.
36. Just T, Stave J, boltze C, Wree A, Kramp B, Gufhoff RF, Pau HW. Laser scanning microscopy of the human larynx mucosa: a preliminary, ex vivo study. Laryngoscope. 2006;116:1136–41.
37. Just T, Stave J, Kreutzer HJ, Guthoff R, Pau HW. Konfokalmikroskopische Untersuchungen des Kehlkopfepithels. Laryngo-Rhino-Otologie. 2007;86:644–8.
38. Boudoux C, Leuin SC, Oh WY, Suter MJ, Desjardins AE, Vakoc BJ, Bouma BE, Hartnick CJ, Tearney GJ. Preliminary evaluation of noninvasive microscopic imaging techniques for the study of vocal fold development. J Voice. 2009;23(3):269–76.
39. Boudoux C, Leuin SC, Oh WY, Suter MJ, Desjardins AE, Vakoc BJ, Bouma BE, Hartnick CJ, Tearney GJ. Optical microscopy of the

pediatric vocal fold. Arch Otolaryngol Head Neck Surg. 2009;135(1):53–64.

40. Su P, Liu Y, Lin S, et al. Efficacy of confocal laser endomicroscopy for discriminating colorectal neoplasms from non-neoplasms: a systematic review and meta-analysis. Color Dis. 2013;15(1):e1–12.
41. Sonn GA, Jones SN, Tarin TV, et al. Optical biopsy of human bladder neoplasia with in vivo confocal laser endomicroscopy. J Urol. 2009; 182:1299–305.
42. Wu K, Liu JJ, Adams W, et al. Dynamic real-time microscopy of the urinary tract using confocal laser endomicroscopy. Urology. 2011;78: 225–31.
43. Tan J, Quinn MA, Pyman JM, et al. Detection of cervical intraepithelial neoplasia in vivo using confocal endomicroscopy. BJOG. 2009;116:1663–70.
44. Thong PS, Olivo M, Kho KW, et al. Laser confocal endomicroscopy as a novel technique for fluorescence diagnostic imaging of the oral cavity. J Biomed Opt. 2007;12:014007.
45. Maitland KC, Gillenwater AM, Williams MD, et al. In vivo imaging of oral neoplasia using a miniaturized fiber optic confocal reflectance microscope. Oral Oncol. 2008; 44:1059–66.
46. Haxel BR, Goetz M, Kiesslich R, Gosepath J. Confocal endomicroscopy: a novel application for imaging of oral and oropharyngeal mucosa in human. Eur Arch Otorhinolaryngol. 2010;267:443–8.
47. Just T, Stave J, Stachs O, et al. Rigid confocal endoscopy of the larynx. In: Wang C-C, editor. Laser scanning, theory and applications. Rijeka, Croatia: InTech; 2011. p. 97–112.
48. Farahati B, Stachs O, Prall F, et al. Rigid confocal endoscopy for in vivo imaging of experimental oral squamous intra-epithelial lesions. J Oral Pathol Med. 2010;39:318–27.
49. Thong PS, Tandjung SS, Movania MM, et al. Toward real-time virtual biopsy of oral lesions using confocal laser endomicroscopy interfaced with embedded computing. J Biomed Opt. 2012;17:056009.

Chapter 31

Nonlinear Microscopy of the Vocal Folds

Mathias Strupler, Romain Deterre, Nadir Goulamhoussen, Fouzi Benboujja, Christopher J. Hartnick, and Caroline Boudoux

Introduction

Many new optical microscopy techniques have recently been investigated to allow better understanding of vocal fold composition. Optical coherence tomography (OCT), which was first demonstrated as a cross-sectional tool to obtain high-resolution virtual sections of the retina [1], was soon adapted to image inner organs through optical fiber-based catheters. This allowed visualization of superficial layers of the oral cavity [2], esophagus [3], bladder [4], and endothelia of arteries [5] and airways [6]. OCT is being applied to laryngeal imaging [7, 8] for cancer detection [9] as well as for vocal fold imaging [10, 11]. More recently, OCT has been used to study the evolution of the lamina propria on porcine specimens [12], pediatric laryngectomy samples [13, 14], and in vivo on infants [15] and neonates [16]. OCT is also used in laryngology as a guiding tool to monitor femtosecond laser microsurgery [17]. While OCT has the potential to noninvasively image the entirety of the lamina propria, it currently lacks the resolution and contrast to visualize cellular components and identify molecular composition of the different areas within the vocal fold.

Another biomedical photonic imaging technique called reflectance confocal microscopy (RCM) provides images with a greater resolution through a property named optical sectioning [18]. Images produced with RCM yield cellular and subcellular details of thick specimen without the processing steps required for histopathological evaluation [19]. Video rate acquisition (tens of images per second) allowed RCM to be applied to ophthalmology [20] and dermatology [21]. The miniaturization of scanning mecha-

Brian J.-F. Wong and Justus Ilgner (eds.), *Biomedical Optics in Otorhinolaryngology: Head and Neck Surgery*, DOI 10.1007/978-1-4939-1758-7_31, © Springer Science+Business Media New York 2016

nisms further allowed RCM to be performed on inner organs such as the colon [22] through fiber optic catheters. An implementation of RCM called spectrally encoded confocal microscopy, or SECM [23, 24], was recently used to image pediatric vocal folds in vivo [13]. RCM and OCT offer complementary view of the vocal fold as the former offers subcellular resolution of superficial layers and the later coarser view of deeper structures [25]. Many groups are therefore attempting to combine both modalities within the same instrument [26, 27], which would contribute to bridging the gap between histopathology and noninvasive imaging. The lack of molecular contrast, however, remains a limiting aspect of these new instruments.

A promising alternative to RCM is nonlinear microscopy, also called multiphoton microscopy [28]. This method relies on nonlinear interactions between light and biological tissues. By nonlinear, we mean that the resulting effect from the interaction does not scale linearly with the light field amplitude. Nonlinear interactions depend on the square, the cube, or even higher powers of the laser irradiance (i.e., the laser power per surface unit). Every tissue is capable of producing some sort of nonlinear interaction—the nonlinearity is becoming significant only when light irradiance reaches tens or hundreds of MW/cm^2. This explains why even if these effects were predicted theoretically in the beginning of the twentieth century, no experimental verification was performed before the discovery of lasers in the 1960s.

In this chapter, we will describe how nonlinear interaction between light and molecules can be utilized to obtain selective intrinsic contrast for macromolecules, such as elastin and collagen, without using exogenous dyes. A large field-of-view (FOV) nonlinear microscope was built to allow multimodal vocal fold imaging. This allows for visualization of one-to-one comparison between nonlinear microscopy images and histology as a step toward integrating this new technique into clinical laryngology practice. While most nonlinear microscopes are still tabletop instruments, research involving specialized optical fibers and microscanning mechanisms very recently allowed nonlinear imaging to be performed through small endoscopic probes [29–31]. In vivo imaging with nonlinear fiberscope was mostly applied to brain imaging [31]. Similar instruments could be developed for laryngology to noninvasively assess the molecular composition of vocal fold structures. The potential of nonlinear microscopy for laryngeal imaging was explored ex vivo [32, 33]. Nonlinear microscopy images of laryngeal tissues were also investigated as a guiding mechanism for laser therapy [34].

Origins of Nonlinear Interactions

The main nonlinear effects exploited in nonlinear microscopy are two-photon excitation fluorescence (2PEF) and second harmonic generation (SHG). The following chapters describe the physical principles involved in nonlinear interaction between light and matter.

Two-Photon Excitation Fluorescence

Figure 1 illustrates a first type of nonlinear interaction based on the absorption of two photons by a molecule. This process may lead to emission of a single fluorescent photon at a different wavelength and is called two-photon excitation fluorescence (2PEF). Linear, one-photon absorption is the contrast mechanism typically used for immunohistochemistry using fluorescent dyes. For linear absorption to occur, the energy of the incoming photon must equal the molecule's transition energy from ground state to excited state. Similarly, for nonlinear, two-photon absorption to occur, the sum of the two photons' energies has to equal the molecule's transition energy. This is a two-step process in which a first interaction with a first photon changes a molecule from its ground state to a virtual state. When in a virtual state and for a very short time, the molecule can absorb another photon. This second intake of energy will change the molecule in a final state. Virtual states have a very short lifetime, in the femtosecond (10^{-15} s) range. Therefore, absorption of a second photon has to take place during the lifetime of the virtual state. The photon flux must therefore be strong enough for two photons to interact with the molecule within this femtosecond timeframe. A detailed explanation of this phenomenon using quantum optics can be found here [35].

Most fluorescent particles have very small nonlinear cross-sections—2PEF is thus only significant when excitation fields reach hundreds of MW/cm^2. To obtain this high irradiance, the excitation laser must be confined in space—using a very high numerical aperture (NA) microscope objective—and in time—using a pulsed laser.

2PEF can excite traditional fluorescent dyes, such as fluorescein. This molecule, which is usually excited at $\lambda_{1PEF} = 490$ nm for 1PEF, can be excited under 2PEF at roughly twice the wavelength, or $\lambda_{2PEF} = 980$ nm.[1] In both circumstances, the emitted fluorescence light will be green light, as shown in Fig. 1, with a peak at

[1] The optimal 2PEF excitation wavelength is typically broader allowing for excitation wavelengths to range from 700 to 1000 nm. This effect is due to the difference in allowed transition between sublevels of the ground and excited states when excited with one or two photons.

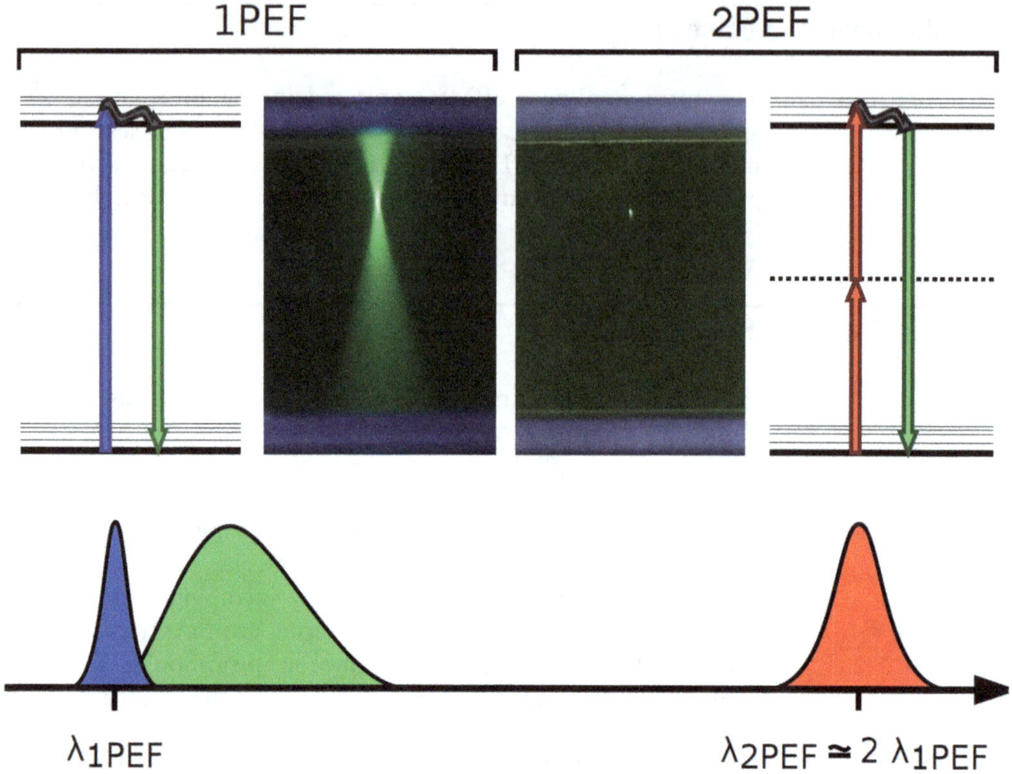

Fig. 1 One-photon (*left*) and two-photon (*right*) excitation fluorescence, or 1PEF and 2PEF, respectively, of a cuvette filled with fluorescein. The 1PEF excitation using a blue laser $\left(\lambda_{1\text{PEF}} = 488\ \text{nm}\right)$ creates an hourglass shape of green fluorescence, while the 2PEF excitation using a near-infrared laser $\left(\lambda_{2\text{PEF}} = 800\ \text{nm}\right)$ yields very localized fluorescence, at the focus of the microscope objective. This interaction requires the quasi-simultaneous absorption of two photons by the molecule

520 nm and approximately the same spectrum. In contrast with 1PEF, 2PEF only excites molecules present at the focus of the microscope objective where the laser irradiance is sufficient for the nonlinear transition to occur. Selective contrast for naturally present fluorescent molecules—such as elastin—is obtained by spectrally filtering light coming back from the sample.

Second Harmonic Generation

A second type of nonlinear interaction is a scattering process called second harmonic generation (SHG). Figure 2 is a schematic of SHG (blue wave) produced with a laser at twice the wavelength. When light shines on any material, including biological tissues, its electromagnetic field will interact with electron clouds within mol-

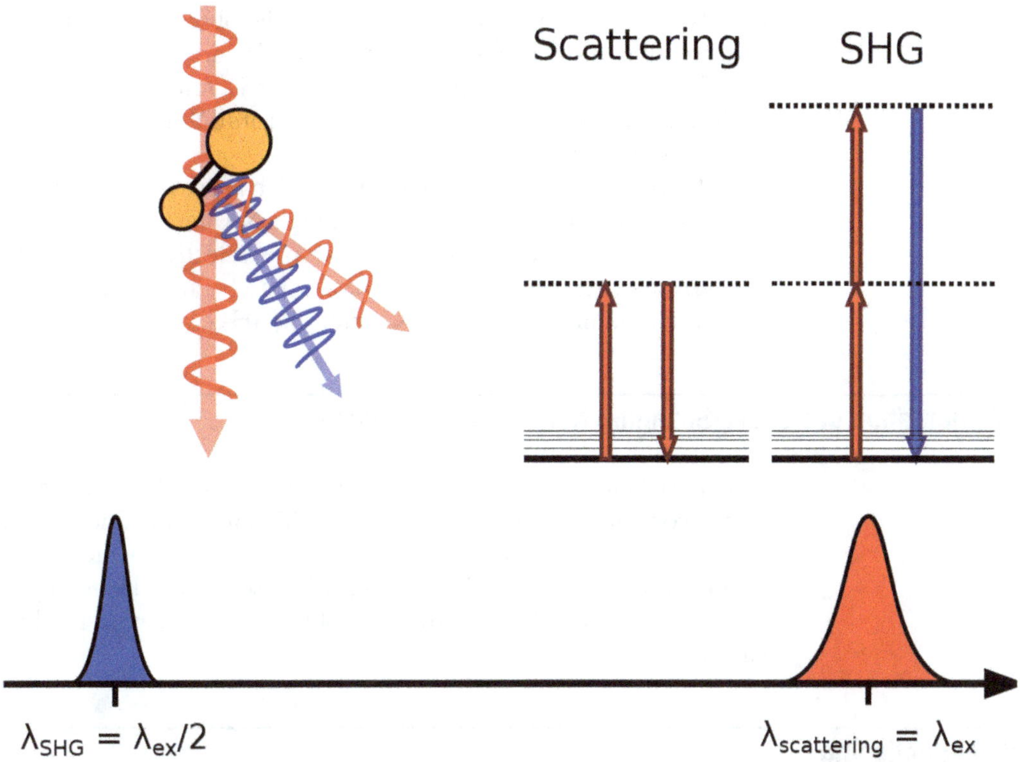

Fig. 2 Generation of second harmonic signal from a non centro-symmetric molecule. Molecules such as collagen, when illuminated under the right conditions, have the property to convert two photons of a given energy into one photon having exactly twice that energy (which corresponds to half the wavelength). This interaction involves scattering of photons through virtual states of the molecule

ecules. The oscillating light field will distort the electron clouds present in the material. This induced motion of electron clouds will in turn create oscillating dipoles that will radiate like antennas. When the excitation field is weak, the electromagnetic field originating from these antennas has rigorously the same wavelength as the excitation field. This phenomenon is called scattering and is the basis for linear imaging techniques such as OCT and RCM. When the excitation field becomes stronger, however, the radiated waveform is a distorted copy of the excitation waveform. This distortion creates harmonics—the same way an acoustic waveform played too loud on a speaker produces a distorted copy of the acoustic wave in which harmonic frequencies appear.

Contrary to fluorescence, second harmonic generation is a coherent process, which means that the electric field radiated by different molecules will interfere. Additionally, second harmonic generation can only occur in materials that do not possess a central symmetry. SHG thus cannot happen in liquids (except for ordered liquids). In fact, in biology, SHG is only observed for highly ordered structures in which many molecules are aligned and all interfere constructively. Such organization is found in collagen molecules arranged in collagen fibers, microtubules in axons, and myosin in muscles.

SHG too requires high irradiance, which is provided by pulsed lasers confined at the focal point of a high NA microscope objective. Intrinsic optical sectioning as well as selective contrast for organized structures will therefore also be characteristic of laser scanning nonlinear microscopes exploiting SHG.

Implementation of a Laser-Scanning Nonlinear Microscope

Nonlinear microscopy is typically implemented as a laser-scanning microscope in a manner similar to RCM. However, due to the nature of the interactions, there are some differences which must be taken into account. This section will describe the key components required to obtaining high-resolution imaging with nonlinear microscopy.

Optical Sectioning

2PEF and SHG signals depend on the square of the excitation irradiance. This differs from conventional one-photon absorption fluorescence signal, which is proportional to the excitation irradiance. This property of nonlinear signals has a huge effect; it creates an intrinsic optical sectioning in nonlinear microscopy that can be seen in Fig. 1. In linear RCM, optical sectioning is obtained by adding a spatial filter (or pinhole) in front of the detector, which rejects out of focus light. In 2PEF or SHG, the nonlinear signal is confined to the focal volume, the only point where laser irradiance is high enough to produce nonlinear interactions. The signal generation in 2PEF is restricted to a small volume. Nonlinear microscopy is a 3D imaging technique allowing precise control over energy deposition in the sample.

Resolution and Penetration Depth

The resolution of nonlinear microscopy is similar to that of RCM, which is on the order of the micrometer or less. It scales with the excitation wavelength and is inversely proportional to the NA of the objective lens. For a given fluorophore, nonlinear microscopy has a slightly coarser resolution, as the illumination wavelength is twice as large. However, this comes with the advantage of greater penetration depth within thick tissue. Nonlinear microscopy uses near-infrared laser, usually with wavelengths between 750 and 950 nm. In this particular window, photons are less scattered and absorbed by biological tissues than photons at visible wavelengths. Therefore, excitation photons penetrate deeper in the tissue. Moreover, because nonlinear effects generate signal only where the laser irradiance is high, excitation photons that are scattered away from the focal point will not produce fluorescence, thus efficiently reducing the background noise in nonlinear microscopy images. Actual penetration depths are highly tissue dependent; in brain, nonlinear microscopy can image about 1 mm deep.

Pulsed Lasers

Spatial confinement of light enhances 2PEF. Another way to increase 2PEF signal without increasing linear absorption is to confine the laser energy in pulses instead of using continuous wave lasers. In fact, it is only after the development of pulsed laser that the first nonlinear scanning microscope was implemented by Denk et al. [36] in 1990. Femtosecond lasers used in nonlinear microscopy are traditionally Titanium:Sapphire lasers [37]. These lasers have pulse duration varying between just a few femtoseconds and hundreds of femtoseconds with repetition rate traditionally close to 80 MHz. Their emission wavelength can be tuned between 750 and 1050 nm and are now integrated into commercially available nonlinear microscopes. Using pulsed lasers, nonlinear microscopy has become an essential tool in neurobiology [38] as well as in oncology [39], in immunology [40], and in developmental biology laboratories [41].

Large FOV Laser-Scanning Nonlinear Microscope

Figure 3 shows a schematic diagram of the large FOV laser-scanning nonlinear microscope developed for vocal fold imaging. Light from a femtosecond Ti–Sapphire laser (shown in red) is scanned onto the sample with a set of two galvanometer-mounted mirrors producing small 512 × 512 pixel images. The sample is further mounted on motorized translation stages to allow large areas (mm × mm) of tissues to be imaged at once. Illumination is performed through a 40×, 0.8NA water immersion microscope objective. Detection for 2PEF, SHG, and RCM images is performed with two filter-equipped PMTs and one avalanche photodiode, respectively. Acquisition and display is performed through a custom software described in greater details in [33].

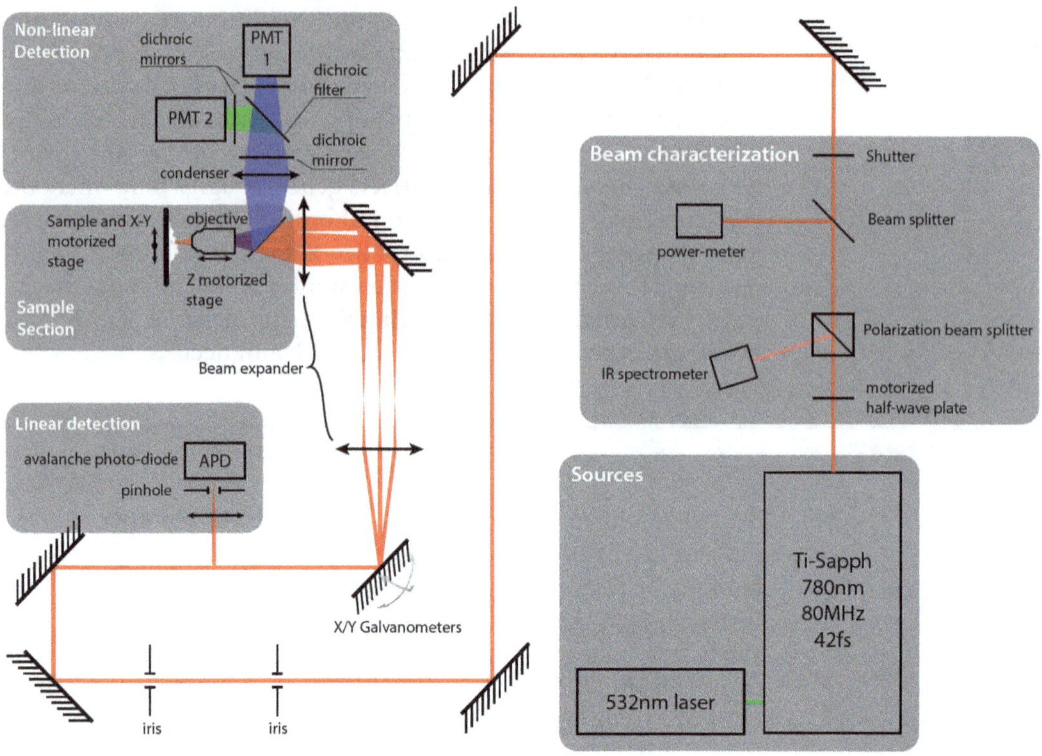

Fig. 3 Schematic diagram of the large FOV nonlinear microscope using a Ti–Sapphire laser for simultaneous excitation of 2PEF, SHG, and RCM

Nonlinear Contrast for Vocal Fold Imaging

Figure 4 shows a section of swine vocal fold imaged using three modalities—RCM, SHG, and 2PEF, simultaneously. The RCM image shows a bright epithelium with brighter nuclei along with a heterogeneous lamina propria, returning overall a lower signal than the epithelium. On the SHG image, however, the epithelium appears to be missing, while signal-rich areas are present in the lamina propria. Finally, under 2PEF, a bright epithelium is clearly visible, but this time, the nuclei are dark—which corresponds to a signal poor region. The lamina propria exhibits a strong signal, but the image pattern is completely different than that from the RCM and SHG images. In this section, we try to provide a preliminary explanation for obtaining contrasting images without exogenous staining.

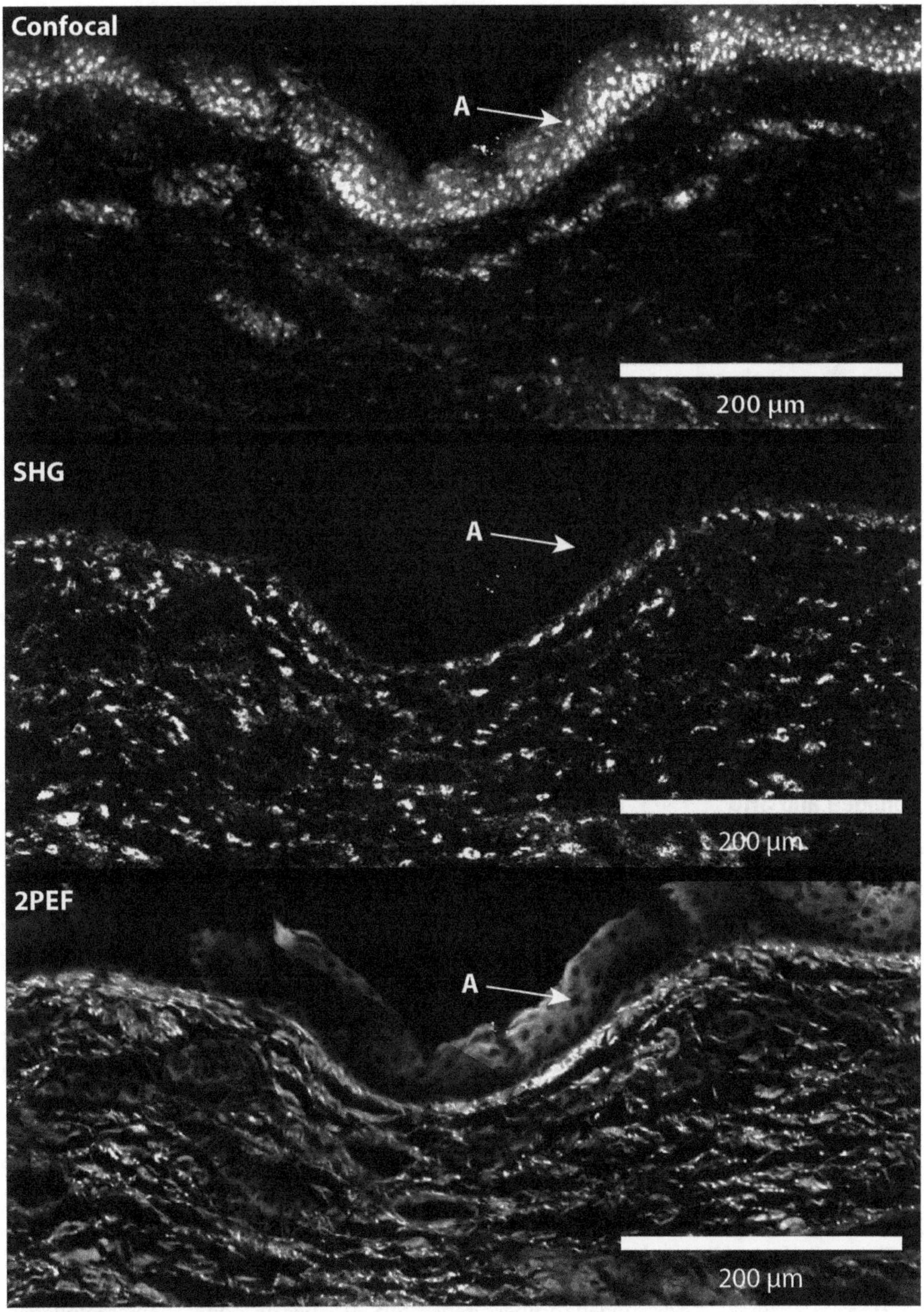

Fig. 4 Images of an unstained swine vocal fold section acquired using confocal microscopy (RCM), SHG, and 2PEF. "A" points at a nucleus within the epithelium

Elastin and 2PEF

Elastin is the main component of elastic fiber and therefore plays a prime role in vertebrate tissue elastic properties [42, 43]. Its distribution and 3D organization is of crucial importance to understand vocal cord properties [44, 45]. As elastin is a fluorescent protein, it can be observed with 2PEF microscopy without staining or preparation. Elastin two-photon absorption spectrum is not well characterized, but its two-photon cross section seems to decrease slowly form 720 to 920 nm [46]. However, other studies point that longer excitation wavelength, such as 860 nm, improves elastin imaging contrast as other intrinsic fluorophores are less exited at these wavelengths [47]. When excited at 800 nm, elastic fibers' fluorescence exhibits two peaks: one around 400 nm, which may correspond to pyridinoline groups, and a stronger one at 480 nm that could originate from the pyridinoline aggregates [48].

The fluorescence signal from elastin molecule is proportional to the number of molecules. However, elastin is not the only endogenous fluorescent protein present in the vocal cords. Therefore, localizing and identifying elastin requires a spectroscopic analysis to separate the elastin fluorescence signal coming from other autofluorescent sources. Another endogenous source of 2PEF includes nicotinamide adenine dinucleotide phosphate [NAD(P)H] and flavoproteins [49, 50].

Collagen and SHG

Collagen is the most abundant protein in mammals and is mainly found in the extracellular matrix. In fact, it consists of a family of more than 23 proteins having in common that they assemble to form triple helices. Type-I collagen, after its secretion by the cell, self-assembles into large fibers. These fibers have extremely high tensile strength and provide structural support to the surrounding tissue, hence their importance in the function of vocal cords. Some collagens do not form fibrils. For example, type-IV collagen assembles into sheets to create basal lamina layers.

As explained before, SHG is only efficient in highly ordered structures. There are just a handful of endogenous structures that generate second harmonic in mammals: collagen fibers, myosin in muscle fibers, and microtubules in axons or when they are aligned during cell mitosis. Therefore, in the lamina propria, SHG arises mostly from collagen. Moreover, only collagen molecules organized in fibers generate SHG, because only then are collagen molecules aligned in the same direction. Collagen IV does not generate SHG due to its sheet structure [51, 52]. Recently, it was shown that the origin of the strong SHG signal in collagen fibers comes from the coherent amplification of the signal generated by all the individual peptide bonds that are tightly packed and aligned in collagen fibers [53].

This makes SHG a very efficient imaging technique for fibrillar collagen with very little background noise and even allows the imaging of individual fibers during their formation [54]. Additionally, because SHG microscopy does not require any sample preparation and can image thick samples, this technique is particularly useful to assess the 3D organization of collagen fibers of intact tissues.

However, because SHG is a coherent process, signal strength depends on the actual molecular arrangement of collagen fibers and is proportional to the square of the number of molecules present in the focal volume. Therefore, it is very difficult to link second harmonic signal strength to a collagen concentration. SHG microscopy is a very sensitive technique to measure fibrotic pathology stages [55, 56]. The sensitivity of SHG to collagen fiber organization was also successfully used to assess extracellular matrix alteration due to cancer [57–59]. Other applications of SHG microscopy of collagen are found in corneal [60–62], musculoskeletal [63, 64], arterial [47, 65, 66], and skin [67–70] studies.

Nonlinear Microscopy of Vocal Fold

Combining various linear (RCM) and nonlinear (2PEF and SHG) effects into a single instrument allows looking at samples from different perspectives, in a manner analogous to using different dyes in histopathological analysis. The key in harnessing this endogenous contrast is to perform one-to-one comparison of nonlinear images with the diagnostic gold standard—histopathology. The task is a large one given the exquisite resolution of nonlinear microscopy. In order to facilitate this comparison, successive sections of vocal folds were cut: some were left unstained for observation under the large FOV nonlinear microscope and other for conventional staining and observation under white light microscopy. Ink marks were placed with a needle at the edges of the samples as fiducial markers between modalities. Figure 5 compares images acquired with the large FOV nonlinear microscope and an H&E stained white light microscopy slide of the same swine vocal fold sample. A composite image created by applying false colors to the RCM (blue), SHG (green), and 2PEF (red) channels highlights the different structures of the vocal fold. In the epithelium (E), endogenous fluorophores present in the cytoplasm result in a moderate 2PEF signal, while nuclei appear as dark structures, which are in contrast very bright in RCM due to their strong scattering properties. The epithelium is completely absent from the

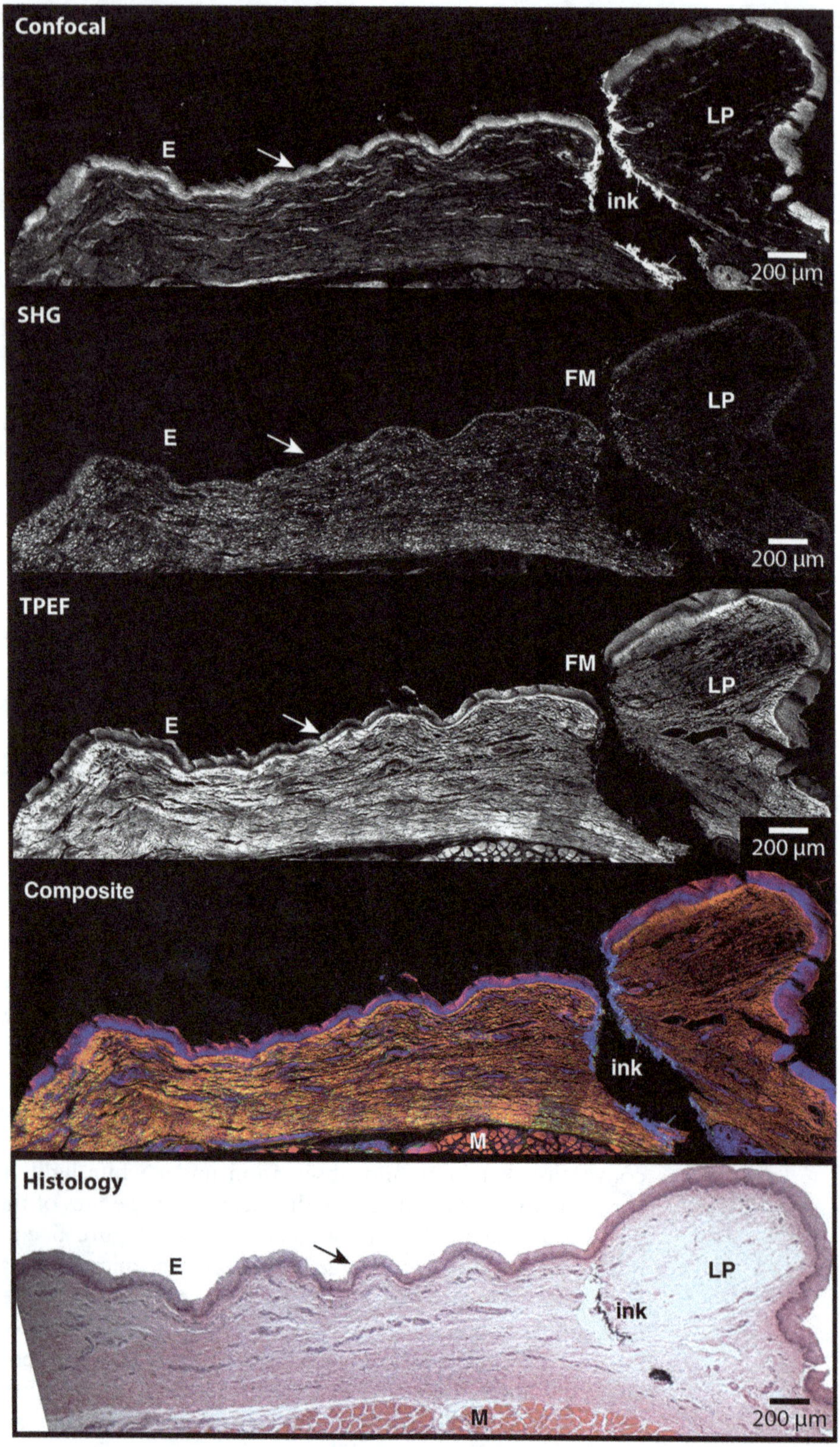

Fig. 5 A section of swine vocal fold imaged confocal microscopy (RCM), SHG, TPEF, and wide field microscopy using hematoxylin and eosin (H&E) staining. A false color composite image was created using confocal (*blue*), SHG (*green*), and 2PEF (*red*) signals. The *arrow* points at the epithelium (E). The entire lamina propria (LP) is imaged down to the muscle layer (M). A needle dipped in India ink was used to create a fiducial marker (FM)

SHG image due to the lack of collagen or other fibrillar structures. At the bottom of the image, the vocalis muscle produces very strong 2PEF signal. In the lamina propria (LP), SHG—from collagen—and 2PEF—from elastin and other endogenous fluorophores—signals are present with intensities varying with depth. The blue signal around the fiducial marker (FM) on the composite image corresponds to a strong RCM signal scattering from the India ink mark.

Figure 6 shows nonlinear microscopy images of a cadaveric adult vocal fold section under SHG (green), 2PEF (red), and a linear combination of both (Composite) compared to an H&E stained histology section. The large FOV nonlinear microscope allowed imaging of a 13×5.5 mm region through an automated mosaicking process. The muscle layer (M) is predominantly red from 2PEF signal from endogenous fluorophores such as NAD(P)H [48]. SHG-rich collagenous structures are seen around the muscle fibers. The lamina propria (LP) alternates between SHG- and 2PEF-rich areas, consistent with varying elastin and collagen concentrations. A zoom-in of the LP region shows an artery in both the SHG and 2PEF images, with strong 2PEF signal within its wall and a strong SHG signal in its outward layer, consistent with the typical elastin and collagen distribution within arterial walls. A large seromucous gland (G) can be seen in the LP. No epithelium was observed on this sample, which could be the result of a prolonged intubation. Arrows point at the India ink needle entry point.

Conclusion

Nonlinear microscopy is becoming one of the most important tools available to life sciences. This powerful three-dimensional technique allows exploration of living organism toward a better understanding of biological processes. The noninvasive nature of nonlinear microscopy, its ability to image deeper into thick tissue along with its submicron resolution, and intrinsic contrast are undeniable assets for the study of vocal folds. The possibility of imaging microstructures (cells and nuclei) as well as macromolecules (such as elastin and collagen) without affecting the integrity of the organ paves the way for a better understanding of vocal folds' normal and pathological conditions. As miniaturization of probes evolves there is no doubt that nonlinear microscopy, either in its current tabletop system or as an endoscope, will become a useful tool in laryngology, along with other biomedical optic imaging modalities such as reflectance confocal microscopy and optical coherence tomography.

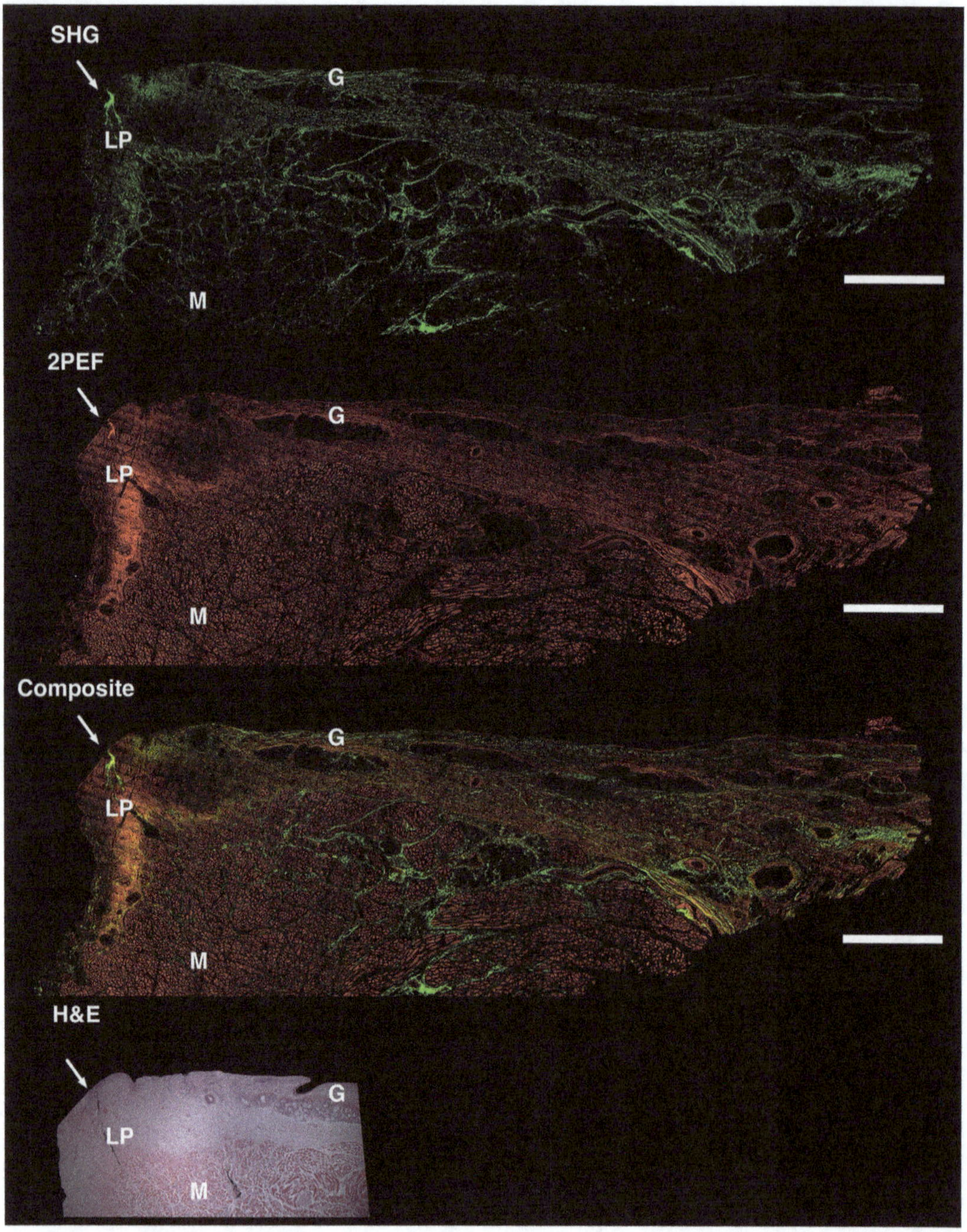

Fig. 6 Nonlinear image (SHG—*green*, 2PEF—*red*, and *Composite*) of a human vocal fold unstained section compared with H&E stained histology section. *Arrow* fiducial marker, *LP* lamina propria, *M* vocalis muscle, *G* seromucous gland. Scale bar: 1 mm

Acknowledgments

The authors would like to thank Dr Amber Beckley, Mr. Étienne de Montigny, Ms. Chloé Gariépy, Mr. Scott Infusino, Pr. Steven Maturo, and Dr. Shilpa Ojha for fruitful discussions. Pr. Boudoux acknowledges funding from the National Sciences and Engineering Research Council of Canada (NSERC) and the Canadian Foundation for Innovation (CFI).

References

1. Huang D, Swanson E, Lin C, et al. Optical coherence tomography. Science. 1991;254(5035):1178–81. doi:10.1126/science.1957169.
2. Ridgway JM, Armstrong WB, Guo S, et al. In vivo optical coherence tomography of the human oral cavity and oropharynx. Arch Otolaryngol Head Neck Surg. 2006;132(10):1074–81. doi:10.1001/archotol.132.10.1074.
3. Bouma BE, Tearney GJ, Compton CC, Nishioka NS. High-resolution imaging of the human esophagus and stomach in vivo using optical coherence tomography. Gastrointest Endosc. 2000;51(4):467–74. doi:10.1016/S0016-5107(00)70449-4.
4. Bus MTJ, Muller BG, de Bruin DM, et al. Volumetric in vivo visualization of upper urinary tract tumors using optical coherence tomography: a pilot study. J Urol. 2013;190(6):2236–42. doi:10.1016/j.juro.2013.08.006.
5. Yabushita H, Bouma BE, Houser SL, et al. Characterization of human atherosclerosis by optical coherence tomography. Circulation. 2002;106(13):1640–5. Available at: http://www.ncbi.nlm.nih.gov/pubmed/12270856. Accessed 12 Mar 2014.
6. Hanna N, Saltzman D, Mukai D, et al. Two-dimensional and 3-dimensional optical coherence tomographic imaging of the airway, lung, and pleura. J Thorac Cardiovasc Surg. 2005;129(3):615–22. doi:10.1016/j.jtcvs.2004.10.022.
7. Wong BJF, Jackson RP, Guo S, et al. In vivo optical coherence tomography of the human larynx: normative and benign pathology in 82 patients. Laryngoscope. 2005;115(11):1904–11. doi:10.1097/01.MLG.0000181465.17744.BE.
8. Kraft M, Glanz H, von Gerlach S, Wisweh H, Lubatschowski H, Arens C. Clinical value of optical coherence tomography in laryngology. Head Neck. 2008;30(12):1628–35. doi:10.1002/hed.20914.
9. Armstrong WB, Ridgway JM, Vokes DE, et al. Optical coherence tomography of laryngeal cancer. Laryngoscope. 2006;116(7):1107–13. doi:10.1097/01.mlg.0000217539.27432.5a.
10. Burns JA, Zeitels SM, Anderson RR, Kobler JB, Pierce MC, de Boer JF. Imaging the mucosa of the human vocal fold with optical coherence tomography. Ann Otol Rhinol Laryngol. 2005;114(9):671–6. Available at: http://www.ncbi.nlm.nih.gov/pubmed/16240928. Accessed 12 Mar 2014.
11. Klein A, Pierce M. Imaging the human vocal folds in vivo with optical coherence tomography: a preliminary experience. Ann Otol Rhinol Laryngol. 2006;115(4):277–84.
12. Boudoux C, Leuin SC, Oh WY, et al. Preliminary evaluation of noninvasive microscopic imaging techniques for the study of vocal fold development. J Voice. 2009;23(3):269–76. Available at: http://dx.doi.org/10.1016/j.jvoice.2007.10.003.
13. Boudoux C, Leuin SC, Oh WY, et al. Optical microscopy of the pediatric vocal fold. Arch Otolaryngol Head Neck Surg. 2009;135(1):53–64. Available at: http://eutils.ncbi.nlm.nih.gov/entrez/eutils/elink.fcgi?dbfrom=pubmed&id=19153308&retmode=ref&cmd=prlinks.
14. Maturo S, Benboujja F, Boudoux C, Hartnick C. Quantitative distinction of unique vocal fold subepithelial architectures using optical coherence tomography. Ann Otol Rhinol Laryngol. 2012;121(11):754–60. Available at: http://www.ncbi.nlm.nih.gov/pubmed/23193909. Accessed 12 Mar 2014.
15. Benboujja F, Rogers D, Infusino S, Strupler M, Hartnick CJ, Boudoux C. A study of vocal fold maturation using optical coherence tomography. San Francisco, CA: SPIE Photonics West; 2014.
16. Ridgway JM, Su J, Wright R, et al. Optical coherence tomography of the newborn airway.

Ann Otol Rhinol Laryngol. 2008;117(5):327–34. Available at: http://www.pubmedcentral.nih.gov/articlerender.fcgi?artid=2871770&tool=pmcentrez&rendertype=abstract. Accessed 12 Mar 2014.

17. Wisweh H, Merkel U. Optical coherence tomography monitoring of vocal fold femtosecond laser microsurgery. European Conference on Biomedical Optics. Munich, Germany; 2007
18. Minsky M. Microscopy apparatus. 1961. Available at: http://www.google.ca/patents/US3013467. Accessed 4 Dec 2013.
19. Pawley J. Handbook of biological confocal microscopy. New York: Springer; 2006.
20. Webb RH, Hughes GW, Delori FC. Confocal scanning laser ophthalmoscope. Appl Opt. 1987;26(8):1492–9. doi:10.1364/AO.26.001492.
21. Gareau DS, Jeon H, Nehal KS, Rajadhyaksha M. Rapid screening of cancer margins in tissue with multimodal confocal microscopy. J Surg Res. 2012;178(2):533–8. doi:10.1016/j.jss.2012.05.059.
22. Hsiung P-L, Hsiung P-L, Hardy J, et al. Detection of colonic dysplasia in vivo using a targeted heptapeptide and confocal microendoscopy. Nat Med. 2008;14(4):454–8. doi:10.1038/nm1692.
23. Tearney GJ, Webb RH, Bouma BE. Spectrally encoded confocal microscopy. Opt Lett. 1998;23(15):1152–4. Available at: http://links.isiglobalnet2.com/gateway/Gateway.cgi?GWVersion=2&SrcAuth=mekentosj&SrcApp=Papers&DestLinkType=FullRecord&DestApp=WOS&KeyUT=000075024400002.
24. Boudoux C, Yun S-H, Oh W, et al. Rapid wavelength-swept spectrally encoded confocal microscopy. Opt Express. 2005;13(20):8214–21.
25. Boudoux C, Benboujja F, Deterre R, Strupler M, Maturo S, Hartnick CJ. Emerging microscopy techniques for pediatric vocal fold evaluation. In: Izdebski K, Yan Y, Ward R, Wong BJF, editors. Normal & Abnormal Vocal Folds Kinematics: High-Speed Digital Phonoscopy (HSDP), Optical Coherence Tomography (OCT) & Narrow Band Imaging (NBI). San Francisco, CA: Pacific Vo.; 2014.
26. Iftimia N, Ferguson RD, Mujat M, et al. Combined reflectance confocal microscopy/optical coherence tomography imaging for skin burn assessment. Biomed Opt Express. 2013;4(5):680–95. doi:10.1364/BOE.4.000680.
27. Kang D, Suter MJ, Boudoux C, et al. Co-registered spectrally encoded confocal microscopy and optical frequency domain imaging system. J Microsc. 2010;239(2):87–91. Availableat:http://doi.wiley.com/10.1111/j.1365-2818.2010.03367.x.
28. Zipfel WR, Williams RM, Webb WW. Nonlinear magic: multiphoton microscopy in the biosciences. Nat Biotechnol. 2003;21(11):1369–77. doi:10.1038/nbt899.
29. Rivera DR, Brown CM, Ouzounov DG, et al. Compact and flexible raster scanning multiphoton endoscope capable of imaging unstained tissue. Proc Natl Acad Sci U S A. 2011;108(43):17598–603. doi:10.1073/pnas.1114746108.
30. Engelbrecht CJ, Johnston RS, Seibel EJ, Helmchen F. Ultra-compact fiber-optic two-photon microscope for functional fluorescence imaging in vivo. Opt Express. 2008;16(8):5556–64. Available at: http://www.ncbi.nlm.nih.gov/pubmed/18542658. Accessed 18 April 2014.
31. Helmchen F, Fee MS, Tank DW, Denk W. A miniature head-mounted two-photon microscope. High-resolution brain imaging in freely moving animals. Neuron. 2001;31(6):903–12. Available at: http://www.ncbi.nlm.nih.gov/pubmed/11580892. Accessed 31 Mar 2014.
32. Miri AK, Tripathy U, Mongeau L, Wiseman PW. Nonlinear laser scanning microscopy of human vocal folds. Laryngoscope. 2012;122(2):356–63. doi:10.1002/lary.22460.
33. Deterre R. Microscopie non-linéaire pour l'imagerie des cordes vocales. 2012.
34. Hoy CL, Everett WN, Yildirim M, Kobler J, Zeitels SM, Ben-Yakar A. Towards endoscopic ultrafast laser microsurgery of vocal folds. J Biomed Opt. 2012;17(3):038002. doi:10.1117/1.JBO.17.3.038002.
35. Boyd RW. Nonlinear optics. San Diego, CA: Acad. Press; 2003. p. 578. Available at: http://books.google.ca/books/about/Nonlinear_Optics.html?id=30t9VmOmOGsC&pgis=1. Accessed 9 Jul 2014.
36. Denk W, Strickler J, Webb W. Two-photon laser scanning fluorescence microscopy. Science. 1990;248(4951):73–6. doi:10.1126/science.2321027.
37. French PMW, Williams JAR, Taylor JR. Femtosecond pulse generation from a titanium-doped sapphire laser using nonlinear external cavity feedback. Opt Lett. 1989;14(13):686. doi:10.1364/OL.14.000686.
38. Denk W. Two-photon scanning photochemical microscopy: mapping ligand-gated ion channel distributions. Proc Natl Acad Sci U S A. 1994;91(14):6629–33. Available at: http://

www.pubmedcentral.nih.gov/articlerender.fcgi?artid=44256&tool=pmcentrez&rendertype=abstract. Accessed 4 Dec 2013.

39. Brown EB, Campbell RB, Tsuzuki Y, et al. In vivo measurement of gene expression, angiogenesis and physiological function in tumors using multiphoton laser scanning microscopy. Nat Med. 2001;7(7):864–8. doi:10.1038/89997.
40. Sipkins DA, Wei X, Wu JW, et al. In vivo imaging of specialized bone marrow endothelial microdomains for tumour engraftment. Nature. 2005;435(7044):969–73. doi:10.1038/nature03703.
41. Squirrell JM, Wokosin DL, White JG, Bavister BD. Long-term two-photon fluorescence imaging of mammalian embryos without compromising viability. Nat Biotechnol. 1999;17(8):763–7. doi:10.1038/11698.
42. Sandberg LB, Soskel NT, Leslie JG. Elastin structure, biosynthesis, and relation to disease states. N Engl J Med. 1981;304:566–79.
43. Debelle L, Tamburro AM. Elastin: molecular description and function. Int J Biochem Cell Biol. 1999;31(2):261–72. doi:10.1016/S1357-2725(98)00098-3.
44. Gray SD, Titze IR, Alipour F, Hammond TH. Biomechanical and histologic observations of vocal fold fibrous proteins. Ann Otol Rhinol Laryngol. 2000;109(1):77–85. Available at: http://europepmc.org/abstract/MED/10651418. Accessed 9 Jul 2014.
45. Moore J, Thibeault S. Insights into the role of elastin in vocal fold health and disease. J Voice. 2012;26(3):269–75. doi:10.1016/j.jvoice.2011.05.003.
46. Breunig HG, Studier H, König K. Multiphoton excitation characteristics of cellular fluorophores of human skin in vivo. Opt Express. 2010;18(8):7857–71. Available at: http://www.ncbi.nlm.nih.gov/pubmed/20588627. Accessed 9 Jul 2014.
47. Boulesteix T, Pena A-M, Pagès N, et al. Micrometer scale ex vivo multiphoton imaging of unstained arterial wall structure. Cytometry A. 2006;69(1):20–6. doi:10.1002/cyto.a.20196.
48. Zipfel WR, Williams RM, Christie R, Nikitin AY, Hyman BT, Webb WW. Live tissue intrinsic emission microscopy using multiphoton-excited native fluorescence and second harmonic generation. Proc Natl Acad Sci U S A. 2003;100(12):7075–80. doi:10.1073/pnas.0832308100.
49. Kierdaszuk B, Malak H, Gryczynski I, Callis P, Lakowicz JR. Fluorescence of reduced nicotinamides using one- and two-photon excitation. Biophys Chem. 1996;62(1–3):1–13. Available at: http://www.ncbi.nlm.nih.gov/pubmed/8962467. Accessed 10 Jul 2014.
50. Huang S, Heikal AA, Webb WW. Two-photon fluorescence spectroscopy and microscopy of NAD(P)H and flavoprotein. Biophys J. 2002;82(5):2811–25. doi:10.1016/S0006-3495(02)75621-X.
51. Strupler M, Pena A-M, Hernest M, et al. Second harmonic imaging and scoring of collagen in fibrotic tissues. Opt Express. 2007;15(7):4054–65. Available at: http://www.ncbi.nlm.nih.gov/pubmed/19532649. Accessed 9 Jul 2014.
52. Pena A-M, Boulesteix T, Dartigalongue T, Schanne-Klein M-C. Chiroptical effects in the second harmonic signal of collagens I and IV. J Am Chem Soc. 2005;127(29):10314–22. doi:10.1021/ja0520969.
53. Deniset-Besseau A, Duboisset J, Benichou E, Hache F, Brevet P-F, Schanne-Klein M-C. Measurement of the second-order hyperpolarizability of the collagen triple helix and determination of its physical origin. J Phys Chem B. 2009;113(40):13437–45. doi:10.1021/jp9046837.
54. Bancelin S, Aimé C, Coradin T, Schanne-Klein M-C. In situ three-dimensional monitoring of collagen fibrillogenesis using SHG microscopy. Biomed Opt Express. 2012;3(6):1446–54. doi:10.1364/BOE.3.001446.
55. Strupler M, Hernest M, Fligny C, Martin J-L, Tharaux P-L, Schanne-Klein M-C. Second harmonic microscopy to quantify renal interstitial fibrosis and arterial remodeling. J Biomed Opt. 2008;13(5):054041.doi:10.1117/1.2981830.
56. Sun W, Chang S, Tai DCS, et al. Nonlinear optical microscopy: use of second harmonic generation and two-photon microscopy for automated quantitative liver fibrosis studies. J Biomed Opt. 2008;13(6):064010. doi:10.1117/1.3041159.
57. Provenzano PP, Eliceiri KW, Campbell JM, Inman DR, White JG, Keely PJ. Collagen reorganization at the tumor-stromal interface facilitates local invasion. BMC Med. 2006;4(1):38. doi:10.1186/1741-7015-4-38.
58. Nadiarnykh O, LaComb RB, Brewer MA, Campagnola PJ. Alterations of the extracellular matrix in ovarian cancer studied by Second Harmonic Generation imaging microscopy. BMC Cancer. 2010;10:94. doi:10.1186/1471-2407-10-94.
59. Zhuo S, Chen J, Wu G, et al. Quantitatively linking collagen alteration and epithelial tumor progression by second harmonic generation

microscopy. Appl Phys Lett. 2010; 96(21):213704. doi:10.1063/1.3441337.

60. Latour G, Kowalczuk L, Savoldelli M, et al. Hyperglycemia-induced abnormalities in rat and human corneas: the potential of second harmonic generation microscopy. Georgakoudi I, ed. PLoS One. 2012;7(11):e48388. doi:10.1371/journal.pone.0048388.

61. Tan H-Y, Sun Y, Lo W, et al. Multiphoton fluorescence and second harmonic generation microscopy for imaging infectious keratitis. J Biomed Opt. 2007;12(2):024013. doi:10.1117/1.2717133.

62. Matteini P, Cicchi R, Ratto F, et al. Thermal transitions of fibrillar collagen unveiled by second-harmonic generation microscopy of corneal stroma. Biophys J. 2012;103(6):1179–87. doi:10.1016/j.bpj.2012.07.055.

63. Donnelly E, Williams RM, Downs SA, Dickinson ME, Baker SP, van der Meulen MCH. Quasistatic and dynamic nanomechanical properties of cancellous bone tissue relate to collagen content and organization. J Mater Res. 2011;21(08):2106–17. doi:10.1557/jmr.2006.0259.

64. Lacomb R, Nadiarnykh O, Campagnola PJ. Quantitative second harmonic generation imaging of the diseased state osteogenesis imperfecta: experiment and simulation. Biophys J. 2008;94(11):4504–14. doi:10.1529/biophysj.107.114405.

65. Le TT, Langohr IM, Locker MJ, Sturek M, Cheng J-X. Label-free molecular imaging of atherosclerotic lesions using multimodal nonlinear optical microscopy. J Biomed Opt. 2007;12(5):054007.doi:10.1117/1.2795437.

66. Zoumi A, Lu X, Kassab GS, Tromberg BJ. Imaging coronary artery microstructure using second-harmonic and two-photon fluorescence microscopy. Biophys J. 2004;87(4):2778–86. doi:10.1529/biophysj.104.042887.

67. König K. Clinical multiphoton tomography. J Biophotonics. 2008;1(1):13–23. doi:10.1002/jbio.200710022.

68. Koehler MJ, Hahn S, Preller A, et al. Morphological skin ageing criteria by multiphoton laser scanning tomography: non-invasive in vivo scoring of the dermal fibre network. Exp Dermatol. 2008;17(6):519–23. doi:10.1111/j.1600-0625.2007.00669.x.

69. Wu S, Li H, Zhang X, Chen WR, Wang Y-X. Character of skin on photo-thermal response and its regeneration process using second-harmonic generation microscopy. Lasers Med Sci. 2014;29(1):141–6. doi:10.1007/s10103-013-1296-3.

70. Yasui T, Takahashi Y, Fukushima S, et al. Observation of dermal collagen fiber in wrinkled skin using polarization-resolved second-harmonic-generation microscopy. Opt Express. 2009;17(2):912–23. Available at: http://www.ncbi.nlm.nih.gov/pubmed/19158906. Accessed 9 Jul 2014.

Chapter 32

Optical Coherence Tomography

Joseph Jing and Zhongping Chen

Introduction

Optical coherence tomography (OCT) is an optical imaging modality that is rapidly gaining adoption for clinical applications. OCT takes advantage of the short coherence length of broadband light sources to perform micrometer scale, cross-sectional imaging of biological tissue [1–3]. OCT was first used clinically in ophthalmology but has since expanded to the fields of cardiology, gastroenterology, urology, and otolaryngology [4]. OCT is analogous to ultrasound B-mode imaging except that it uses light rather than sound to achieve axial resolutions of 1–15 μm. The high spatial resolution of OCT enables noninvasive in situ "optical biopsy" and provides immediate and localized diagnostic information to better aid physicians in the diagnosis and treatment of diseases. Functional extensions have also been developed to further add physiological contrast to OCT imaging. Doppler OCT (D-OCT) combines the Doppler principle with OCT to obtain high-resolution tomographic images and calculate the velocity of moving constituents. Optical coherence elastography utilizes an applied external force to measure the mechanical properties of tissue. In this chapter, we will review the principles behind OCT and discuss the innovations in OCT that have dramatically increased imaging speeds and sensitivity. Functional extensions to OCT will then be described. Lastly, a few recent applications of OCT imaging in otolaryngology will be highlighted.

Brian J.-F. Wong and Justus Ilgner (eds.), *Biomedical Optics in Otorhinolaryngology: Head and Neck Surgery*,
DOI 10.1007/978-1-4939-1758-7_32, © Springer Science+Business Media New York 2016

Principles Behind OCT

Time-Domain OCT

OCT utilizes coherent gating to discriminate single scattered photons from multiple scattered photons. OCT is based on a Michelson interferometer with a broadband light source (Fig. 1). Light from a source is split into a reference path and a sample path. The reference path light, after reflecting from the reference mirror, interferes with the backscattered light from the sample, and an interference pattern or fringe is formed and detected by a photodetector. If a highly coherent source such as a monochromatic light source is used, then interference will be present over a large range of reference and sample path length differences (Fig. 2a). However, if a low-coherence source such as a broadband light source is used, then an interference pattern is only observed when the reference and sample path lengths are matched to within the coherence length of the source (Fig. 2b). By scanning or changing the reference arm path length and recording the subsequent interference fringe intensity, a map of scattering particles can be formed as an A-scan. OCT designs that incorporate this type of depth scanning are known as time-domain (TD) systems. Translating the probing sample beam laterally across the sample to acquire multiple A-scans creates an image or B-scan. Therefore, the axial resolution of an OCT system is directly determined by the coherence

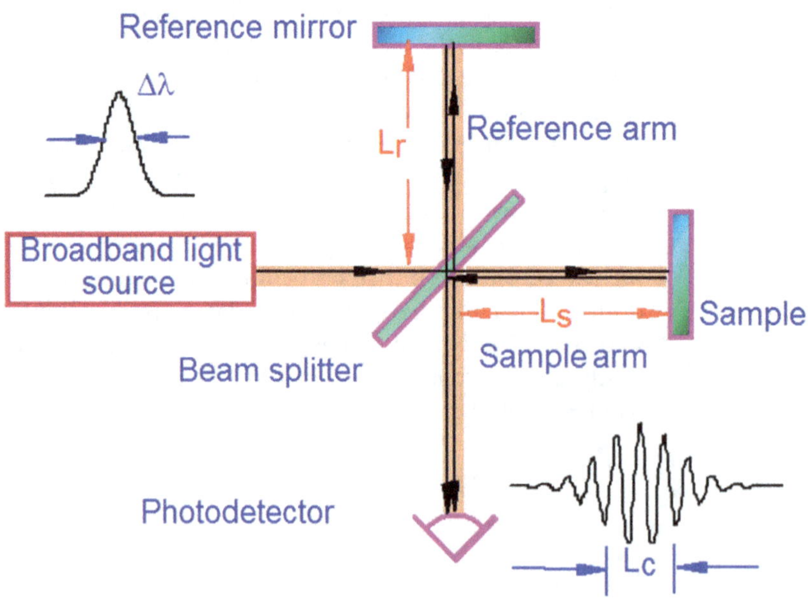

Fig. 1 Schematic of OCT system consists of a free space Michelson interferometer with a partially coherent light source

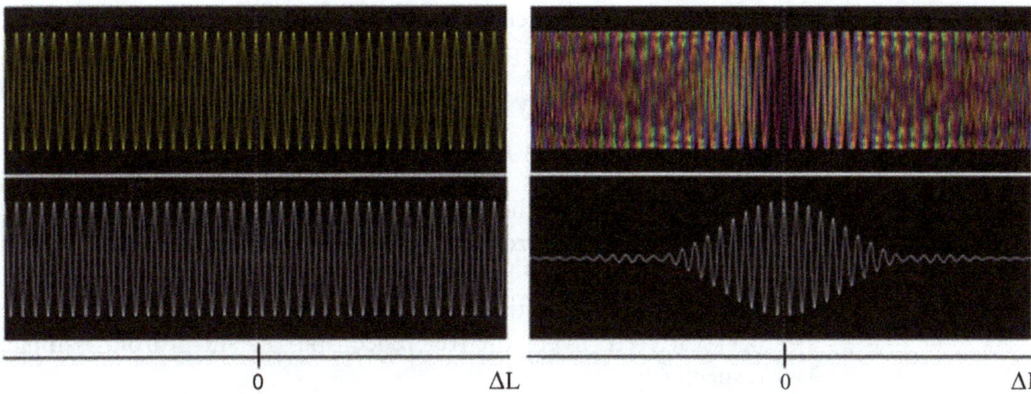

Fig. 2 Fringe (*bottom*) formed from interference of waves (*top*) with single wavelength (*left*) and multiple wavelengths (*right*). ΔL is the difference in path length between reference and sample arms

length of the light source calculated by Eq. (1), where λ_0 and $\Delta\lambda$ are the center wavelength and bandwidth of the source, respectively. The lateral resolution is decoupled from the axial resolution and is determined by the numerical aperture of the objective lens used to focus the light and the beam diameter incident on the objective.

$$L_c = \frac{\tau_c}{2} c = \frac{2 \ln 2}{\pi} \frac{\lambda_0^2}{\Delta\lambda} \tag{1}$$

To illustrate the coherence gating of the broadband light source, we consider the interference fringe generated in the Michelson interferometer with a broadband light source. Let us denote $U(t)$ as a complex-valued analytical signal of a stochastic process representing the field amplitude emitted by a low-coherent light source and $\bar{U}(\nu)$ as the corresponding spectral amplitude at optical frequency ν. The amplitude of a partially coherent light source coupled into the interferometer at time t can be written as a harmonic superposition:

$$U(t) = \int_{\infty}^{0} \bar{U}(\nu) e^{2\pi i \nu t} d\nu \tag{2}$$

Because the stochastic process of a partially coherent light source is stationary, cross-spectral density of $\bar{U}(\nu)$ satisfies

$$\langle \bar{U}^*(\nu) \bar{U}(\nu') \rangle = S_o(\nu) \delta(\nu - \nu') \tag{3}$$

where $S_o(\nu)$ is the source power spectral density and $\delta(n)$ is the Dirac delta function. Assuming that light couples equally into the reference arm and sample arm with spectral amplitude of $\bar{U}_0(\nu)$, the light coupled back to the detectors from the reference, $\bar{U}_r(\nu)$, and sample, $\bar{U}_s(\nu)$, is given by Eqs. (3) and (4), respectively:

$$\bar{U}_r(v) = e^{2\pi i v(2L_r + L_d)/c} K_r e^{i\alpha_r} \bar{U}_0(v) \quad (4)$$

$$\bar{U}_s(v) = e^{2\pi i v(2L_s + L_d)/c} K_s e^{i\alpha_s} \bar{U}_0(v) \quad (5)$$

where L_r and L_s are the optical path lengths from the beam splitter to the reference mirror and sample, respectively, L_d is the optical path length from the beam splitter to the detector, and $K_r(v)e^{i\alpha_r(v)}$ and $K_s(v)e^{i\alpha_s(v)}$ are the amplitude reflection coefficients of light backscattered from the reference mirror and turbid sample, respectively.

If we translate the reference mirror to change the time delay (τ) between light in the reference and sample paths, the total power detected at the interferometer output is given by a time average of the squared light amplitude:

$$I_d = \langle | U_s(t) + U_r(t) |^2 \rangle. \quad (6)$$

Combining harmonic expansions for $U_s(t)$ and $U_r(t)$ and applying Eq. (2) when computing a time average, the total power detected is a sum of three terms representing reference (I_r), sample (I_s), and the interference fringe intensity ($\Gamma_{OCT}(\nu)$),

$$I_d = I_r + I_s + \Gamma_{OCT}(\tau), \quad (7)$$

where explicit expressions for each term are

$$I_r = \int_{\infty}^{0} S_o(v) | K_r(v) |^2 \, dv \quad (8)$$

$$I_s = \int_{\infty}^{0} S_o(v) | K_s(v) |^2 \, dv \quad (9)$$

$$\Gamma_{OCT}(\tau) = \int_{\infty}^{0} 2S_o(v) K_r(v) K_s(v) \cos[2\pi v\tau + \alpha_s(v) - \alpha_r(v)] dv, \quad (10)$$

where τ is the time delay determined by the optical path length difference between light traveled in the sample and reference arms:

$$\tau = \frac{2}{c}(L_s - L_r). \quad (11)$$

In the case where K_s, K_r, α_s, and α_r are spectrally independent over the source spectrum, the interference fringe term $\Gamma_{OCT}(\tau)$ is simplified to

$$\Gamma_{OCT}(\tau) = 2K_r K_s \int_{\infty}^{0} S_o(v) \cos[2\pi v\tau] dv. \quad (12)$$

Fourier-Domain OCT

Since the introduction of OCT in the 1990s, OCT has evolved from early time domain to Fourier domain systems. In a time-domain OCT system, the source is typically a superluminescent diode (SLD), and the photodetector is a single element photovoltaic detector. Depth in the sample is probed sequentially by rapidly changing the reference path length either by translating the reference mirror or through the use of a rapid-scanning optical delay (RSOD) line. The data processing consists of detecting the envelope of the detected fringe pattern corresponding to interference. In Fourier-domain OCT (FD-OCT), the reference arm is kept stationary, and the interference spectrum is measured as a function of frequency or wavelength which allows for simultaneous measurement of backscattered photons from all depths. Therefore, the OCT signal can be written as a superposition of fields generated from different path length delays:

$$\Gamma_{\mathrm{OCT}} \propto \sum_{n} K_{\mathrm{r}} K_{\mathrm{s},n} S_{\mathrm{o},n}(v) \cos[2\pi v \tau_n]. \tag{13}$$

Note the differences between Eqs. (12) and (13). In TD-OCT, the photodiode detects the contributions of all frequencies, while in FD-OCT, each frequency fringe is detected separately and the resulting fringe signal is a summation of these individual fringes. From Eq. (13), it is also evident that there exists a Fourier transform relationship between the OCT backscatter location and the fringe spectrum:

$$\Gamma_{\mathrm{OCT}}(z) = \mathcal{F}^{-1}\{\Gamma_{\mathrm{OCT}}(v)\} \tag{14}$$

where z is the path length difference between reference and sample arms. The Fourier transform of a real signal is conjugate symmetric which results in mirror terms. Removal of these mirror terms typically involves ensuring that the zero path length delay between the reference arm and sample arm is outside of the sample. Various schemes including incorporating acousto-optic modulators, electro-optic modulators, and complex 3×3 couplers have been developed to remove the complex mirror artifact.

FD-OCT has been implemented in two different schemes: a spectrometer-based design [5, 6] displayed in Fig 3a and a swept laser source-based design [7, 8] shown in Fig 3b. Both methods share similar sensitivity and speed benefits as compared to traditional time-domain-based OCT systems. In a spectrometer-based OCT system, the photodetector in Fig. 1 is replaced with a spectrometer and a line scan camera, and the reference arm is replaced with a static mirror. The interference fringe is passed through the spectrometer which spatially disperses the different wavelengths of light onto different pixels of the line scan camera. In a swept laser source-based OCT system, a wavelength swept laser is used as the light source, and the interference pattern is detected by a

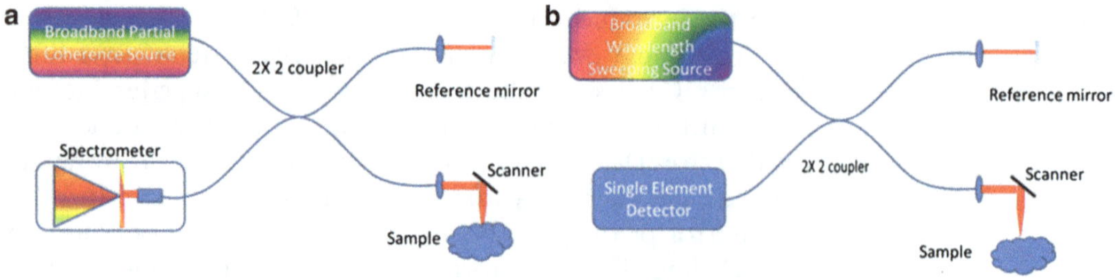

Fig. 3 Schematic of spectrometer-based OCT system (**a**) and swept source OCT system (**b**)

photodetector as a function of time in order to separate the spectral information. The development of high-speed line scan cameras and high-speed swept source lasers has led to 2–3 orders of magnitude increase in imaging speed. At the same time, FD-OCT systems have been shown to have significantly improved signal-to-noise ratios (SNR) as compared to TD-OCT systems.

Doppler OCT

Doppler OCT (D-OCT) combines the Doppler principle with OCT to obtain high-resolution tomographic images of static and moving constituents simultaneously in highly scattering biological tissues [9, 10]. When backscattered light from a moving particle interferes with the reference beam, a Doppler frequency shift occurs in the resulting interference fringe. The first two-dimensional measurement of this frequency shift was first reported in 1997 [9, 10]. These early approaches used a spectrogram method either via a short-time fast Fourier transformation (STFFT) or wavelet transformation to determine the power spectrum of the measured fringe signal. Although spectrogram methods allow for simultaneous imaging of in vivo tissue structure and flow velocity, velocity sensitivity is directly coupled with both spatial resolution and imaging speed; increased velocity sensitivity requires a larger time window which decreases both spatial resolution and imaging speed.

Phase-resolved D-OCT was developed to overcome these limitations [11]. This method uses the phase change between sequential A-line scans for velocity image reconstruction. Phase-resolved D-OCT decouples spatial resolution and velocity sensitivity in flow images and increases imaging speed by more than two orders of magnitude. The significant increase in scanning speed and velocity sensitivity makes it possible to image in vivo tissue microcirculation in human skin [11–13]. Combining the high-speed and high-sensitivity FD-OCT with the phase-resolved method has been demonstrated by a number of groups [14–16]. The dynamic range of phase-resolved D-OCT depends on the speed of the line scans; therefore, FD Doppler OCT has an advantage over time-domain methods in terms of both imaging speed and dynamic range.

In phase-resolved D-OCT, the Doppler frequency shift Δf is obtained by measuring the phase difference between sequential

A-scans. The phase information of the fringe signal can be determined from the complex analytical signal *Aj,z*, where *Aj,z* is the complex OCT signal at the *j*th A-scan and a depth of *z*. The Doppler frequency shift Δf can be expressed as

$$\Delta f = \frac{1}{2\pi}\frac{d\phi}{dt} = \frac{\Delta\phi}{2\pi T} = \frac{1}{2\pi\Delta T}[\tan^{-1}(\frac{\text{Im}(A_{j+1,z})}{\text{Re}(A_{j+1,z})}) - \tan^{-1}(\frac{\text{Im}(A_{j,z})}{\text{Re}(A_{j,z})})], \quad (15)$$

where ΔT is the time difference between *j*th A-scan and (j+1)th A-scan. In a time-domain D-OCT system, the complex analytical signal *Aj,z* is determined through analytical continuation of the measured interference fringes function by use of a Hilbert transformation. In Fourier-domain ODT systems, the complex signal *Aj,z* is directly obtained through the Fourier transformation of the acquired interference fringe. Velocity can be calculated as

$$\Delta f = \frac{2v \cdot \cos(\theta)}{\lambda_0} \quad (16)$$

where θ is the angle between the incident light and the velocity direction and λ_0 is the center wavelength of the light source.

Alternatively, the phase change can also be calculated by cross-correlation [11]. In addition, averaging can improve the signal-to-noise ratio [11, 17]. Averaging could be performed in both lateral and depth directions and Eq. (15) becomes

$$\bar{f} = \frac{1}{(2\pi \cdot \Delta T)} \cdot \arctan\{\frac{\sum_{J}^{j=1}\sum_{N}^{z=1}[\text{Im}(A_{j+1,z})\text{Re}(A_{j,z}) - \text{Im}(A_{j,z})\text{Re}(A_{j+1,z})]}{\sum_{J}^{j=1}\sum_{N}^{z=1}[\text{Re}(A_{j,z})\text{Re}(A_{j+1,z}) + \text{Im}(A_{j+1,z})\text{Im}(A_{j,z})]}\} \quad (17)$$

where J is the number of A-lines that are averaged, and N is the number of depth points that are averaged. The choice of J and N is dependent on application. Generally, a larger J and N will increase SNR, however, will also increase the computation time and decrease resolution.

Figures 4a–d are OCT structure images of the flow phantom pumped at 20 µl/min, 40 µl/min, 60 µl/min, and 80 µl/min, respectively. Figures 4e–h are phase-resolved D-OCT images of the flow phantom pumped at 20 µl/min, 40 µl/min, 60 µl/min, and 80 µl/min, respectively. It should be noted that the phase is wrapped in Fig. 4h. It can be clearly seen from the D-OCT images that the Doppler frequency shift increases with increasing pumping speed.

In addition to the Doppler shift, Doppler variance can also be used to map flow. Doppler variance has the benefit of being less sensitive to the pulsatile nature of blood flow and the incidence angle which allows for better discrimination of transverse flow

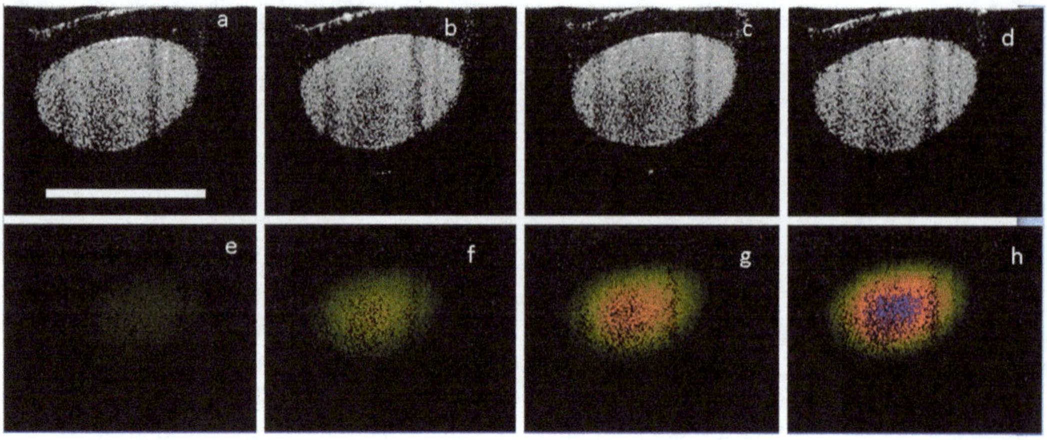

Fig. 4 **(a)**, **(b)**, **(c)**, and **(d)** are OCT structure images of the flow phantom pumped at, respectively, 20 μl/min, 40 μl/min, 60 μl/min, and 80 μl/min; **(e)**, **(f)**, **(g)**, and **(h)** are D-OCT images of the flow phantom pumped at, respectively, 20 μl/min, 40 μl/min, 60 μl/min, and 80 μl/min. Scale bar, 500 μm

velocity. If σ denotes the standard deviation of the Doppler spectrum, the Doppler variance σ^2 can be obtained [12]:

$$\sigma^2 = \frac{\int (f - \bar{f})^2 P(f)df}{\int P(f)df} \overline{f^2} - \bar{f}^2 \quad (18)$$

where $\bar{f}$ is the Doppler frequency and $P(f)$ is the power spectrum of the Doppler frequency shift. Using the autocorrelation theory, the variance can be expressed as

$$\sigma^2 = \frac{1}{(2\pi \cdot \Delta T)^2}\left[1 - \frac{\left|\sum_{J}^{j=1}\sum_{N}^{z=1}(A_{j+1,z}A^*_{j,z})\right|}{\sum_{J}^{j=1}\sum_{N}^{z=1}(A_{j,z}A^*_{j,z})}\right] \quad (19)$$

where Aj,z^* is the complex conjugate of Aj,z, J is the number of A-lines that are averaged, and N is the number of depth points that are averaged.

Recently, another approach has been applied to calculate Doppler variance [18]. The variance acquired via Eq. (19) relies on the summation of multiple correlation calculations across either time or space and is thus dependent on both the amplitude and phase terms of the complex OCT data. This approach shows excellent results when the phase stability of the system is high; however, in a phase instable situation, the calculated variance will be greatly skewed by the abrupt change in phase terms. Eq. (19) can be modified slightly to remove this phase dependence and solely rely on the intensity values of the correlation data as shown in Eq. (20).

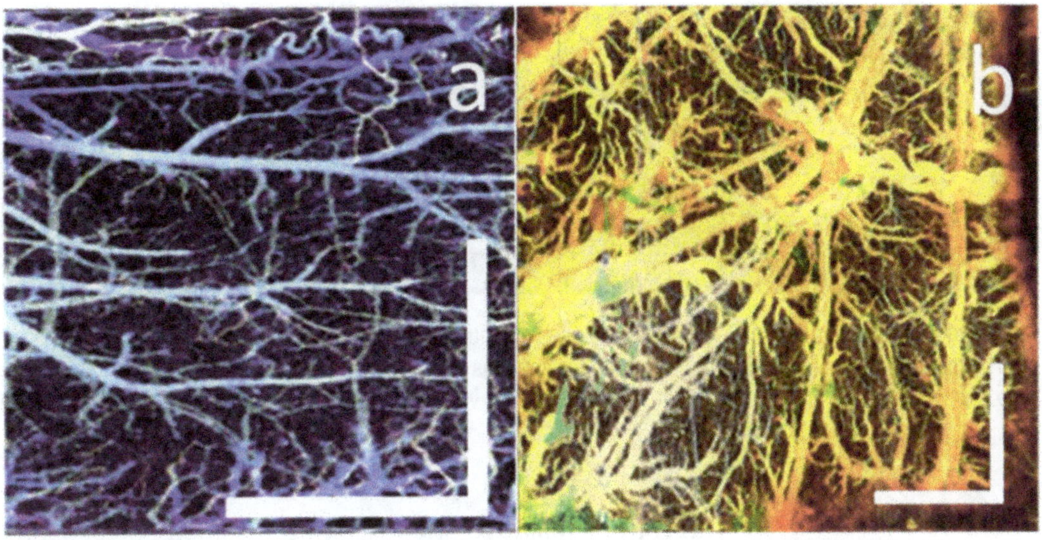

Fig. 5 D-OCT imaging of microvasculature. (**a**) Microvasculature of mouse cerebral cortex. (**b**) Microvasculature of rat cerebral cortex. Scale bar, 1 mm

$$\sigma^2 = \frac{1}{(2\pi \cdot \Delta T)^2}[1 - \frac{\sum_{J}^{j=1}\sum_{N}^{z=1} |(A_{j+1,z}A^*_{j,z})|}{\sum_{J}^{j=1}\sum_{N}^{z=1}(A_{j,z}A^*_{j,z})}] \tag{20}$$

Figure 5 shows a representative maximum intensity projection D-OCT image of vasculature from the cerebral cortex of a mouse and rat. These images were acquired utilizing a swept source FD-OCT system, taking advantage of the higher sensitivity to allow visualization of the smaller microvasculature in addition to the larger vessels.

Optical Coherence Elastography

Mechanical properties can be important indicators of tissue health such as in cancer where tumors typically have a significantly different stiffness than surrounding tissue. Elastography has been utilized in the study of laryngeal cancer and has shown to be a valuable tool for improving classification of malignancy [19–21]. Optical coherence elastography (OCE) is a functional extension of OCT in which a mechanical map of tissue stiffness can be determined. An external force or load is applied to a sample in order to create a mechanical deformation. The resulting displacement caused by the load is quantified by OCT measurements, and by relating the displacement with the known deformation force, various properties such as strain, stiffness, and Young's modulus can be calculated. The earliest demonstration of OCT utilized a piezoelectric actuator to physically compress a sample and quantified the deformation via cross-correlation of sequential OCT images [22].

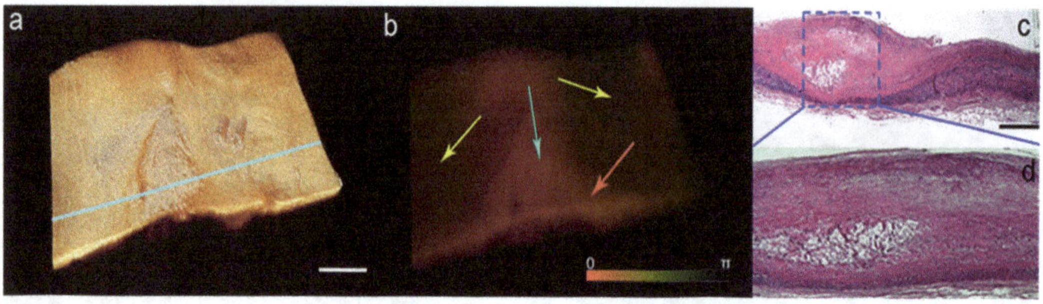

Fig. 6 **(a)** OCT structural. (**b**) ARF-OCE phase images of a human cadaver coronary artery under 500-Hz, 350-mV AM modulated excitation; an atherosclerotic lesion was identified as the *red* region corresponding to the *blue* box in (**c**). (**c**) The histological image. (**d**) The close-up view of the atherosclerotic lesion. Scale bar, 1 mm

Recently, a phase-resolved acoustic radiation force optical coherence elastography (PR-ARF-OCE) method was developed to evaluate the elastic properties of tissue [23]. This method utilizes a chirped acoustic radiation force to produce excitation along the sample's axial direction and phase-resolved D-OCT to measure the vibration of the sample. ARF-OCE has the advantage of combining a high-repetition excitation force with the high-sensitivity displacement detection of phase-resolved D-OCT. Figure 6 shows the ex vivo 3D images of an atherosclerotic human coronary artery obtained with the phase-resolved ARF-OCE. The OCT intensity image, shown in Fig. 6a, provides a general morphological view of the tissue, but provides no obvious evidence of the presence of atherosclerosis. The ARF-OCE image in Fig. 6b shows a strong vibration phase contrast between the normal and plaque regions. The red-colored region indicated by the blue arrow in the ARF-OCE image is characterized by smaller phase changes which correspond to smaller vibration amplitudes and therefore represent stiffer tissue. The stronger vibration regions representing softer tissue (dark area) are indicated by yellow arrows. The transition between plaque and normal regions appears orange in color (indicated by the red arrow) and is characterized by intermediate elasticity which corresponds with the histology image in Fig 6c.

OCT Imaging in Otolaryngology

OCT has been successfully utilized in a variety of medical fields including cardiology, gastroenterology, and, most prominently, ophthalmology. While OCT has been utilized in otolaryngology in the past, the recent development of novel high-speed light sources in addition to improved light delivery schemes has created a renewed interest in using OCT to study various clinical disorders.

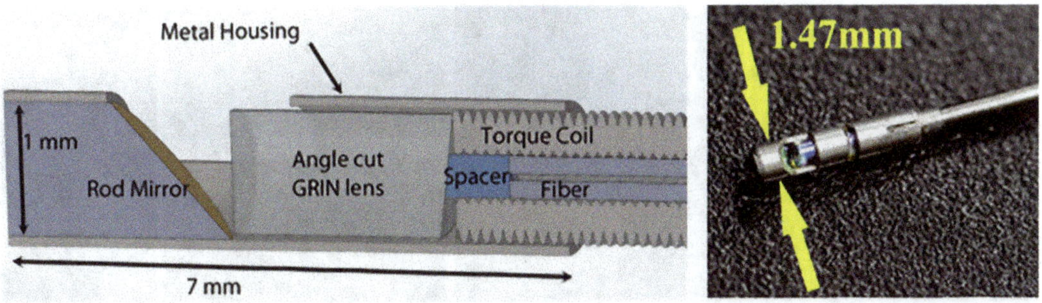

Fig. 7 A photograph of and the schematic of OCT imaging probe tip. This probe features an angle cut gradient index (GRIN) lens and a rod mirror both 1 mm in diameter, secured in a 7-mm-long stainless steel metal housing that is soldered to the stainless torque coil for protection of the optical components. A single-mode SMF-28 fiber inside the torque coil is used to carry the laser beam, and the length of spacer determines the working distance of the probe. The maximum diameter of the imaging probe is 1.47 mm

Flexible fiber optic imaging probes have been developed for a wide range of uses in the study of internal tissues and organs which would be otherwise unreachable. Scanning of the tissue can be achieved through various approaches including proximal rotation of the probe, utilization of a distal rotational motor, or via a complex piezoelectric scan pattern. Figure 7 shows a representative example of a proximal rotation OCT probe with an outer diameter of 1.47 mm. A single-mode optical fiber couples light from an external source to a gradient index (GRIN) lens and an angled rod mirror to focus the OCT beam out radially. The focal length of the probe is controlled by adjusting the length of a spacer in between the GRIN lens and the optical fiber. A stainless steel tube with a window is utilized to house the lens and mirror elements, while a hollow torque coil provides durability and protection for the entire length of optical fiber. Radial scanning is achieved by rotating the entire probe body via an external rotational motor coupled to a fiber optic rotary joint. During imaging, sterility is maintained by inserting the entire OCT probe into a sealed-off protective sheath, typically made from some form of transparent plastic polymer.

Utilizing OCT to image tissue morphology in the airway is a growing field of interest. Obstruction in the upper airway can often cause reductions in breathing or gas exchange efficiency and lead sleep disorders. Traditional imaging diagnosis has been accomplished using computed tomography (CT) and magnetic resonance imaging (MRI). However, both CT and MRI have drawbacks that preclude their expansive use in obstructive airway diagnosis such as ionizing radiation, procedure cost, and ease of access to equipment. Early OCT studies of the airway utilizing fiber scanning probes successfully imaged lumens with diameters of up to 30–40 mm by utilizing TD-OCT setups with long reference scans which limited their frames rates to 1–5 Hz [24, 25]. Ridgway et al.

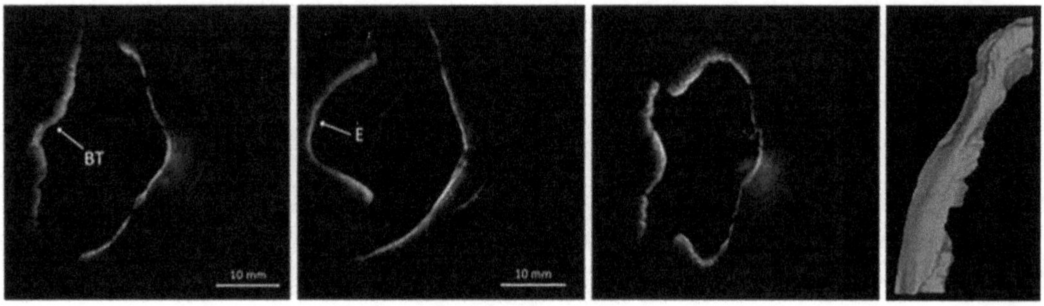

Fig. 8 In vivo OCT images of human upper airway: *BT* Base of tongue, *E* Epiglottis, *SP* Soft palate, 3D rendering of stacked OCT images of airway from larynx to nasal cavity

have reported on utilizing OCT to characterize subsurface tissue trauma in the subglottis of neonatal patients requiring prolonged endotracheal intubation [26]. FD-OCT approaches have also been adopted by utilizing acousto-optic modulators (AOMs) to remove complex conjugate artifacts and double the achievable imaging range [27–29]. Imaging rates of 50 Hz utilizing a rotational probe have been demonstrated allowing for complete imaging of the airway lumen from the larynx to the nostril in 16 s [30]. Figure 8 shows three cross-sectional slices from an adult airway acquired in vivo during a clinical visit. From the series of slices, a three-dimensional volume is created by stacking the slices along the translational pullback path and allows for a better visualization of areas of airway obstruction.

Vocal fold dynamics have been widely imaged using laryngeal video-stroboscopy and high-speed video cameras and linked with vocal fold health and pathology [31–33]. Although video-stroboscopy provides an excellent method to dynamically assess the vocal folds, only surface information of the vocal folds is provided; therefore, the subsurface health of the vocal folds remains largely unknown. Differentiation between benign polyps and malignant lesions in the vocal folds can require a biopsy which can result in permanent damage or alternation of an individual's voice. The integrity of the basement membrane in the vocal folds has been shown to be a hallmark of laryngeal cancer. Various studies have utilized OCT to study the vocal folds. Yu et al. utilized a handheld dynamic focusing probe in combination with a swept source OCT system to image the tissue structure of vibrating human vocal cords in vivo at an imaging speed of 40 Hz (Fig 9) [34]. The average vibration frequency was calculated based on the number of complete vibration cycles per frame. Liu et al. later demonstrated a phase-resolved Doppler OCT approach to calculate the localized vocal fold velocity distribution in an ex vivo porcine larynx [35]. Comparison of the phase change between adjacent A-lines allows for the calculation of vibration

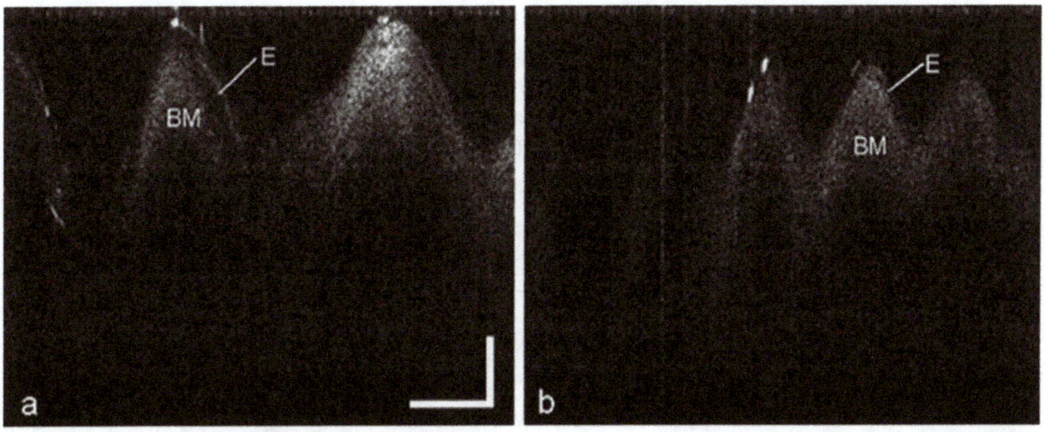

Fig. 9 Vibrating vocal cord with different frequencies: (**a**) ~120 Hz and (**b**) ~200 Hz. *E* Epithelium, *BM* Basement Membrane. Scale bar represents 500 μm

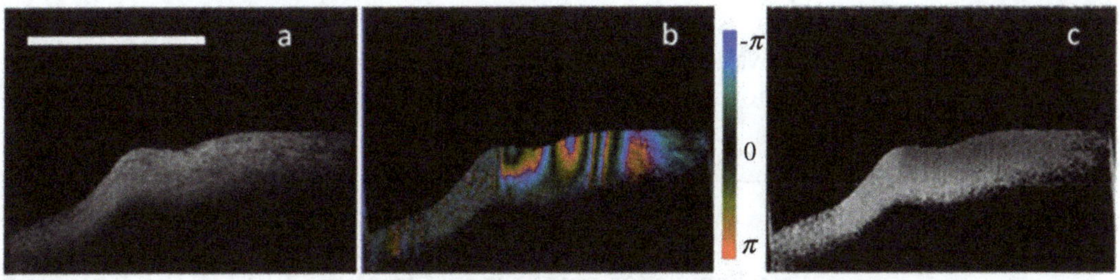

Fig. 10 OCT images of a vibrating vocal fold with frequency of ~ 1.1 Hz. (**a**) B-mode OCT structure image, (**b**) B-mode color Doppler OCT image, and (**c**) B-mode Doppler variance OCT image. Scale bar represents 500 μm

velocity in the axial or vertical direction, while the variance between the adjacent A-lines allows for determination of the lateral or horizontal velocity (Fig. 10).

Recently, two semiconductor-based swept lasers have been introduced that open new possibilities for OCT imaging in otolaryngology. New swept vertical cavity surface-emitting lasers (VCSELs) utilize a tunable microelectromechanical system (MEMS) dielectric mirror to tune the wavelength by varying the cavity length of the laser. The short cavity length also ensures single-mode operation with a very narrow instantaneous linewidth which allows for a significant increase in maximum imaging range. Potsaid et al. have reported an imaging range of greater than 50 mm at an imaging speed of 150 kHz with no loss of OCT sensitivity over the entire range [36]. In endoscopic imaging, these lasers offer both the ability to increase imaging speed and image larger lumen diameters. Akinetic lasers utilize Vernier-tuned distributed Bragg reflectors (VT-DBRs) to selectively tune wavelength [37]. These lasers utilize changes in current density which selectively changes the index of refraction or effective length of the laser cavity as well as tunes the reflectivity of the Vernier mirrors to a specific wavelength. Similarly to VCSEL sources, these VT-DBR lasers also ensure single-mode operation and narrow instantaneous linewidth to achieve a large maximum imaging range. In addition, since these sources do not rely on mechanical tuning, they offer significant improvements in terms of phase stability for increased phase-resolved D-OCT vibration measurements.

Summary

OCT is a rapidly developing imaging technology with many potential applications in the field of otolaryngology. OCT provides rapid morphological information based on inherent tissue scattering properties, and functional OCT methods can also provide various complementary physiological measurements. The high-resolution capabilities of OCT allow for precise quantitative measurements such as tissue layer thickness and displacement dynamics. Innovations in laser sources and probe designs will further expand the potential for OCT imaging in otolaryngology.

Acknowledgment

We acknowledge grant support from the BEST IGERT program funded by the National Science Foundation DGE-1144901, the National Institutes of Health (R01EB-10090, R01EY-021519, R01HL-105215, R01HL-103764, P41EB-015890), the Air Force Office of Scientific Research (FA9550-10-1-0538), and the Beckman Laser Institute Endowment. Dr. Chen has a financial interest in OCT Medical Imaging, Inc., which, however, did not support this work.

References

1. Huang D, et al. Optical coherence tomography. Science. 1991;254(5035):1178–81.
2. Izatt JA, et al. Micrometer-scale resolution imaging of the anterior eye in vivo with optical coherence tomography. Arch Ophthalmol. 1994;112(12):1584–9.
3. Fercher AF. Optical coherence tomography. J Biomed Opt. 1996;1:157–73.
4. Drexler W, Fujimoto JG, editors. Optical coherence tomography: technology and applications. Berlin: Springer; 2008.
5. Fercher AF, et al. Measurement of intraocular distances by backscattering spectral interferometry. Opt Commun. 1995;117:43–8.
6. Wojtkowski M, et al. In vivo human retinal imaging by Fourier domain optical coherence tomography. J Biomed Opt. 2002;7:457–63.
7. Chinn SR, Swanson EA, Fujimoto JG. Optical coherence tomography using a frequency-tunable optical source. Opt Lett. 1997;22:340–2.
8. Golubovic B, et al. Optical frequency-domain reflectometry using rapid wavelength tuning of a Cr4+: forsterite laser. Opt Lett. 1997;22(22):1704–6.
9. Chen Z, et al. Noninvasive imaging of in vivo blood flow velocity using optical Doppler tomography. Opt Lett. 1997;22(14):1119–21.

10. Izatt JA, et al. In vivo bidirectional color Doppler flow imaging of picoliter blood volumes using optical coherence tomography. Opt Lett. 1997;22:1439–41.
11. Zhao Y, et al. Phase-resolved optical coherence tomography and optical Doppler tomography for imaging blood flow in human skin with fast scanning speed and high velocity sensitivity. Opt Lett. 2000;25(2):114–6.
12. Zhao Y, et al. Doppler standard deviation imaging for clinical monitoring of in vivo human skin blood flow. Opt Lett. 2000;25: 1358–60.
13. Zhao Y, et al. Three-dimensional reconstruction of in vivo blood vessels in human skin using phase-resolved optical Doppler tomography. IEEE J Sel Top Quantum Electron. 2001;7:931–5.
14. Leitgeb RA, et al. Real-time assessment of retinal blood flow with ultrafast acquisition by color Doppler Fourier domain optical coherence tomography. Opt Express. 2003;11: 3116–21.
15. Wang L, et al. Frequency domain Phase-resolved optical Doppler and Doppler variance tomography. Opt Commun. 2004;242:345–7.
16. Zhang J, Chen Z. In vivo blood flow imaging by a swept laser source based Fourier domain optical Doppler tomography. Opt Express. 2005;13:7449–57.
17. Yang VX, et al. Improved phase-resolved optical Doppler tomography using the Kasai velocity estimator and histogram segmentation. Opt Commun. 2002;208:209–14.
18. Liu G, et al. Intensity-based modified Doppler variance algorithm: application to phase instable and phase stable optical coherence tomography systems. Opt Express. 2011;19(12): 11429–40.
19. Koudounarakis E, et al. Synchronous multifocal medullary and papillary thyroid microcarcinoma detected by elastography. Int J Surg Case Rep. 2014;5(1):5–7.
20. Fodor D. The utility of elastography and CEUS for the differentiation between benign and malignant cervical lymphadenopathy. Three cases report. Med Ultrason. 2013;15(1):63–6.
21. Lyshchik A, et al. Thyroid gland tumor diagnosis at US elastography. Radiology. 2005;237(1):202–11.
22. Schmitt JM. OCT elastography: imaging microscopic deformation and strain of tissue. Opt Express. 1998;3(6):199–211.
23. Qi W, et al. Phase-resolved acoustic radiation force optical coherence elastography. J Biomed Opt. 2012;17(11):110505.
24. Armstrong J, et al. In vivo size and shape measurement of the human upper airway using endoscopic longrange optical coherence tomography. Opt Express. 2003;11(15): 1817–26.
25. Lau B, et al. Imaging true 3D endoscopic anatomy by incorporating magnetic tracking with optical coherence tomography: proof-of-principle for airways. Opt Express. 2010; 18(26):27173–80.
26. Ridgway JM, et al. Optical coherence tomography of the newborn airway. Ann Otol Rhinol Laryngol. 2008;117(5):327–34 (Cover story).
27. Zhang J, Nelson JS, Chen Z. Removal of a mirror image and enhancement of the signal-to-noise ratio in Fourier-domain optical coherence tomography using an electro-optic phase modulator. Opt Lett. 2005;30(2):147–9.
28. Yun S, et al. Removing the depth-degeneracy in optical frequency domain imaging with frequency shifting. Opt Express. 2004;12(20): 4822–8.
29. Davis AM, Choma MA, Izatt JA. Heterodyne swept-source optical coherence tomography for complete complex conjugate ambiguity removal. J Biomed Opt. 2005;10(6):064005.
30. Jing J, et al. High-speed upper-airway imaging using full-range optical coherence tomography. J Biomed Opt. 2012;17(11):110507.
31. Patel R, Dailey S, Bless D. Comparison of high-speed digital imaging with stroboscopy for laryngeal imaging of glottal disorders. Ann Otol Rhinol Laryngol. 2008;117(6):413–24.
32. Lohscheller J, et al. Phonovibrography: mapping high-speed movies of vocal fold vibrations into 2-D diagrams for visualizing and analyzing the underlying laryngeal dynamics. IEEE Trans Med Imaging. 2008;27(3):300–9.
33. Lohscheller J, Eysholdt U. Phonovibrogram visualization of entire vocal fold dynamics. Laryngoscope. 2008;118(4):753–8.
34. Rubinstein M, et al. Office-based dynamic imaging of vocal cords in awake patients with swept-source optical coherence tomography. J Biomed Opt. 2009;14(6):064020.
35. Liu G, et al. Imaging vibrating vocal folds with a high speed 1050 nm swept source OCT and ODT. Opt Express. 2011;19(12):11880–9.
36. Potsaid B, et al. MEMS tunable VCSEL light source for ultrahigh speed 60kHz–1MHz axial scan rate and long range centimeter class OCT imaging. 2012.
37. Bonesi M, et al. Akinetic all-semiconductor programmable swept-source at 1550 nm and 1310 nm with centimeters coherence length. Opt Express. 2014;22(3):2632–55.

Chapter 33

Optical Coherence Tomography for the Middle and Inner Ear

Justus Ilgner, Tino Just, Csaba Farkas, Achim Lenenbach, and Martin Westhofen

Introduction

With the advent of operating microscopes in the early 1950s and the continuous development of prosthetic materials, functional restoration of hearing, whenever impaired sound conduction is the leading phenomenon, became a reliable treatment modality in the hands of otologic surgeons. For diagnostic purposes, a variety of functional tests form the repertoire from which the diagnosis for the underlying disease process is made. However, in most cases the cause for conductive hearing loss can only be concluded indirectly from a variety of audiometric findings. Direct visualization of the pathologic process is one need which has not yet been fully met. At present, magnetic resonance imaging and computed tomography images provide resolutions in the range of 300 μm. CT scans are mostly used to detect bony abnormalities as soft tissue differentiation is limited. Over recent years, Flat Panel CT, Cone Beam CT, and Digital Volume Tomography are about to increase resolution for middle and inner ear structures, but these imaging techniques cannot be used with contrast agents. On the other hand, MRI imaging is undergoing a continuous evolution process with higher field strengths, enabling soft tissue differentiation within middle ear structures for the detection of chronic middle ear inflammation involving epithelial growth, i.e., cholesteatoma. However, MRI scanners with field strengths of 7.5–10 T are required, which are not yet available for clinical routine.

OCT for the middle and inner ear faces considerable advantages as well as challenges: The tympanic membrane is readily accessible in humans, while the penetration of near infrared light

Brian J.-F. Wong and Justus Ilgner (eds.), *Biomedical Optics in Otorhinolaryngology: Head and Neck Surgery*,
DOI 10.1007/978-1-4939-1758-7_33, © Springer Science+Business Media New York 2016

does not require any transduction medium as in ultrasound. Therefore, structures within the air-filled middle ear cavity are readily visible. The imaging process can be noninvasive, and the size of structures under investigation meets the range suitable for OCT. Imaging devices can be built in small, compact units. They can be coupled to existing devices, as the operating microscope or a handheld otoscope, and can be operated by the clinician or operating surgeon himself who can also interpret the results. OCT provides visible results in real-time, making it suitable for quality control, e.g., in the operating theater. The change of refraction index between air and liquid, when facing an open inner ear, e.g., during stapes surgery, is not an obstacle for OCT, as long as image distortion along the *z* axis is taken into account and, if necessary, corrected by image processing. On the down side, however, in-vivo imaging of nonanesthetized subjects can suffer from movement artifacts, which can be overcome by increasing image acquisition rates. Imaging through an intact tympanic membrane can attenuate the signal and create artifacts, if the TM is sclerotic or thickened, making visualization of middle ear structures difficult or impossible. Finally, penetration depth through solid bone is limited, requiring a direct line of sight to the region of interest in most cases. Middle ear ossicles or overhanging parts of the outer ear canal can obstruct the scanning beam. Yet there are numerous approaches considering the use of OCT either as an imaging modality on its own or as an adjunct in functional investigations of the middle ear, which have the potential to widen the diagnostic spectrum of otologists in clinical routine over the next decades.

OCT in Experimental Middle and Inner Ear Imaging: Ex Vivo and In Vivo

Pitris and coworkers [1] were one of the first to apply OCT to middle ear imaging in general. In an ex vivo experiment using four human temporal bones from cadavers, they employed a TD-OCT scanner with a probe introduced next to the outer ear canal, in 15 mm distance to the closed tympanic membrane. Acquisition time of one B-image took between 10 and 30 s. While the authors noticed shadowing effects of solid structures, as middle ear ossicles, and resolution loss by the closed tympanic membrane, they were still able to identify and label middle ear structures. They concluded that OCT has the advantage of using air, as well as fluids/soft tissues as a transduction medium, thereby making it suitable for middle ear imaging in real time. Probes could be built compact and adapted to any kind of instrument used in otology.

Just et al. [2–4] specifically aimed to characterize the oval niche and the stapes footplate. In a first experiment, they used an

SD-OCT system producing 1000 A-lines per second, which was coupled to a conventional operating microscope. First results could differentiate layers (bone and cartilage) within the stapes footplate. Furthermore, the elastic suspension of the stapes footplate could be identified, although anatomical variations in some cases, as an overhanging facial nerve, might prevent this. Following stapes perforation by CO_2 laser, the outline of the vestibulum was visualized through the open footplate by OCT. The authors also noted that while working on the open vestibulum, resulting images required depth correction along the z-axis, as the refraction index in an air-filled middle ear (1.0) is different from the inner ear filled with fluids, i.e., perilymph and endolymph (1.33).

Subhash and coworkers [5] proposed a system for ultra-high sensitive optical microangiography, which they used to visualize blood flow in the cochlea of mice. Their system is based on an SD-OCT scanner acquiring 47,000 A-scans per second, resulting in high-resolution B-scans at a rate of 300 frames per second. Their system is sensitive for flow velocities between 4.0 μm/s and 30 mm/s, making it suitable for physiological blood flow rates down to capillary level. They were able to create 3D volumetric images of blood flow in the basal, middle, and apical turn of the mouse cochlea, depicting inner ear structures as the modiolus, stria vascularis, Reissner's membrane, and basilar membrane and visualizing blood flow in the stria vascularis in particular using the phase difference between adjacent B-scans. Resolution is sufficiently high in order to subsegment different areas of the cochlea from three-dimensional reconstruction, thereby enabling the measurement of blood flow in different cochlear structures separately.

In another experiment by the same workgroup [6], phase-sensitive SD-OCT was used to detect sound induced motions of middle ear structures, thereby using the SD-OCT system as a middle ear vibrometer. From a human temporal bone cadaver, structural B-scan images were taken and compared to vibrational images visualizing the velocity of different areas of the tympanic membrane as well as of the middle ear ossicles. Using this method, which was applied through the closed tympanic membrane, the authors propose the setup to diagnose different causes of conductive hearing loss directly and noninvasively.

Cho et al. [7] also combined an SD-OCT scanner with a surgical microscope for imaging middle ear and inner ear structures in mice through the closed tympanic membrane. In their experiment, they also created models of different clinical situations, e.g., middle ear effusion, remaining effusion after paracentesis and suction, tympanic membrane perforation, and compared these to OCT imaging results. In their view, the advantage of SD-OCT lies in imaging and 3D image reconstruction of middle ear structures in vivo which is now possible in real-time.

Chang et al. [8] in a recent study were able to use an OCT system to simultaneously visualize sound induced motions of the tympanic membrane and middle ear ossicles in three-dimensional reconstruction of three temporal bones from chinchilla cadavers. They examined pure tone frequencies of 800, 1910, and 3050 Hz. Their OCT system produces 15,000–20,000 A-lines per second, while the number of A-scans divided by the pure tone frequency under examination results in the number of different phases displayed by the system. Sensitivity for tympanic membrane movement was 0.5 nm and 5 nm for the stapes footplate, as all measurements were performed through the closed tympanic membrane. Different motion and phase-related features could be identified for (a) normal middle ear structures, (b) stapes fixation, and (c) interruption of the incudo-stapedial joint. As for future perspectives, the authors see the potential to differentiate between different causes of conductive hearing loss directly in an outpatient setting using their system.

With similar intention, Burkhardt and coworkers [9] presented a Doppler OCT system to analyze human temporal membrane motion by acoustic chirps over a frequency range between 400 Hz and 6400 Hz. They used a Frequency-Domain OCT system with a center wavelength of 1300 nm ± 160 nm. Lateral resolution was calculated at 9 μm and axial resolution at 13 μm. Measuring the tympanic membrane with 512 Motion(M)-scans in z axis at a rate of 60 kHz over a grid of 25 × 25 points, 8.5 ms were required for one scan to render one full tympanic membrane scan over 625 points within 5.3 s. By means of the setup, tympanic membrane motion showed an increasing complexity and falling amplitude with rising frequency. Resonance frequency of the human tympanic membrane was observed at 1062 Hz, while amplitude maxima were observed to shift over different spots with varying frequency. Their setup, however, employed a human temporal bone model, although the authors see the possibility to adapt it for clinical use with reasonable effort.

OCT in Clinical Middle and Inner Ear Imaging

One of the first to use OCT in clinical settings, Heermann and coworkers [10] coupled a TD-OCT scanner to an operating microscope and used it under sterile conditions while performing microsurgery of the middle ear. They employed the OCT system in B-Mode in five cases of tympanoplasty type III, i.e., restoration of the tympanic membrane, the malleus, the incus, and—in some cases—the stapes suprastructure following chronic inflammation of the middle ear, as well as five cases of stapes surgery, in which the stapes is fixed by a sclerotic change of the elastic ring supporting it to the inner ear capsule. In both operations, OCT was mainly used to measure the length of the prosthesis which is critical for reestablishing sound transmission in the best possible way. The authors concluded that optical measurement of distances in the inner ear were preferable over mechanical measurement, as the latter always carries the risk of destruction to the remaining middle ear chain, particularly breaking the stapes footplate. The authors stated that B-mode imaging through a closed tympanic membrane were impossible due to methodological restrictions. Although this may apply to cases of tympanosclerosis or extreme scarring, in cases of healthy, semi-transparent tympanic membranes this hypothesis was proven otherwise by later authors.

Djalilian et al. [11, 12] employed a TD-OCT-system in an outpatient setting in order to characterize healthy tympanic membranes and to differentiate these from distinct pathological processes. In 10 patients, they were able to delineate the physiological trilaminar structure of the tympanic membrane with an outer squamous layer, middle fibrous layer, and medial cuboidal epithelium. This trilaminar structure could be differentiated from atrophic areas of the tympanic membrane with only one thin layer visible. Furthermore, hyperkeratosis of the tympanic membrane, a tympanosclerotic plaque, and cholesteatoma could be seen, although in these three cases, penetration depth of the infrared light is limited and therefore prevents further differentiation in depth, as well as judging the extent of chronic inflammatory process as in cholesteatoma. Image acquisition rate was 1 Hz, making it suitable for the practical use in an outpatient department with a total examination time of 3 min for each patient.

In the aforementioned studies by Just et al. [2–4], imaging of the oval window niche in human temporal bones was transferred to an operative setting in eight patients undergoing stapes surgery. In these patients, the sclerotic changes to the elastic suspension of the stapes footplate, as well as the footplate itself were contrasted against their results obtained from healthy temporal bones ex vivo. Scanning speed allowed imaging in B-mode in real time, although three-dimensional reconstruction of the data required some image postprocessing and could not be realized in an operative setting. However, scan resolution allowed online characterization of shape and extent of sclerotic changes encountered in otosclerosis patients. As a practical aspect, the use of the SD-OCT scanner extended the total duration of surgery by 5–10 min.

In 2012, Nguyen et al. [13] from S. Boppart's workgroup set out to detect bacterial biofilm attached to the inner layer of the tympanic membrane of patients with chronic otitis media (COM)/otitis media with effusion (OME). The general hypothesis is that bacteria whose number per volume exceeds a certain threshold can produce a thick layer of mucopolysaccharides which is impenetrable by macrophages, lymphocytes, etc. as well as by antibiotics. Nguyen et al. aimed to detect this layer optically. They used two methods, low coherence interferometry (LCI) and optical coherence tomography, either as a stand-alone method (LCI) or in combination, using a custom built hand-held device similar to an office otoscope. From a total of 20 individuals, 13 patients with clinical signs of COM and seven healthy controls, 18,537 LCI scans and 742 OCT images were taken. Biofilm was defined as a thick and highly scattering signal up to a depth of 400 μm (200 μm average) behind the tympanic membrane, while the TM itself showed two distinct peaks about 90 μm apart, related to the outer and inner epithelial layer. As many LCI scans per ear were taken, the specificity for the presence of biofilm was such that normal ears had a low percentage of abnormal scans (<11 %), while ears with presence of biofilm had an abnormal scan rate of >37 %. Therefore, the authors set the threshold of biofilm diagnosed with LCI/OCT at a rate of abnormal scans of >25 % per ear resulting in a sensitivity of 68 % and specificity of 98 %. According to the authors, the low sensitivity can be explained by patchy areas of biofilm that result in normal and abnormal scans at the same time in one ear.

In a consecutive study [14], the workgroup of Nguyen and Boppart compared the presence of biofilm assessed by OCT to acoustic effects on the tympanic membrane induced by biofilm. They found that in cases with the presence of biofilm confirmed by OCT, tympanic membranes showed certain features of acoustic resistance and power reflectance that could be differentiated from normal tympanic membranes and potentially also from TM in chronic otitis media with effusion. However, the authors also state that three-dimensional reconstruction of OCT images could help identifying the extent of biofilm and its local effects of TM movement, while in this study local effects were difficult to assess as only two-dimensional images were available.

OCT in Conjunction with Other Experimental Methods

McCaughey and coworkers [15] used a TD-OCT scanner to compare the shape of bone ablated by two different lasers, an Er:YAG laser (2940 nm) and a femtosecond laser (1053 nm) ex vivo. Other means of characterization were light microscopy and scanning electron microscopy (SEM). Although penetration depth of OCT was extremely limited in bone, the ablation depth was easily quantified as well as ablation margins characterized without mechanically cross-sectioning of the specimen, thereby avoiding preparation artifacts.

The question which thermal alterations affect the perilymph during CO_2 laser stapedotomy was addressed by Just and coworkers in 2010 [16]. In this context of an ex vivo experiment, the shape and thickness of the stapes footplate as well as the shape of the CO_2 laser-induced footplate perforation were addressed. To achieve this, the shape of the footplate was reconstructed three-dimensionally using data from the SD-OCT scanning system described in [2–4]. The OCT data confirmed perforation diameters between 490 and 550 μm with an unevenly shaped "crystallization zone" and evenly shaped, unaffected bone. No significant correlation was found between the thickness of the stapes footplate and the perforation diameter.

Just et al. [17] also examined tympanic membrane movement by using a film patch with integrated strain gauge. In this context, two different types of film patch with integrated strain gauge were attached to tympanic membranes in vitro. The SD-OCT system described in [2–4] was employed to (a) assess the thickness of tympanic membranes under investigation in vitro and in vivo and (b) evaluate whether the film patch was tightly attached to the tympanic membrane surface during pressure changes, leaving no gaps between the membrane and the film patch.

Own Experience

In a research project conducted jointly be the Fraunhofer Institute for Laser Technology (ILT) and the Department of Otorhinolaryngology, Plastic Surgery of the Head and Neck, RWTH Aachen, we aimed to evaluate the use of OCT for otologic diagnosis in an outpatient setting. The objective was to create an additional tool for the otologist to (i) confirm/refine the clinical diagnosis made by otomicroscopy for preoperative patients and to (ii) follow up patients postoperatively for early detection of recurrent disease, e.g., cholesteatoma.

A time-domain OCT system with a low-coherent super luminescent diode light source with a center wavelength of 1310 nm was coupled to the front lens of a microscope via a micromanipulator (Figs. 1 and 2). The micromanipulator allows adjustment of the scan direction and the field of view of about 1 × 1 mm minimum to 2 × 3 mm maximum. The system creates 200 A-lines per second in an x/y matrix of 100 × 100 scans, resulting in a total scan time of 50 s for one volumetric scan. As the field of view in x/y direction is variable so is the transverse resolution of the system. The axial resolution is 10 μm, with a comparatively large scan range along the z-axis of 9 mm. This range was necessary in order to achieve one scan ranging from the tympanic membrane to the medial wall of the middle ear, e.g., the promontory and structures in between (Table 1).

A standard resolution CCD camera was incorporated in the system to monitor areas under scan and to document the clinical

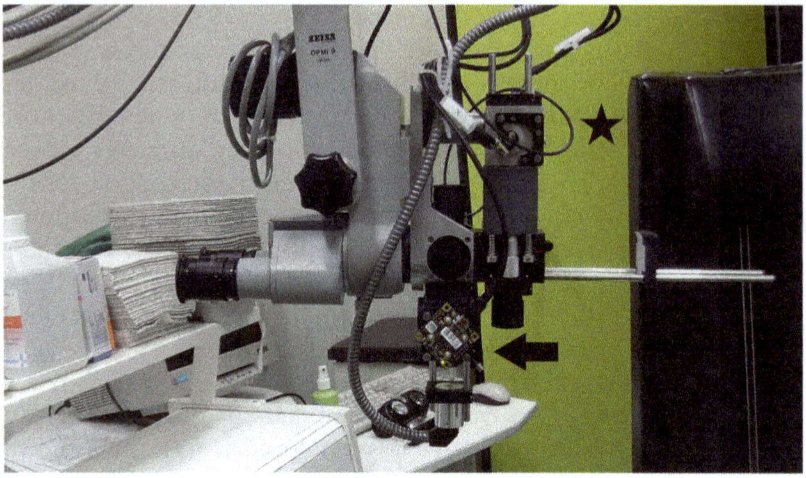

Fig. 1 Oto-Microscope (Zeiss OPMI9) in outpatient department with micromanipulator attached including *x*/*y* scanner drive (*star*) and CCD camera (*arrow*). The guide rails to the right are attached for calibration purposes only

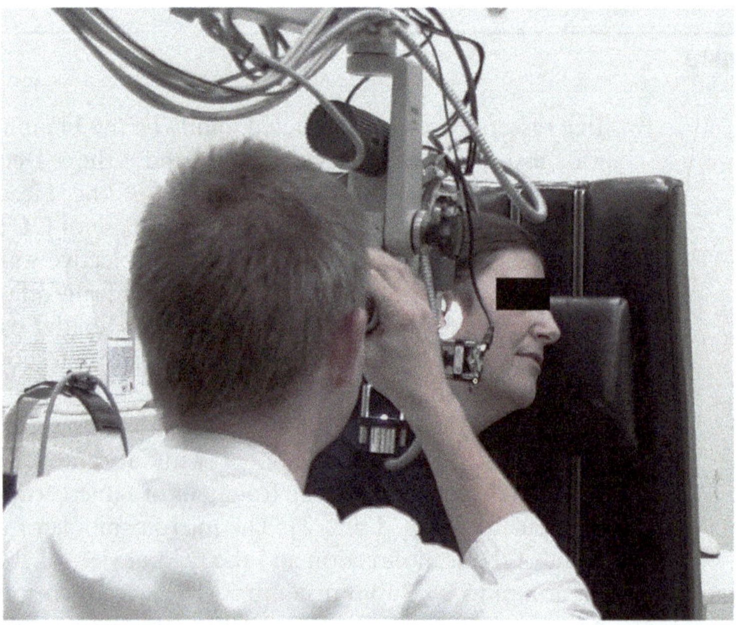

Fig. 2 Setup in outpatient department for examination of the *right ear*

aspect as seen through the microscope (Fig. 3). The tympanic membrane, posterior wall of the outer ear canal, and the umbo (tip of the malleus inserting at the center of the tympanic membrane) were always visible and considered as reference structures, while the promontory, round window membrane, long incus process, and stapes suprastructure were regarded as target structures (Fig. 4). The aim was to visualize target structures through an intact

Table 1
Optical coherence tomography for the middle and inner ear

Investigator	Year	OCT system	Wavelength	Transverse resolution	Axial resolution	Image acquisition rate	Setting	Material/patients	Purpose
Pitris et al. [1]	2001	TD-OCT	1310 nm ± 50 nm	10–20 μm	15 μm	10–30 s for 1 B-frame	Experimental	Four human temporal bones	Feasibility study
Heermann et al. [10]	2002	TD-OCT	975 nm ± 36 nm	30 μm	12 μm	200 A-lines/s ≥ 1 B-frame/s	Clinical, intraoperative	Ten patients	Distance measurement for stapes/PORP/TORP prosthesis
Djalilian et al. [11, 12]	2008	TD-OCT	1310 nm	10 μm	7 μm	1 B-frame/s	Clinical, out-patient	Ten patients	Tympanic membrane characterization
Just et al. [2–4]	2009	SD-OCT	830 nm	23 μm	12 μm	1,000 A-lines/s ≥ 1 B-frame/s	Experimental	Five human temporal bones	Oval niche characterization
							Clinical, intraoperative	Eight patients	Oval niche and vestibular imaging in tympanoplasty and stapes surgery
McCaughey et al. [15]	2009	TD-OCT	1310 nm	<50 μm	10–20 μm	1 B-frame/s	Experimental	Human bone specimen	Evaluation of Femtosecond laser ablation of bone
Just et al. [16]	2010	SD-OCT	830 nm	23 μm	12 μm	1000 A-lines/s ≥ 1 B-frame/s	Experimental	Human stapes	Thermographic measurement of heat deposition in CO_2 laser stapedotomy, stapes and perforation morphology
Subhash et al. [5]	2011	SD-OCT	1300 nm ± 28 nm	16 μm	13 μm	47,000 A-lines/s ≥ 300 B-frames/s	Experimental	Mouse cochlea	Vascular imaging and blood flow velocity measurement

Table 1
(continued)

Investigator	Year	OCT system	Wavelength	Transverse resolution	Axial resolution	Image acquisition rate	Setting	Material/patients	Purpose
Just et al. [17]	2011	SD-OCT	840 nm	24 μm	12 μm	1000 A-lines/s ≥ 1 B-scan/s	Experimental	Three human temporal bones	Tympanic membrane characterization, attachment of film strain gauge
Subhash et al. [6]	2012	PS-SD-OCT	1300 nm ± 28 nm	16 μm	13 μm		Experimental	Two human temporal bones	Vibrational measurement of ossicular chain under 500 Hz/65 dB stimulus
Nguyen et al. [13]	2012	SD-OCT and LCI	830 nm ± 70 nm (OCT) 940 nm ± 70 nm (LCI)	30 μm (LCI)	3.1 μm (OCT) 4 μm (LCI)	70,000 A-lines/s ≥ 1000 scans/s (LCI) 70 B-frames/s (OCT)	Clinical, out-patient	Four healthy individuals, sixteen patients	Bacterial biofilm detection on tympanic membrane
Nguyen et al. [14]	2013	SD-OCT	830 nm ± 70 nm		3.1 μm	70,000 A-lines/s ≥70 B-frames/s (OCT)	Clinical, out-patient	One healthy individual, five patients	Assessment of acoustic effects of bacterial biofilm on human TM
Chang et al. [8]	2013	PS-SD-OCT	1220 nm–1350 nm tunable	25 μm	12 μm	18,000 A-lines/s	Experimental	Three chinchilla temporal bones	Vibrational measurement of ossicular chain physiological and pathological conditions
Cho et al. [7]	2014	SD-OCT	870 nm ± 65 nm	30.2 μm	8.7 μm		Experimental	Five mice	Middle ear characterization under physiological and pathological conditions

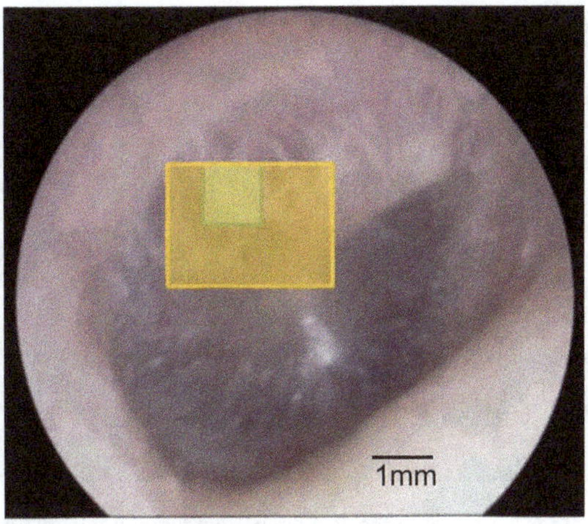

Fig. 3 OCT scan area varying from 1 × 1 mm (*light green square*) up to 2 × 3 mm (*yellow rectangle*) in relation to tympanic membrane size (*right ear*)

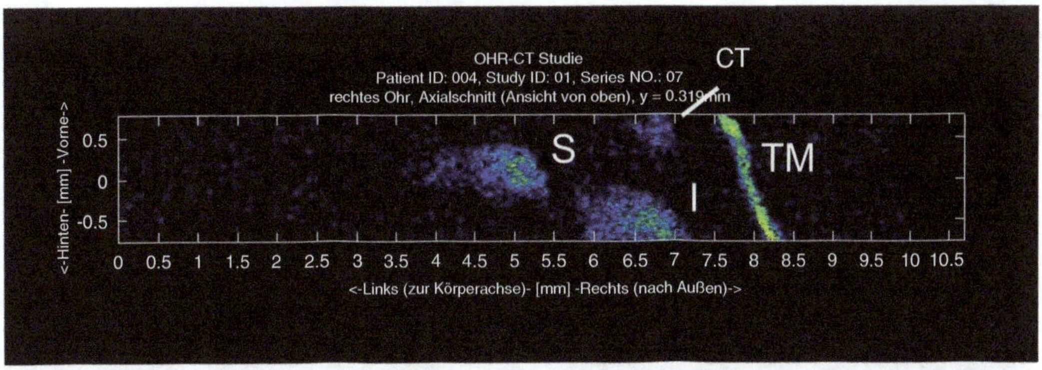

Fig. 4 OCT scan of a healthy right ear (outer ear canal to the right) showing outlines of tympanic membrane (TM), chorda tympani (CT), long incus process (I), and stapes head (S) (Image by C. Farkas and A. Lenenbach, Fraunhofer Institute of Laser Technology, Aachen)

tympanic membrane in 18 healthy individuals and 13 patients with varying pathology. In 56 scans of healthy individuals, the promontory could be identified in 35 scans, the long incus process in 21, round window membrane in 8, and stapes suprastructure in 4. Of 26 scans performed in patients, the identification of aforementioned structures was possible in 3, 1, 3, and 0 scans, respectively. Although results in patients seem disappointing considering the identification of structures for the middle ear, it has to be mentioned that the anatomy was largely altered by the underlying pathological process itself and by the following surgery. Secondly, although thickened tympanic membranes following tympanoplasty are absorbing and scattering most of the infrared light, alterations in the near field close to the tympanic membrane could be seen (Figs. 5 and 6).

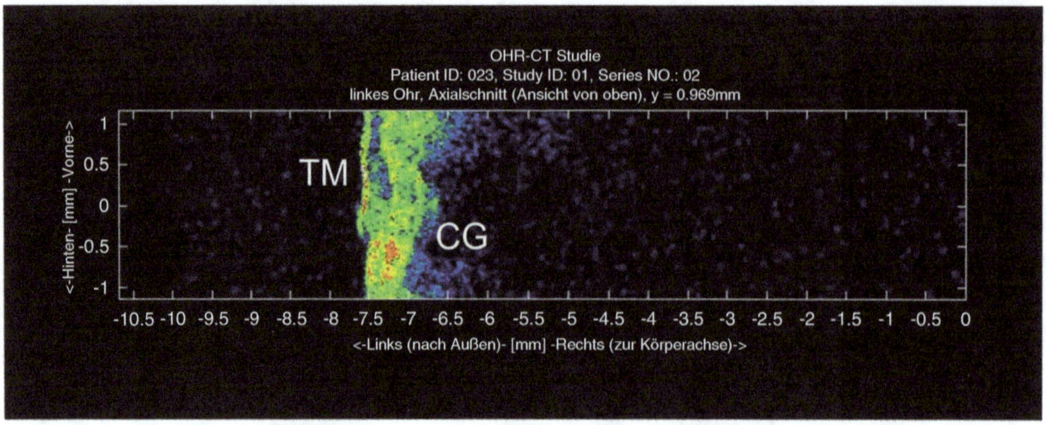

Fig. 5 OCT scan of a left ear (outer ear canal to the *left*) showing a tympanoplasty type I (i.e., tympanic membrane repair only) in postoperative follow-up. Tympanic membrane (TM) with edge of former perforation, supported by cartilage graft (CG) (Image by C. Farkas and A. Lenenbach, Fraunhofer Institute of Laser Technology, Aachen)

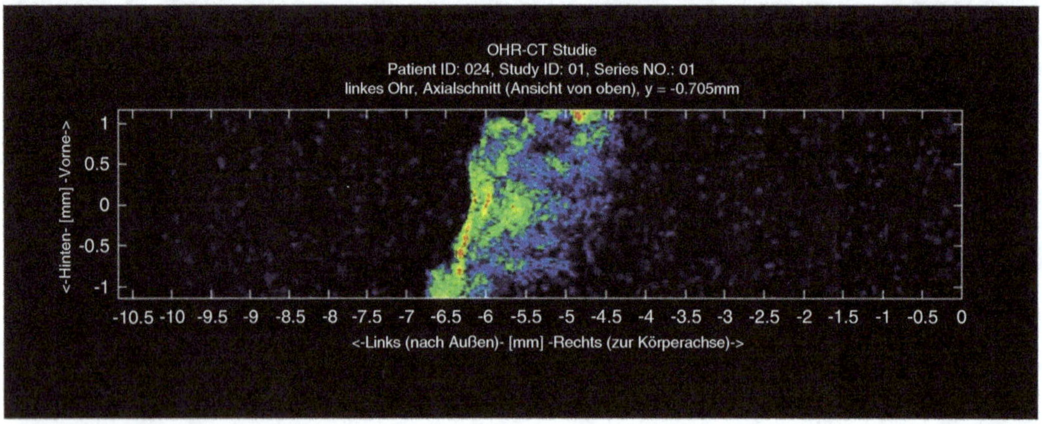

Fig. 6 OCT scan of a left ear (outer ear canal to the *left*) showing a pars tensa cholesteatoma: Note the cloudy structure of >2 mm thickness (Image by C. Farkas and A. Lenenbach, Fraunhofer Institute of Laser Technology, Aachen)

With scanning speed of 200A-lines per second, patients had to keep still for 50 s in order to reduce motion-related artifacts as good as possible. On the other hand, patients readily accepted the use of OCT, as the examination was conducted within the normal course of otomicroscopy and did not create any discomfort whatsoever. Consequently, OCT has the potential to become a powerful imaging modality in the hands of the otologist, bridging the gap between experimental research and everyday clinical use.

Acknowledgements

This study was conducted jointly by Dipl.-Ing. Csaba Farkas and Dr.-Ing Achim Lenenbach, both Fraunhofer Institute for Laser Technology (ILT), Aachen, and the author. OCT system and equipment including custom-built scanner, micromanipulator, and CCD monitoring camera were built, adjusted, and operated by the ILT, while examination of healthy individuals as well as patients was performed by the author.

References

1. Pitris C, Saunders KT, Fujimoto JG, Brezinski ME. High-resolution imaging of the middle ear with optical coherence tomography: a feasibility study. Arch Otolaryngol Head Neck Surg. 2001;127:637–42.
2. Just T, Lankenau E, Hüttmann G, Pau HW. Intraoperative application of optical coherence-tomography (OCT) for visualization of the oval window niche. Laryngorhinootologie. 2009;88:168–73.
3. Just T, Lankenau E, Hüttmann G, Pau HW. Optical coherence tomography of the oval window niche. J Laryngol Otol. 2009;123:603–8.
4. Just T, Lankenau E, Hüttmann G, Pau HW. Optical coherence tomography in middle ear surgery. HNO. 2009;57:421–7.
5. Subhash HM, Davila V, Sun H, Nguyen-Huynh AT, Shi X, Nuttall AL, Wang RK. Volumetric in vivo imaging of microvascular perfusion within the intact cochlea in mice using ultra-high sensitive optical microangiography. IEEE Trans Med Imaging. 2011;30: 224–30.
6. Subhash HM, Nguyen-Huynh A, Wang RK, Jacques SL, Choudhury N, Nuttall AL. Feasibility of spectral-domain phase-sensitive optical coherence tomography for middle ear vibrometry. J Biomed Opt. 2012;17:060505.
7. Cho NH, Jang JH, Jung W, Kim J. In vivo imaging of middle-ear and inner-ear microstructures of a mouse guided by SD-OCT combined with a surgical microscope. Opt Express. 2014;22(8):8985–95.
8. Chang EW, Cheng JT, Röösli C, Kobler JB, Rosowski JJ, Yun SH. Simultaneous 3D imaging of sound-induced motions of the tympanic membrane and middle ear ossicles. Hear Res. 2013;304:49–56. doi:10.1016/j.heares.2013.06.006.
9. Burkhardt A, Kirsten L, Bornitz M, Zahnert T, Koch E. Investigation of the human tympanic membrane oscillation ex vivo by Doppler optical coherence tomography. J Biophotonics. 2014;7:434–41.
10. Heermann R, Hauger C, Issing PR, Lenarz T. Application of optical coherence tomography (OCT) in middle ear surgery. Laryngorhinootologie. 2002;81:400–5.
11. Djalilian HR, Ridgway J, Tam M, Sepehr A, Chen Z, Wong BJ. Imaging the human tympanic membrane using optical coherence tomography in vivo. Otol Neurotol. 2008; 29:1091–4.
12. Djalilian HR, Rubinstein M, Wu EC, Naemi K, Zardouz S, Karimi K, Wong BJ. Optical coherence tomography of cholesteatoma. Otol Neurotol. 2010;31:932–5.
13. Nguyen CT, Jung W, Kim J, Chaney EJ, Novak M, Stewart CN, Boppart SA. Noninvasive in vivo optical detection of biofilm in the human middle ear. Proc Natl Acad Sci USA. 2012;109:9529–34.
14. Nguyen CT, Robinson SR, Jung W, Novak MA, Boppart SA, Allen JB. Investigation of bacterial biofilm in the human middle ear using optical coherence tomography and acoustic measurements. Hear Res. 2013;301: 193–200.
15. McCaughey RG, Sun H, Rothholtz VS, Juhasz T, Wong BJ. Femtosecond laser ablation of the stapes. J Biomed Opt. 2009;14:024040.
16. Just T, Specht O, Ovari A, Langnau E, Schmidt W, Pau HW. Thermographic investigations during stapedotomy using a CO2 laser. Laryngorhinootologie. 2010;89:549–55.
17. Just T, Zehlicke T, Specht O, Sass W, Punke C, Schmidt W, Lankenau E, Behrend D, Pau HW. Detection of tympanic membrane movement using film patch with integrated strain gauge, assessed by optical coherence tomography: experimental study. J Laryngol Otol. 2011;125:467–73.

Chapter 34

Optical Coherence Tomography of the Oral Cavity and Pharynx: Normative Anatomy and Benign Processes

Giriraj K. Sharma and Brian J.-F. Wong

Introduction

At present, otolaryngologists have limited options for in vivo diagnosis of head and neck pathology. Workup of suspicious lesions of the OC or pharynx begins with a systematic office-based head and neck examination. With assistance of a headlamp or flashlight, the surgeon can quickly examine the OC to assess a patient's general health status and identify suspicious lesions. Visual assessment and digital palpation of the lips, buccal mucosa, gingiva, teeth, retromolar trigone, tongue, and floor of mouth are performed in a systematic manner to assess for textural and structural irregularities, color, and odor. Next, the tongue is relaxed or depressed with a tongue blade to visually examine the oropharynx (OP) for mucosal color, structural integrity, antero-posterior and lateral dimensions, tonsillar symmetry, and uvula movement and symmetry. Examination of the nasopharynx (NP), hypopharynx, and larynx requires an indirect mirror exam or can be performed by flexible fiber-optic nasopharyngoscopy. A significant limitation, however, to visual inspection, flexible, or rigid endoscopy is that these examinations only permit subjective evaluation of surface tissues. At present, surgeons lack a practical diagnostic modality which allows for in vivo high-resolution imaging of subepithelial tissue in the event of suspicious oral or pharyngeal lesions. Computed tomography (CT) and magnetic resonance (MR) imaging do not have adequate resolution to differentiate between benign and malignant lesions. Furthermore, both procedures may require sedation for pediatric patients and CT carries the risk of ionizing radiation. The only way to definitively differentiate between benign, premalignant, and malignant lesions is histopathological analysis of excised tissue. This is an invasive

Brian J.-F. Wong and Justus Ilgner (eds.), *Biomedical Optics in Otorhinolaryngology: Head and Neck Surgery*,
DOI 10.1007/978-1-4939-1758-7_34, © Springer Science+Business Media New York 2016

procedure, associated with patient morbidity, cost, poor coverage of at-risk tissue, and, in many cases, a delayed diagnosis of advanced-stage lesions.

A variety of inflammatory lesions and benign pathology may occur in the OC and pharynx. Tumors of the OC and OP are generally grouped together, with the OC being a more common site for benign pathology. These include inflammatory hyperplasias (e.g., fibroma, pyogenic or giant cell granuloma, and benign lymphoid hyperplasia), hamartomas (e.g., lymphangioma, hemangioma, neurofibroma, granular cell tumor, and lipoma), benign epithelial tumors (e.g., pleomorphic adenoma), benign tumors of the bone, benign odontogenic tumors, and cysts. Additional benign oral conditions include candidiasis, aphthous ulcers, recurrent herpes labialis, erythema migrans, lichen planus, and hyperkeratosis [1]. Dysplastic lesions include leukoplakia (white), erythroplakia (red), or mixed white-red epithelial lesions. Leukoplakias develop in 1–4 % of the population, with a reported 0.13–33 % of these lesions undergoing malignant transformation [2, 3]. Erythroplakias carry risk for malignant conversion in up to 85 % of lesions [3]. Benign tumors of the NP are rare and occur more commonly in children and young adults. These include developmental tumors (e.g., teratomas), ectodermal tumors (e.g., papillomas and adenomatous polyps), mesodermal tumors (e.g., juvenile angiofibroma, fibromyxomatous polyps, osteomas, and fibrous dysplasia), and benign salivary gland tumors [4]. Tumors of the NP have a capacity for undetected growth and expansion, often leading to a delay in the onset of symptoms which, combined with the diagnostic inaccessibility of the NP, often results in delayed diagnosis.

Anatomy

The OC has several functions including the sense of taste, mastication, and deglutition and is involved in vocalization and respiration. The OC is bounded anteriorly at the vermilion border of the lip, laterally by the cheeks and tonsillar pillars, and extends posteriorly to the hard–soft palate junction (superior boundary) and circumvallate papillae (inferior boundary). Oral mucosa consists of stratified squamous epithelium and underlying connective tissue (lamina propria) which are separated by a basal lamina. The lamina propria is divided into a papillary layer (superficial) and a more fibrous layer (deep). Classifications of oral mucosa are based upon location and function, including masticatory mucosa (keratinized stratified squamous epithelium), lining mucosa (non-keratinized stratified squamous epithelium), and specialized mucosa in the regions of the taste buds. OCT images of normal buccal mucosa (non-keratinized stratified squamous epithelium) are depicted in Fig. 1. In contrast, the lips contain keratinized epithelium, as noted by a distinct contrast difference in the epithelial layer in Fig. 2. Figure 3 depicts OCT images of the normal floor of the mouth.

The pharynx participates in vocalization, digestive, and respiratory functions and is divided into three anatomical sections: the NP, OP, and laryngopharynx. The NP is bounded anteriorly by the choanae, superiorly by the body of the sphenoid bone (base of skull), laterally by the Eustachian tube orifices, and posteriorly by the superior constrictor muscles. Nasopharyngeal soft tissue is composed of various epithelial (keratinized and non-keratinized squamous, pseudostratified, ciliated, and columnar), glandular, and lymphoid tissues. The OP is posterior to the OC and is bounded by the soft palate superiorly and hyoid bone inferiorly. Posterior and lateral boundaries are formed by the muscular pharyngeal wall (superior and middle constrictors). The laryngopharynx or hypopharynx is

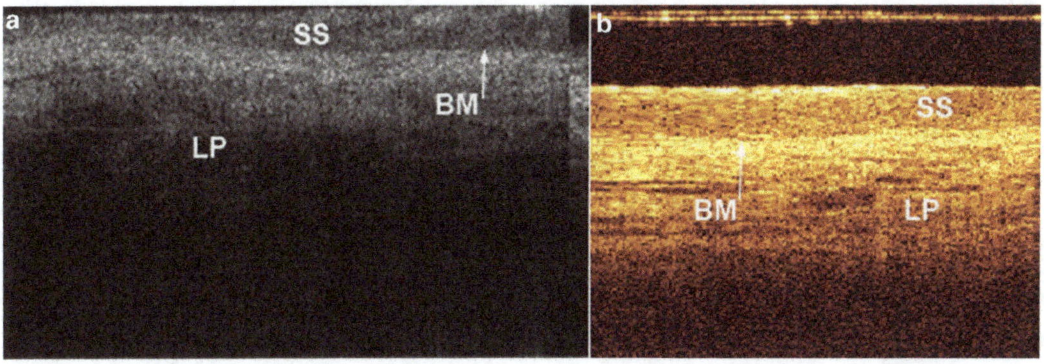

Fig. 1 OCT images of normal buccal mucosa acquired from a university-built TD-OCT system (**a**) and a commercially available system (**b**). *SS* non-keratinized stratified squamous epithelium, *BM* basement membrane, *LP* lamina propria

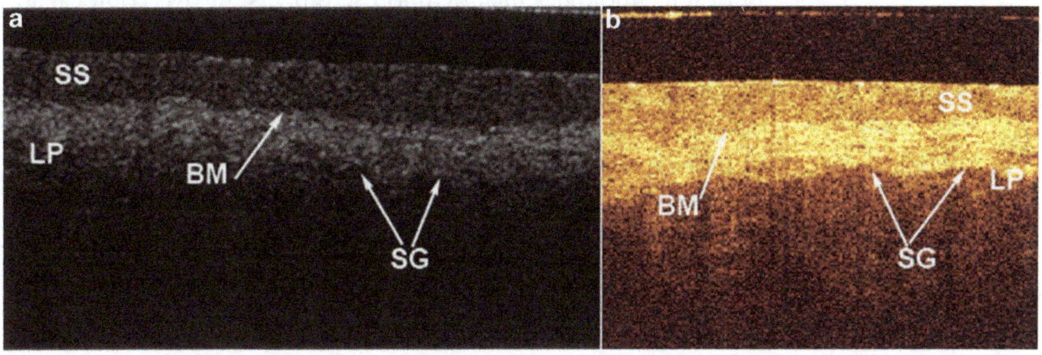

Fig. 2 OCT images of normal lip mucosa acquired from a research TD-OCT system (**a**) and a commercially available system (**b**). *SS* keratinized stratified squamous epithelium, *BM* basement membrane, *LP* lamina propria, *SG* seromucinous glands

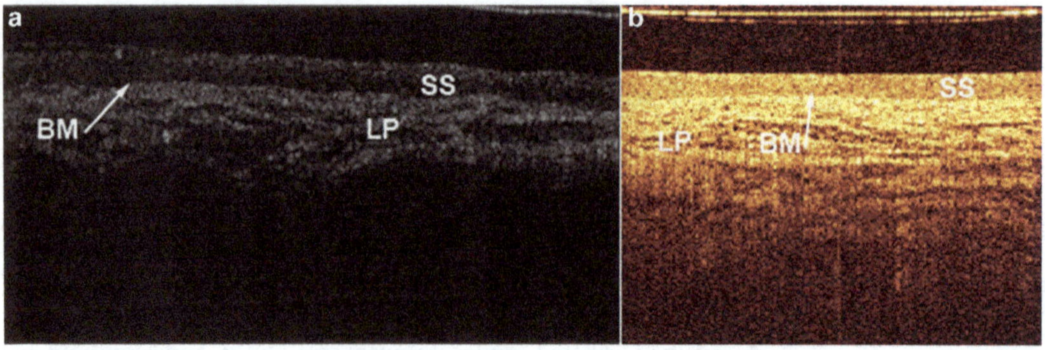

Fig. 3 OCT images of normal floor of mouth acquired from a research TD-OCT system (**a**) and a commercially available system (**b**). *SS* keratinized stratified squamous epithelium, *BM* basement membrane, *LP* lamina propria

the caudal most section of the pharynx and lies inferior to the epiglottis and is bounded laterally by the aryepiglottic folds. The laryngopharynx communicates inferiorly with the esophagus (posteriorly) and larynx (anteriorly). The OP and laryngopharynx are lined by non-keratinized stratified squamous epithelium.

Principles of OCT

In the last 10 years, substantial research in optical diagnostics has increased our understanding of the relationship between the optical and biologic properties of tissues. By detecting alterations in light–tissue interaction, optical technologies can provide real-time assessment of tissue structure and physiologic state at a molecular level. Furthermore, optical diagnostics have the potential to identify early precancerous changes which are frequently undetectable by visual examination. Current noninvasive or minimally invasive optical technologies include photosensitizers, in vivo confocal and multiphoton imaging microscopy, spectroscopy (e.g., Raman spectroscopy, elastic scattering spectroscopy, and fluorescence spectroscopy), and OCT. While the benefits of optical diagnostics vary with each technology, common advantages over histopathological examination include a real-time diagnosis, decreased morbidity, and cost. Furthermore, certain optical imaging modalities (e.g., spectroscopy) offer objective data analysis which may reduce diagnostic subjectivity commonly associated with the interpretation of tissue samples.

OCT is a light-based imaging modality which is based upon principles of low coherence interferometry [5, 6]. A near-infrared light source (e.g., laser or superbright light emitting diode) is split into two paths culminating in a mirror (reference arm) and biological tissue (sample arm), respectively. Back-reflected light from the reference and sample arms is recombined and detected to construct interference profiles (A-lines) as a function of tissue depth. Individual and adjacent A-lines are combined to form a three-dimensional (3D), cross-sectional images of tissue. OCT is able to provide real-time images with resolution up to 10–15 μm and optical penetration depth up to 1–2 mm [5]. Two major types of OCT systems include time domain OCT (TD-OCT) and frequency or "Fourier" domain OCT (FD-OCT). FD-OCT is an advanced generation technology which offers improved signal-to-noise ratio and higher imaging speeds and diagnostic sensitivity compared to TD-OCT [7–9]. Long-range or "anatomic" OCT (LR-OCT) systems were later developed to allow for extended range imaging (axial range up to 25 mm) without sacrifice of resolution [10, 11].

Various OCT systems have been developed to allow for tissue scanning in a linear or radial fashion. Most in vivo OCT imaging of the OC or pharynx is accomplished using a fiber-optic probe which is placed in direct contact or near-contact with mucosal tissue. OCT sample arms may be housed in a rigid handheld instrument for intraoral or transoral imaging, integrated with the instrument channel of a flexible endoscope or applied to the pharynx in a flexible, transparent endoscopic catheter. Early TD-OCT systems had scan rates up to 1 kHz, axial resolution between 10 and 20 μm, and lateral resolution between 10 and 25 μm [12–17]. Later, swept source FD-OCT systems offered a substantial leap in scan rate (up to 100 kHz) and resolution (<10 μm) [18–22]. While the majority of OCT systems described in the literature are custom-built for research purposes, several TD-OCT and FD-OCT systems are available for commercial use including the United States Food and Drug Administration-approved Niris TD-OCT system (Imalux Corp., Cleveland, OH).

Diagnostic OCT of Mucosal Lesions

Animal and Ex Vivo Studies

In 2005, Wilder-Smith's group conducted in vivo OCT of oral premalignant and malignant lesions in hamster cheek pouch models [14]. OCT was combined with optical Doppler tomography (ODT) to image the epithelial and subepithelial layers of buccal mucosa as well as the structural integrity of the basement membrane. Several additional studies have reported OCT imaging epithelial and subepithelial structures with close correlation with histological samples in a hamster cheek pouch model [23–27].

In 2010, a group of researchers based at the University College London Hospital used a swept-source FD-OCT microscope (Michelson Diagnostics EX1301 OCT Microscope V1.0) to perform ex vivo OCT of suspicious oral lesions immediately following excisional or incisional biopsy [21]. Thirty-four oral lesions were analyzed for (1) architectural changes in keratin, epithelial, and subepithelial layers, and identification of basement membrane, and (2) compared with histopathological results. While OCT data demonstrated distinct zones of normal and altered architectural changes, resolution was inadequate to identify exactly changes in pathologic tissue and, consequently, diagnosis and differentiation between dysplastic and malignant tissues was not possible. Additional reports of ex vivo OCT on human OC/OP tissues are included for review [28–31].

Clinical Studies

Select reports have focused solely on OCT imaging of normal, healthy mucosa of the OC/OP [12, 19, 32]. In 1998, Feldchtein et al. (Nizhny Novgorod, Russia) first reported in vivo OCT of hard and soft tissue of the oral cavity [12]. They used a dual wavelength TD-OCT system consisting of two superluminescent diodes operating at $\lambda_1 = 830$ nm and $\lambda_2 = 1280$ nm, respectively. Dual infrared beams with resolution of 17 μm (830 nm) and 22 μm (1280 nm) were aimed at masticatory, lining, and specialized oral mucosa to conduct transverse scanning. Single transverse scans were completed in 2–5 s, with simultaneous recording of OCT data from both signals. Differences in epithelial and lamina propria thickness were noted from different oral mucosa subtypes. The presence of keratin in the epithelium was also shown to reduce light penetration to underlying tissue layers, thus causing difficulty in distinguishing epithelium from lamina propria and submucosa in keratinized tissues. Later, Prestin et al. used OCT to measure epithelial thickness within the OC in 143 subjects [32]. Their data demonstrated varying epithelial thickness depending on location within the OC and provided a reference standard for differentiating normal from dysplastic tissue.

Numerous studies have evaluated in vivo OCT of benign or premalignant lesions of the OC and pharynx [15, 17, 20, 21, 33–35]. In 2006, Ridgway et al. imaged the OC and OP in 41 patients during operative endoscopy [15]. A TD-OCT system (central wavelength $\lambda = 1310$ nm, lateral and axial resolution ~10 μm) was used with a handheld fiber-optic probe (Fig. 4a) housed in a rigid, hollow metal tube (Fig. 4b). The probe was positioned manually or with endoscopic guidance and consisted of a gradient refractive index (GRIN) lens (1 mm diameter, 0.23 pitch) coupled with a right-angle prism to focus and reflect the OCT signal at 90. Their OCT data demonstrated normal microstructures, including keratinized epithelium, papillae, ducts, glands, and blood vessels, and benign pathologic features including mature scar, granulation tissue, mucous cysts, and leukoplakia.

A research team led by Betz and Kraft has been a forerunner in evaluating OCT in the diagnosis of lesions of the upper aerodigestive tract. Recently, they published multiple reports of in vivo imaging of OC anatomy and premalignant lesions using the Niris OCT imaging system (Imalux Corp.) [32, 35]. Their studies

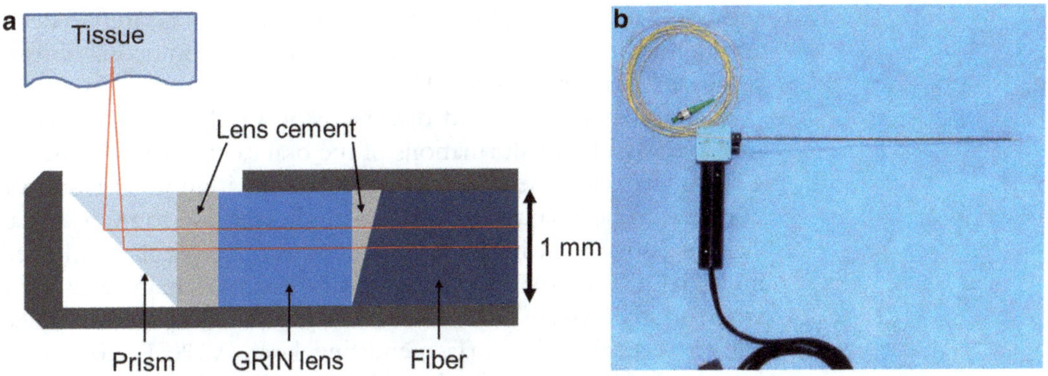

Fig. 4 Schematic of distal apparatus of endoscopic OCT probe (**a**) and rigid, hollow metal tubing for handheld, transoral application of OCT probe (**b**) constructed by Ridgway et al. [15]. *GRIN* gradient index refractive lens

reported that OCT-based differentiation between noninvasive and invasive lesions could be performed with 88.9 % sensitivity and 89.0 % specificity. Comparative analysis of OCT images from hyperplastic and dysplastic lesions demonstrated a statistically significant difference in intensity profiles of the epithelial layer between the two groups.

Other Oral Lesions and Dental Pathologies

Pharyngeal or oral mucositis (OM) is a toxic effect of chemotherapy and head and neck irradiation. At present, there is no means to predict the onset and severity of OM, thus limiting options for preventive and treatment measures. Early studies demonstrated OCT-based early detection and quantification of radiation- and chemotherapy-induced OM in mouse and hamster models [36, 37]. In 2007, Wilder-Smith et al. first reported OCT of chemotherapy-induced OM in human subjects [16]. Following commencement of chemotherapy, oral mucosa structure was longitudinally evaluated using a TD-OCT system (central wavelength $\lambda = 1310$ nm, axial resolution 10 μm) and a handheld fiber-optic probe. Their results demonstrated early and progressive changes in epithelial and subepithelial tissue thickness and integrity, prior to clinical manifestation of disease. The same group later reported TD-OCT of oral mucosa in 48 patients undergoing chemotherapy [38]. Using the Niris OCT system (Imalux Corp.), they demonstrated a higher sensitivity of detection for OM using OCT than using the gold standard OM assessment scale. Additional reports of OCT-based diagnosis of oral mucositis or postradiation changes are described in the literature [39–41]. Lee et al. performed swept-source OCT of healthy OC mucosa and oral submucosal fibrosis and noted decreases in both epithelial thickness and standard deviation of A-mode scan intensity in mucosa with submucosal fibrosis compared to normal tissue [18].

There has been limited discussion on OCT of microvasculature and vascular malformations of the oral cavity [20, 22, 33, 37, 42]. In vivo assessment of microcirculation within OC tissues has potential to be a valuable diagnostic indicator due to the vascular change associated with pathologic lesions. Choi et al. conducted in vivo OCT of OC and nasal cavity microvasculature using a swept-source system (central wavelength $\lambda = 1300$ nm) coupled with a vertical cavity surface-emitting laser (VCSEL, coherence length ≥ 50 mm; Thorlabs, Inc. Newton, NJ, USA) [22]. A handheld probe (Thorlabs) was mounted in a positioning stage for oral and nasal cavity imaging. Side imaging (90° projection of OCT signal) and forward imaging (0° projection) scan modes were used to image circumferential or lateral wall tissues (e.g., buccal mucosa and nasal mucosa) and frontal regions (e.g., labial mucosa), respectively. Volumetric structural OCT images of oral and nasal cavity tissues were obtained to map blood perfusion. Additional studies have used ODT to detect functional blood flow within oral cavity tissue [37, 42]. ODT is a functional extension of OCT that measures phase change secondary to Doppler frequency shift of light backscattered from moving red blood cells within a blood vessel. Recently, speckle variance of OCT signal has been studied to analyze large blood vessels of the OC [33, 41].

Lastly, structural imaging of dental tissues has been evaluated using OCT. In 1997, Colston et al. first reported OCT of in vitro porcine periodontal tissues [43]. A transverse-scanning TD-OCT system (central wavelength $\lambda = 1310$ nm, resolution ~20 μm) coupled with a He–Ne laser (633 nm wavelength) was used to scan enamel–cementum and gingiva–tooth interfaces. OCT data were correlated with histological sections to demonstrate internal tooth and soft tissue structural relationships which are critical in the diagnosis of periodontal disease. Additional, early studies of TD-OCT imaging of dental structure are described [12, 44–46]. While this chapter does not cover OCT of dental structures, select articles on OCT applications in diagnostic evaluation and therapeutic monitoring in dentistry are included for review purposes [47–57].

Long-Range OCT

Upper airway obstruction is a frequently diagnosed condition among adult and pediatric patients and has potential for severe long-term sequela if untreated. A variety of pathologic conditions may be causative of upper airway obstruction including anatomic obstruction (e.g., deviated septum, stenosis, thickened palate, and collapse of aryepiglottic folds), tumors, tonsillar and/or adenoidal hypertrophy, and congenital diseases (e.g., choanal atresia). Quantitative measurements of the pharyngeal lumen enable construction of virtual computational airway models to evaluate airflow. This information may help surgeons identify regions of airway stenosis, predict outcomes of medical or surgical intervention, and ultimately improve the management of OSA. At present, laryngoscopy and bronchoscopy remain the gold standard for diagnosis of upper airway obstructive disease, but only provide semiquantitative information on pharyngeal morphology. CT and MRI have been shown to provide quantitative upper airway dimensions; however, these techniques are associated with the need for sedation in children and ionizing radiation exposure (CT) and are limited by respiratory motion artifacts and long imaging times [58, 59].

LR-OCT or "anatomical" OCT is a minimally invasive endoscopic technique used to quantitatively assess the size and shape of the upper airway. Advantages of LR-OCT include high patient safety, portability, low cost, and long permissible patient exposure times given that OCT uses nonionizing radiation. In 2003, Armstrong et al. (Western Australia) first reported in vivo endoscopic LR-OCT of the upper airway in human subjects [10]. Using a frequency domain LR-OCT system (central wavelength $\lambda = 1325$ nm, axial resolution 17.4 μm), their group achieved long-range imaging (axial range 26 mm) using an endoscopic probe inserted through a transparent, distally sealed naso-esophageal catheter. The probe was rotated (3.75 Hz) to acquire stationary and continuous (0.2 mm/s pullback) cross-sectional images from the esophagus and pharynx. Further LR-OCT studies by the same group (Western Australia) demonstrated high correlation between LR-OCT and CT-derived measurements of pharyngeal cross-sectional area [60]. With the evolution of frequency domain technology, LR-OCT of the pharynx has been performed at helical scanning speeds up to 30 Hz [61] and axial imaging range up to 20 mm [11] in order to acquire three-dimensional volumetric images of the airway. LR-OCT images of select anatomic levels of the adult upper airway are depicted in Fig. 5. Additional reports of LR-OCT to quantitatively evaluate pharyngeal size and shape are described in the literature [11, 61–65].

OCT Limitations

The primary limitation of OCT is the optical penetration depth in biological tissue. Current OCT systems offer a maximum penetration depth of 1–2 mm. Achieving adequate signal penetration is imperative to differentiate between benign, premalignant, and malignant processes of the OC and pharynx. OCT diagnostic sensitivity is thus limited in the event of larger, exophytic lesions with high depths. Furthermore, OCT signal absorption and/or

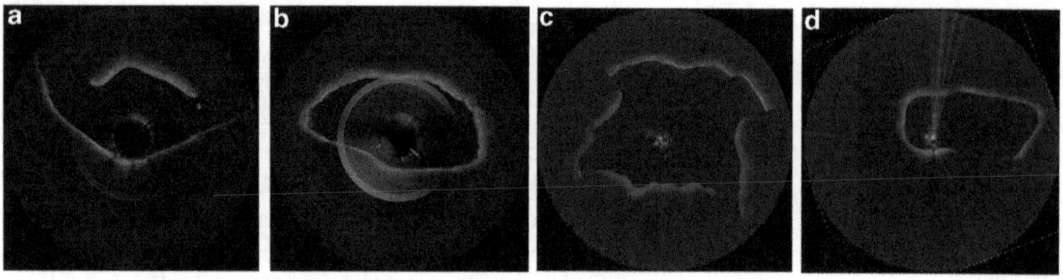

Fig. 5 Long-range OCT images of the tip of epiglottis (**a**), base of tongue (**b**), adenoids (**c**), and choana (**d**) from an adult upper airway. All OCT images are displayed in polar coordinates, with anterior tissues at the top of the image

scattering by tissues such as cartilage and bone results in distal shadows on cross-sectional images and further limits the diagnostic sensitivity in mixed hard–soft tissues. Additional factors which may limit image quality for in vivo imaging include physician hand tremor, patient movement, and equipment vibrations; such movements translate to reverberating effects on measured optical backscattering and can result in image distortion or stretching. Lastly, although advanced FD-OCT systems offer a peak resolution of approximately 10 μm, this precludes tissue diagnosis at the cellular level. Hence, OCT cannot provide definitive differentiation between premalignant and malignant lesions, necessitating histologic analysis of excised tissue.

Malignancy

In 2014, an estimated 42,440 new cases of oral cavity and pharyngeal cancer will be diagnosed in the United States [66]. A majority of these cancers are squamous cell carcinomas, which are preceded by dysplastic lesions including white (leukoplakia), red (erythroplakia), or mixed epithelial lesions. These lesions may progress to cancer, with erythroplakia (51 %) lesions more likely to undergo malignant transformation than leukoplakia (5 %) [2, 3]. Fundamental to long-term survival is early diagnosis and routine follow-up with the otolaryngologist for close monitoring of disease. Optical diagnostics holds promise for minimally invasive, cost-effective, and early detection of malignant lesions in the head and neck. While OCT resolution limits preclude the definitive diagnosis of malignant lesions, OCT may be used as an adjunct imaging modality to guide biopsy decisions and localize subclinical disease. A thorough review of OCT research in the diagnosis of malignant lesions in the upper aerodigestive tract is described elsewhere in this text.

References

1. Lian T. Benign tumors and tumor-like lesions of the oral cavity. In: Robbins K, Haughey B, editors. Cummings otolaryngology head & neck surgery. Philadelphia, PA: Mosby Elsevier; 2010. p. 1287–93.
2. Reibel J. Prognosis of oral pre-malignant lesions: significance of clinical, histopathological, and molecular biological characteristics. Crit Rev Oral Biol Med. 2003;14(1):47–62.
3. Walsh T, et al. Clinical assessment to screen for the detection of oral cavity cancer and potentially malignant disorders in apparently healthy adults. Cochrane Database Syst Rev. 2013;11:CD010173.
4. Tan L, Loh T. Benign and malignant tumors of the nasopharynx. In: Robbins K, Haughey B, editors. Cummings otolaryngology head & neck surgery. Philadelphia, PA: Mosby Elsevier; 2010. p. 1348–58.
5. Huang D, et al. Optical coherence tomography. Science. 1991;254(5035):1178–81.
6. Fercher AF. Optical coherence tomography—development, principles, applications. Z Med Phys. 2010;20(4):251–76.
7. Beaurepaire E, et al. Full-field optical coherence microscopy. Opt Lett. 1998;23(4):244–6.
8. Choma M, et al. Sensitivity advantage of swept source and Fourier domain optical coherence tomography. Opt Express. 2003;11(18): 2183–9.
9. Yun S, et al. High-speed optical frequency-domain imaging. Opt Express. 2003;11(22): 2953–63.
10. Armstrong J, et al. In vivo size and shape measurement of the human upper airway using endoscopic longrange optical coherence tomography. Opt Express. 2003;11(15):1817–26.
11. Jing J, et al. High-speed upper-airway imaging using full-range optical coherence tomography. J Biomed Opt. 2012;17(11):110507.
12. Feldchtein F, et al. In vivo OCT imaging of hard and soft tissue of the oral cavity. Opt Express. 1998;3(6):239–50.
13. Feldchtein F, et al. Endoscopic applications of optical coherence tomography. Opt Express. 1998;3(6):257–70.
14. Wilder-Smith P, et al. Noninvasive imaging of oral premalignancy and malignancy. J Biomed Opt. 2005;10(5):051601.
15. Ridgway JM, et al. In vivo optical coherence tomography of the human oral cavity and oropharynx. Arch Otolaryngol Head Neck Surg. 2006;132(10):1074–81.
16. Kawakami-Wong H, et al. In vivo optical coherence tomography-based scoring of oral mucositis in human subjects: a pilot study. J Biomed Opt. 2007;12(5):051702.
17. Wilder-Smith P, et al. In vivo diagnosis of oral dysplasia and malignancy using optical coherence tomography: preliminary studies in 50 patients. Lasers Surg Med. 2009;41(5):353–7.
18. Lee CK, et al. Diagnosis of oral submucous fibrosis with optical coherence tomography. J Biomed Opt. 2009;14(5):054008.
19. Ozawa N, et al. In vivo imaging of human labial glands using advanced optical coherence tomography. Oral Surg Oral Med Oral Pathol Oral Radiol Endod. 2009;108(3):425–9.
20. Ozawa N, et al. Evaluation of oral vascular anomalies using optical coherence tomography. Br J Oral Maxillofac Surg. 2009;47(8): 622–6.
21. Jerjes W, et al. In vitro examination of suspicious oral lesions using optical coherence tomography. Br J Oral Maxillofac Surg. 2010;48(1):18–25.
22. Choi WJ, Wang RK. In vivo imaging of functional microvasculature within tissue beds of oral and nasal cavities by swept-source optical coherence tomography with a forward/side-viewing probe. Biomed Opt Express. 2014;5(8):2620–34.
23. Dong H, et al. Quantitative analysis on tongue inspection in traditional Chinese medicine using optical coherence tomography. J Biomed Opt. 2008;13(1):011004.
24. Graf RN, Brown WJ, Wax A. Parallel frequency-domain optical coherence tomography scatter-mode imaging of the hamster cheek pouch using a thermal light source. Opt Lett. 2008;33(12):1285–7.
25. Graf RN, et al. Detecting precancerous lesions in the hamster cheek pouch using spectroscopic white-light optical coherence tomography to assess nuclear morphology via spectral oscillations. J Biomed Opt. 2009;14(6):064030.
26. Hammer-Wilson MJ, et al. Detection of vesicant-induced upper airway mucosa damage in the hamster cheek pouch model using optical coherence tomography. J Biomed Opt. 2010;15(1):016017.
27. Park J, et al. A dual-modality optical coherence tomography and fluorescence lifetime imaging microscopy system for simultaneous morphological and biochemical tissue characterization. Biomed Opt Express. 2010;1(1):186–200.

28. Hamdoon Z, et al. Structural validation of oral mucosal tissue using optical coherence tomography. Head Neck Oncol. 2012;4:29.
29. Adegun OK, et al. Quantitative analysis of optical coherence tomography and histopathology images of normal and dysplastic oral mucosal tissues. Lasers Med Sci. 2012;27(4): 795–804.
30. Adegun OK, et al. Quantitative optical coherence tomography of fluid-filled oral mucosal lesions. Lasers Med Sci. 2013;28(5):1249–55.
31. Hamdoon Z, et al. Optical coherence tomography in the assessment of suspicious oral lesions: an immediate ex vivo study. Photodiagn Photodyn Ther. 2013;10(1):17–27.
32. Prestin S, et al. Measurement of epithelial thickness within the oral cavity using optical coherence tomography. Head Neck. 2012;34(12):1777–81.
33. Davoudi B, et al. Noninvasive in vivo structural and vascular imaging of human oral tissues with spectral domain optical coherence tomography. Biomed Opt Express. 2012;3(5):826–39.
34. Lee CK, et al. Diagnosis of oral precancer with optical coherence tomography. Biomed Opt Express. 2012;3(7):1632–46.
35. Volgger V, et al. Evaluation of optical coherence tomography to discriminate lesions of the upper aerodigestive tract. Head Neck. 2013;35(11):1558–66.
36. Muanza TM, et al. Evaluation of radiation-induced oral mucositis by optical coherence tomography. Clin Cancer Res. 2005;11(14): 5121–7.
37. Wilder-Smith P, et al. In vivo imaging of oral mucositis in an animal model using optical coherence tomography and optical Doppler tomography. Clin Cancer Res. 2007;13(8):2449–54.
38. Calantog A, et al. A prospective study to assess in vivo optical coherence tomography imaging for early detection of chemotherapy-induced oral mucositis. Lasers Surg Med. 2013;45(1):22–7.
39. Gladkova ND, et al. Potential of optical coherence tomography for diagnosing mucositis in cancer of the nasal cavity and throat in the course of radio- and chemoradiotherapy. Vopr Onkol. 2006;52(4):443–7.
40. Maslennikova AV, et al. Use of optical coherence tomography for prognosis of the severity of oral mucositis. Vopr Onkol. 2009;55(5): 572–9.
41. Davoudi B, et al. Optical coherence tomography platform for microvascular imaging and quantification: initial experience in late oral radiation toxicity patients. J Biomed Opt. 2013;18(7):76008.
42. Otis LL, et al. Quantifying labial blood flow using optical Doppler tomography. Oral Surg Oral Med Oral Pathol Oral Radiol Endod. 2004;98(2):189–94.
43. Colston BW, et al. Optical coherence tomography for diagnosing periodontal disease. Proc SPIE. 1997;2973:216–20. Lasers in Dentistry III.
44. Colston Jr BW, et al. Imaging of hard- and soft-tissue structure in the oral cavity by optical coherence tomography. Appl Opt. 1998;37(16):3582–5.
45. Warren JA, et al. Imaging and characterization of dental structure using optical coherence tomography. Opt Soc Am: Tech Dig Ser. 1998;6:128.
46. Baek JH, et al. Optical approach to the salivary pellicle. J Biomed Opt. 2009;14(4):044001.
47. Baumgartner A, et al. Polarization-sensitive optical coherence tomography of dental structures. Caries Res. 2000;34(1):59–69.
48. Fried D, et al. Imaging caries lesions and lesion progression with polarization sensitive optical coherence tomography. J Biomed Opt. 2002; 7(4):618–27.
49. Chen Y, et al. Characterization of dentin, enamel, and carious lesions by a polarization-sensitive optical coherence tomography system. Appl Opt. 2005;44(11):2041–8.
50. de Melo LS, et al. Evaluation of enamel dental restoration interface by optical coherence tomography. J Biomed Opt. 2005;10(6): 064027.
51. Gimbel C. Optical coherence tomography diagnostic imaging. Gen Dent. 2008;56(7): 750–7. Quiz 758–9, 768.
52. Kang H et al. Imaging early demineralization with PS-OCT. Proc SPIE Int Soc Opt Eng. 2010;7549. http://www.ncbi.nlm.nih.gov/pubmed/22399835
53. Park KJ, Schneider H, Haak R. Assessment of interfacial defects at composite restorations by swept source optical coherence tomography. J Biomed Opt. 2013;18(7):076018.
54. Chan KH, et al. A method for monitoring enamel erosion using laser irradiated surfaces and optical coherence tomography. Lasers Surg Med. 2014;46(9):672–8.
55. Nee A, et al. Longitudinal monitoring of demineralization peripheral to orthodontic brackets using cross polarization optical coherence tomography. J Dent. 2014;42(5):547–55.
56. Nakajima Y, et al. Detection of occlusal caries in primary teeth using swept source optical coherence tomography. J Biomed Opt. 2014;19(1):16020.

57. Marcauteanu C, et al. Quantitative evaluation of dental abfraction and attrition using a swept-source optical coherence tomography system. J Biomed Opt. 2014;19(2):21108.
58. Arens R, et al. Linear dimensions of the upper airway structure during development: assessment by magnetic resonance imaging. Am J Respir Crit Care Med. 2002;165(1):117–22.
59. Abramson Z, et al. Age-related changes of the upper airway assessed by 3-dimensional computed tomography. J Craniofac Surg. 2009;20 Suppl 1:657–63.
60. Armstrong JJ, et al. Quantitative upper airway imaging with anatomic optical coherence tomography. Am J Respir Crit Care Med. 2006;173(2):226–33.
61. Wijesundara K, et al. Quantitative upper airway endoscopy with swept-source anatomical optical coherence tomography. Biomed Opt Express. 2014;5(3):788–99.
62. Leigh MS, et al. Anatomical optical coherence tomography for long-term, portable, quantitative endoscopy. IEEE Trans Biomed Eng. 2008;55(4):1438–46.
63. Walsh JH, et al. Evaluation of pharyngeal shape and size using anatomical optical coherence tomography in individuals with and without obstructive sleep apnoea. J Sleep Res. 2008;17(2):230–8.
64. Walsh JH, et al. Effect of body posture on pharyngeal shape and size in adults with and without obstructive sleep apnea. Sleep. 2008; 31(11):1543–9.
65. Cisonni J, et al. Effect of the velopharynx on intraluminal pressures in reconstructed pharynges derived from individuals with and without sleep apnea. J Biomech. 2013;46(14): 2504–12.
66. Society AC. Cancer facts & figures 2014. Atlanta: American Cancer Society; 2014.

Chapter 35

Optical Coherence Tomography of the Larynx: Normative Anatomy and Benign Processes

Giriraj K. Sharma and Brian J.-F. Wong

Introduction

In patients presenting to the otolaryngologist with throat or voice complaints, a comprehensive laryngeal examination is necessary. While no standardized diagnostic workup applies to all laryngology patients, each established technique has advantages and limitations. In the awake, office-based head and neck examination, the most commonly used technique to evaluate the larynx is indirect mirror laryngoscopy. While efficient and least invasive of all examination techniques, this method does not allow for image capture and is limited to a surface view of laryngeal tissues. Flexible fiberoptic or rigid endoscopy with or without videostroboscopy allows for indirect evaluation of the larynx, but is also restricted to a superficial examination of laryngeal lesions. Conventional imaging modalities such as computed tomography (CT), magnetic resonance imaging (MRI), and ultrasound have limited spatial resolution, precluding their ability to characterize subepithelial microanatomy and structural integrity of the vocal folds. Without a precise assessment of depth of penetration and integrity of the basement membrane, surgeons cannot differentiate between benign and malignant lesions of the larynx in patients presenting with identical symptoms. At present, the gold standard for the assessment of malignant processes is microlaryngoscopy with excisional biopsy. This invasive technique is associated with increased healthcare costs, risks of general anesthesia and, most importantly, risk of disruption of vocal fold structure resulting in permanent dysphonia. Hence, there exists a need for a less invasive diagnostic modality which can assess the microanatomy of laryngeal tissues, while preserving the structural integrity of the vocal folds.

Brian J.-F. Wong and Justus Ilgner (eds.), *Biomedical Optics in Otorhinolaryngology: Head and Neck Surgery*,
DOI 10.1007/978-1-4939-1758-7_35, © Springer Science+Business Media New York 2016

Anatomy

The layered microstructure of the vocal fold was described by Hirano et al. based on images from a scanning electron microscope [1]. This information formed the basis of the "body-cover" theory of voice production. At the luminal surface, the superficial "cover" consists of stratified squamous epithelium and the superficial (SLP) layer of the lamina propria (LP), as depicted in Fig. 1. Immediately below, the "transition zone" contains the intermediate and deep layers of the LP (combining to form the vocal ligament), while the deeper "body" contains the thyroarytenoid muscle. During phonation, as air flows through the larynx and tension develops within the vocal folds, the contrasting properties of the "cover" and "body" cause a functional separation of these layers and vibration at different rates [1, 2]. Penetrating laryngeal lesions which disrupt the mucosal "cover" or cause tissue loss can disrupt the "body-cover" model, affect VF vibrational parameters, and may lead to significant changes in voice quality.

OCT is capable of characterizing the layered microstructure of the larynx with optical penetration (approximately 1–2 mm) just short of the vocalis muscle. In a cross-sectional image, gray-scale representations of individual tissue layers are based upon their respective backscattering properties. The vocal folds have a weakly scattering epithelium while the SLP, known as Reinke's space, has a loosely organized fibrous composition. Deeper layers of the LP

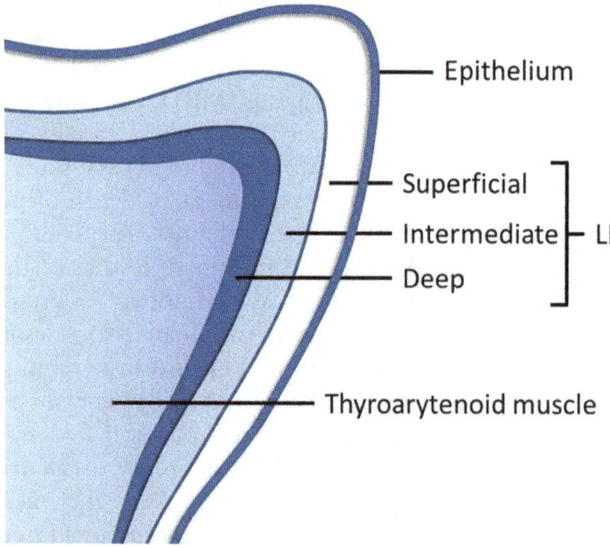

Fig. 1 Cross-sectional schematic of true vocal fold, depicting the epithelium and superficial layer of the lamina propria (LP, "cover"), intermediate and deep layers of the LP ("transition zone"), and the thyroarytenoid muscle ("body")

can be differentiated based on their varying density of collagen and elastic fibers. Hence, OCT can assess depth of penetration of laryngeal lesions and basement membrane and SLP integrity, thus offering a noninvasive means to differentiate benign versus malignant lesions of the larynx.

Principles of OCT

OCT uses a spectrally broadband light source coupled with a low coherence interferometer (e.g., Michelson) to produce high-resolution images of biological tissue. Light from an optical source is split into two arms: a "sample" arm (containing the tissue of interest) and a "reference" arm (stationary or moving mirror). Light back-reflectance from the "sample" is dependent on unique optical backscattering coefficients of biological tissue layers. Both optical paths are recombined and detected to form an interference profile as a function of tissue depth. As the sample beam is scanned across the tissue surface, adjacent depth profiles (A-lines) are compiled to construct two-dimensional or 3-D images with micrometer resolution (~10 μm), millimeter depth (1–2 mm), and video-rate imaging speed [3, 4].

The two principal OCT schemes are time domain OCT (TD-OCT) and frequency or "Fourier" domain OCT (FD-OCT). In 1991, Fujimoto's group published the first report of real-time low coherence tomographic imaging in a biological system [3]. Using a super luminescent diode as a light source, their TD-OCT system used a "reference" beam back-reflected from a moving mirror coupled with a Michelson interferometer to construct an interference pattern. In vitro, cross-sectional images of the retina and coronary artery were produced by mechanically adjusting the distance to the "reference," thereby limiting the image acquisition speed [3]. At the turn of the century, Fercher's group developed the first FD-OCT systems [5, 6]. FD-OCT uses a wavelength-swept light source and with a stationary reference arm to acquire information in the spectral domain, per Fourier transform of the combined spectra at the output of the interferometer. FD-OCT provides improved signal-to-noise ratio, increased image acquisition rates, and higher sensitivity compared to TD-OCT [7–9]. Long-range or "anatomic" OCT (LR-OCT), first pioneered in 2003 by Sampson as a derivative of TD-OCT, and later as version of FD-OCT, extends the axial imaging range of traditional systems without sacrificing resolution [10, 11].

Variations in OCT Technology

Polarization-sensitive OCT (PS-OCT) enhances the diagnostic potential of conventional OCT by recording both the intensity and birefringence of backscattered light. Birefringent tissue (e.g., collagen, muscle, cartilage) changes the polarization state of reflected light to provide an additional degree of contrast and specificity to fibrous tissue layers. In imaging the vocal folds, increased collagen content in the vocal ligament can be contrasted with the relatively acellular, overlying SLP [12–14]. Furthermore, PS-OCT allows for differentiation between areas of vocal fold scarring and normal epithelium.

In 1993, the first in vivo OCT studies were completed independently by groups at the Massachusetts Institute of Technology (MIT, Boston, MA) and Medical University of Vienna (Vienna, Austria) to image the retina [15, 16]. Later, the introduction of endoscopic OCT systems led to applications in cardiology and gastroenterology [17–21]. Further evolution into ultrahigh-resolution OCT (2–3 μm axial resolution) and spectral domain OCT has expanded the diagnostic potential of OCT within ophthalmology [5, 22–24]. Comprehensive review of OCT principles and research in biomedical interferometry are described in the literature [4, 24, 25].

Evolution of OCT in Laryngology

OCT research within laryngology traverses ex vivo and in vivo imaging in animal and human models. Given the range of applications and imaging techniques (pediatric vs. adult airways, office-based vs. intraoperative imaging, static vs. vibrating vocal folds), OCT systems and optical probe design have evolved to optimize functionality and data quality.

The first systems developed for in vivo scanning of the human larynx utilized near-contact endoscopic probes [19, 26]. These TD-OCT systems (central wavelength $\lambda = 830$ nm, 30 nm bandwidth) integrated the OCT sampling arm into standard endoscopic devices for transverse scanning (30 cm/s) along the plane of laryngeal tissue to identify mucosal structural changes in precancerous and cancerous states. Future iterations of these systems led to the Niris Imaging System (Imalux Corp., Cleveland, OH) which was the only commercially available OCT system for imaging of the upper aerodigestive tract (UADT). Designed as a portable TD-OCT system, this unit includes a 2.7 mm diameter probe to acquire real-time 2D images (200×200 pixels) with a maximum frame rate of 0.7 Hz. The Niris spatial depth resolution is 10–20 μm with scanning depth of 1.5 mm; lateral resolution is 25 μm with lateral scanning range of 1.5–2.5 mm [27]. In 2010, Rubinstein et al. used the Niris system to obtain intraoperative images of normal laryngeal tissue, transition zones, and pathology [27]. A flexible probe held within a modified suction handpiece was inserted through a surgical laryngoscope for controlled, accurate positioning at the area of interest (Fig. 2). The same year, Brenner's group used the Niris system to identify layered tissue microstructure of recurrent respiratory papillomatosis in the trachea [28].

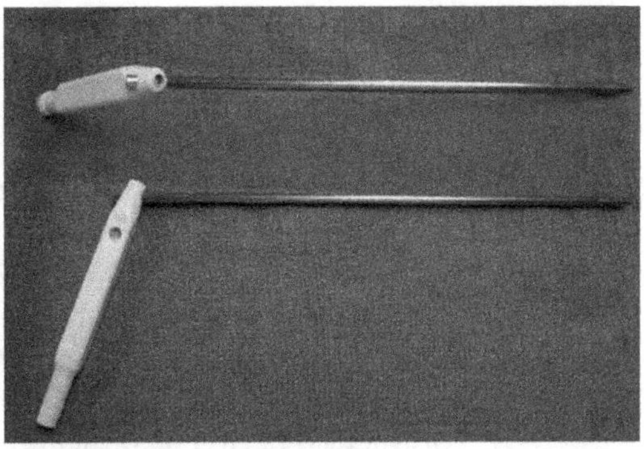

Fig. 2 Specially designed handheld device coupled with NIRIS OCT system to guide a flexible probe into the larynx [27]

At present, most laryngeal imaging has been accomplished using research systems designed and constructed in-house, customized for specific applications of interest. Imaging systems can be adapted for short- or long-range imaging and stationary or rotational scanning. Sampling probe designs may vary in outer diameter, focal length, and direction of light propagation (0° vs 90°).

Ex Vivo Studies

With the advent of faster, minimally invasive OCT systems, research has trended towards in vivo OCT imaging of the human larynx. However, much of our understanding of OCT-based visualization of laryngeal microstructure is derived from studies on harvested tissue. Ex vivo OCT in animal and human models has served to provide anatomical standards for normal laryngeal microanatomy and lay the foundation for OCT-based differentiation of benign versus malignant processes. Furthermore, direct comparison of OCT images with corresponding histological section allows scientists to measure OCT sensitivity and understand limitations associated with the technology and image quality.

Human Studies

In 2004, Bibas et al. used PS-OCT to image 10 tissue samples from a single human postlaryngectomy specimen in both longitudinal (B-scan) and transverse/*en-face* (C-scan) modes. Stacks of C-scans were used to construct 3D images to identify reflectivity patterns within the layered microstructure and to correlate OCT with histological sections [29]. Similarly, de Boer's group used conventional OCT and PS-OCT to image human cadaveric larynges to identify patterns of optical backscattering and tissue birefringence associated with the layered microstructure of normal laryngeal mucosa [30]. These reports helped to establish standards for OCT-based visualization of laryngeal microanatomy and provided a framework for future OCT data analysis.

Animal Studies

A team led by Luerssen, Lubatschowski, Ptok, and colleagues has been a forerunner in investigating OCT applications in laryngology since the early 2000s. In 2005, Luerssen et al. performed high-resolution TD-OCT (central wavelength $\lambda = 1350$ nm, 5 μm axial resolution) of porcine larynges with an optical fiber tip in direct contact with sample tissue. Their data demonstrated a clear distinction between epithelium and underlying LP, as well as direct correlation of layered microstructure with histologic section [31]. Additional trials by this group in porcine and primate models using high-resolution or fiber-based systems (5–10 μm resolution) in contact mode have been described [32–34]. In these reports, the authors report OCT-based identification of mucosal substructure, laryngeal mucosa micrometry, and comparable sensitivity to histological examination.

Injury to laryngeal mucosa secondary to gastroesophageal reflux, prolonged endotracheal intubation, or laser therapy for VF lesions triggers a wound healing cascade which, if undiagnosed, terminates in granulation and fibrosis. However, occult subepithelial pathology cannot be identified by operative endoscopy or CT/MRI. Multiple ex vivo animal studies have demonstrated OCT capability of identifying laryngeal and subglottic histopathology following simulated morphologic injury to the VF or subglottis [35–37]. Karamzadeh et al. studied OCT of a variety of simulated subglottic injuries (collagen injection, dehydration, rehydration/edema, and repeated intubation) in harvested rabbit larynges [35]. Larynges were suspended vertically in an OCT imaging stage with a probe positioned over the cricoid cartilage to acquire images vertically, in a cephalocaudal direction. OCT-based micrometry of mucosal tissues demonstrated an increase in LP thickness following submucosal injury, as well as unique signal intensity patterns correlating with levels of subepithelial collagen or edema [35].

Operative treatment of glottic lesions is often limited by the surgeon's inability to precisely gauge the depth of disease. Given the critical interaction of adjacent layers of the laryngeal mucosa during phonation, the "body cover" model must be respected during excision of glottic lesions to prevent vocal fold scarring or permanent dysphonia. In 2007, Wisweh et al. performed simultaneous OCT and femtosecond laser (fs-laser) cutting on extracted porcine larynges [38]. An OCT system developed by Optimec Ltd. (Nizhny Novgorod, Russia) with 15 μm spatial resolution was used to identify sites of therapy and provides a reference for positioning the sample; the OCT scanner was swiveled out prior to fs-laser ablation at defined volumes and depths. This was the first report which investigated the potential of OCT as an intraoperative imaging tool to guide laryngeal microsurgery.

Clinical Studies

Intraoperative Imaging

In the operative setting, the larynx is exposed under direct laryngoscopy and visualized with an operating microscope and flexible or rigid endoscope (0°–90°). Intraoperative OCT of the larynx has been studied using a flexible endoscopic probe or a probe integrated with an operative microscope. In 1997, Sergeev et al. reported the first in vivo imaging of the larynx. Under direct laryngoscopy, a flexible sampling arm was advanced through the working channel of a standard endoscope and positioned 5–7 mm away from the tissue of interest. The distal fiber tip was swung by a galvanometric plate to image healthy laryngeal tissue and differentiate epithelium and LP based on optical scattering properties [19].

In 2005, Wong et al. reported laryngeal OCT during surgical endoscopy in 82 patients using a custom-built handheld probe. A flexible sampling fiber encased in a transparent, flexible plastic sheath was supported by an outer metal tube (2 mm diameter) and manually guided through the laryngoscope for near-contact or gentle contact imaging of laryngeal mucosa (axial resolution 9 μm, depth 2.6 mm). Images were analyzed for epithelial thickness, layered structure of the mucosa, and microstructural features (e.g., glands, microvasculature). Benign pathology, including Reinke's edema, papillomatosis, polyps, mucous cysts, and granulation tissue were identified based on unique patterns of signal backscattering [39]. In 2008, Kraft et al. used a commercial, contact-mode OCT device (Optimec Ltd.; central wavelength $\lambda = 980$ nm, 15 μm spatial resolution) to compare the diagnostic accuracy of microlaryngoscopy with OCT compared with microlaryngoscopy alone in a series of 217 benign and malignant laryngeal lesions [40]. They found that microlaryngoscopy and OCT provided an accurate diagnosis in 93 % of benign lesions and had a higher sensitivity (78 %) than microlaryngoscopy alone (66 %) in predicting epithelial dysplasia; specificity and accuracy were comparable in both methods.

Additional reports on OCT under direct laryngoscopy or microlaryngoscopy have been described [27, 40–46]. Later, spectral domain systems boasting faster imaging speeds (up to 18.5 frames/s) demonstrated improved efficiency and allow for 3D endoscopic imaging [47]. While imaging through endoscope working channels or handheld probes allow for contact or near-contact imaging, certain factors have been found to limit image quality. Motion artifact due to the movement of the probe tip, enhanced by surgeon's hand tremor, can significantly affect OCT image quality given its high-resolution scale. Furthermore, placement of a probe within the laryngoscope limits the surgeon's visualization of the operative field and interferes with insertion and manipulation of microlaryngeal instruments [48]. To answer this challenge, Vokes et al. first described a hands-free noncontact OCT system, with the sampling probe integrated with a surgical microscope. They integrated a custom built TD-OCT system with a novel interface device attached to an operating microscope by acrylic housing. The interface device consisted of a lens to adjust the focal length of the OCT beam, a galvanometer-mounted mirror to allow for coronal scanning and a second fixed mirror to redirect the path of light towards the sample tissue. Image frames were acquired at 1.6 mm depth and 6 mm width, with axial resolution of approximately 7 μm [48]. Additional reports of OCT integrated with microlaryngoscopy have been described in the literature [49, 50].

Office-Based Imaging

OCT probes can be affixed to flexible or rigid endoscopes to perform awake, office-based laryngeal imaging. Conjoining the sampling arm with a flexible endoscope allows for imaging (contact or near-contact) with a fixed working distance from the vocal folds, easier manipulation of the instrument, and a side-view of the vocal cords. However, direct contact with the vocal folds may precipitate severe cough, gagging or, in rare cases, laryngospasm. In rigid endoscopes cantilevered in the oropharynx approximately 5–8 cm above the vocal folds, LR-OCT systems can scan the larynx in a less invasive manner which may be better tolerated by patients. However, this method requires manual adjustment of the working distance with any movement.

In 2005, Luerssen et al. first described laryngeal OCT in awake patients under local anesthesia. A fiber-based endoscopic system (Institute of Applied Physics, Nizhny Novgorod, Russia) acquired images with the distal end of the sampling probe (2 mm diameter) in direct contact with laryngeal tissues. OCT data demonstrated clear distinction between epithelial mucosa and the loose, subepithelial collagenous tissue of the LP [31]. Additional studies by Luerssen's group describe a laryngoscope-integrated OCT probe for noncontact, transoral imaging with a low-profile design to optimize practicality and patient comfort [32–34]. Figure 3 demonstrates OCT images from healthy false vocal folds (supraglottic tissues), acquired from a research system (Fig. 3a) and a commercially available system (Fig. 3b). This data demonstrates respiratory epithelium, consisting of pseudostratified columnar epithelium with mucous-secreting goblet cells and ciliae. In contrast, OCT of the healthy true vocal folds depict nonkeratinized, stratified squamous epithelium (Fig. 4).

Chen and Wong's group constructed a TD-OCT system with a sampling probe fixed onto a laryngoscope to perform transoral, noncontact OCT [51]. This first-generation system had a slow scanning mechanism (1 frame/s) and produced images with significant motion artifact secondary to patient movement (breathing, swallowing, and reflexes) and physician hand tremor. Later, the same research group developed an FD-OCT system with a "double barrel" handheld carriage integrating a gradient-index (GRIN) lens-based probe

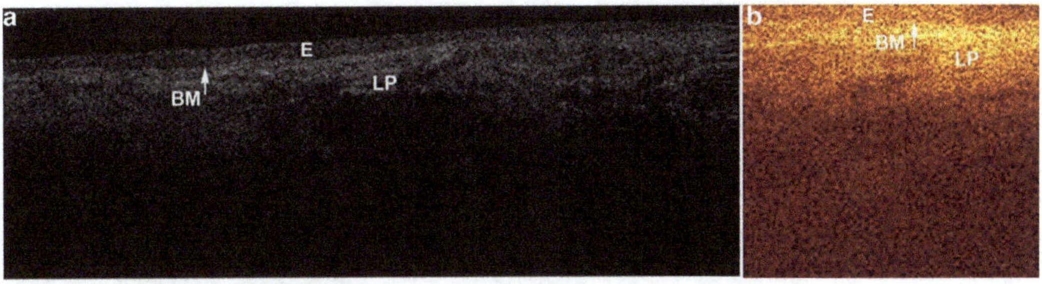

Fig. 3 OCT images of the normal false vocal folds acquired from a research OCT system (**a**) and a commercially available OCT system (**b**). *E* Epithelium (psuedostratified columnar), *BM* basement membrane locus, *LP* lamina propria

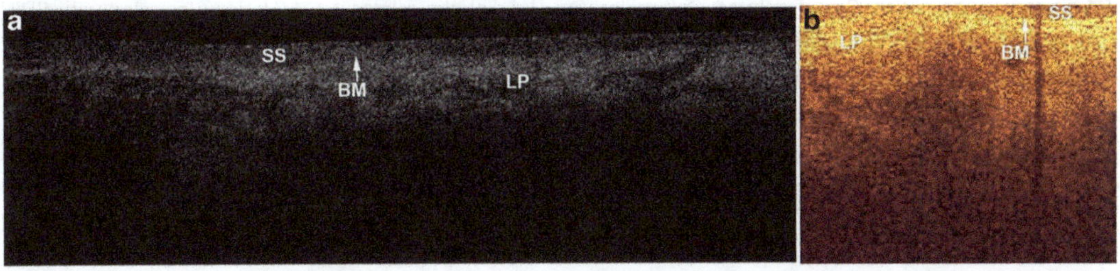

Fig. 4 OCT images of the normal true vocal fold acquired from a research OCT system (**a**) and a commercially available OCT system (**b**). *SS* stratified squamous epithelium, *BM* basement membrane locus, *LP* lamina propria

and rigid video endoscope. This instrument acquired cross-sectional images at 8 frames/s, thus reducing the degree of motion artifact [52]. Further pushing the frontier in dynamic imaging of the VF, a swept source (central wavelength $\lambda = 1310$ nm) FD-OCT system was designed (Fig. 5a) and constructed to acquire transoral endoscopic images of the larynx at 40 frames/s using an enhanced long GRIN lens-based probe integrated with a rigid endoscope in a similar double-barrel apparatus (Fig. 5b) [53]. Lubatschowski's group integrated a swept-source FD-OCT system with a rigid laryngoscope for noncontact OCT and synchronous video imaging of the vocal folds through a singular beam path [54]. Their compact imaging apparatus offered a more practical and well-tolerated means for transoral office-based imaging of the vocal folds. These noncontact, transoral endoscopic systems were the first to provide synchronous OCT and video imaging of the larynx during respiration and phonation without the use of topical anesthesia. Furthermore, noncontact imaging prevents morphometric distortion which may result from direct tissue compression from the tip of the probe. Awake, office-based OCT offers comparable results to contact or near-contact OCT during surgical endoscopy, however, with lower axial resolution (20 μm). Limitations of these modified laryngoscope-based systems include

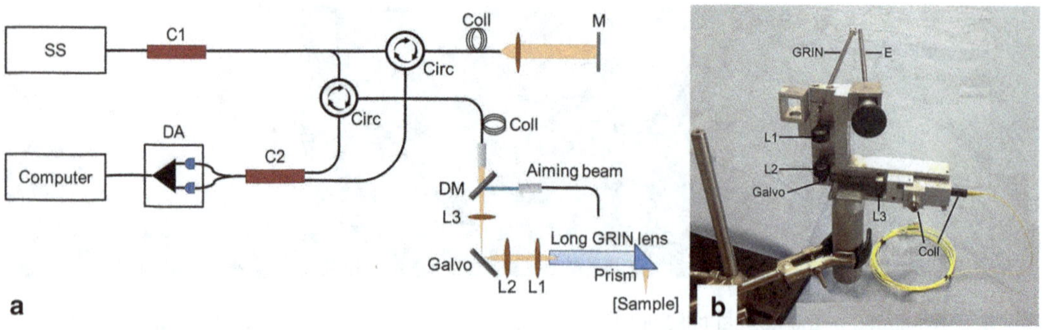

Fig. 5 Schematic diagram of gradient index (GRIN) lens rod-based dynamic focusing swept-source OCT system (**a**). Handheld "double barrel" carriage with integrated OCT probe and rigid endoscope for transoral imaging of the larynx. *SS* swept light source (central wavelength $\lambda = 1310$ nm), *C1* 1×2 coupler, *C2* 2×2 coupler, *DA* differential amplifier, *Circ* circulator, *Coll* collimator, *DM* dichotic mirror, *L1*, *L2* lenses (coupled with GRIN lens to form an optical ballast and produce an optical relay within the reference arm), *L3* focusing lens, *Galvo* galvanometer, *M* mirror, *E* rigid endoscope

motion artifact caused by patient movement during the exam (e.g., breathing, swallowing, reflexes) and physician's hand tremor. Furthermore, because the endoscope-OCT systems were cantilevered within the limited space of the pharynx, an extended focal length (compared to systems integrated with surgical endoscopes) was required for laryngeal imaging, limiting the lateral resolution and signal intensity [31, 32, 51, 55]. Currently, long-range swept source systems are being designed for high-speed transoral imaging without compromise of resolution.

In 2006, Klein et al. described laryngeal OCT and PS-OCT in awake subjects using a probe integrated with a flexible transnasal endoscope. The OCT probe, encased in Teflon tubing, was advanced through the operating channel of the endoscope until the distal end was visible and placed in contact with the glottic mucosal surface. Images were analyzed for epithelial micrometry, gray-scale intensity variation secondary to birefringent tissue (i.e., collagen content), and unique features of benign processes (e.g., papilloma, cysts, scarring) [41]. Additional reports of awake, office-based, flexible endoscopic OCT are described in the literature [56].

Vocal Fold Vibration

Vocal fold vibration has been widely studied under normal and pathologic circumstances using laryngeal videostroboscopy and high-speed video. Lohscheller et al. utilized phonovibrography to translate vocal fold vibration frequency, velocity, and acceleration into 2D diagrams for visualization and analysis [57, 58]. In examination of patients with laryngeal lesions, clinicians routinely correlate endoscopic findings with characteristics of vocal fold vibration noted on stroboscopy. This information helps to predict the consequence of lesions or interventions on phonation. However, the diagnostic sensitivity and specificity of endoscopy with videostroboscopy is low, as examination is limited to a surface view of the vocal folds. Thus, noninvasive diagnostic technology is needed to characterize the laryngeal mucosal wave in 3D during phonation. Correlation of high-resolution cross-sectional OCT images with vibratory characteristics of the laryngeal mucosa (e.g., frequency, amplitude) may lead to better understanding of how lesions or interventions affect the mechanical properties of laryngeal mucosal tissue and alter phonation.

In 2006, Luerssen's group first reported in vivo TD-OCT (central wavelength $\lambda = 1300$ nm) of the vocal folds during phonation [32]. A fiber-based OCT probe was integrated into a beam path of a laryngoscope to capture images in noncontact mode with a scanning rate of 10 Hz (resolution 10–20 μm). By measuring oscillation peaks in relation to scanning time, they were able to calculate vibrational frequency. Later, Yu et al. used a swept-source FD-OCT system to image vocal fold oscillation at 40 frames/s [53]. The higher frame rate allowed for minimization of motion artifact and dynamic vibration of the vocal folds. In seated, non-anesthetized patients, an OCT probe attached to a laryngoscope was inserted through the oral cavity and centered above the larynx. Their device allowed for dual-channel endoscopic and video-rate OCT imaging of the vocal folds. In both studies, vibration parameters such as frequency and amplitude were calculated from individual OCT frames. In 2011, Wong and Chen's group demonstrated OCT and optical Doppler tomography (ODT) of vibrating focal folds using a swept-source FD-OCT system (center wavelength $\lambda = 1050$ nm) with an imaging speed of 100 frames/s [59]. Their system extended the limit for high-speed functional OCT with image frames rate near that of physiologic fundamental frequencies (females 200 Hz, males 120 Hz).

Typically, however, imaging speeds of OCT systems are insufficient to directly capture vocal fold oscillation in the audio frequency range. To answer this challenge, Chang et al. reported motion-triggered laser scanning to capture four-dimensional (4D) images of vibrating ex vivo calf larynges [60]. Their modified OCT system acquired multiple A-lines over a single oscillation cycle at a frequency of 100 Hz before shifting to the adjacent transverse location. This method of data acquisition allows for temporal and spatial registration of A-lines to yield phase-aligned snapshots of tissue oscillation over a complete vibratory cycle. Hence, the imaging frequency range is determined by the A-line rate (up to 200 kHz) instead of the OCT system frame rate. Additional studies of triggered laser scanning of vibrating laryngeal tissue are reported in the literature [61].

Neonatology and Pediatrics

Anatomy

The neonatal and adult larynges differ significantly in both structural and microanatomic aspects. In the newborn airway, the larynx sits higher up and more anteriorly while the circumferential cricoid results in a cross-sectional narrowing of the airway at the subglottis [62]. Newborn VF mucosa consists of a uniform, monolayered LP composed of ground substances (hyaluronic acid, fibronectin, fibroblasts, collagenous and elastic fibers), less fibrous components, and no vocal ligament [63]. During the adolescent years, the LP matures into a layered microstructure. The delicate mucosa of the newborn larynx, coupled with the unique anatomical configuration of the airway, make the newborn laryngeal and subglottic tissues susceptible to injury following long-term intubation or gastroesophageal reflux.

Boseley et al. used pediatric cadaveric larynges to describe the maturation of the vocal fold. They noted a differentiation from the monolayered LP into a bilaminar structure beginning by 2 months of age. Transition into a trilaminar structure occurs between ages 1 and 5 years, with full maturation into the adult molecular composition occurring around age 13 [64]. However, it is unknown exactly when these transitions occur and thus difficult to estimate at what age microsurgical techniques can be used without affecting phonation. OCT's ability to evaluate the subepithelial microstructure of the pediatric larynx can allow clinicians to assess stage of laryngeal development and develop individualized treatment plans.

Future Applications

Given the unique anatomical configuration of the neonatal airway, patients requiring long-term endotracheal intubation and mechanical ventilation are at risk for subglottic mucosal injury. In managing neonates with suspected subglottic stenosis, pediatric otolaryngologists do not have means to comprehensively evaluate the airway without subjecting patients to general anesthesia and further airway instrumentation. Direct laryngoscopy and bronchoscopy is the gold standard for diagnosis of SGS [65]. However, this procedure may lead to further mucosal abrasion (removal and reinsertion of endotracheal tube, endoscope contact with airway mucosa) and is limited to a view of surface anatomy. Furthermore, risks of general anesthesia in patients with preexisting cardiopulmonary insufficiencies must be considered. These factors, combined, often lead to a delay in diagnosis of SGS and increased morbidity. Thus, there exists a need for a less invasive imaging modality which can characterize the subepithelial tissue of the subglottis and identify precursors to subglottic stenosis.

OCT Studies

In 2007, Ridgway et al. were the first to use OCT to image the pediatric upper aerodigestive tract. Using a fiber-based OCT system, they imaged 15 pediatric patients during operative endoscopy at various airway landmarks with a flexible, handheld probe positioned manually or with endoscopic guidance. Layered microstructure of normal laryngeal and subglottic tissue and distinct pathologic changes (mature scar, granulation tissue, edema, ulceration) were identified on OCT and correlated with endoscopic photographs [66]. The following year, the same group conducted in vivo OCT of the larynx in intubated neonates to identify tissue microstructure of the larynx, subglottis, and proximal trachea. This data provided a framework for using OCT to identify subepithelial injury at the subglottis in neonates under long-term intubation [67].

Boudoux et al. conducted ex vivo imaging of both pediatric and porcine larynges using FD-OCT, spectrally encoded confocal microscopy, and full-field optical coherence microscopy followed by comparison with histologic section. They noted that the combined application of OCT with confocal microscopy allows for comprehensive evaluation of subepithelial microstructure and cellular and subcellular components of the vocal folds. Combined, these modalities may allow for longitudinal analysis of vocal fold development and differentiation [68, 69].

OCT Limitations

The primary limitation of OCT imaging of the larynx is the depth of signal penetration. Current OCT systems offer optical penetration depths of up to 1–2 mm. As benign and malignant processes are differentiated by depth of invasion and disruption of the basement membrane, achieving adequate signal penetration is critical to providing a definitive diagnosis of laryngeal pathology. Larger, exophytic lesions of greater than 2 mm depth cannot be identified to their full extent, limiting the diagnostic sensitivity of OCT. Furthermore, certain tissue interfaces (e.g., cartilage, bone) with high optical scattering or absorption properties impede photon penetration and cast a distal shadow within A-lines, further limiting diagnostic sensitivity in such tissues. Additional factors which limit image quality include physician hand tremor and patient movement during office-based OCT, or equipment vibrations which may all translate into image distortion of far greater magnitude. Lastly, the OCT resolution limit (approximately 10 μm) precludes evaluation of laryngeal microanatomy at the cellular level. This degree of microanatomical analysis is fundamental for differentiation between dysplastic, precancerous, and cancerous lesions, necessitating formal histopathologic analysis for a definitive diagnosis of malignancy.

At present, near-contact sampling probes offer the best OCT image resolution, clarity, and diagnostic sensitivity. This method of imaging requires general anesthesia for OCT under microlaryngoscopy or adequate topical anesthesia for awake, office-based laryngeal OCT. However, office-based near-contact imaging may not be well tolerated by all patients, given the risk of paroxysmal airway reactions such as coughing, gagging, or choking. While these reactions may be self-limiting and the incidence of true laryngospasm is rare, noncontact imaging may cause discomfort or anxiety to some patients. Current efforts are focused on developing full range OCT systems using vertical-cavity surface-emitting lasers (VCSEL), which may ultimately allow for transoral imaging of the vocal cords from a sampling arm cantilevered in the oropharynx while maintaining current spatial resolution.

Malignancy

OCT has been shown to provide detailed microanatomical information about the laryngeal epithelial layer and integrity of the BM and LP [29–31]. By identification of small foci of BM breakdown, OCT can identify premalignant or invasive cancerous lesions with high sensitivity [70, 71]. In 1997, Sergeev et al. were the first to study normal and cancerous tissue of the larynx and reported a "loss of normal tissue stratification in tumors" [19]. Later, Shakhov et al. conducted TD-OCT in 26 patients with small laryngeal squamous cell carcinomas. Similarly, they described a stratification of layered tissue within mucosa of the healthy larynx, the disappearance of which signifies pathologic changes [26]. Further OCT studies on premalignant and malignant lesions of the larynx are illustrated and reviewed elsewhere in this text [39, 43, 70].

References

1. Hirano M. Morphological structure of the vocal cord as a vibrator and its variations. Folia Phoniatr (Basel). 1974;26(2):89–94.
2. Titze IR, Jiang J, Drucker DG. Preliminaries to the body-cover theory of pitch control. J Voice. 1988;1(4):314–9.
3. Huang D, et al. Optical coherence tomography. Science. 1991;254(5035):1178–81.
4. Fercher AF. Optical coherence tomography—development, principles, applications. Z Med Phys. 2010;20(4):251–76.
5. Fercher AF, et al. Measurement of intraocular distances by backscattering spectral interferometry. Opt Commun. 1995;117:43–8.
6. Wojtkowski M, et al. In vivo human retinal imaging by Fourier domain optical coherence tomography. J Biomed Opt. 2002;7(3):457–63.
7. Beaurepaire E, et al. Full-field optical coherence microscopy. Opt Lett. 1998;23(4):244–6.
8. Yun S, et al. High-speed optical frequency-domain imaging. Opt Express. 2003;11(22): 2953–63.
9. Choma M, et al. Sensitivity advantage of swept source and Fourier domain optical coherence tomography. Opt Express. 2003;11(18): 2183–9.
10. Armstrong J, et al. In vivo size and shape measurement of the human upper airway using endoscopic longrange optical coherence tomography. Opt Express. 2003;11(15):1817–26.
11. Jing J, et al. High-speed upper-airway imaging using full-range optical coherence tomography. J Biomed Opt. 2012;17(11):110507.
12. de Boer JF, et al. Two-dimensional birefringence imaging in biological tissue by polarization-sensitive optical coherence tomography. Opt Lett. 1997;22(12):934–6.
13. de Boer JF, Milner TE. Review of polarization sensitive optical coherence tomography and Stokes vector determination. J Biomed Opt. 2002;7(3):359–71.
14. Kuo WC, et al. Polarization-sensitive optical coherence tomography for imaging human atherosclerosis. Appl Opt. 2007;46(13):2520–7.

15. Fercher AF, et al. In vivo optical coherence tomography. Am J Ophthalmol. 1993;116(1): 113–4.
16. Swanson EA, et al. In vivo retinal imaging by optical coherence tomography. Opt Lett. 1993;18(21):1864–6.
17. Tearney GJ, et al. Scanning single-mode fiber optic catheter-endoscope for optical coherence tomography. Opt Lett. 1996;21(7):543–5.
18. Tearney GJ, et al. In vivo endoscopic optical biopsy with optical coherence tomography. Science. 1997;276(5321):2037–9.
19. Sergeev A, et al. In vivo endoscopic OCT imaging of precancer and cancer states of human mucosa. Opt Express. 1997;1(13):432–40.
20. de Feyter PJ, Nieman K. New coronary imaging techniques: what to expect? Heart. 2002;87(3):195–7.
21. Sivak Jr MV, et al. High-resolution endoscopic imaging of the GI tract using optical coherence tomography. Gastrointest Endosc. 2000;51(4 Pt 1):474–9.
22. Drexler W. Ultrahigh-resolution optical coherence tomography. J Biomed Opt. 2004;9(1): 47–74.
23. Drexler W, et al. In vivo ultrahigh-resolution optical coherence tomography. Opt Lett. 1999;24(17):1221–3.
24. Yaqoob Z, Wu J, Yang C. Spectral domain optical coherence tomography: a better OCT imaging strategy. Biotechniques. 2005;39(6 Suppl):S6–13.
25. Drexler W, Fujimoto JG. In: Drexler W, Fujimoto JG, editors. Introduction to Optical Coherence Tomography Optical coherence tomography: technology and applications. New York: Springer; 2008; 1–45.
26. Shakhov AV, et al. Optical coherence tomography monitoring for laser surgery of laryngeal carcinoma. J Surg Oncol. 2001;77(4):253–8.
27. Rubinstein M, et al. Optical coherence tomography of the larynx using the Niris system. J Otolaryngol Head Neck Surg. 2010; 39(2):150–6.
28. Colt HG, et al. Multimodality bronchoscopic imaging of recurrent respiratory papillomatosis. Laryngoscope. 2010;120(3):468–72.
29. Bibas AG, et al. 3-D optical coherence tomography of the laryngeal mucosa. Clin Otolaryngol Allied Sci. 2004;29(6):713–20.
30. Burns JA, et al. Imaging the mucosa of the human vocal fold with optical coherence tomography. Ann Otol Rhinol Laryngol. 2005;114(9):671–6.
31. Luerssen K, et al. Optical characterization of vocal folds with optical coherence tomography. Photon Ther Diagn. 2005;5686:328–32.
32. Lurssen K, et al. Optical characterization of vocal folds using optical coherence tomography—art. no. 60781O. Photon Ther Diagn II. 2006;6078:O781.
33. Lurssen K, et al. Optical coherence tomography in the diagnosis of vocal folds. HNO. 2006;54(8):611–5.
34. Lueerssen K, et al. Optical characterization of vocal folds by OCT-based laryngoscopy—art. no. 64241O. Photon Ther Diagn III. 2007;6424:O4241.
35. Karamzadeh AM, et al. Characterization of submucosal lesions using optical coherence tomography in the rabbit subglottis. Arch Otolaryngol Head Neck Surg. 2005;131(6): 499–504.
36. Nassif NA, et al. Measurement of morphologic changes induced by trauma with the use of coherence tomography in porcine vocal cords. Otolaryngol Head Neck Surg. 2005;133(6): 845–50.
37. Torkian BA, et al. Noninvasive measurement of ablation crater size and thermal injury after CO2 laser in the vocal cord with optical coherence tomography. Otolaryngol Head Neck Surg. 2006;134(1):86–91.
38. Wisweh H, et al. Optical coherence tomography monitoring of vocal fold femtosecond laser microsurgery—art. no. 663207. Ther Laser Appl Laser-Tissue Interact III. 2007; 6632:63207.
39. Wong BJ, et al. In vivo optical coherence tomography of the human larynx: normative and benign pathology in 82 patients. Laryngoscope. 2005;115(11):1904–11.
40. Kraft M, et al. Clinical value of optical coherence tomography in laryngology. Head Neck. 2008;30(12):1628–35.
41. Klein AM, et al. Imaging the human vocal folds in vivo with optical coherence tomography: a preliminary experience. Ann Otol Rhinol Laryngol. 2006;115(4):277–84.
42. Foster MC, et al. Association of subcutaneous and visceral adiposity with albuminuria: the Framingham Heart Study. Obesity (Silver Spring). 2011;19(6):1284–9.
43. Kraft M, et al. Significance of optical coherence tomography in the assessment of laryngeal lesions—art. no. 68421O. Photon Ther Diagn IV. 2008;6842:O8421.
44. Zhu Y, et al. Discovery and characterization of sulfoxaflor, a novel insecticide targeting sap-feeding pests. J Agric Food Chem. 2011; 59(7):2950–7.
45. Lima LH, et al. A new dual port cutter system for vitrectomy surgery. Retina. 2010;30(9): 1515–9.

46. Norwood KW, et al. Traumatic brain injury in children and adolescents: surveillance for pituitary dysfunction. Clin Pediatr (Phila). 2010;49(11):1044–9.
47. Kim KH, et al. In vivo 3D human vocal fold imaging with polarization sensitive optical coherence tomography and a MEMS scanning catheter. Opt Express. 2010;18(14): 14644–53.
48. Walker SE, et al. Racial/ethnic discrepancies in the metabolic syndrome begin in childhood and persist after adjustment for environmental factors. Nutr Metab Cardiovasc Dis. 2012;22(2): 141–8.
49. Wilhelm-Leen ER, et al. Vitamin D deficiency and frailty in older Americans. J Intern Med. 2010;268(2):171–80.
50. Krishnamoorthy G, et al. Electrokinetic lab-on-a-biochip for multi-ligand/multi-analyte biosensing. Anal Chem. 2010;82(10): 4145–50.
51. Guo S, et al. Office-based optical coherence tomographic imaging of human vocal cords. J Biomed Opt. 2006;11(3):30501.
52. Guo S, et al. Gradient-index lens rod based probe for office-based optical coherence tomography of the human larynx. J Biomed Opt. 2009;14(1):014017.
53. Yu L, et al. Office-based dynamic imaging of vocal cords in awake patients with swept-source optical coherence tomography. J Biomed Opt. 2009;14(6):064020.
54. Wisweh H, et al. A laryngoscope for office-based imaging of human vocal folds using OCT. Proc SPIE. 2009;7372.
55. Easter B, et al. The impact of music on the PACU patient's perception of discomfort. J Perianesth Nurs. 2010;25(2):79–87.
56. Sepehr A, et al. Optical coherence tomography of the larynx in the awake patient. Otolaryngol Head Neck Surg. 2008;138(4):425–9.
57. Lohscheller J, et al. Phonovibrography: mapping high-speed movies of vocal fold vibrations into 2-D diagrams for visualizing and analyzing the underlying laryngeal dynamics. IEEE Trans Med Imaging. 2008;27(3):300–9.
58. Lohscheller J, Eysholdt U. Phonovibrogram visualization of entire vocal fold dynamics. Laryngoscope. 2008;118(4):753–8.
59. Liu G, et al. Imaging vibrating vocal folds with a high speed 1050 nm swept source OCT and ODT. Opt Express. 2011;19(12):11880–9.
60. Chang EW, Kobler JB, Yun SH. Triggered optical coherence tomography for capturing rapid periodic motion. Sci Rep. 2011;1:48.
61. Kobler JB, et al. Dynamic imaging of vocal fold oscillation with four-dimensional optical coherence tomography. Laryngoscope. 2010;120(7): 1354–62.
62. Holinger PH, et al. Subglottic stenosis in infants and children. Ann Otol Rhinol Laryngol. 1976;85(5 Pt.1):591–9.
63. Sato K, Hirano M, Nakashima T. Fine structure of the human newborn and infant vocal fold mucosae. Ann Otol Rhinol Laryngol. 2001;110(5 Pt 1):417–24.
64. Boseley ME, Hartnick CJ. Development of the human true vocal fold: depth of cell layers and quantifying cell types within the lamina propria. Ann Otol Rhinol Laryngol. 2006; 115(10):784–8.
65. Holinger LD. Diagnostic endoscopy of the pediatric airway. Laryngoscope. 1989;99(3):346–8.
66. Ridgway JM, et al. Imaging of the pediatric airway using optical coherence tomography. Laryngoscope. 2007;117(12):2206–12.
67. Ridgway JM, et al. Optical coherence tomography of the newborn airway. Ann Otol Rhinol Laryngol. 2008;117(5):327–34.
68. Boudoux C, et al. Optical microscopy of the pediatric vocal fold. Arch Otolaryngol Head Neck Surg. 2009;135(1):53–64.
69. Boudoux C, et al. Preliminary evaluation of noninvasive microscopic imaging techniques for the study of vocal fold development. J Voice. 2009;23(3):269–76.
70. Armstrong WB, et al. Optical coherence tomography of laryngeal cancer. Laryngoscope. 2006;116(7):1107–13.
71. Hughes OR, et al. Optical and molecular techniques to identify tumor margins within the larynx. Head Neck. 2010;32(11):1544–53.

Chapter 36

Optical Coherence Tomography of Malignancies of the Head and Neck

Giriraj K. Sharma, Marc Rubinstein, Christian Betz, and Brian J.-F. Wong

Introduction

In 2014, The American Cancer Society estimates over 42,000 new cases of oral and pharyngeal cancer, and over 12,000 new cases of laryngeal cancer will be diagnosed in the United States [1]. The majority of these malignancies are head and neck squamous cell carcinomas (HNSCC), a particularly aggressive form of cancer, for which tobacco and alcohol use are major risk factors. Despite novel molecular targeting therapies (e.g., epidermal growth factor receptor), expanded roles for chemotherapy (e.g., neoadjuvant treatment for laryngeal cancer), and new irradiation techniques (e.g., hyperfractionated radiotherapy), the long-term survival rates for advanced-stage HNSCC remain low [2, 3]. Between 2004 and 2010, 65 % of the newly diagnosed cancers of the oral cavity (OC) and pharynx were advanced-stage tumors (regional or distant metastasis); 40 % of laryngeal cancers were in advanced stage [4]. One explanation for the delayed diagnosis of head and neck cancer is that many early stage cancerous lesions are subtle and do not demonstrate clinical characteristics of advanced lesions including ulceration, induration, pain or associated cervical lymphadenopathy [5]. Furthermore, premalignant lesions are often undetectable to the naked eye and are highly heterogeneous in presentation, frequently mimicking benign or reactive conditions. Hence, a practical and accurate imaging modality which may improve the incidence of early stage diagnosis and allow for screening of head and neck cancer is needed.

Diagnostic evaluation of head and neck cancer patients begins with a thorough history and physical examination. The head and neck examination includes visual and digital assessment of hard

Brian J.-F. Wong and Justus Ilgner (eds.), *Biomedical Optics in Otorhinolaryngology: Head and Neck Surgery*, DOI 10.1007/978-1-4939-1758-7_36, © Springer Science+Business Media New York 2016

and soft tissues within the OC and oropharynx (OP). Examination of the pharynx and larynx may be accomplished with an indirect mirror examination or, for more comprehensive evaluation, with transnasal flexible laryngoscopy. Panendoscopy (bronchoscopy, esophagoscopy, and direct laryngoscopy) is often performed for a more thorough preoperative assessment and tumor staging. All aforementioned diagnostic techniques provide information on the color and surface pattern of mucosal tissue only and therefore are unable to detect subepithelial pathology. Computed tomography (CT), positron emission tomography CT (PET-CT), and magnetic resonance (MR) imaging are commonly used imaging modalities in the management of head and neck cancer. However, these technologies lack adequate spatial resolution to differentiate between benign, premalignant, and malignant lesions at the substructural or cellular level. Screening of the OC for cancerous lesions may be attempted with toluidine blue staining, fluorescence staining, exfoliative cytology, and brush biopsy [6]. However, these tests lack standardized methodology, have variable reported diagnostic sensitivity and specificity, or lack randomized controlled trials.

Histopathological analysis of excised tissue remains the gold standard of care for achieving a definitive diagnosis of suspicious lesions. However, office-based or operative biopsy is not a pragmatic option for routine screening. A single lesion may require multiple biopsies to avoid overlooking the most dysplastic region of pathology. Biopsy is also associated with patient morbidity and may pose risk for long-term speech or swallowing sequela. Hence, a less invasive imaging modality which can delineate mucosal substructure in vivo, identify tumor margins and screen for occult foci of pathology has the potential to improve the management of head and neck cancer patients.

Principles of OCT

OCT is a minimally invasive imaging modality which combines nonionizing near-infrared light with principles of low coherence interferometry [7]. A light source (e.g., laser or superbright light emitting diode) is split into a reference arm (mirror) and a sample arm (biological sample). Back-reflected light from each path is recombined and detected to construct a two-dimensional reflectivity profile (A-line) as a function of tissue depth with up to 2 mm optical penetration. Adjacent A-lines are combined to yield high-resolution (~10 μm), 3D cross-sectional images of tissue. Early OCT systems were developed using a time-domain (TD-OCT) configuration. Later, OCT systems based on Fourier-domain (FD-OCT) detection were constructed, either with a spectrometer configuration (spectral-domain OCT) or a frequency-swept source (swept-source OCT). FD-OCT systems spectrally resolve the interference signal to measure the echo time delay of backscattered light. The advantages of FD-OCT over TD-OCT include faster imaging speeds, higher sensitivity, and greater resolution [8–10]. Polarization-sensitive OCT (PS-OCT) augments conventional OCT by detecting changes in the polarization state of reflected light [11, 12].

OCT imaging of laryngeal tissue can be accomplished in contact or near-contact modes using an endoscopic probe during operative microlaryngoscopy or office-based upper-airway endoscopy. Some research groups have evaluated long-range imaging of the vocal folds by integrating OCT sampling arms with operative microscopes, while others have adapted handheld laryngoscopes for transoral endoscopic OCT imaging of the larynx.

Oral and Pharyngeal Cancer

The OC and pharynx are the most common sites for neoplasm of the head and neck. Precancerous lesions include leukoplakia (white), erythroplakia (red), mixed red-white lesions, and verrucous hyperplasia. Leukoplakias develop in 1–4 % of the population, with malignant transformation in approximately 0.13–33 % of these lesions [13, 14]. Up to 85 % of erythroplakias carry risk for malignant transformation [14]. Accurate differentiation between benign, premalignant and malignant pathology requires assessment of the structure and integrity of the epithelium and subepithelial layers. Potential applications of OCT in the management of oral and pharyngeal cancer include identification of transition zones between different histological states (e.g., definition of tumor margins to guide therapy), evaluation of basement membrane integrity for suspicious lesions and longitudinal monitoring of disease progression. Figure 36.1 depicts OCT images from normal and cancerous tissue of the floor of the mouth, acquired by Betz's group (Munich, Germany) using a commercially available system. A loss of layered substructural integrity is noted in cancer tissue, secondary to the downgrowth of malignant epithelial cells and breakdown of the basement membrane. The transition zone between both regions is demonstrated in Fig. 2 using a research TD-OCT system.

Animal and Ex Vivo Studies

The hamster cheek model is frequently used to evaluate OCT of premalignant and malignant lesions followed by image correlation with histological section [15–24]. In 2004, Matheny et al. reported in vivo and, following excision, in vitro OCT (central wavelength $\lambda = 1310$ nm) and optical Doppler tomography (ODT) of induced dysplasia and malignancies in hamster cheek pouches [16]. Their OCT images of dysplastic lesions demonstrated epithelial thickening

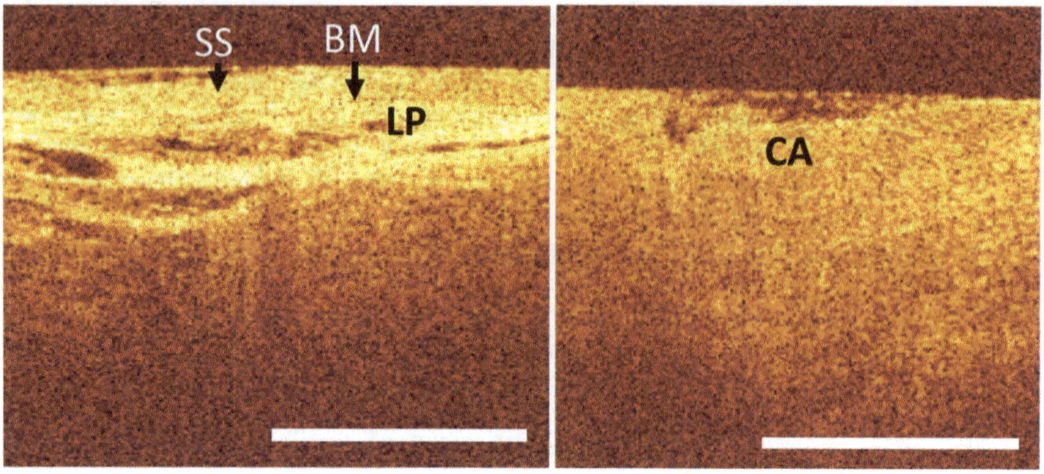

Fig. 1 OCT images of normal epithelial tissue (**a**) and squamous cell carcinoma (**b**) from the floor of the mouth, acquired from a commercially available system. *SS* nonkeratinized stratified squamous epithelium, *BM* basement membrane, *LP* lamina propria, *CA* cancer. *White bar*=1000 μm

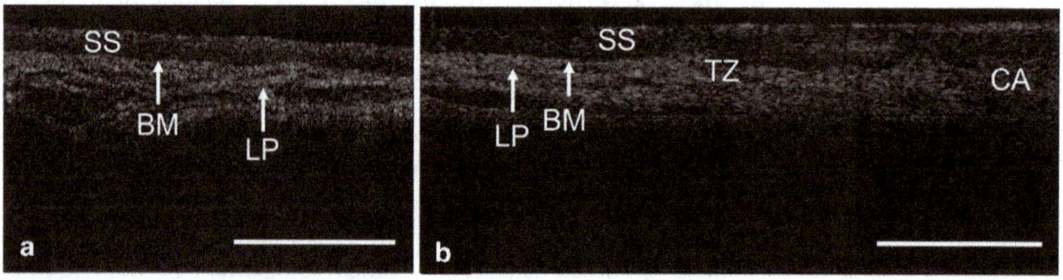

Fig. 2 OCT images of normal epithelial tissue (**a**) and the transition zone (**b**) between normal tissue and squamous cell carcinoma of the floor of mouth, acquired from a research system. *SS* nonkeratinized stratified squamous epithelium, *BM* basement membrane, *LP* lamina propria, *TZ* transition zone, *CA* cancer. *White bar*=1000 μm

into the underlying connective tissue; cancerous regions appeared to have higher levels of scattering and absorption, thus reducing the overall optical penetration depth in these tissues. In 2011, Ahn et al. performed longitudinal in vivo FD-OCT (center wavelength $\lambda=1310$ nm) to image the development of carcinogenesis including epithelial migration, loss of basement membrane integrity, and subepithelial invasion [23]. Multiple reports of OCT of precancerous and cancerous lesions of the human OC in the immediate ex vivo phase have allowed for diagnostic sensitivity and specificity measurement by direct comparison with histopathology [25–29].

Clinical Studies

In vivo OCT evaluation of normal human OC/OP mucosa is described in the literature [30–34]. These reports have helped establish standards for OCT-based identification of substructural tissue layers within the OC and OP and provide a reference for differentiating noncancerous from cancerous lesions. In vivo human studies have demonstrated the efficacy of OCT in differentiating premalignant and malignant lesions of the OC/pharynx [35–39]. In 2006, Ridgway et al. imaged normal and pathologic lesions within the OC and OP in 41 patients using a TD-OCT system (central wavelength $\lambda = 1310$ nm) and a flexible endoscopic probe mechanically supported in a rigid, stainless steel cylinder [36]. Their OCT images of histologically proven oral cancer depicted ablation of subepithelial tissue and a progressive loss of layering and basement membrane integrity at tumor margins. Tsai et al. performed in vivo swept-source FD-OCT in 32 patients to evaluate OC lesions at different oncologic stages [37]. By computing the lateral variation of multiple A-line parameters (standard deviation of signal intensity fluctuation, exponential decay constant, epithelial thickness), their image analysis offered objective diagnostic indicators to differentiate between premalignant and malignant lesions.

Field Cancerization

Field cancerization describes the process in which an invasive cancer within a mucosal surface is surrounded by multiple molecular lesions with cancer-associated genetic or epigenetic alterations [40, 41]. With high resolution and high diagnostic sensitivity, OCT has the unique capability of identifying transition zones between normal and cancerous subepithelial tissue and the potential to detect subclinical pathologic foci [18, 23, 25]. Tsai et al. used a swept-source FD-OCT system (central wavelength $\lambda = 1310$ nm, axial resolution 8 μm) to image OC cancer ex vivo and analyzed the lateral variation of A-scan profiles across the margin of lesions [25]. Intensity decay constants were calibrated by plotting exponential fitting curves of OCT signal intensity as a function of tissue depth. Their data showed a decreasing trend of the decay constant as the A-line scan point moved across the margin from normal to abnormal tissue. Secondly, they analyzed the fluctuation extent (standard deviation) of OCT signal intensity in A-scans; this parameter increased significantly as the A-line scan point was moved across the transition zone from normal to abnormal tissue. Hence, OCT has potential as a screening tool for identifying margins of disease, satellite foci, or neighboring secondary tumors within the upper aerodigestive tract.

Laryngeal Cancer

The larynx is the second most common site for malignancy in the upper aerodigestive tract, with over 12,000 new cases annually in the United States [1]. Approximately 85–95 % of malignant laryngeal tumors are squamous cell carcinomas (SCC) [42]. The layered microanatomy of the vocal fold is described in the literature and reviewed elsewhere in this text [43]. While excisional biopsy remains the gold standard for diagnosis of suspicious lesions, this procedure may result in soft tissue deficits and/or vocal fold scarring, both events which may adversely affect postoperative voice quality [44]. OCT offers a less invasive means of acquiring an "optical biopsy" to assess the structural architecture of the vocal fold. Similar to applications in the OC/pharynx, OCT of laryngeal precancerous or cancerous lesions would allow for delineation of tumor margins to guide laser therapy or excisional biopsy, evaluation of basement membrane integrity and penetration depth for suspicious lesions, and monitoring of disease progression. The transition zone between normal laryngeal epithelial tissue and SCC is marked by a gradual loss of basement membrane, which separates the optically distinct stratified squamous epithelium and lamina propria (Fig. 3). OCT of laryngeal SCC demonstrates a lack of clear epithelial borders, without delineation of a basement membrane (Fig. 4).

comprehensive review of research in OCT imaging of vocal fold anatomy and vibrational parameters is provided in an alternate chapter in this text. Select laryngeal OCT studies in porcine and primate models are included here for review purposes [45–48]. These reports provided a basis for understanding OCT-based delineation of the layered microstructure of the vocal fold. Additional reports of OCT in human *ex vivo* larynx specimens are described [49, 50].

Clinical Applications

In 1997, Sergeev et al. first reported in vivo endoscopic OCT of healthy and cancerous laryngeal tissues under direct laryngoscopy in the operating room [51]. Their TD-OCT system (central wavelength $\lambda = 830$ nm, scanning rate 30 cm/s) included a flexible sampling arm integrated into the working channel of a standard

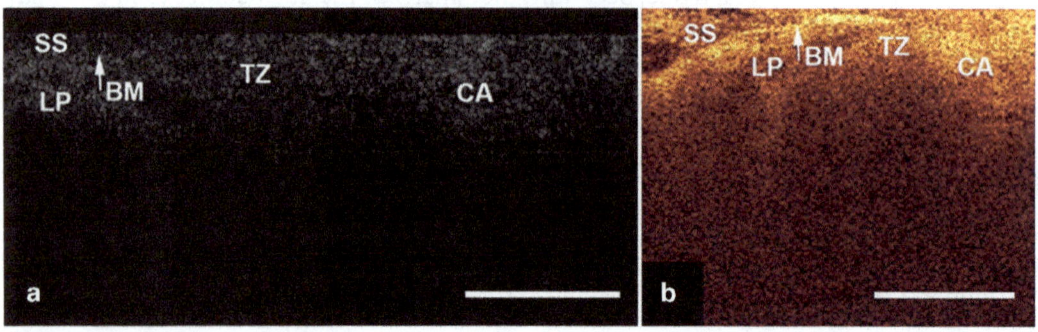

Fig. 3 OCT image of the transition zone between normal epithelium and squamous cell carcinoma of the true vocal fold, acquired from a research system (**a**) and a commercially available system (**b**). *SS* stratified squamous epithelium, *LP* lamina propria, *BM* basement membrane, *TZ* transition zone, *CA* cancer. *White bar* = 1000 µm

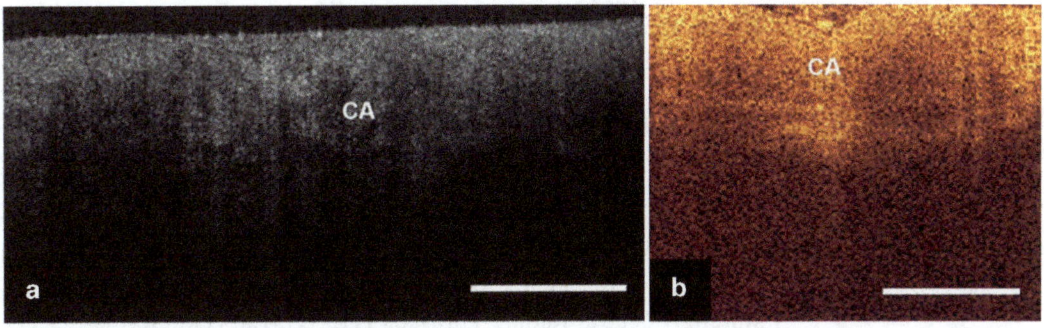

Fig. 4 OCT images of squamous cell carcinoma of the true vocal folds, acquired from a research system (**a**) and a commercially available system (**b**). *CA* cancer. *White bar*=1000 μm

endoscope. The distal fiber tip was positioned 5–7 mm away from the tissue of interest and swung by a galvanometric plate to scan tissue in a lateral motion with a 2 mm wide optical beam. Their results contrasted healthy and cancerous laryngeal tissue using OCT, revealing a disruption of substructural anatomy and a greater degree of optical backscattering and vascularization in tumor tissue. Similar experiments of tandem OCT-endoscopy of the larynx have been described for operative and office-based settings [52, 53].

Multiple groups have performed OCT of laryngeal cancer during microlaryngoscopy and operative endoscopy by manually inserting a fiber-based probe through the lumen of a surgical laryngoscope or mechanically integrating the probe with a laryngoscope [54–60]. In 2001, Shakhov et al. used endoscopic TD-OCT to identify laryngeal tumor margins during microlaryngoscopy and transoral laser surgery [54]. They noted that OCT allowed for identification of tumor margins up to 3 mm beyond the margins visually identified under microlaryngoscopy. Kraft et al. prospectively compared the intraoperative diagnosis of 217 laryngeal lesions including 41 precancerous and 46 malignant lesions using microlaryngoscopy with and without OCT; all diagnoses were confirmed with histopathology [57]. During microlaryngoscopy, the surgeon used a handheld applicator to apply the probe in direct contact with laryngeal tissue. They determined that microlaryngoscopy with OCT yielded a correct diagnosis in 93 % of malignant lesions and correctly predicted the exact grade of dysplasia in 71 % of lesions. Microlaryngoscopy with OCT presented a higher sensitivity than microlaryngoscopy alone in predicting invasive tumor growth (93 % vs. 87 %) and epithelial dysplasia (78 % vs. 66 %).

Vokes et al. first described OCT integrated with a surgical microscope to conduct hands-free, noncontact imaging of the vocal cords in 10 patients, including five cases of laryngeal SCC [61]. The fiber terminus of their sampling arm was positioned

40 cm from laryngeal tissue, limiting the lateral resolution (50 μm) as a result of diffraction. Nonetheless, their OCT images delineated the epithelium-lamina propria border and provided cross-sectional images to a depth of 1.6 mm. The integrated, hands-free OCT-microscope system offered multiple advantages compared to handheld contact or near-contact OCT probes: (1) minimizing of motion artifact, (2) eliminating OCT instrumentation in the body of a laryngoscope and, as a result, (3) offering surgeons an improved field of view. Just et al. integrated a commercially available FD-OCT system (Spectral Radar; Thorlabs HL AG, Lubeck, Germany; central wavelength $\lambda = 840$ nm) with the camera port of an operating microscope to image suspicious laryngeal lesions during microlaryngoscopy [60]. By adjusting the zoom on their OCT-microscope system they were able to control the size of the lateral imaging field (2–8 mm). They noted additional advantages over endoscope-based OCT systems, including a longer working distance and visualization of the scanning plane with a pilot beam which allowed for unobstructed, precise localization of biopsy sites.

In 2005, Luerssen et al. first reported office-based OCT of normal vocal cords using a contact endoscopic probe [45]. Later generations of office-based OCT systems included integration of the sampling arm with a handheld rigid laryngoscope [48, 62]. With an increasing number of laryngeal diagnostic and therapeutic procedures being conducted in office-based settings, OCT of the laryngeal airway in the awake patient has considerable utility for monitoring lesions, real-time identification of pathologic margins and guidance for office-based excisional biopsy or laser therapy.

OCT Limitations

While advanced generations of OCT technology have led to higher resolution, imaging speeds, and diagnostic sensitivity, a number of factors preclude OCT to serve as an independent diagnostic imaging modality. A primary limitation of OCT in the diagnosis of cancer is the optical penetration depth. Achieving adequate signal penetration to assess basement membrane integrity is critical to differentiating dysplastic lesions such as hyperkeratosis from malignancy. Most research and commercial systems report a maximum imaging depth of 2 mm. Larger, exophytic lesions which exceed OCT signal range cannot be identified and require biopsy for confirmation of diagnosis. Secondly, despite the ability to delineate substructural features, most OCT systems lack adequate resolution to resolve cellular (e.g., cellular maturation) and subcellular features (e.g., nuclear pleomorphism). Hence, OCT may not adequately and independently differentiate subtle lesions such as benign dysplasia and carcinoma-in-situ where invasion is not present. Ultra-high resolution OCT systems (axial resolution 1–5 μm) may offer promise for cellular resolution. Lastly, technical issues such as motion artifact (minimized with video-rate imaging speeds), probe stabilization, probe signal strength, and imaging range may all affect OCT image quality.

References

1. American Cancer Society. Cancer facts & figures 2014. Atlanta: American Cancer Society; 2014.
2. Haddad RI, Shin DM. Recent advances in head and neck cancer. N Engl J Med. 2008;359(11):1143–54.
3. Pulte D, Brenner H. Changes in survival in head and neck cancers in the late 20th and early 21st century: a period analysis. Oncologist. 2010;15(9):994–1001.
4. Howlader N, Noone AM, Krapcho M, Garshell J, Miller D, Altekruse SF, Kosary CL, Yu M, Ruhl J, Tatalovich Z, Mariotto A, Lewis DR, Chen HS, Feuer EJ, Cronin KA. Surveillance, Epidemiology, and End Results Program (SEER) Cancer Statistics Review, 1975–2011. 2014 [2014 Sept 10; 2014 Sept 20]. Available from: http://seer.cancer.gov/csr/1975_2011/.
5. Mashberg A, Feldman LJ. Clinical criteria for identifying early oral and oropharyngeal carcinoma: erythroplasia revisited. Am J Surg. 1988;156(4):273–5.
6. Lingen MW, et al. Critical evaluation of diagnostic aids for the detection of oral cancer. Oral Oncol. 2008;44(1):10–22.
7. Huang D, et al. Optical coherence tomography. Science. 1991;254(5035):1178–81.
8. de Boer JF, et al. Improved signal-to-noise ratio in spectral-domain compared with time-domain optical coherence tomography. Opt Lett. 2003;28(21):2067–9.
9. Choma M, et al. Sensitivity advantage of swept source and Fourier domain optical coherence tomography. Opt Express. 2003;11(18): 2183–9.
10. Leitgeb R, Hitzenberger C, Fercher A. Performance of fourier domain vs. time domain optical coherence tomography. Opt Express. 2003;11(8):889–94.
11. de Boer JF, et al. Two-dimensional birefringence imaging in biological tissue by polarization-sensitive optical coherence tomography. Opt Lett. 1997;22(12):934–6.
12. de Boer JF, Milner TE. Review of polarization sensitive optical coherence tomography and Stokes vector determination. J Biomed Opt. 2002;7(3):359–71.
13. Reibel J. Prognosis of oral pre-malignant lesions: significance of clinical, histopathological, and molecular biological characteristics. Crit Rev Oral Biol Med. 2003;14(1):47–62.
14. Walsh T, et al. Clinical assessment to screen for the detection of oral cavity cancer and potentially malignant disorders in apparently healthy adults. Cochrane Database Syst Rev. 2013;11, CD010173.
15. Wilder-Smith P, et al. In vivo optical coherence tomography for the diagnosis of oral malignancy. Lasers Surg Med. 2004;35(4):269–75.
16. Matheny ES, et al. Optical coherence tomography of malignancy in hamster cheek pouches. J Biomed Opt. 2004;9(5):978–81.
17. Wilder-Smith P, et al. Noninvasive imaging of oral premalignancy and malignancy. J Biomed Opt. 2005;10(5):051601.
18. Hanna NM, et al. Feasibility of three-dimensional optical coherence tomography and optical Doppler tomography of malignancy in hamster cheek pouches. Photomed Laser Surg. 2006;24(3):402–9.
19. Graf RN, Brown WJ, Wax A. Parallel frequency-domain optical coherence tomography scatter-mode imaging of the hamster cheek pouch using a thermal light source. Opt Lett. 2008;33(12):1285–7.
20. Graf RN, et al. Detecting precancerous lesions in the hamster cheek pouch using spectroscopic white-light optical coherence tomography to assess nuclear morphology via spectral oscillations. J Biomed Opt. 2009; 14(6):064030.
21. Kim CS, et al. Enhanced detection of early-stage oral cancer in vivo by optical coherence tomography using multimodal delivery of gold nanoparticles. J Biomed Opt. 2009;14(3): 034008.
22. Park J, et al. A dual-modality optical coherence tomography and fluorescence lifetime imaging microscopy system for simultaneous morphological and biochemical tissue characterization. Biomed Opt Express. 2010;1(1):186–200.
23. Ahn YC, et al. Multimodality approach to optical early detection and mapping of oral neoplasia. J Biomed Opt. 2011;16(7):076007.
24. Pande P, et al. Automated classification of optical coherence tomography images for the diagnosis of oral malignancy in the hamster cheek pouch. J Biomed Opt. 2014;19(8):086022.

25. Tsai MT, et al. Delineation of an oral cancer lesion with swept-source optical coherence tomography. J Biomed Opt. 2008;13(4):044012.
26. Jerjes W, et al. In vitro examination of suspicious oral lesions using optical coherence tomography. Br J Oral Maxillofac Surg. 2010;48(1):18–25.
27. Adegun OK, et al. Quantitative analysis of optical coherence tomography and histopathology images of normal and dysplastic oral mucosal tissues. Lasers Med Sci. 2012;27(4): 795–804.
28. Hamdoon Z, et al. Structural validation of oral mucosal tissue using optical coherence tomography. Head Neck Oncol. 2012;4:29.
29. Hamdoon Z, et al. Optical coherence tomography in the assessment of suspicious oral lesions: an immediate ex vivo study. Photodiagnosis Photodyn Ther. 2013;10(1):17–27.
30. Feldchtein F, et al. In vivo OCT imaging of hard and soft tissue of the oral cavity. Opt Express. 1998;3(6):239–50.
31. Ozawa N, et al. In vivo imaging of human labial glands using advanced optical coherence tomography. Oral Surg Oral Med Oral Pathol Oral Radiol Endod. 2009;108(3):425–9.
32. Prestin S, et al. Measurement of epithelial thickness within the oral cavity using optical coherence tomography. Head Neck. 2012; 34(12):1777–81.
33. Lee CK, et al. Diagnosis of oral precancer with optical coherence tomography. Biomed Opt Express. 2012;3(7):1632–46.
34. Volgger V, et al. Evaluation of optical coherence tomography to discriminate lesions of the upper aerodigestive tract. Head Neck. 2013;35(11):1558–66.
35. Chen SF, et al. Oral cancer diagnosis with optical coherence tomography. Conf Proc IEEE Eng Med Biol Soc. 2005;7:7227–9.
36. Ridgway JM, et al. In vivo optical coherence tomography of the human oral cavity and oropharynx. Arch Otolaryngol Head Neck Surg. 2006;132(10):1074–81.
37. Tsai MT, et al. Effective indicators for diagnosis of oral cancer using optical coherence tomography. Opt Express. 2008;16(20):15847–62.
38. Tsai MT, et al. Differentiating oral lesions in different carcinogenesis stages with optical coherence tomography. J Biomed Opt. 2009;14(4):044028.
39. Wilder-Smith P, et al. In vivo diagnosis of oral dysplasia and malignancy using optical coherence tomography: preliminary studies in 50 patients. Lasers Surg Med. 2009;41(5):353–7.
40. Slaughter DP, Southwick HW, Smejkal W. Field cancerization in oral stratified squamous epithelium; clinical implications of multicentric origin. Cancer. 1953;6(5):963–8.
41. Braakhuis BJ, et al. A genetic explanation of Slaughter's concept of field cancerization: evidence and clinical implications. Cancer Res. 2003;63(8):1727–30.
42. Barnes L, Tse L, Hunt JL, Brandwein-Gensler M, Urken M, Slootweg P, Gale N, Cardesa A, Zidar N, Boffetta P. Tumours of the hypopharynx, larynx and trachea: introduction. In: Eveson J, Barnes L, Reichart P, Sidransky D, editors. World health organization classification of tumours. Pathology and genetics of head and neck tumours. Lyon, France: IARC Press; 2005. p. 111–7.
43. Hirano M. Morphological structure of the vocal cord as a vibrator and its variations. Folia Phoniatr (Basel). 1974;26(2):89–94.
44. Zeitels SM. Premalignant epithelium and microinvasive cancer of the vocal fold: the evolution of phonomicrosurgical management. Laryngoscope. 1995;105(3 Pt 2):1–51.
45. Luerssen K, et al. Optical characterization of vocal folds with optical coherence tomography. Photon Ther Diagn. 2005;5686:328–32.
46. Lurssen K, et al. Optical characterization of vocal folds using optical coherence tomography—art. no. 60781O. Photon Ther Diagn II. 2006;6078:O781.
47. Lurssen K, et al. Optical coherence tomography in the diagnosis of vocal folds. HNO. 2006;54(8):611–5.
48. Lueerssen K, et al. Optical characterization of vocal folds by OCT-based laryngoscopy—art. no. 64241O. Photon Ther Diagn III. 2007;6424:O4241.
49. Bibas AG, et al. 3-D optical coherence tomography of the laryngeal mucosa. Clin Otolaryngol Allied Sci. 2004;29(6):713–20.
50. Burns JA, et al. Imaging the mucosa of the human vocal fold with optical coherence tomography. Ann Otol Rhinol Laryngol. 2005;114(9):671–6.
51. Sergeev A, et al. In vivo endoscopic OCT imaging of precancer and cancer states of human mucosa. Opt Express. 1997;1(13):432–40.
52. Klein AM, et al. Imaging the human vocal folds in vivo with optical coherence tomography: a preliminary experience. Ann Otol Rhinol Laryngol. 2006;115(4):277–84.
53. Sepehr A, et al. Optical coherence tomography of the larynx in the awake patient. Otolaryngol Head Neck Surg. 2008;138(4):425–9.

54. Shakhov AV, et al. Optical coherence tomography monitoring for laser surgery of laryngeal carcinoma. J Surg Oncol. 2001;77(4):253–8.
55. Armstrong WB, et al. Optical coherence tomography of laryngeal cancer. Laryngoscope. 2006;116(7):1107–13.
56. Kraft M, et al. Technique of optical coherence tomography of the larynx during microlaryngoscopy. Laryngoscope. 2007;117(5):950–2.
57. Kraft M, et al. Clinical value of optical coherence tomography in laryngology. Head Neck. 2008;30(12):1628–35.
58. Kraft M, et al. Significance of optical coherence tomography in the assessment of laryngeal lesions—art. no. 68421O. Photo Ther Diagn IV. 2008;6842:O8421.
59. Rubinstein M, et al. Optical coherence tomography of the larynx using the Niris system. J Otolaryngol Head Neck Surg. 2010;39(2):150–6.
60. Just T, et al. Optical coherence tomography allows for the reliable identification of laryngeal epithelial dysplasia and for precise biopsy: a clinicopathological study of 61 patients undergoing microlaryngoscopy. Laryngoscope. 2010;120(10):1964–70.
61. Vokes DE, et al. Optical coherence tomography-enhanced microlaryngoscopy: preliminary report of a noncontact optical coherence tomography system integrated with a surgical microscope. Ann Otol Rhinol Laryngol. 2008;117(7):538–47.
62. Guo S, et al. Office-based optical coherence tomographic imaging of human vocal cords. J Biomed Opt. 2006;11(3):30501.

Chapter 37

Early Detection and Diagnosis of Oral Premalignant Squamous Mucosal Lesions

Nadarajah Vigneswaran and Adel K. El-Naggar

Background

Head and neck squamous cell carcinoma (SCC) arises from the squamous mucosal lining of the oral cavity, oropharynx, and larynx and is the sixth most common cancer with an estimated 500,000 new cases diagnosed annually worldwide [1]. SCC of the oral cavity accounts for ~15 % of all head and neck malignancies, leading to 7000 deaths per year in the USA [2, 3]. Risk factors for oral SCC include smoking and chewing tobacco, betel quid, heavy alcohol consumption, and chewing. Recently, a new category of SCC that typically affects the oropharyngeal mucosa and caused by human papillomavirus (HPV) has been recognized [4]. The tongue is the most common site for oral cancer among European and US populations, accounting for 40–50 % of oral cancers [2, 5], and the buccal mucosa is the most common site of the Indian subcontinent due to betel quid/tobacco chewing habits [5]. In the Indian subcontinent and neighboring countries, oral cancer ranks first in prevalence among all cancers in males and third in females [5]. In south-central Asia, oral cancer is one of the three most common types of cancer. Recent epidemiologic data shows sharp increases in the incidence of oral cancer reported in European countries, and to a lesser extent, the USA. Morbidity and mortality from oral cancer are strongly dependent on the stage at diagnosis, with the average survival rate decreasing from 80 %, when the tumors are limited to the primary site, to 50 % for tumors with regional metastatic disease and to 30 % for metastatic disease [2, 3]. In the USA, there has been only marginal improvement in the 5-year survival rates for oral cancer since 1975.

Brian J.-F. Wong and Justus Ilgner (eds.), *Biomedical Optics in Otorhinolaryngology: Head and Neck Surgery*, DOI 10.1007/978-1-4939-1758-7_37, © Springer Science+Business Media New York 2016

Early diagnosis of oral cancer significantly reduces treatment-related morbidity and improves overall long-term survival [6, 7]. Patients with oral cancers are at risk of developing second primary tumors and one-fourth of all oral cancer-related deaths are caused by second primary tumors [8]. Moreover, in developing countries, oral cancer patients tend to be diagnosed at a later stage than in developed countries. Early detection one of the best effective means to improve survival and quality of life for oral cancer patients worldwide. Therefore, close surveillance of patients who were successfully treated for oral cancer is critical for early detection of recurrences and/or second primaries. It is widely realized that screening high-risk populations and the early detection of oral cancer and its precursors are critical to combat this cancer.

The stated objectives of the International Agency for Research on Cancer, American Cancer Society, and WHO is to reduce by one third of the predicted 15 million cancer cases by detecting and treating these cancers at their preneoplastic levels [9]. Oral cancer is an ideal subject for this strategy for the following reasons: (1) oral cavity provides easy access for clinical inspection and (2) oral cancer development is preceded by visible mucosal changes [10]. The goal of oral cancer screening is to predict potentially pregresive early lesions and to provide more timely interventions to reduce morbidity and mortality.

Screening for Oral Cancer Individuals risks for developing oral cancer are determined based on the length of tobacco and alcohol use. Oral cancer screening is based on a practitioner assessment of asymptomatic individual to determine if he or she is likely to have an oral cancer or its precursors [11]. Screening for oral cancer can be population based, or through screening of patients attending a healthcare provider on routine visits [12].

An effective screening program must address three critical issues: (1) Do early detection and intervention improve outcome? (2) Is the screening test practical and reproducible? (3) Feasibility and cost of implementing a screening program [13]. Oral cancer is an ideal target for early detection screening. Therefore, the detection of early lesions by clinical examination in high-risk patients may lead to substantial reduction in the incidence of oral SCC. The United States Preventive Services Task Force (USPSTF) recently concluded that for adults 18 years or older attending a primary care setting, the "current evidence is insufficient to assess the balance of benefits and harms of screening for oral cancer in asymptomatic adults." There is, however, strong and empirical evidence for the efficacy of oral cancer screening that is further supported by the input from clinical specialists who deal with the diagnosis and treatment of oral cancer in the USA. Accordingly, *Evidence-Based Clinical Recommendations Regarding Screening for Oral Squamous*

Cell Carcinomas, published by the American Dental Association (ADA) Council on Scientific Affairs, supports routine visual and tactile examination for oral cancer screening and its precursors in high-risk patients [11]. For successful programs, therefore, all oral healthcare professionals should be knowledgeable of the oral cancer risk factors, its precursors, and their mimics in order to perform an effective oral cancer screening. Moreover, although clinical examination and histologic assessment of the abnormal lesions remain the main methods for screening and early diagnosis of oral cancer, these methods are not widely available and costly for an effective screening program. New noninvasive tools for rapid and affordable screening and early diagnosis are emerging. Accordingly, the combined application of these new techniques with conventional methods will lead to substantial improvement in this field.

Oral Cancer Precursors

Similar to common solid epithelial malignancies, oral squamous cell carcinoma development is a multistep process often preceded by precursors which are commonly known as precancerous or premalignant lesions. The expert working group of WHO Collaborating Center for Oral Cancer and Precancer on the terminology, definitions, and classifications recently recommended the use of the term “potentially malignant disorder (PMD)” that includes premalignant lesions and conditions that have increased risk for malignant transformation [14]. Premalignant lesions are defined as morphologically altered oral mucosae in which oral cancer is more likely to develop and include leukoplakia, erythroplakia, and palatal keratoses [14, 15]. Premalignant conditions are oral cavity states that are associated with a substantially increased risk for oral cancer and include actinic keratosis, oral submucous fibrosis, and lichen planus [14].

Risk factors including tobacco and alcohol abuse are commonly associated with the development of white (leukoplakia) or red (erythroplakia) patches or plaques. Although the majority of leukpllakia are non-progressive a subset of these lesions often progress and develop invasive squamous carcinoma. Currently, there are no known precursor lesions for HPV-associated oropharyngeal cancer [16].

Premalignant Lesions

(a) **Leukoplakia:** Leukoplakia is the most common and best-known clinically recognizable oral mucosal abnormalities PMD, accounting for 85 % of all oral premalignant lesions (Figs. 1, 2, 3 and 6). On visual basis, leukoplakia is defined as

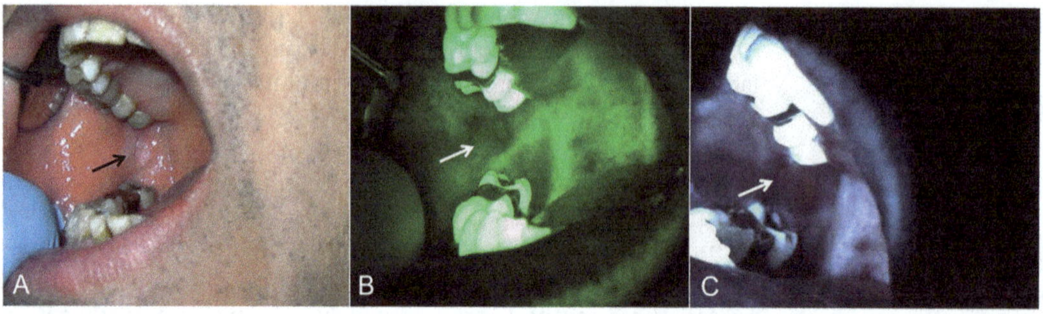

Fig. 1 Comparison of an oral mucosal lesion with images of two commercially available tissue autofluorescence visualization devices. (**a**) Physical appearance by oral examination leukoplakia (*arrow* posterior buccal mucosa). (**b**) Autofluorescence visualization (*arrows*) using VELscope and (**c**) Identafi 3000 visualization of loss of fluorescence (*dark area*)

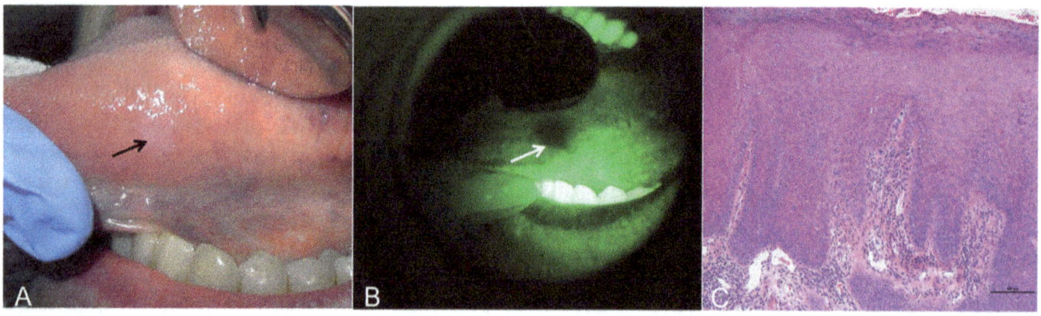

Fig. 2 (**a**) Faintly visible leukoplakia (*arrow*) in the left lateral surface of the tongue. (**b**) Autofluorescence imaging of the same lesion using VELscope with loss of fluorescence (*arrow*). (**c**) Mild hyperkeratotic dysplasia on microscopic examination (×100)

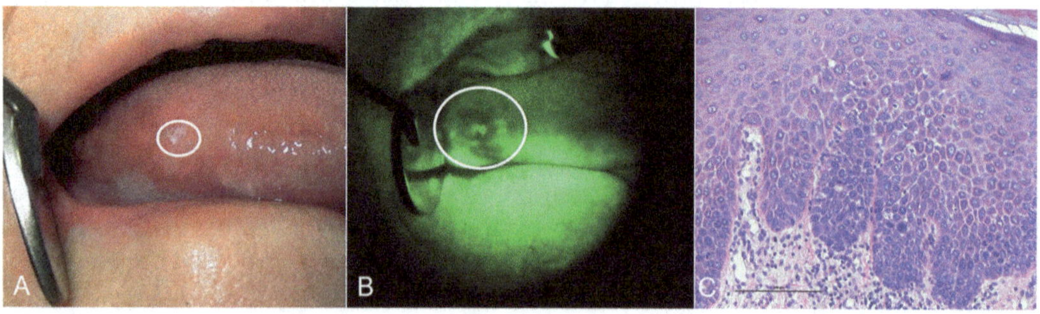

Fig. 3 (**a**) Localized leukoplakia (*white circle*) in the right posterior lateral surface of the tongue. (**b**) Autofluorescence imaging of the same lesion using VELscope demonstrates loss of fluorescence extending to a larger area (*white circle*) beyond that seen on visual examination. (**c**) Moderate dysplasia by microscopic examination (×100)

Table 1
Clinical conditions with overlapping gross features with leukoplakia

Reactive and infectious	Hereditary conditions	Systemic diseases
Frictional keratosis	Leukoedema	Lichen/lichenoid lesions
Dentifrice desquamation	Hereditary benign/dyskeratosis	Hairy leukoplakia (AIDS)
Nicotine stomatitis	White sponge nevus	Lupus erythematosus
Smokeless tobacco keratosis	Dyskeratosis congenita	O
Submucous fibrosis	O	O
Hyperplastic candidiasis	O	O

a white patch or plaque that cannot be rubbed off and cannot be diagnosed clinically or histopathologically to any specific disease [17]. Hereditary-, reactive-, infectious-, and immune-mediated disorders presenting as intraoral white patches or plaques mimicking leukoplakia are listed in Table 1 [17]. Therefore, leukoplakic lesions that persist for more than 1 month despite conventional treatment should be subjected to histologic evaluation. The risk of malignant transformation of leukoplakias varies markedly and is dependent on the following factors:

- Etiology (smoking and/or alcohol use versus idiopathic)
- Clinical presentation
- Location
- The presence and degree of dysplasia

In rare instances, patients may present with leukoplakia without history of known risk factors and is considered as idiopathic leukoplakia. [18].

Leukoplakias most frequently occur at a single site (localized leukoplakia) and are more common in men and are associated with smoking. Localized leukoplakias presenting at a single site have two distinct clinical forms, namely, homogenous and nonhomogenous types, which are classified based on their visual appearance. Homogenous leukoplakias are uniformly white flat (patch) or slightly raised (plaque) lesions and exhibit a low malignant transformation risk. Nonhomogenous leukoplakias have a verrucous/granular surface, with or without red zones (speckled leukoplakia or erythroleukoplakia), and have a higher risk for malignant transformation than homogenous leukoplakias. The intraoral site of the leukoplakia is a critical factor in determining its malignant transformation risk. In the USA and other Western countries, leukoplakias in

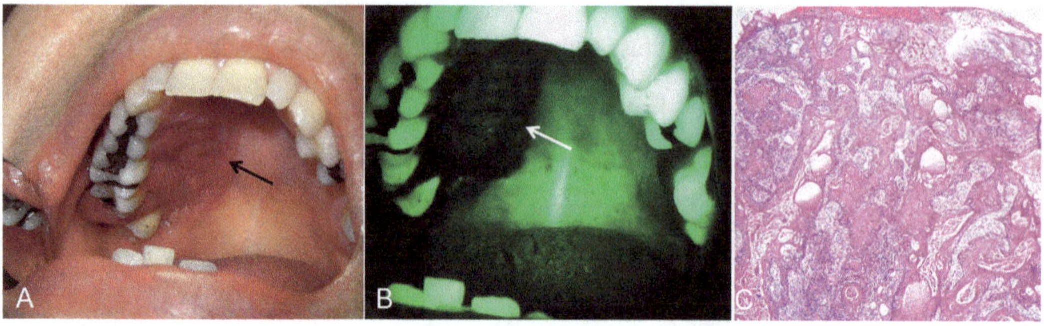

Fig. 4 (**a**) Erythroplakia (*arrow*) of the right hard palate. (**b**) Autofluorescence imaging of the same lesion by VELscope, complete loss of fluorescence in the lesion (*arrow*). (**c**) Invasive squamous carcinoma by microscopic examination (×100)

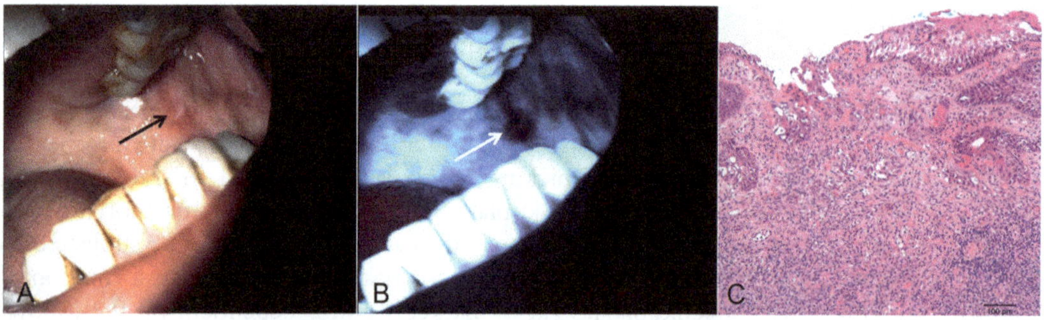

Fig. 5 (**a**) Oral submucous fibrosis with a focal erythroplakia (*arrow*) in the left posterior buccal mucosa. (**b**) Tissue autofluorescence imaging of the same lesion by Identafi 3000, complete loss of fluorescence at the erythroplakia (*arrow*) in contrast to adjacent mucosa affected by submucous fibrosis with enhanced fluorescence. (**c**) Superficially invasive squamous carcinoma by microscopic examination (×100)

the floor of the mouth, soft palate, and lateral/ventral surfaces of tongue have the highest risk for malignant transformation. Overall, 9–37 % of leukoplakias are expected to show either dysplasia or carcinoma in situ and/or invasive carcinoma at the time of biopsy.

(b) **Erythroplakia:** Erythroplakia is definitely a preinvasive phase of oral mucosal lesions. It presents as a well-defined red, raised velvety plaque that cannot be characterized clinically as any other disease (Figs. 4, 5 and 7) [17]. Oral mucosal conditions that may clinically resemble erythroplakia are listed in Table 2. Erythroplakias frequently occur in older adults in the floor of the mouth, ventral tongue, and soft palate. Frequently, erythroplakias are associated with adjacent leukoplakias (erythroleukoplakia) in geographic and multifocal oral leukoplakia. For accurate diagnosis, biopsies must be taken from the erythroplakic areas. Histopathologically, full thickness dysplasia of the squamous epithelium must be present.

Table 2
Clinical conditions mimicking erythroplakia

Reactive and infectious	Neoplastic/others	Systemic disorders
Erythematous candidiasis	Hemangioma	Atrophic lichen planus
Allergic contact mucositis	Kaposi's sarcoma, plaque form	Lupus erythematosus
Erythema migrans, tongue	Telangiectasia/purpose	Mucous membrane pemphigoid

Premalignant Conditions

(a) **Proliferative verrucous leukoplakia:** A rare clinical condition characterized by multifocal, proliferative, and progressive biological course. PVL commonly begins as a simple keratosis that eventually becomes verrucous and multifocal involving large contiguous sites [19]. PVL is more common in elderly women, frequently involves the gingiva, and is not associated with either smoking or alcohol abuse. PVL tends to be persistent and frequently recurs even after surgical removal. PVL are high-risk lesions as almost 60–100 % evolve into carcinoma over 10–20 years. Moreover, PVL generally lacks specific morphologic features, including the classical microscopic features of epithelial dysplasia, making PVL specifically a clinical diagnosis. Clinically and microscopically, PVL may mimic the plaque variant of lichen planus because of its multifocal involvement and frequent presentation of lichenoid inflammation in the biopsy [20]. Definitive diagnosis depends on a keen observation of lesional progression and close communication between clinicians and pathologists.

(b) **Oral submucous fibrosis(OSF):** OSF is considered a premalignant condition that is more prevalent among the South Asian population with the highest incidence in the Indian subcontinent (Fig. 5). OSF is a chronic, progressive condition characterized by diffuse mucosal rigidity due to dense fibrosis within the lamina propria and might extend into the underlying skeletal muscle. It is caused by chewing betel quid containing the areca nut. The extent and severity of this disorder are dependent on the amount of areca nut in the betel quid and duration and frequency of this habit. Oral submucous fibrosis frequently involves the buccal mucosa, tongue, and soft palate. The affected mucosal surfaces appear pale and blanching marble-like with focal areas of atrophy and erythema (Fig. 5). Patients are commonly present with trismus, burning sensation, and xerostomia; difficulties in speech, mastication, and swallowing are experienced at the advanced stages. The incidence of malignant transformation of this condition is 8–12 % over the period of 10–15 years [21].

(c) **Oral lichen planus:** Lichen planus is the most common chronic autoimmune inflammatory disorder of oral mucosa that affects 1–2 % of middle-aged adults. It is more common among females and tends to have multifocal lesions, often bilateral and symmetric in distribution. It frequently involves buccal mucosa, gingiva, and tongue. Based on the clinical presentation, the following clinical variants of lichen planus are recognized:

- *Reticular variant (classic pattern)*: White striations and/or papules, asymptomatic, occur frequently in the buccal mucosa.
- *Plaque variant:* Thick white plaque clinically resembling leukoplakia, asymptomatic, occurs frequently in the dorsal surface of the tongue.
- *Erythematous/erosive variant:* Diffuse red areas with focal areas of mucosal erosions and atrophy are painful and frequently occur in the gingiva (desquamative gingivitis).
- *Ulcerative/bullous variant:* Diffuse red and white patches with a central, chronic, nonhealing ulcer are frequently seen in the lateral and ventral surfaces of the tongue and buccal mucosa.

The malignant potential of oral lichen planus, although controversial, is considered to be low with a rate of 1 % over a 5-year period [22]. Oral lichenoid dysplasia may exhibit a chronic inflammatory cell infiltrate consisting of mostly lymphocytes that resembles the chronic inflammation seen in lichen planus; however, it has accompanying epithelial cellular alterations consistent with dysplasia [23, 24]. Moreover, the plaque variant of lichen planus and PVL may also share similar clinical and microscopic features, leading to a misdiagnosis of lichen planus [19].

(d) **Fanconi anemia and dyskeratosis congenita:** Fanconi anemia (FA; MIM 227650) and dyskeratosis congenita (DC; MIM 30500,127550, 224230) are two hereditary cancer syndromes that predispose to oral cancer at an early age. FA is a chromosomal instability disorder inherited as an autosomal or X-chromosomal recessive trait due to germ line mutations in one of 15 FA genes involved in the DNA repair pathway, resulting in increased risks for bone marrow failure, leukemia, and solid malignancies [25]. Oral cancer is the most frequently diagnosed solid cancer in FA patients. The risk of oral cancer among FA patients is 800-fold higher than in the general population and occurs at a younger age (median age, 27 years) than the general population [26, 27]. Frequent oral screenings in FA patients for premalignant lesions are essential to try and reduce morbidity from OSCC. Similar to FA, DC is also an inherited bone marrow failure disorder caused by defects in telomere maintenance [28]. Oral cancer is the most common solid malignancy seen in patients with DC. The tongue is the most common site for oral cancer in both FA and DC patients [29]. Hence, semiannual examination for oral cancer is recommended for both FA and DC patients beginning at a very young age.

Methods for Screening and Diagnosis of Potentially Malignant Disorders of Oral Mucosa

PMD of oral mucosa is considered as class I lesions, in contrast to other benign oral mucosal mimics PMD that are defined as class II lesions (Tables 1 and 2) are the potentially progressive lesion [30]. The oral cavity is the site of the highest prevalence for the presence of confounding lesions compared to other anatomic sites [17]. In that context, screening is not a confirmatory test for the presence of cancer or its precursor, while diagnosis by histopathologic examination of tissue is a case-finding test in individual with suspected PMD [30]. Studies of screening (detection) and diagnosis (case finding) of oral cancer and its precursors have been frequently used interchangeably which may lead to blurring the distinction between the oral cancer screening and diagnostic aids to properly assess their respective effectiveness.

Screening

Oral cancer screening by conventional oral examination under white light by a trained oral healthcare provider remains the main acceptable practice (Table 3). The gold standard for establishing the diagnosis (case finding) of oral cancer and its precursors also continues to be based on tissue sampling of suspected PMD using a scalpel biopsy for microscopic examination (Table 3). Although conventional oral examination has been shown to have a high discriminatory ability in distinguishing normal and abnormal oral mucosal patterns [31], the majority of the oral mucosal lesions detected through COE in asymptomatic patients are considered class II lesions. Visual oral examination is known for poor sensitivity and specificity in discriminating class I lesions from class II lesions leading to either delay in the diagnosis of class I lesions or unnecessary biopsies of innocuous class II lesions (Table 4) [32]. Such examination is frequently aided by the use of a dye toluidine blue. **Toluidine blue** is a vital dye that has been used in the oral cavity for decades to improve visibility of lesions during visual

Table 3
Current screening and diagnosis of potentially malignant oral mucosa lesions

Screening and diagnosis of potentially malignant disorders of oral mucosa
Screening: Evaluation of an asymptomatic high-risk individuals for presence of PMD
Current: Clinical oral examination
Adjunctive optical devices:
• Reflectance based
• Autofluorescence based
Diagnosis:
Standard: histopathologic examination
Adjunctive predictive markers:
• LOH
• TP53 mutations • DNA aneuploidy

Table 4
Sensitivity and specificity of currently available screening and detection techniques for oral cancer and its precursors

Diagnostic reliability	Oral examination	Toluidine blue	Optical imaging	
			Tissue reflectance	Tissue autofluorescence
Sensitivity	60–93 %	38–98 %	0–100 %	50–100 %
Specificity	31–99 %	9–93 %	0–75 %	15–74 %

exam. A recent review of the performance of visual exam with toluidine blue sensitivity ranged from 38 to 98 %, while specificity varied from 9 to 93 % [9]. In general, examination with toluidine blue is associated with low specificity, and this has prevented toluidine blue from becoming a standard component of early oral cancer detection efforts in the USA.

Community-based dentists and physicians do not have the clinical training and experience to distinguish PMD from their mimics; hence, many of these patients need to be referred to a specialist for scalpel biopsy for a definitive diagnosis. Referring patients with PMD to specialist centers is confounded by a long waiting time and significant diagnostic delays [33]. Therefore, the development of an oral cancer screening device that can reliably discriminate PMDs from their mimics, as an alternative to visual examination by specialists, will not only eliminate unnecessary biopsies but also facilitate early detection in high-risk populations for developing oral cancer.

Optical Screening Aids Based on Tissue Reflectance and Autofluorescence

Optical imaging techniques are currently being developed as adjunct to conventional oral examination for noninvasive and instantaneous detection of PMD [9, 34, 35]. Devices for optical scanning of oral cavity are increasingly used in community dental clinics as adjuncts to standard oral examination for oral cancer screening. Detail descriptions of the optical oral cancer screening devices and their efficacy and limitations are reviewed in several published reports [9, 30]. The ViziLite (Zila Pharmaceuticals, Inc., Phoenix, AZ) is a disposable chemiluminescent light source that illuminates tissue with blue light to detect abnormal changes in the oral cavity. Initial studies conducted by Epstein et al. and Kerr et al. indicated that the ViziLite could potentially aid in detection of oral premalignant lesions by improving brightness and sharpness [9]. However, other studies have reported that ViziLite does not aid in the identification of oral lesions [9]. These studies concluded that ViziLite examination could not discriminate between benign or inflammatory and premalignant or malignant oral lesions.

Commercially available autofluorescence-based oral cancer screening devices include VELscope® (Visually Enhanced Lesion Scope; LED Dental Inc., White Rock, BC, Canada), Identafi 3000 (DentalEZ group, Malvern, PA, USA), and OralID (OralID, Houston, Texas, USA). All optical devices employ a special light source to illuminate oral mucosal surfaces with either blue/violet light (VELscope, 400–460 nM) or blue light (Identify and OralID, 405 nM). Oral epithelium and stroma absorb high-energy photons (short wavelength, 400–460 nm visible light) for excitation and emit a green (VELscope) or blue (Identify and OralID) fluorescence spectra at longer wavelengths (Fig. 1) [17]. The examiner can directly view the autofluorescence emitted by the normal tissue with the use of a longpass to block the reflected light. Epithelial fluorescence is produced by NADH, FAD, and keratin, whereas stromal florescence is primarily derived from collagen fibers with cross-links and elastin. Tissue autofluorescence emission can be affected by absorption and scattering of the excitation light by oxy- and deoxyhemoglobin and enlarged and crowded cellular nuclei. Alterations in the optical properties of oral mucosal pathoses reflect the changes in their metabolic, biochemical, and structural properties. Normal oral mucosa emits a pale green or blue autofluorescence, whereas lesional mucosa shows loss of autofluorescence and appears dark (Fig. 1). The majority of PMDs display loss of autofluorescence due to their altered metabolic activity and cellular and tissue architecture and appear dark brown or black compared to adjacent healthy tissue with blue or green fluorescence (Figs. 1–5).

Tissue autofluorescence imaging is a valuable method to screen and detect PMD with subtle mucosal changes or those that appear clinically occult on white light examination (Fig. 2). Fluorescence visualization is also very useful for discerning the extent of a lesion involvement, selecting optimal biopsy sites, and aiding intraoperative surgical margins (Fig. 3). Loss of tissue autofluorescence is not observed in benign and nonneoplastic oral mucosal lesions which frequently exhibit fluorescence spectra similar to the adjacent uninvolved mucosa (Fig. 6). Tissue autofluorescence visualization is more effective than conventional oral examination in finding suspicious oral mucosal lesions; however, it demonstrates a low specificity in discriminating high-risk PMD from low-risk lesions due to the higher rate of false positivity associated with benign inflammatory, ulcerative, highly vascular, and pigmented oral mucosal lesions (Figs. 7 and 8). Although rare, autofluorescence visualization may yield false-negative results in highly keratinized (i.e., proliferative verrucous leukoplakia) or fibrotic (i.e., oral submucous fibrosis) PMD because of the enhanced autofluorescence produced by the thick surface keratin or excess stromal collagen deposition (Figs. 5 and 9). Oral mucosal lesions with surface bacterial and fungal (i.e., candidosis) colonization may exhibit an altered red-to-orange autofluorescence impeding the interpretation of their visual fluorescent examination test results (Fig. 10). Understanding how tissue factors alter the fluorescence spectra and its limitations is critical for proper use of tissue autofluorescence imaging devices in clinical practice (Table 5). Similarly, awareness of the clinical conditions with overlapping imaging spectrum is critical to proper differential diagnostic evaluation.

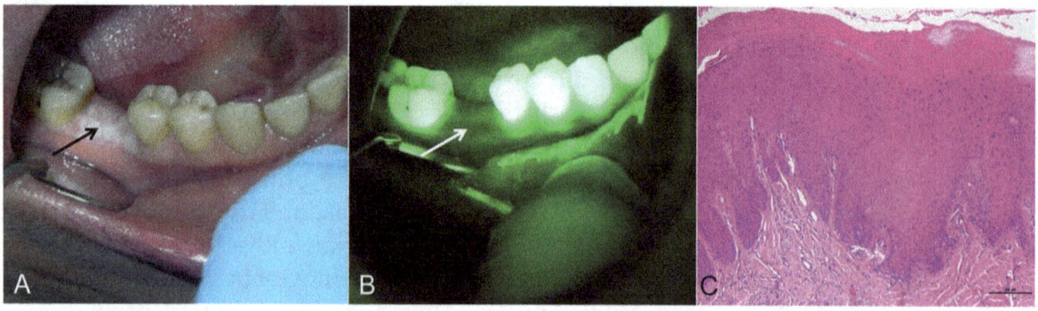

Fig. 6 (**a**) Leukoplakia-like (*arrow*) in the right edentulous mandibular alveolar mucosa. (**b**) VELscope imaging of the same lesion with no loss of fluorescence (*arrow*). (**c**) Epithelial hyperplasia and hyperkeratosis by microscopic examination (×100)

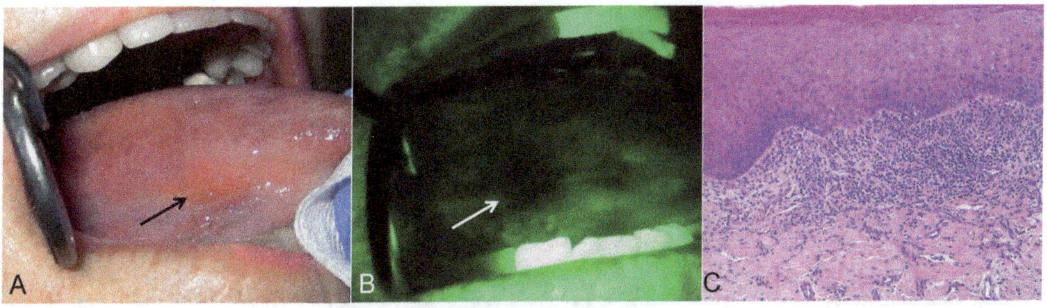

Fig. 7 (**a**) Visual examination reveals an erythroplakia (*arrow*) of the right lateral surface of the tongue. (**b**) VELscope imaging of the lesion shows loss of fluorescence as a false-positive reading. (**c**) Hyperplasia and hyperkeratosis with chronic lichenoid mucositis without dysplasia (×100)

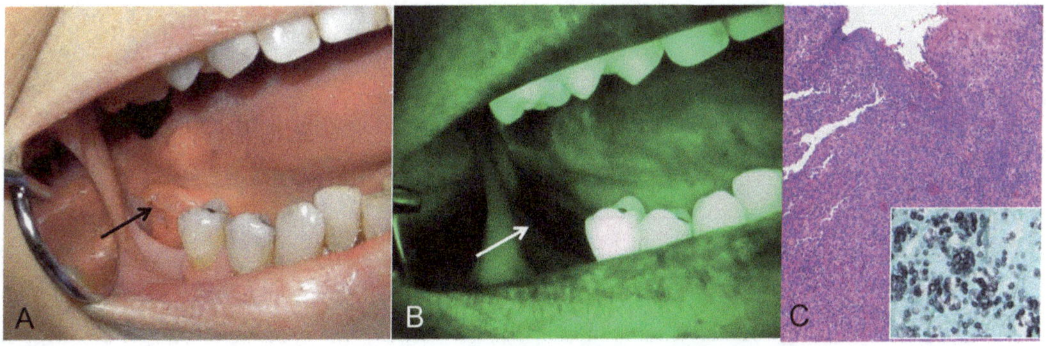

Fig. 8 (**a**) A nonhealing ulcer (*arrow*) in the right floor of the mouth clinically suspicious for cancer. (**b**) VELscope imaging of the same lesion shows (*arrow*) loss of fluorescence as a false-positive reading. (**c**) Microscopic examination of the ulcer showed histoplasmosis (×200)

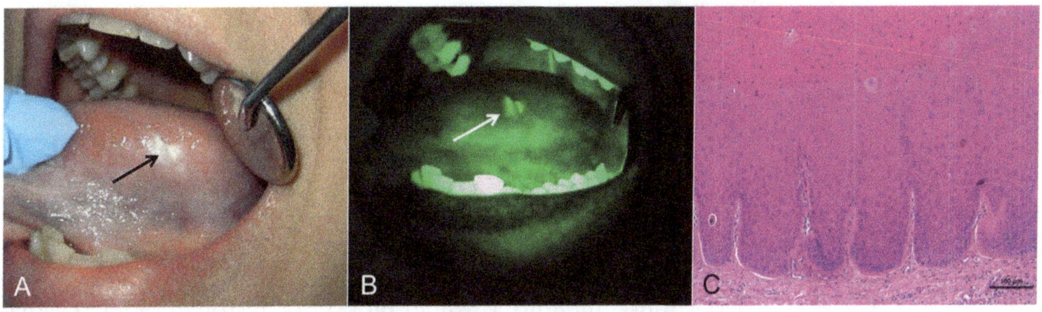

Fig. 9 (**a**) Leukoplakia (*arrow*) of the left posterior lateral tongue. (**b**) VELscope imaging revealing (*arrow*) no loss of fluorescence as a false-negative reading. (**c**) Microscopic examination of the leukoplakia showed epithelia hyperkeratosis and hyperplasia with mild dysplasia (×100)

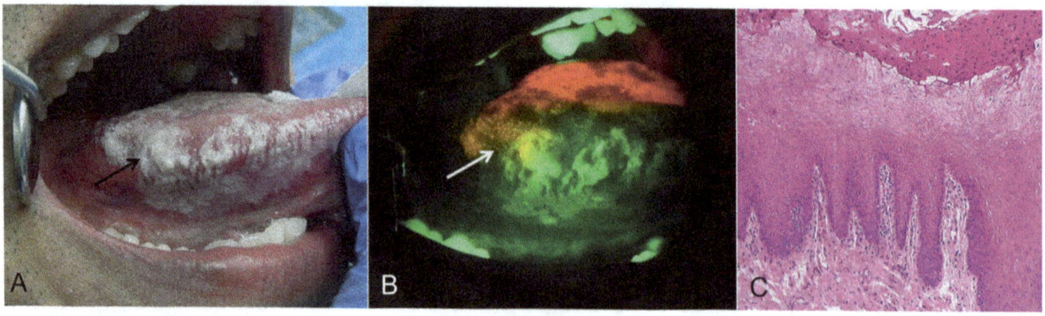

Fig. 10 Porphyrin-related red-to-orange autofluorescence due to surface bacterial/fungal (candidosis) colonization. (**a**) A leukoplakia in the lateral and ventral surface of the tongue in an HIV-positive male. (**b**) VELscope imaging of the same lesion demonstrates red-to-orange autofluorescence. (**c**) Microscopic examination of the leukoplakia showed epithelial hyperkeratosis and hyperplasia without dysplasia (×100). Ancillary histochemical and immunohistochemical studies confirmed the diagnosis of oral hairy leukoplakia and candidiasis

Table 5
Effects of tissue changes in autofluorescence

Histologic assessment	Autofluorescence feature
Epithelial hyperplasia	No change
Dysplasia	Complete or partial loss
Invasive carcinoma	Complete loss
Verruciform hyperkeratosis	No change or increase
Infectious	Complete or partial loss
Vascular lesions	Complete or partial loss
Submucous fibrosis	Enhanced
Amalgam pigmentation (tattoo)	Complete loss
Focal melanosis	Complete loss
Hairy leukoplakia/candidiasis	Red-to-orange spectrum

Diagnosis of Oral Epithelial Dysplasia

PMDs must undergo a scalpel biopsy for histopathologic evaluation. This is central to the assessment of the potential malignant transformation risk and the appropriate therapeutic management. Microscopically, these lesions may demonstrate epithelial hyperplasia and hyperkeratosis, various stages of dysplasia, and invasive SCC (Fig. 11). As oral epithelial dysplasia is a microscopic diagnosis of precancer, without a specific clinical appearance, this term should

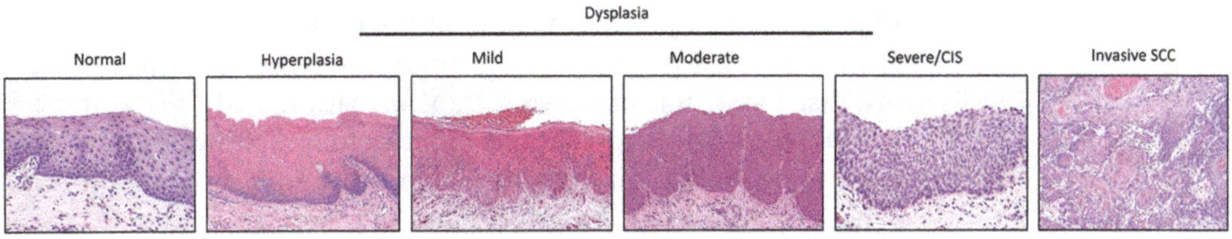

Fig. 11 Multistep progression oral squamous cell carcinoma with corresponding histopathologic findings of hyperplasia, dysplasias of different severities, and invasive squamous cell carcinoma

not be used as a clinical description. Pathologically the term "epithelial atypia" is not synonymous with oral epithelial dysplasia and its use should be restricted to epithelial changes not meeting the definition of dysplasia. An example of "epithelial atypia" is reactive and regenerative epithelial changes associated with inflammation adjacent to an ulcer. Hence, the use of the term "epithelial atypia" as a microscopic diagnosis for PMD may lead to confusion and should be avoided.

Both cellular and architectural alterations of the oral squamous epithelium are evaluated for grading oral epithelial dysplasia. However, microscopic evaluation of these features unexperienced professional combo subjective and associated with significant inter- and intra-observer variations in grading oral epithelial dysplasia. The malignant transformation rate of oral epithelial dysplasia varies considerably, ranging from 6 to 50 % (mild dysplasia, 0–5 %; moderate dysplasia, 3–15 %; severe dysplasia: 7–50 %) [36], that a significant proportion of benign hyperkeratoses without dysplasia have progressed to cancer. This may suggest a tendency for underdiagnosing dysplasia in PVL patients secondary to the lack of specific cytological features associated with dysplasia.

Although pathologic diagnosis of oral epithelial dysplasia may not imply definitive progression to cancer, it is the only reliable method for identifying potentially progressive PMD. Histologic grading of oral epithelial dysplasia, therefore, remains the standard method to determine the presence of cellular dysplasia prognosis and to make treatment recommendation for these lesions. Currently, there are no reliable and reproducible molecular or genetic biomarkers that are superior to the diagnosis alone of oral epithelial dysplasia in predicting malignant transformation risks to carcinoma. Although, p53 mutations, loss of heterozygosity (LOH), and DNA ploidy analysis have been reported to predict the malignant transformation risk of PMD, neither of these techniques have been adopted in the clinical practice [37]. Loss of heterozygosity at chromosome 3p and/or chromosome 9p increases the malignant transformation risk of oral epithelial dysplasias by 22.6-fold compared to dysplastic lesions with 3p and 9p retention.

Oral epithelial dysplasias with additional loss of heterozygosity on chromosome arms 4q and chromosome 17p reveal a 41.7-fold increased risk for malignant transformation [38]. In summary, PMD with dysplasias should be carefully followed or excised depending on the clinical situation, on the site of the lesion (high versus low-risk sites), and associated risk factors.

In summary, detection of oral cancer at its precursor level is of great clinical significance in reducing the oral cancer-related mortality and morbidity. Visual examination by an experienced clinician followed by biopsy is the current standard of care for detection of oral cancer or its precursors. However, visual examination cannot discriminate epithelial alterations specific for malignant progression from nonneoplastic oral mucosal alterations. Hence, new optical imaging devices are being developed for noninvasive and instantaneous detection of potentially malignant oral mucosal lesions in a highly sensitive and specific manner. Unlike visual examination, optical imaging techniques are sensitive in detecting biochemical, metabolic, and architectural alterations of neoplastic progression and hence are valuable for early detection of oral malignancies.

References

1. Ferlay J, Shin HR, Bray F, Forman D, Mathers C, Parkin DM. Estimates of worldwide burden of cancer in 2008: GLOBOCAN 2008. Int J Cancer. 2010;127(12):2893–917.
2. Chen AY, Myers JN. Cancer of the oral cavity. Dis Mon. 2001;47(7):275–361.
3. Marur S, Forastiere AA. Head and neck cancer: changing epidemiology, diagnosis, and treatment. Mayo Clin Proc. 2008;83(4):489–501.
4. Vidal L, Gillison ML. Human papillomavirus in HNSCC: recognition of a distinct disease type. Hematol Oncol Clin North Am. 2008; 22(6):1125–42. vii.
5. Warnakulasuriya S. Global epidemiology of oral and oropharyngeal cancer. Oral Oncol. 2009;45(4–5):309–16.
6. Dolan RW, Vaughan CW, Fuleihan N. Symptoms in early head and neck cancer: an inadequate indicator. Otolaryngol Head Neck Surg. 1998;119(5):463–7.
7. Vernham GA, Crowther JA. Head and neck carcinoma--stage at presentation. Clin Otolaryngol Allied Sci. 1994;19(2):120–4.
8. Day GL, Blot WJ. Second primary tumors in patients with oral cancer. Cancer. 1992; 70(1):14–9.
9. Shin D, Vigneswaran N, Gillenwater A, Richards-Kortum R. Advances in fluorescence imaging techniques to detect oral cancer and its precursors. Future Oncol. 2010;6(7): 1143–54.
10. Scott SE, Grunfeld EA, McGurk M. The idiosyncratic relationship between diagnostic delay and stage of oral squamous cell carcinoma. Oral Oncol. 2005;41(4):396–403.
11. Rethman MP, Carpenter W, Cohen EE, et al. Evidence-based clinical recommendations regarding screening for oral squamous cell carcinomas. J Am Dent Assoc. 2010;141(5): 509–20.
12. Brocklehurst P, Kujan O, Glenny AM, et al. Screening programmes for the early detection and prevention of oral cancer. Cochrane Database Syst Rev. 2010;11:CD004150.
13. Rose G, Barker DJ. Epidemiology for the uninitiated. Screening. Br Med J. 1978;2(6149): 1417–8.
14. Warnakulasuriya S, Johnson NW, van der Waal I. Nomenclature and classification of potentially malignant disorders of the oral mucosa. J Oral Pathol Med. 2007;36(10):575–80.
15. van der Eb MM, Leyten EM, Gavarasana S, Vandenbroucke JP, Kahn PM, Cleton FJ. Reverse smoking as a risk factor for palatal cancer: a cross-sectional study in rural Andhra Pradesh, India. Int J Cancer. 1993;54(5):754–8.
16. Caporaso NE. Why precursors matter. Cancer Epidemiol Biomarkers Prev. 2013;22(4):518–20.
17. Vigneswaran N, Williams MD. Epidemiologic trends in head and neck cancer and aids in diagnosis. Oral Maxillofac Surg Clin North Am. 2014;26(2):123–41.

18. Napier SS, Speight PM. Natural history of potentially malignant oral lesions and conditions: an overview of the literature. J Oral Pathol Med. 2008;37(1):1–10.
19. Gillenwater AM, Vigneswaran N, Fatani H, Saintigny P, El-Naggar AK. Proliferative verrucous leukoplakia (PVL): recognition and differentiation from conventional leukoplakia and mimics! Head Neck. 2013;36(11):1662–8.
20. Gillenwater AM, Vigneswaran N, Fatani H, Saintigny P, El-Naggar AK. Proliferative Verrucous Leukoplakia (PVL): a review of an elusive pathologic entity! Adv Anat Pathol. 2013;20(6):416–23.
21. Zain RB, Ikeda N, Gupta PC, et al. Oral mucosal lesions associated with betel quid, areca nut and tobacco chewing habits: consensus from a workshop held in Kuala Lumpur, Malaysia, November 25–27, 1996. J Oral Pathol Med. 1999;28(1):1–4.
22. Eisen D. The clinical features, malignant potential, and systemic associations of oral lichen planus: a study of 723 patients. J Am Acad Dermatol. 2002;46(2):207–14.
23. Lovas JG, Harsanyi BB, ElGeneidy AK. Oral lichenoid dysplasia: a clinicopathologic analysis. Oral Surg Oral Med Oral Pathol. 1989;68(1):57–63.
24. Zhang L, Cheng X, Li Y, et al. High frequency of allelic loss in dysplastic lichenoid lesions. Lab Invest. 2000;80(2):233–7.
25. Levitus M, Joenje H, de Winter JP. The Fanconi anemia pathway of genomic maintenance. Cell Oncol. 2006;28(1-2):3–29.
26. Kutler DI, Auerbach AD, Satagopan J, et al. High incidence of head and neck squamous cell carcinoma in patients with Fanconi anemia. Arch Otolaryngol Head Neck Surg. 2003;129(1):106–12.
27. Masserot C, Peffault de Latour R, Rocha V, et al. Head and neck squamous cell carcinoma in 13 patients with Fanconi anemia after hematopoietic stem cell transplantation. Cancer. 2008;113(12):3315–22.
28. Bessler M, Wilson DB, Mason PJ. Dyskeratosis congenita. FEBS Lett. 2010;584(17):3831–8.
29. Scheckenbach K, Wagenmann M, Freund M, Schipper J, Hanenberg H. Squamous cell carcinomas of the head and neck in Fanconi anemia: risk, prevention, therapy, and the need for guidelines. Klin Padiatr. 2012;224(3): 132–8.
30. Lingen MW, Kalmar JR, Karrison T, Speight PM. Critical evaluation of diagnostic aids for the detection of oral cancer. Oral Oncol. 2008;44(1):10–22.
31. Moles DR, Downer MC, Speight PM. Meta-analysis of measures of performance reported in oral cancer and precancer screening studies. Br Dent J. 2002;192(6):340–4. discussion 32.
32. Epstein JB, Guneri P, Boyacioglu H, Abt E. The limitations of the clinical oral examination in detecting dysplastic oral lesions and oral squamous cell carcinoma. J Am Dent Assoc. 2012;143(12):1332–42.
33. Epstein JB, Sciubba JJ, Banasek TE, Hay LJ. Failure to diagnose and delayed diagnosis of cancer: medicolegal issues. J Am Dent Assoc. 2009;140(12):1494–503.
34. Rana M, Zapf A, Kuehle M, Gellrich NC, Eckardt AM. Clinical evaluation of an autofluorescence diagnostic device for oral cancer detection: a prospective randomized diagnostic study. Eur J Cancer Prev. 2012;21(5): 460–6.
35. Schwarz RA, Gao W, Redden Weber C, et al. Noninvasive evaluation of oral lesions using depth-sensitive optical spectroscopy. Cancer. 2009;115(8):1669–79.
36. Speight PM. Update on oral epithelial dysplasia and progression to cancer. Head Neck Pathol. 2007;1(1):61–6.
37. Mithani SK, Mydlarz WK, Grumbine FL, Smith IM, Califano JA. Molecular genetics of premalignant oral lesions. Oral Dis. 2007; 13(2):126–33.
38. Zhang L, Poh CF, Williams M, et al. Loss of heterozygosity (LOH) profiles--validated risk predictors for progression to oral cancer. Cancer Prev Res (Phila). 2012;5(9):1081–9.

Chapter 38

Image-Guided Surgery by OCT and Other Optical Imaging Modalities

Waseem Jerjes, Ahmed A. Sultan, and Colin Hopper

It has been proposed that one of the possible applications of optical diagnostics is to guide the clinician to undertake accurate intervention when managing tissue pathology. The ability to provide an instant optical signature of pathological lesions or margins will help in identifying changes occurring at cellular and subcellular levels which can be invaluable for decision-making and treatment planning and aid in predicting the disease behaviour and overall prognosis. The mapping of tumour margins using optical techniques has not been fully explored. The applications of this technology can be useful to many body areas including the head and neck with the upper aerodigestive tract and skin [1–3].

The gold standard for pathological tissue removal remains surgery. Radiotherapy while used as primary treatment for some conditions, is usually advocated to deal with any positive margins and can be also employed as a neoadjuvant intervention. When it comes to skin cancer, Mohs micrographic surgery has been employed with impressive success rates but it requires special set-up, training, and maintenance. This procedure requires the clinician and the pathologist working side by side to assess every single piecemeal resection. This procedure has the advantage of being guided by a pathologist [1–3].

Photodynamic therapy has achieved success in managing tissue disease in the head and neck as well as skin. The depth of effect depends on the photosensitiser used and the light properties as well as the availability of oxygen in the pathological tissue [1–3].

Brian J.-F. Wong and Justus Ilgner (eds.), *Biomedical Optics in Otorhinolaryngology: Head and Neck Surgery*,
DOI 10.1007/978-1-4939-1758-7_38, © Springer Science+Business Media New York 2016

Optical Guidance of Treatment Modalities

Optical biopsy can be acquired from the suspicious legion or the tissue margin at the time of biopsy or intervention (i.e. surgery, radiotherapy, laser or photodynamic therapy). Optical biopsy techniques (in vitro and in vivo clinical trials data) have the advantage of being non-invasive (results in no tissue loss), provide instant diagnosis, and are cost-effective. They can also be used to assess the photosensitiser concentration if photodynamic therapy is the treatment modality. The tumour mapping ability of optical modalities has not been fully explored as yet [1–3].

In cancer surgery, this technique can facilitate tumour-specific targeting which can potentially result in margin-free tumour and improved survival. Many factors may affect the use of optical biopsy as a guiding modality in clinical procedures that has been discussed by Keereweer et al. [4] including:

- Accuracy of the optical signature as it can be complicated by optical tissue properties
- The optical signature and its correlation with the clinical presentation
- The practicality of implementing optical image-guided procedure and potential improvement in patient's care
- Clinicians' knowledge gap when it comes to optical diagnostics and its influence on decision-making

The authors concluded that despite all the limitations to the intrinsic capacity of the optical techniques, optical biopsy can be a very powerful intraoperative tool in guiding the future oncologic procedures and leading to improve prognosis and quality of life [4]. The same group suggested that optical imaging has the potential of bridging the gap between radiology and surgery by providing real-time visualization of the tumour, thereby allowing for image-guided intervention. An example here was the use of near-infrared light spectrum which offers two essential advantages: increased tissue penetration of light and an increased signal-to-background ratio of contrast agents; this is one of many advantages of the optical techniques in this field [5].

Optical Coherence Tomography: Case Study

A study by Hamdoon et al. investigated the role of optical coherence tomography (OCT) in lesion (squamous cell carcinoma) mapping, assisting the surgeon to correctly deliver photodynamic therapy (PDT) and monitor the outcome. Optical coherence tomographic images were acquired pretreatment to assess tumour extent and margins to enable guidance of the PDT. Tomographic images taken post-PDT up to 6 months revealed complete response to the treatment and no recurrence. It is proposed that OCT-guided PDT is one of the promising approaches to efficiently discriminate between tumour involved and noninvolved margins as it can potentially reduce untoward healthy tissue necrosis and provides an encouraging monitoring of the healing process. The case is presented here.

A 56-year-old Caucasian male was referred for suspected basal cell carcinoma of the right infraorbital region. An incisional biopsy revealed a well-differentiated squamous cell carcinoma (SCC). A neck ultrasound examination confirmed no nodal disease. The patient declined wide surgical excision with local flap reconstruction and elected to undergo photodynamic therapy. Intravenous mTHPC (0.05 mg/kg) was administered 48 h prior to skin illumination to allow the maximum accumulation of the photosensitiser in the tissue. On day two, the VivoSight OCT scanner with hand-held probe was used to map the tumour margins precisely. OCT scanning was performed centrally and then swept out peripherally toward the visible margin. This manoeuvre enabled demarcation between the central active lesional zone and peripheral questionable zones. The "light delivery" part of the PDT took place under local anaesthesia in an outpatient setting. A 652 nm diode laser was used to illuminate the pathological area [6] (Fig. 1).

In the follow-up period, OCT was used to monitor the healing process. Multiple large dark spaces occupying the epidermis and part of the dermis were identified 4 weeks post-PDT. These spaces represented necrotic tumour clusters. OCT identification of the interface between the tumour and uninvolved tissue was based on a clear delineation of the thin bright groove, thus enabling the clinician to accurately assess the wound depth. In the third month post-PDT, the progress of wound healing was characterized by further useful morphological information which could be derived from the epidermis and dermis. However, structures represented by the interface between epidermis and dermis were difficult to differentiate at that stage. The image contrast was compromised by immature collagen matrices (associated with early wound healing) which in turn increased signal reflective index (proliferative phase); thus, the effective imaging depth and contrast decreased. The authors suggested that OCT is a technique that can monitor lesions more precisely and accurately so obviating many of the previous shortcomings of PDT follow-up and monitoring process and proposed the development of OCT-guided fine needle aspiration cytology (FNAC) for more accurate monitoring and mapping [6] (Fig. 1).

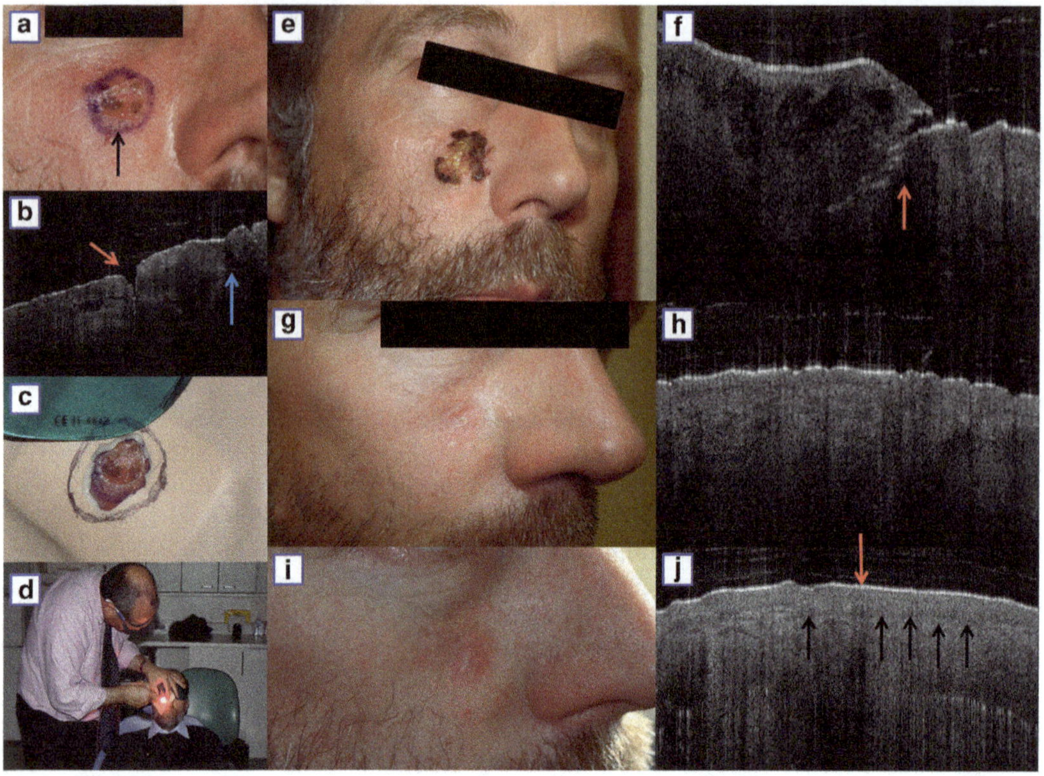

Fig. 1 (**a**) SCC of the infraorbital area with the visible margin (*black arrow*). (**b**) OCT image showing vertical crater which represents the clinical visible tumour margin (*red arrow*); there is a vertical cleft showing non-visible actual damage beyond the margin (blue arrow). (**c** and **d**) After mapping the real margins by OCT, custom-made template was constructed and followed by PDT illumination. (**e** and **f**) 4 weeks post-PDT, the OCT image showing vertical cleft with multiple empty spaces which indicate necrotic changes (*red arrow*). (**g** and **h**) 3 months post-PDT, healing with granulation tissue formation which can be seen clearly in the OCT image with slight poor differentiation in skin layer as the area is in state of healing. (**I** and **J**) 6 months post-PDT, the OCT image showing early differentiation of epidermal and dermal layers with distinctive dermo-epidermal junction (*black arrows*) and very thin stratum corneum layer (*red arrow*). The figure is adapted from authors' own article: Hamdoon Z, Jerjes W, Upile T, Hopper C. Optical coherence tomography-guided photodynamic therapy for skin cancer: case study. Photodiagnosis Photodyn Ther. 2011 Mar;8(1):49–52

Discussion

OCT-guided laser hyperthermia with passively tumour-targeted gold nanoparticles has been developed by Sirotkina et al. [7]. Bifunctional plasmon resonant nanoparticles have been used with OCT diagnostics and laser heating at the wavelength of 810 nm. The resultant OCT images showed that the accumulation of gold nanoparticles in the tumour invading into the skin was maximal 4–5 h after intravenous injection. Laser hyperthermia was employed at the maximum nanoparticle accumulation and led to apoptosis and inhibited tumour growth by 104 % on the 5th day after treatment [7].

Optical imaging is experiencing marked technologic advances which resulted in new capabilities to biomedical research and is edging toward clinical use. Optical diagnostics is developing from imaging of structures and morphology into the visualization of the individual biologic processes underlying disease and could potentially contribute to more accurate diagnostics and improved patient's care. A review by Taruttis and Ntziachristos into the translation of macroscopic optical imaging—including fluorescence-guided surgery and endoscopy, intravascular fluorescence imaging, diffuse fluorescence and optical tomography and multispectral optoacoustics (photoacoustics)—for applications ranging from tumour resection and assessment of atherosclerotic plaques to dermatologic and breast examinations has reached this conclusion [8].

References

1. Upile T, Jerjes W, Sterenborg HJ, El-Naggar AK, Sandison A, Witjes MJ, Biel MA, Bigio I, Wong BJ, Gillenwater A, MacRobert AJ, Robinson DJ, Betz CS, Stepp H, Bolotine L, McKenzie G, Mosse CA, Barr H, Chen Z, Berg K, D'Cruz AK, Stone N, Kendall C, Fisher S, Leunig A, Olivo M, Richards-Kortum R, Soo KC, Bagnato V, Choo-Smith LP, Svanberg K, Tan IB, Wilson BC, Wolfsen H, Yodh AG, Hopper C. Head & neck optical diagnostics: vision of the future of surgery. Head Neck Oncol. 2009;1:25.
2. Upile T, Jerjes WK, Sterenborg HJ, Wong BJ, El-Naggar AK, Ilgner JF, Sandison A, Witjes MJ, Biel MA, van Veen R, Hamdoon Z, Gillenwater A, Mosse CA, Robinson DJ, Betz CS, Stepp H, Bolotine L, McKenzie G, Barr H, Chen Z, Berg K, D'Cruz AK, Sudhoff H, Stone N, Kendall C, Fisher S, MacRobert AJ, Leunig A, Olivo M, Richards-Kortum R, Soo KC, Bagnato V, Choo-Smith LP, Svanberg K, Tan IB, Wilson BC, Wolfsen H, Bigio I, Yodh AG, Hopper C. At the frontiers of surgery: review. Head Neck Oncol. 2011;3(1):7.
3. Jerjes WK, Upile T, Wong BJ, Betz CS, Sterenborg HJ, Witjes MJ, Berg K, van Veen R, Biel MA, El-Naggar AK, Mosse CA, Olivo M, Richards-Kortum R, Robinson DJ, Rosen J, Yodh AG, Kendall C, Ilgner JF, Amelink A, Bagnato V, Barr H, Bolotine L, Bigio I, Chen Z, Choo-Smith LP, D'Cruz AK, Gillenwater A, Leunig A, MacRobert AJ, McKenzie G, Sandison A, Soo KC, Stepp H, Stone N, Svanberg K, Tan IB, Wilson BC, Wolfsen H, Hopper C. The future of medical diagnostics: review paper. Head Neck Oncol. 2011;3:38.
4. Keereweer S, Van Driel PB, Snoeks TJ, Kerrebijn JD, Baatenburg de Jong RJ, Vahrmeijer AL, Sterenborg HJ, Löwik CW. Optical image-guided cancer surgery: challenges and limitations. Clin Cancer Res. 2013;19(14):3745–54.
5. Keereweer S, Sterenborg HJ, Kerrebijn JD, Van Driel PB, Baatenburg de Jong RJ, Löwik CW. Image-guided surgery in head and neck cancer: current practice and future directions of optical imaging. Head Neck. 2012;34(1): 120–6.
6. Hamdoon Z, Jerjes W, Upile T, Hopper C. Optical coherence tomography-guided photodynamic therapy for skin cancer: case study. Photodiagnosis Photodyn Ther. 2011;8(1): 49–52.
7. Sirotkina MA, Elagin VV, Shirmanova MV, Bugrova ML, Snopova LB, Kamensky VA, Nadtochenko VA, Denisov NN, Zagaynova EV. OCT-guided laser hyperthermia with passively tumor-targeted gold nanoparticles. J Biophotonics. 2010;3(10–11):718–27.
8. Taruttis A, Ntziachristos V. Translational optical imaging. AJR Am J Roentgenol. 2012;199(2): 263–71.

Chapter 39

Narrow Band Imaging of the Upper Aerodigestive Tract

Christoph Arens and Susanne Voigt-Zimmermann

Introduction

Endoscopy of the upper aerodigestive tract (UADT) has been influenced by different innovations over the last two decades. The use of chip-on-the-tip rigid or flexible endoscopes was a change in endoscopic function. The next step was the increase of resolution as well as the introduction of high-definition (HD) imaging especially in flexible endoscopes. 4K resolution is almost ready to take the next step. Additionally, endoscopic imaging techniques, e.g., Narrow Band Imaging (NBI), autofluorescence, optical coherence tomography, a.o., have been developed to get more details about the pathological changes besides normal white light endoscopy.

These imaging techniques are divided in horizontal and vertical imaging techniques. While horizontal imaging techniques look primarily at the surface, vertical images focus on pathological changes underneath the surface. NBI belongs to the horizontal imaging techniques looking at superficial changes of the epithelium and the underlying vessels. In combination with HD, NBI is a powerful endoscopic imaging technique offering a better contrasted picture especially for the assessment of vascular changes. Therefore, it is suitable for the detection of early lesions—either benign or malignant.

Narrow Band Imaging Endoscopy

2004 NBI endoscopy was introduced in the diagnostic workup of the UADT by Muto et al. [1]. At that time it had already proven to be a useful imaging tool in other endoscopic areas, e.g., gastroenterology [2–4] and pulmonology [5].

Brian J.-F. Wong and Justus Ilgner (eds.), *Biomedical Optics in Otorhinolaryngology: Head and Neck Surgery*,
DOI 10.1007/978-1-4939-1758-7_39, © Springer Science+Business Media New York 2016

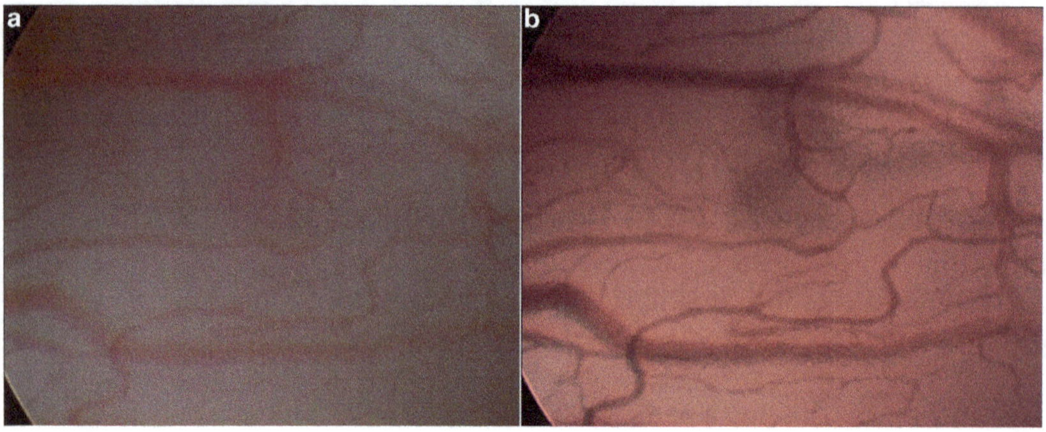

Fig. 1 Contact endoscopy of the left vocal fold in white light and NBI mode. Different vessel types can be recognized. Superficial vessels are sharply demarcated and contrasted. Deeper vessels are *blurred*. Intracapillary papillary loops are not visible

NBI is a noninvasive imaging technique which can be applied to in- and outpatients during endoscopy by pressing a button, immediately switching from white light to NBI. It enhances the visualization of epithelial and subepithelial microvascular structure and lesions. Especially small lesions can be detected much easier compared to normal white light endoscopy alone.

Compared to white light, superficial epithelial lesions can be detected much better especially due to a more intensive fluorescence of keratin in leukoplakia. Keratotic lesions can be looked at specifically, including their surrounding margins, offering more detailed information about the character of the lesion. Epithelial thickening can be detected much easier. Furthermore, this optical imaging enhancement tool focuses on subepithelial vessels and their different sizes and shapes (Fig. 1).

In oral and oropharyngeal squamous cell carcinoma, Piazza et al. described a sensitivity, specificity, positive, negative predictive values, and accuracy for HDTV white light endoscopy (WLE) of 51 %, 100 %, 100 %, 87 %, and 68 %, respectively, while for HDTV NBI figures were 96 %, 100 %, 100 %, 93 %, and 97 %, respectively [6] (Figs. 2, 3, and 4).

Kraft et al. [7] reported that NBI with WLE showed a significantly higher sensitivity (97 % vs 79 %) and accuracy (97 % vs 90 %) than WLE alone in identifying laryngeal cancer and its precursor lesions. In contrast, the specificity (96 % vs 95 %) was essentially equal for both imaging techniques.

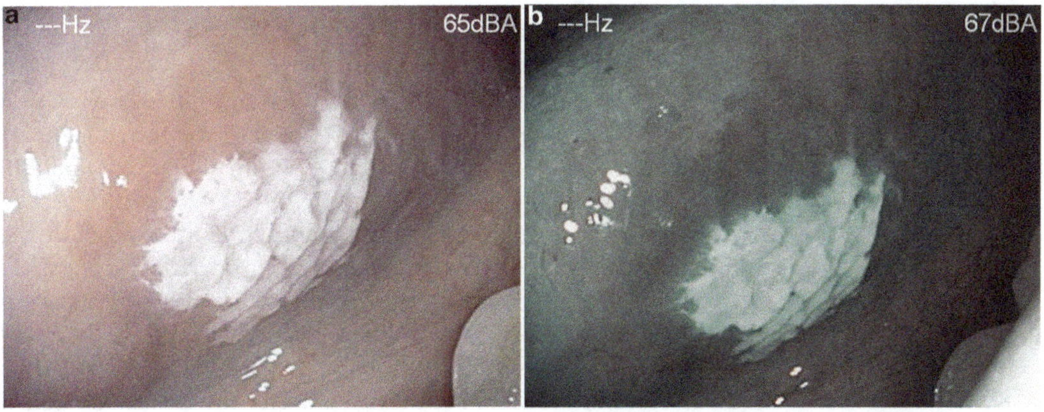

Fig. 2 Sharply delineated leukoplakia of the left tongue. Normal vascular pattern without any vascular atypia can be noticed

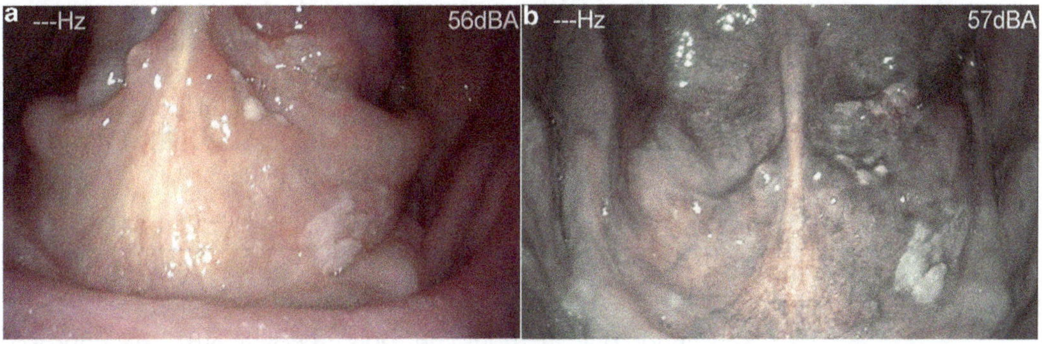

Fig. 3 An unregular spotted leukoplakia of the left floor of the mouth can be observed. Vascular atypia can be detected in the NBI. Histologic assessment revealed a squamous cell carcinoma with a diameter of 5 mm

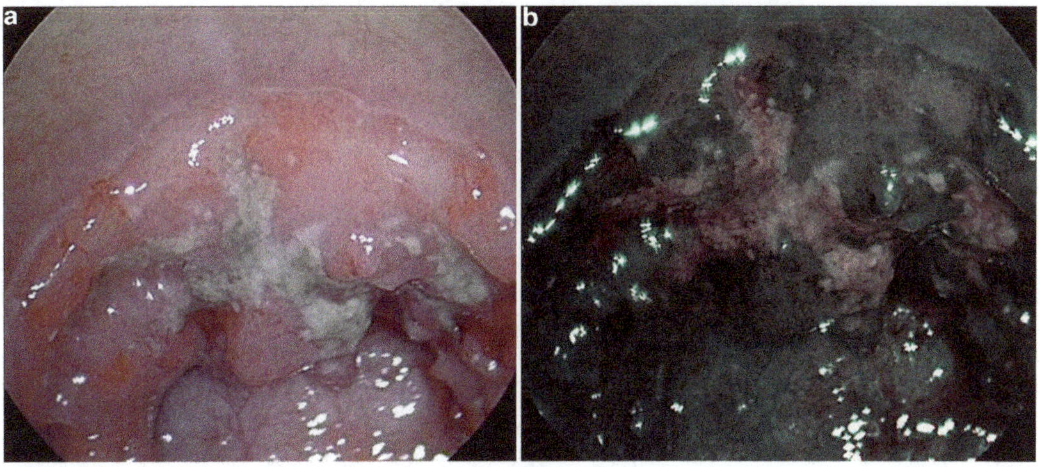

Fig. 4 Bilateral oropharyngeal carcinoma of the soft palate with ulceration and anterior extension to the hard palate. Chaotic tumor growth with irregular vascular pattern and shape

NBI Equipment

The technical equipment consists of a xenon light source with a special NBI filter narrowing the wavelength of emitted light to 400–430 nm (center wavelength at 415 nm) and 525–555 nm (center wavelength at 540 nm).

Additionally, a high-definition camera in combination with a rigid endoscope (0°–120°) and/or a flexible videoendoscope (30–90 cm length and max. 4 mm in diameter) with chip-on-the-tip technology and a video system unit is needed.

Both wavelengths have special characteristics. 415 nm represents blue light and penetrates about 400 μm into the tissue. In normal mucosa the light beam hits the underlying connective tissue. It leads to better contrasted endoscopic pictures secondary to the corresponding peak absorption spectrum of hemoglobin by enhancement of capillary vessels. The green light centered at the longer wavelength of 540 nm can penetrate deeper into the connective tissue resulting in endoscopic visualization of the submucosal vascular plexus. Additionally, keratin present in leukoplakias is a potential fluorophore emitting bright white light from the epithelial surface, leading to a better depiction of these epithelial changes in contrast to the surrounding green epithelium.

Epithelial Changes in NBI

New endoscopic methods and tools especially NBI have improved the endoscopic diagnosis leading to an early depiction of epithelial but also vascular lesions of the UADT. Therefore, a more differentiated knowledge and assessment of epithelial as well as vascular lesions resulted in a more precise diagnostic workup and therapy [6, 8–18].

Epithelial tumors of the UADT are grouped in papilloma, epithelial dysplasia, and squamous cell carcinoma. These tumors differ in vascular changes, the expression of epithelial changes, as well as the connective tissue architecture being important in the process of preoperative differential diagnosis.

Thin, non-keratinized, stratified squamous epithelium of the larynx and hypopharynx allows good endoscopic visualization of fine vascular lesions during the development of precancerous and cancerous lesions. Especially typical intraepithelial papillary capillary loops (IPCLs) of recurrent respiratory papillomatosis (RRP) (Fig. 5) can be detected by NBI.

In the upper aerodigestive tract, we differentiate between two different epithelial layers—respiratory and squamous cell epithelium. Respiratory epithelium may become metaplastic and change in the lower differentiated squamous cell epithelium. This epithe-

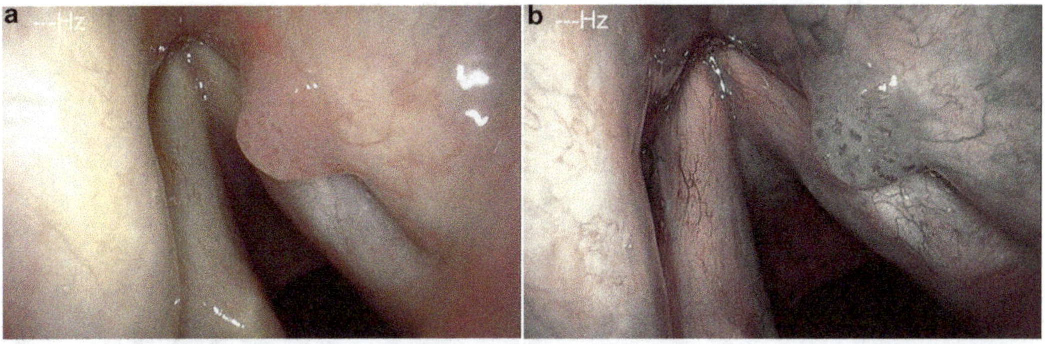

Fig. 5 Recurrent respiratory papillomatosis of the ventricular fold. Typical intracapillary papillary loops can be better detected with NBI. Scars can be detected on both vocal folds with a typical vascular pattern after papilloma surgery

lial change may also result in the development of squamous cell cancer. During NBI endoscopy, an epithelial defect or ulceration can easily be detected by bright red color which is sharply demarcated by the green color of the surrounding tissue covered by epithelium.

In NBI endoscopy, epithelial thickening primarily leads to a darker green appearance of the NBI picture in contrast to the more reddish-green color in normal epithelium. This development is followed by a leukoplakia which contains the fluorophore keratin. The color of the "leukoplakia" becomes more whitish and less transparent leading to the observation of vessel breaks ("umbrella effect"). Leukoplakia is a descriptive term which represents epithelial lesions from hyperkeratosis up to squamous cell cancer. In combination with vascular changes, epithelial lesions can be much better classified by NBI in contrast to white light alone.

In earlier stages leukoplakias are still transparent and have a sharp and regular edge (Fig. 6). Additionally, they present with a more round to oval shape and mostly have a smooth surface. When leukoplakias become dysplastic, they develop an irregular shape and edge. Furthermore, the surface is inhomogeneous and diverse. In carcinoma in situ as well as microinvasive cancer, the epithelial lesion may have a spot-like appearance and goes along with typical vascular changes which will be described in the next section (Figs. 7 and 8). Besides the endoscopic picture of the epithelial lesion during NBI examination, the absence of the mucosal wave during stroboscopy may give additional information about the nature of the lesion. In a progressing lesion, the character of the squamous cell carcinoma is characterized by a recognizable change of the surface and shape secondary to the increase of tumor volume and ulceration (Fig. 9).

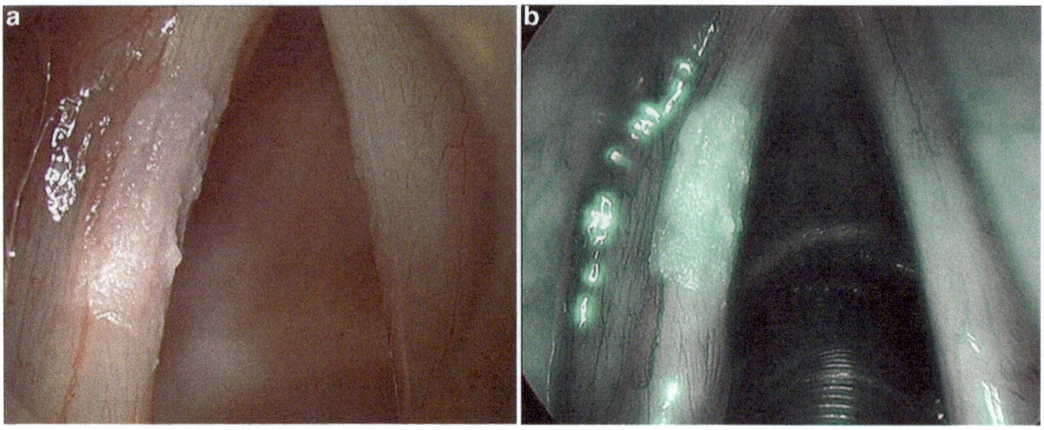

Fig. 6 Homogenous and sharp demarcated leukoplakia of the left vocal fold. Only ectatic vessels on the border can be recognized, which are partially interrupted by the leukoplakia (umbrella effect). Histologically it was diagnosed as a hyper- and parakeratosis

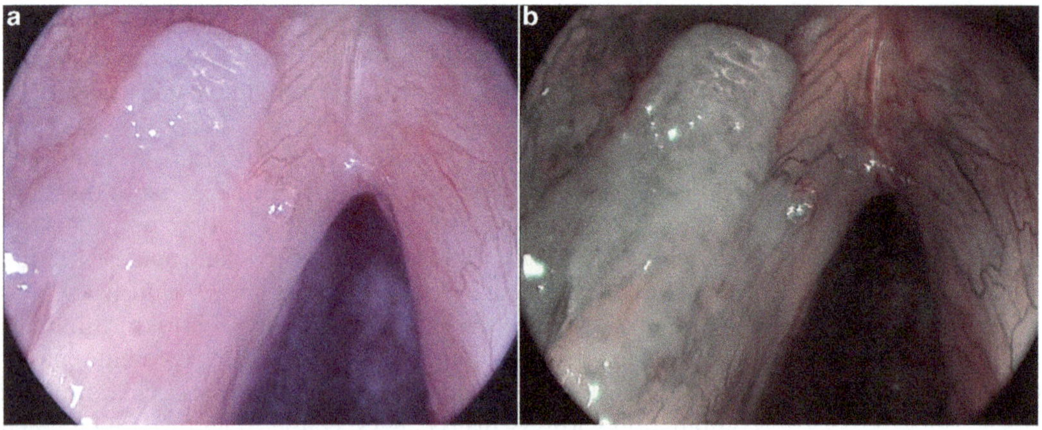

Fig. 7 Carcinoma in situ besides acanthosis and hyper-parakeratosis of the left vocal fold. Capillary loops are more present in the NBI

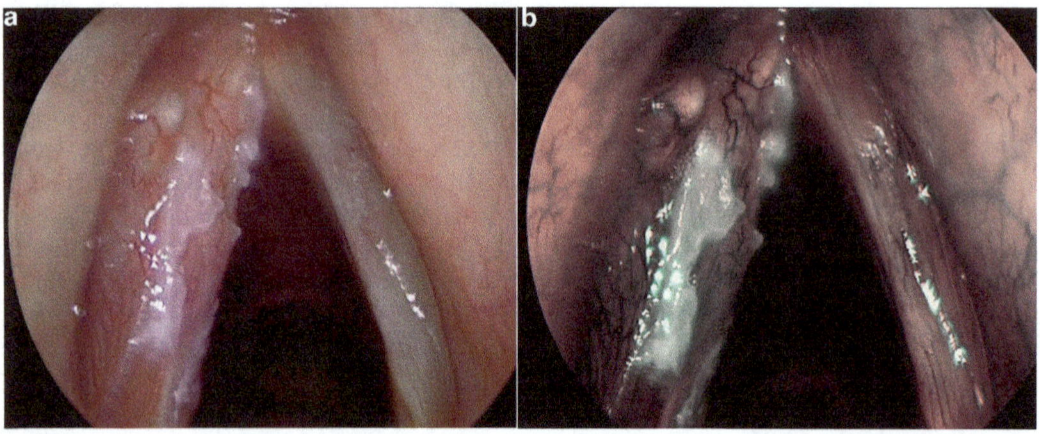

Fig. 8 Spotted irregular leukoplakia of the left vocal fold in combination with dysplastic vessels and increase of volume representing T1a carcinoma of the vocal fold

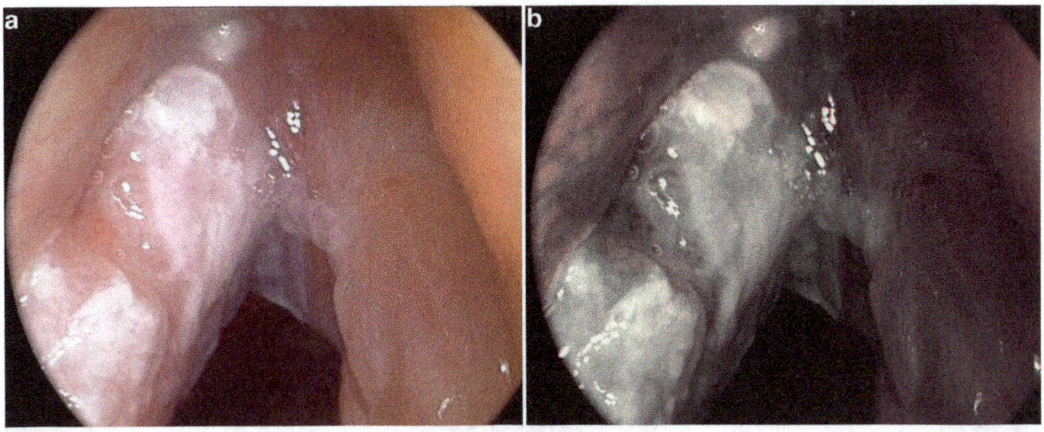

Fig. 9 T2 carcinoma of the left vocal fold with subglottic extension

Vascular Lesions in NBI

Two groups of vascular lesions can be differentiated-longitudinal and perpendicular. While horizontal vascular lesions are primarily reactive due to ongoing mechanical, chemical, or other external stress factors, vertical lesions develop by a stimulus of the epithelium itself.

Ni et al. [19] have transferred a model coined as "IPCLs" (intraepithelial papillary capillary loops) for the classification of vascular changes of the esophagus seen during NBI examination to precancerous and cancerous lesions of the vocal folds. Kumagai et al. [20] already stated that vessels of the mucosa show characteristic changes according to the invasion depth of cancer. This classification is widely used in gastroenterological endoscopic diagnosis [21, 22] but implies some disadvantages and may not simply be transferred to the description of vascular pattern of the UADT. Additionally the term "papillary loops" is misleading, because regular mucosa of the UADT rarely contains papillary loops (Fig. 1).

Longitudinal Vascular Changes

In the beginning of the pathogenesis of vascular changes, blood vessels often appear enlarged and/or ectatic, especially in inflammation. Ongoing reactive processes and external stimuli lead to angiogenesis and the formation of new vascular structures. Vessels become more visible. The increase of the vessel size is associated with further branching of vessels and anastomoses. These changes may lead to an increased visible vascular density and diameter followed by an increased reddish appearance under white light and a darker green appearance under NBI.

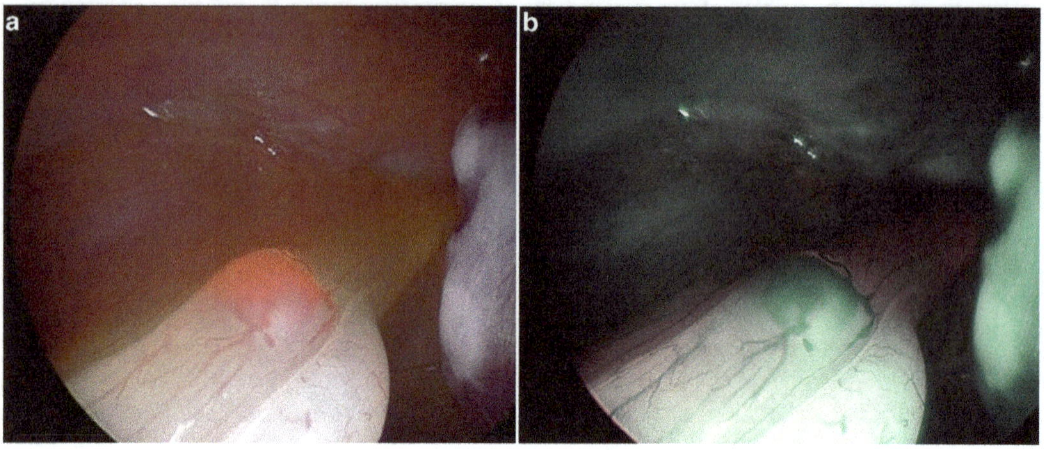

Fig. 10 Myxoid polyp in statu nascendi with a convolute on top of the left vocal fold. Vessels are better contrasted and can be detected much easier in the NBI

Consideration of such precursor changes of vascular diseases, e.g. vessel ectasia, meander, increasing number and branching of vessels, and change of direction, may lead to more differentiated prognostic statements and adequate therapeutic decisions.

The mentioned vascular changes type I and type II of the IPCL classification [19] correlate to these early vascular changes described. They are primarily induced by mechanical stress on the vessel walls and are typically localized at point of the strongest mechanical forces. The initial changes in the blood vessels are beginning signs of future manifest vascular diseases especially in the vocal folds, like varices, convolutes, polyps (Fig. 10), and hemorrhages.

Perpendicular Vascular Lesions

Perpendicular vascular lesions are characterized by the development of intraepithelial papillary capillary vessel loops (IPCLs) developing secondary to an epithelial stimulus. In HPV-related recurrent respiratory papillomatosis, these loops can endoscopically be recognized as real loops embedded in a three-dimensional warty structure. In contrast precancerous lesions show symmetrical arranged dot-like loops which represent the tip of the loop under the epithelium arising from deeper layers of the mucosa. These typical changes can be detected by NBI.

Perpendicular vessel changes in papillomas, precancerous or cancerous lesions, are induced by an epithelial stimulus. Not only the vessel but also the surrounding tissue is altered by this stimulus. In RRP typical morula-like "warty" changes develop. They may be uni- or bilateral, multicentric, and exophytic with a glassy convex surface, similar to raspberries. There seems to be a local immunological deficit. The epithelial infection stimulus in the underlying connective tissue seems to initiate angiogenesis and a transformation of the connective tissue. Squamous cell carcinoma can also be caused by "high-risk" HPV [23]. Lukes et al. [24] and Tjon Pian Gi et al. [25] highlight that the changes of IPCL and the epithelial surface are essential for differential diagnosis in endoscopic imaging of RRP. Typical features, like central vessel loops in each morula-like bulge usually help to distinguish RRPs from high-grade dysplasia or SCCs.

In the development of precancerous and cancerous lesions, the reddish-appearing effect of an erythroplakia is caused by an increased density of subepithelial vascular structure secondary to neoangiogenesis in combination with a thin and atrophic epithelium. As already described before, leukoplakia is like a chameleon which resembles epithelial changes from benign epithelial thickening to cancerous lesions.

In context of carcinogenesis, perpendicular vascular changes (IPCL) may be recognized during endoscopy at the border of the leukoplakia described above. The combination of a leukoplakia as well as its perilesional vascular changes can give a hint to the character of the disease. Benign hyperkeratotic lesions may go along with vessel ectasia but do not present any kind of vascular loops. These epithelial lesions are reactive and may regress spontaneously. In most cases these lesions are transparent and vessel may be detected underneath the leukoplakia.

As the epithelium becomes dysplastic, the leukoplakia becomes more irregular in shape and size. Longitudinal vascular changes like vessel ectasia transform into perpendicular vascular lesions. Loops become visible in the periphery of the leukoplakia. These loops occur primarily as typical dots representing the top of the loop. In early stages the loops are still visible in a regular symmetrical pattern. When cancer develops, the vascular loops and the epithelial lesion become completely irregular. The irregular tumor surface and shape are caused by vascular malnutrition secondary to chaotic neoangiogenesis (Fig. 11).

NBI, especially in combination with high-definition imaging, is a useful and effective imaging technique in the diagnosis and therapy of pathological changes of the UADT. Especially small lesions characterized by vascular changes can be detected much earlier in contrast to normal white light. It is also suitable for the early diagnosis of papilloma, precancerous and cancerous lesions [6, 17, 19]. NBI can also be used during papilloma or cancer surgery for detection of superficial surgical margins.

NBI in combination with contact endoscopy during microlaryngoscopy, so called "compact endoscopy" [26], allows us to detect and classify different types of IPCL. Using this technique we are able to distinguish between papilloma, mild or moderate

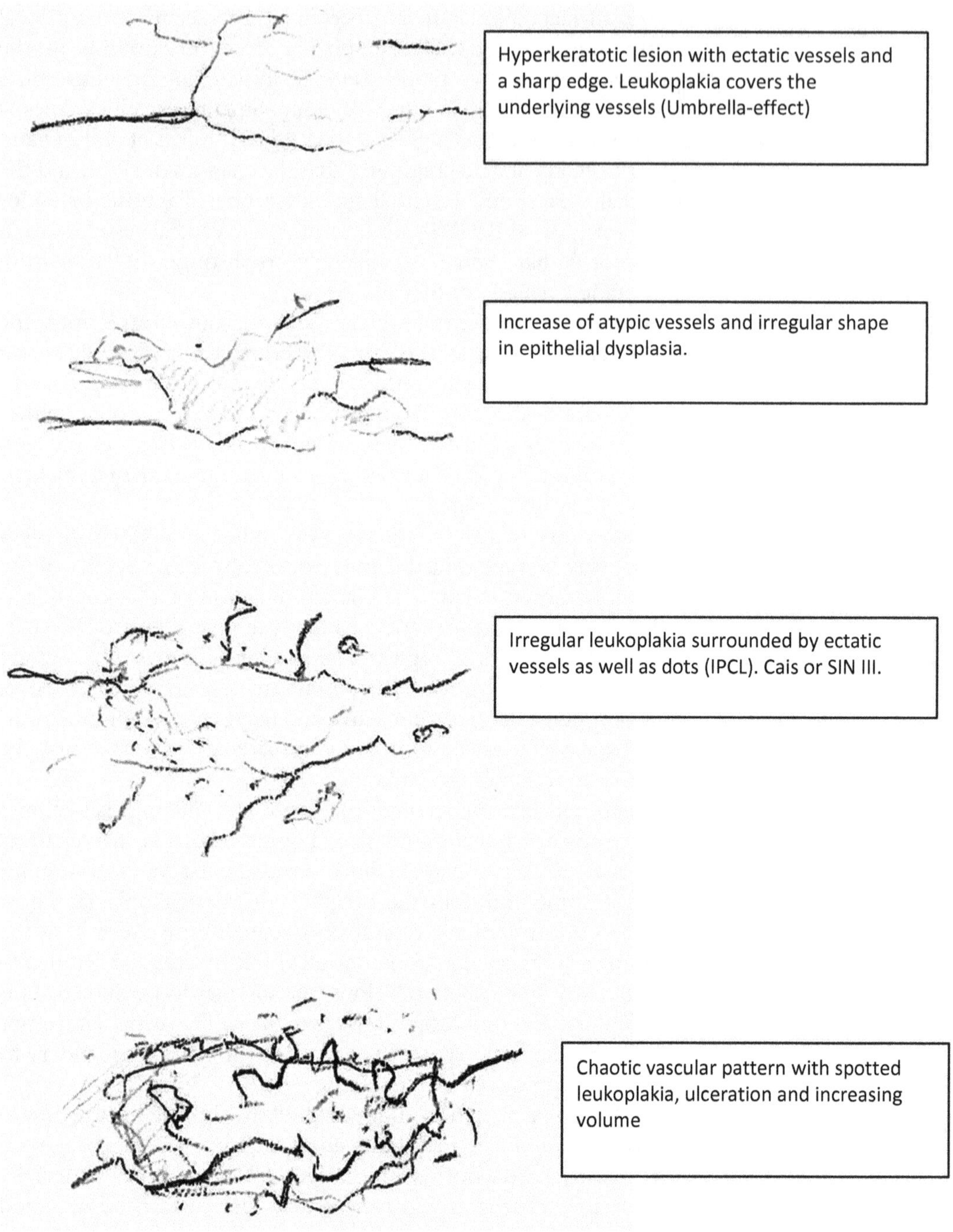

Fig. 11 Sketch of the development of epithelial cancerization with typical vascular and epithelial pattern

epithelial dysplasia, SIN III, and microinvasive cancer (Figs. 12, 13, 14, and 15).

Therefore, vascular lesions play a significant role in the endoscopic workup of lesions of the UADT. New endoscopes in

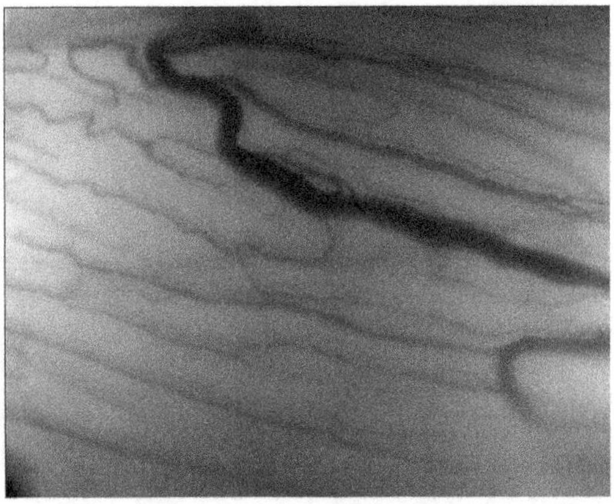

Fig. 12 Regular vascular pattern with an ectatic vessel. The underlying tissue of Reinke's space appears homogeneously green (compact endoscopy)

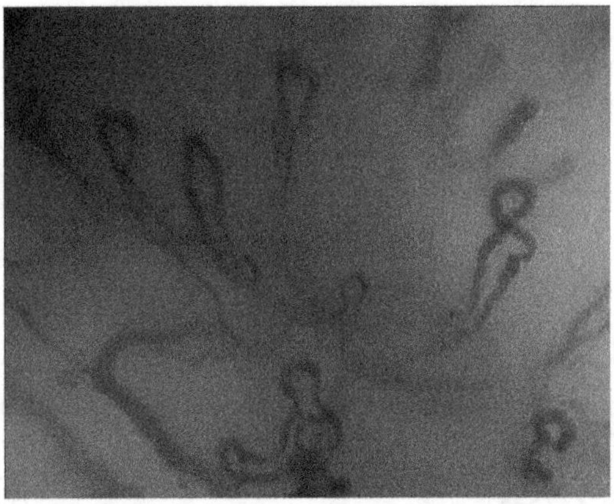

Fig. 13 Papilloma with typical symmetrical IPCL (compact endoscopy)

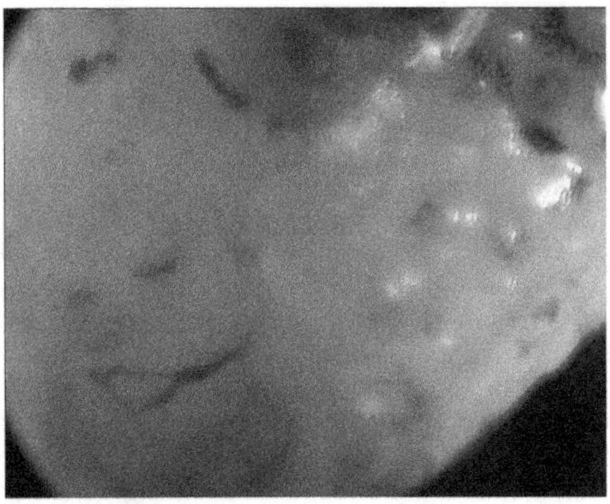

Fig. 14 Papillary cancerization of the left vocal fold. Different colors express the diverse thickness of the squamous cell epithelium. The IPCLs are irregular, asymmetrical with different shapes and sizes (compact endoscopy)

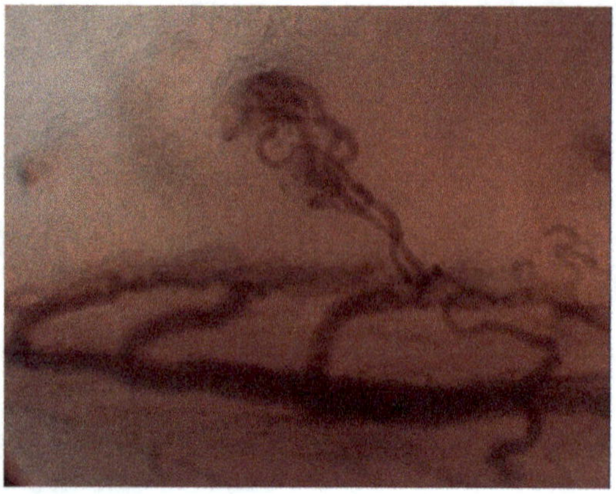

Fig. 15 Microinvasive cancer with deep irregular ectatic vessels and a typically curled IPCL (compact endoscopy)

combination with HD or even 4K imaging as well as NBI permit a detailed observation of the mucosal surface allowing the diagnosis of superficial pathologies with a high probability to anticipate the correct histological examination during preoperative stage. NBI as a new endoscopic tool for rigid as well as flexible endoscopy may be an early step on the way in performing an "optical biopsy."

References

1. Muto M, Nakane M, Katada C, et al. Squamous cell carcinoma in situ at oropharyngeal and hypopharyngeal mucosal sites. Cancer. 2004;101:1375–81.
2. Gono T, Yamazaki K, Doguchi N, et al. Endoscopic observation of tissue by narrow-band illumination. Opt Rev. 2003;10:211–5.
3. Sano Y, Kobayashi M, Hamamoto Y, et al. New diagnostic method based on color imaging using narrow band imaging (NBI) system for gastrointestinal tract. Gastrointest Endosc. 2001;53:AB125.
4. Yoshida T, Inoue H, Usui S, Satodate H, et al. Narrow-band imaging system with magnifying endoscopy for superficial esophageal lesion. Gastrointest Endosc. 2004;59:288–95.
5. Shibuya K, Hoshino H, Chiyo M, Iyoda A, et al. High magnification bronchovideoscopy combined with narrow band imaging could detect capillary loops of angiogenic squamous dysplasia in heavy smokers at high risk for lung cancer. Thorax. 2003;58:989–95.
6. Piazza C, Cocco D, Del Bon F, Mangili S, et al. Narrow band imaging and high definition television in evaluation of oral and oropharyngeal squamous cell cancer: a prospective study. Oral Oncol. 2010;46:307–10.
7. Kraft M, Fostiropoulos K, Gürtler N, Arnoux A, Davaris N, Arens C. Value of narrow band imaging in the early diagnosis of laryngeal cancer. Head Neck. 2016;38(1):15–20. doi: 10.1002/hed.23838.
8. Chu PY, Tsai TL, Tai SK, Chang SY. Effectiveness of narrow band imaging in patients with oral squamous cell carcinoma after treatment. Head Neck. 2012;34:155–61.
9. Ho CY, Lee YL, Chu PY. Use of narrow band imaging in evaluation of possible nasopharyngeal carcinoma. Am J Rhinol Allergy. 2011; 25:107–11.
10. Katada C, Nakayama M, Tanabe S, et al. Narrow band imaging for detecting superficial oral squamous cell carcinoma: a report of two cases. Laryngoscope. 2007;117:1596–9.
11. Lin YC, Watanabe A, Chen WC, et al. Narrowband imaging for early detection of malignant tumors and radiation effect after treatment of head and neck cancer. Arch Otolaryngol Head Neck Surg. 2010;136: 234–9.

12. Nonaka S, Saito Y. Endoscopic diagnosis of pharyngeal carcinoma by NBI. Endoscopy. 2008;40:347–51.
13. Takano JH, Yakushiji T, Kamiyama I, et al. Detecting early oral cancer: narrowband imaging system observation of the oral mucosa microvasculature. Int J Oral Maxillofac Surg. 2010;39:208–13.
14. Ugumori T, Muto M, Hayashi R, Hayashi T, Kishimoto S. Prospective study of early detection of pharyngeal superficial carcinoma with the narrowband imaging laryngoscope. Head Neck. 2009;31:189–94.
15. Wang WH, Lin YC, Lee KF, Weng H. Nasopharyngeal carcinoma detected by narrow-band imaging endoscopy. Oral Oncol. 2011;47:736–41.
16. Watanabe A, Tsujie H, Taniguchi M, Hosokawa M, Fujita M, Sasaki S. Laryngoscopic detection of pharyngeal carcinoma in situ with narrowband imaging. Laryngoscope. 2006;116:650–4.
17. Watanabe A, Taniguchi M, Tsujie H, Hosokawa M, et al. The value of narrow band imaging endoscope for early head and neck cancers. Otolaryngol Head Neck Surg. 2008;138:446–51.
18. Yang SW, Lee YS, Chang LC, Hwang CC, Chen TA. Diagnostic significance of narrowband imaging for detecting high-grade dysplasia, carcinoma in situ, and carcinoma in oral leukoplakia. Laryngoscope. 2012;122:2754–61.
19. Ni XG, He S, Xu ZG, et al. Endoscopic diagnosis of laryngeal cancer and precancerous lesions by narrow band imaging. J Laryngol Otol. 2011;125:288–96.
20. Kumagai Y, Inoue H, Nagai K, et al. Magnifying endoscopy, stereoscopic microscopy, and the microvascular architecture of superficial esophageal carcinoma. Endoscopy. 2002;34:369–75.
21. Inoue H, Honda T, Nagai K, et al. Ultra-high magnification endoscopic observation of carcinoma in situ of the esophagus. Dig Endosc. 1997;9:16–8.
22. Inoue H, Kaga M, Sato Y, Sugaya S, Kudo S. Magnifying endoscopy diagnosis of tissue atypia and cancer invasion depth in the area of pharyngo-esophageal squamous epithelium by NBI enhanced magnification image: IPCL pattern classification. In: Cohen J, editor. Advanced digestive endoscopy: comprehensive atlas of high resolution endoscopy and narrowband imaging. New York, NY: Blackwell Publishing; 2007. p. 49–66.
23. Zaravinos A. An updated overview of HPV-associated head and neck carcinomas. Oncotarget. 2014;5(12):3956–69.
24. Lukes P, Zabrodsky M, Lukesova E, et al. The role of NBI HDTV magnifying endoscopy in the prehistologic diagnosis of laryngeal papillomatosis and spinocellular cancer. Biomed. Res. Int. 2014;7 pages. doi: 10.1155/2014/285486.
25. Tjon Pian Gi REA, Halmos GB, et al. Narrow band imaging is a new technique in visualization of recurrent respiratory papillomatosis. Laryngoscope. 2012;122:1826–30.
26. Arens C, Voigt-Zimmermann S. Contact endoscopy of the vocal folds in combination with narrow band imaging (compact endoscopy). Laryngorhinootologie. 2015;94(3):150–2.

Index

A

B

C

Brian J.-F. Wong and Justus Ilgner (eds.), *Biomedical Optics in Otorhinolaryngology: Head and Neck Surgery*, DOI 10.1007/978-1-4939-1758-7, © Springer Science+Business Media New York 2016

D

E

F

G

H

M

Q

R

S

T

U

V

W

Y

GPSR Compliance
The European Union's (EU) General Product Safety Regulation (GPSR) is a set of rules that requires consumer products to be safe and our obligations to ensure this.

If you have any concerns about our products, you can contact us on

ProductSafety@springernature.com

In case Publisher is established outside the EU, the EU authorized representative is:

Springer Nature Customer Service Center GmbH
Europaplatz 3
69115 Heidelberg, Germany

www.ingramcontent.com/pod-product-compliance
Lightning Source LLC
LaVergne TN
LVHW082006200926
848481LV00010B/2813
9781493979660